Praise for David France's

How to Survive a Plague

"Important and powerfully written. . . . Inspiring, uplifting and necessary reading. . . . [France has] a novelist's eye for telling details and a poet's gift for indelible images." —*Financial Times*

"Flawless. Masterfully written, impeccably researched, and full of feeling for the living and dead heroes of the AIDS movement. . . . [There's] no better person to write this book." —*Newsday*

"The definitive book on AIDS activism." —*San Francisco Chronicle*

"Heroic and heartbreaking and [full of] magnificent history throughout, *How to Survive a Plague* is one of the great tales of our time." —Carl Bernstein

"France delivers a monumental punch in the gut; his book is as moving and involving as a Russian novel. . . . An intimate, searing memoir and a vivid, detailed history." —*The Washington Post*

"Masterful. . . . A salient reminder of what can be achieved by citizens who remain unbowed and unbroken." —*The Economist*

"Formidable in scope and profoundly humane." —Alexandra Schwartz, *The New Yorker*

"A truly American story. . . . A powerful reminder of what happens when ideology is put before humanity." —*Newsweek*

"Substantial and elegantly written." —*The Boston Globe*

"A must-read for a new generation of empowered patients, informed medical practitioners, and challenged caregivers—lest history repeat itself." —*Publishers Weekly* (starred review)

"David France is uniquely positioned to bear witness to the science and politics of the AIDS epidemic, its deeply personal impact, and the activists who refused to be silenced by it."
—Rebecca Skloot, author of
The Immortal Life of Henrietta Lacks

"Subtle and searing. . . . [France] uses his privileged access to put us in the heart of the action, or more usually, inaction."
—*The Observer*

"Essential. . . . An extraordinary book. . . . A sweeping social history, a bracing act of in-depth journalism, and a searingly honest memoir all at once."
—*Slate*

"A great and an important book, and we owe David France an enormous debt of gratitude for writing it."
—Richard Russo, author of *Everybody's Fool*

"Unflinching, brutally honest. . . . A must-read."
—*Library Journal* (starred review)

"This superbly written chronicle will stand as a towering work in its field, the best book on the pretreatment years of the epidemic since Randy Shilts's *And the Band Played On* (1987), which it corrects in places."
—*The Sunday Times* (London)

"An incredibly thorough people's history. . . . There's no question these stories will serve as useful models for the ongoing fight for LGBTQ rights in this country."
—*The Stranger*

"A masterpiece of intimate storytelling with moral purpose."
—Andrew Solomon

"Spectacular and soulful."
—*Booklist* (starred review)

"A sweeping social history, a bracing act of in-depth journalism, and a searingly honest memoir all at once."
—*Slate*

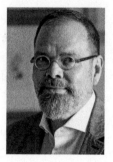

David France

How to Survive a Plague

David France is the author of *Our Fathers*, a book about the Catholic sexual abuse scandal, which Showtime adapted into a film. He coauthored *The Confession* with former New Jersey governor Jim McGreevey. He is a contributing editor for *New York* and has written as well for *The New York Times*. His documentary film *How to Survive a Plague* was an Oscar finalist, won a Directors Guild Award and a Peabody Award, and was nominated for two Emmys, among other accolades.

www.davidfrance.com

ALSO BY DAVID FRANCE

Our Fathers: The Secret Life of the Catholic Church in an Age of Scandal

Bag of Toys

How to Survive a Plague

The Story
of How Activists
and Scientists
Tamed AIDS

·

David France

Vintage Books
A Division of Penguin Random House LLC
New York

FIRST VINTAGE BOOKS EDITION, OCTOBER 2017

Copyright © 2016 by David France

All rights reserved. Published in the United States by Vintage Books,
a division of Penguin Random House LLC, New York, and in Canada by
Random House of Canada, a division of Penguin Random House Canada
Limited, Toronto. Originally published in hardcover in the United States by
Alfred A. Knopf, a division of Penguin Random House LLC, New York, in 2016.

Vintage and colophon are registered trademarks of Penguin Random House LLC.

The Library of Congress has cataloged the Knopf edition as follows:
Names: France, David, author.
Title: How to survive a plague : the inside story of how citizens and science tamed AIDS
/ by David France.
Description: First edition. | New York : Alfred A. Knopf, 2016. |
Includes bibliographical references and index.
Identifiers: LCCN 2016010685
Subjects: LCSH: HIV-positive persons—New York (State)—New York. | AIDS
activists—New York (State)—New York. | AIDS (Disease)—Research—New York
(State)—New York. | AIDS (Disease)—Treatment—New York (State)—New York. |
BISAC: HEALTH & FITNESS / Diseases / AIDS & HIV. | HISTORY / Social
History. | HISTORY / United States / 20th Century.
Classification: LCC RA643.84.N7 F73 2016 | DDC 362.19697/920097471—dc23
LC record available at https://lccn.loc.gov/2016010685

Vintage Books Trade Paperback ISBN: 978-0-307-74543-9
eBook ISBN: 978-0-451-49330-9

Author photograph © Ken Schles
Book design by Iris Weinstein

www.vintagebooks.com

Printed in the United States of America
10 9 8 7 6 5 4

Grief is a sword, or it is nothing.

PAUL MONETTE

CONTENTS

How to Survive a Plague

The Memorial Service

The experience of death, which had bound them together a quarter century ago, unexpectedly reunited them on an unseasonably warm January afternoon in 2013. They made their way down East Thirty-second Street in Manhattan just after two o'clock, wending sedately toward the stark black doorway of the Cutting Room, a performance space hosting the memorial service for Spencer Cox, one of the country's most recognizable AIDS activists. Long before the glass doors swung open, a line stretched down the block. Taxicabs deposited luminaries from the worlds of science and medicine, of theater, advertising, and media, of activism, art, and academia, people from all over the United States, from Europe and Africa. Many of them were hollow cheeked and balanced on canes or on one another, slowed by age or disease or a reluctance to reenter the community of the grieving. Even the nimble among them wore haunted expressions. If you knew what to look for, you saw in their faces the burden of a shared past, the years and years of similar services. This was what survivors of the plague looked like.

The crowd swelled to five hundred. Some among them were adorned in mementos: faded protest buttons or T-shirts with militant slogans. This was the generation that fought AIDS from the dawn of the global pandemic. Most had been members or supporters of the AIDS Coalition to Unleash Power, or ACT UP—the radical protest organization that started in New York City but went on to count 148 chapters in 19 countries, with perhaps 10,000 members at its peak. The movement collapsed in the mid-1990s, when the advent of effective medicine finally staunched much of the dying. In the decades since then, it had seemed that the menace had receded, at least in America. But death convoked them once again.

Few people personified the epidemic's long history in America more than Cox. A college dropout, he was just twenty years old when he got

3

his grim diagnosis. Given only a few months to live, he threw himself into ACT UP, becoming a central player in the movement's Treatment + Data Committee, where patients and their advocates puzzled through the science of virology, chemistry, and immunology. Their insights won them audiences with researchers in the deepest corridors of science—audiences, then respect, then working partnerships; it was the first time patients had joined in the search for their own salvation. Cox, a consummate networker, illustrated the developing science by submitting his own health complications to the scrutiny of reporters. In his drive to give the disease a face, he kept no aspect of his life with HIV offstage—not his rapid viral mutations, his enlarging lymph nodes, the humiliating and painful diarrhea that regularly sidelined him, or the cruel complication that turned his left eye cloudy and useless.

That was how I first met him. In the winter of 1988, he brought me his latest laboratory results to help describe how certain experimental drugs were thought to work, and how, in fact, they routinely failed. We met in a dark coffee shop late in the morning. Short and smooth faced with dark eyes and floppy black hair, he arrived Brando style in industrial work boots, jeans tight as a sunburn, and a black leather bomber jacket over a white T-shirt—the uniform of ACT UP. His youth disarmed me. He looked like a teenager, not yet able to grow a beard. But he displayed a researcher's grasp of his own cellular tapestry and a facility for rendering complex immunological principles into everyday language. He was anything but self-pitying. Reaching into a canvas army surplus bag, he spun a sheath of his lab results across the table, accompanied by a line from Bette Davis that was lost on me. Until recently, Cox had learned much of what he knew from the movies, especially those of the 1940s and '50s, or the theater, which had been the subject of his aborted education.

Over the ensuing years, he became a principal source for much of my AIDS reporting, and among the most effective treatment advocates in the field. But his seminal achievement came in the area of biostatistics. It was Cox who conceived the drug trial innovations that in record time helped to bring to market the therapies that stopped HIV from being an automatic death sentence. He claimed no credit for this, and until shortly before his death only a few insiders were aware that a self-taught person with AIDS—by training an actor—had made this history-changing contribution.

Since that stunning breakthrough in 1996, the new treatments had reached millions of people worldwide, returning to them the promise of a near-normal life-span. Some had been just breaths away from their own deaths. But after a few weeks on treatment they rose from their hospital beds and, against all reasonable expectation, went home to resume an ordinary life. So dramatic was their resurrection that stupefied doctors began calling it the Lazarus effect.

And yet the pharmaceutical marvels Cox fought so hard to bring into existence failed him in the end. His infection proved to be resistant to many drug combinations. The country's best doctors tinkered with "salvage" regimens specifically for him, accomplishing numerous barely-in-time rescues. For over half his life Cox careened from one medical trauma to another, maintaining his darkly comic facade, though in recent years he had grown weary. The last time I saw him he spoke of feeling run-down. When he checked into the hospital a few weeks later, his viral load was overbearing and his T-cell count, which had been in the healthy range, had sunk to just thirty, putting him at risk for a host of fatal infections. Doctors diagnosed hypoglycemia and severe pneumonia. By the following Tuesday, forty-four years old but wracked and worn as a guerrilla commandant, he died from multiple complications of AIDS.

So went the global AIDS pandemic in its fourth decade. A precise number of the dead can't be fixed, as the majority have fallen in areas of sub-Saharan Africa unknown to doctors or census takers. At the time of Cox's death, the body count was as high as forty million, which is nearly twice the devastation of the bubonic plague that threatened humankind in the fourteenth century. In the United States, the official count was 658,507 dead by the end of 2012—an approximate figure, despite its ring of precision. In the early years especially, many people were declared dead from other causes in order to spare the relatives from stigma or because doctors mistook the symptoms. Or the deceased went down as suicide statistics instead, having chosen pills or bullets or the high-rise window over the inevitable.

Though so much has changed, so much is still the same. Around the globe two million people still die from AIDS every year because the cost of the effective medicines—under a dollar a day—is prohibitive. In America, where the price is fifty times higher, a federal law provided the treatment to indigent patients since 1987, adopted under intense lobbying by gay leaders, though access to the medicine was spotty nonetheless, because a prescription was required and many could not afford to visit a doctor. The year Cox died, 13,711 other Americans were claimed by AIDS. As in the epidemic's very first year, most belonged to communities that were stigmatized, marginalized, feared, or hated. Cox had begun his journey through the plague as a gay man at a time when most Americans supported laws criminalizing homosexuality. He finished his life entirely dependent upon social services for his day-to-day living, and on probation for a criminal conviction after a descent into common drug addiction.

Few of his old colleagues knew about Cox's last days. The members of ACT UP had drifted far apart in recent years. Even Cox's old HIV-positive support group, men who had relied upon one another in the way one does in wartime and made a blood vow to be at one another's side when the time came, scattered once AIDS went from a mostly fatal disease to a condition that could for the most part be managed. "When we realized we weren't going to die," said David Barr, who convened the support group, "instead we all got sick of each other."

That could not have been foreseen at the support group's height. In the epic struggle for survival that consumed the plague years, these men—Barr, an attorney by training; Peter Staley, a former bond trader; Gregg Bordowitz, an experimental filmmaker; Derek Link, a onetime bookstore clerk; Mark Harrington, a film archivist—were among the recognized generals, the architects and administrators of the movement's public health strategy. Successive presidential administrations sought their insights, and Nobel Prize winners adopted their critiques. Global pharmaceutical companies succumbed to their demands, at first out of fear of guerrilla protests and later out of respect for their minds. Embracing their reputations for arrogance, insolence, and prominence, they had jokingly called themselves "the HIVIPs." That anyone with HIV had a chance for an ordinary life was thanks to the work they did.

Yet their extraordinary journeys had rendered them mostly unprepared for an ordinary life. In countless ways, survival, unexpected as it was, proved as hard to adjust to as the plague itself. Many in the at-risk communities shared this paradox, whether or not they'd been infected themselves. Nobody left those years uncorrupted by what they'd witnessed, not only the mass deaths—100,000 lost in New York City alone, snatched from tightly drawn social circles—but also the foul truths that a microscopic virus had revealed about American culture: politicians who welcomed the plague as proof of God's will, doctors who refused the victims medical care, clergymen and often even parents themselves who withheld all but a shiver of grief. Such betrayal would be impossible to forget in the subsequent years. As when the gates of Auschwitz were thrown open at last, this new era only made it possible to finally grasp the hideousness of what came before. "So for us," wrote Primo Levi about his own liberation, "even the hour of victory rang out grave and muffled, and filled our souls with joy and yet with a painful sense of prudency so that we should have liked to wash our consciences and our memories clean from the foulness that lay upon them; and also with anguish, because we felt that this should never happen, that now nothing could ever happen good and pure enough to rub out our past, and that the scars of the outrage would remain within us forever, and in the memories of those who saw it, and in the places where it occurred and in the stories that we should tell of it."

The burden of memory was something Cox spoke about with deep insight. Sensing its toll on the mental health of survivors, he formed a new organization to bring attention to the second crucible. In our "hour of victory," depression and isolation were expanding problems. So was a syndrome labeled "survivor's guilt," an idea that bound those who remained more to the dead than to the living. Add to this the unrecognized health consequences common among those diagnosed in the 1980s—including rapid aging issues, and an onslaught of end-of-life cancers and conditions. Cox saw all of this coming. He issued white papers and penned op-eds, but despite those efforts, he was unable to spark the interest of researchers or funders, much less of the generation of gays who never experienced the plague. His new organization withered, and he sank deep into his own depression and isolation.

I remained closer to him than most of his friends over his final year. In our last conversation, he bitterly complained that the community that inherited the advances he helped wrought, who lived integrated lives as gay citizens, who went on to fight for marriage equality and against discrimination in the military, whether or not they'd been infected, had abandoned his generation and forgotten the events that had shaped them. He felt erased, his suffering—which in the past had enlightened the public and challenged science—suddenly insignificant. His new policy was to talk as little about his personal health as possible. It wasn't until after he died that I learned that Cox, a regular poster on the website Gawker, used the nom de plume "French Twist 40" to describe his agony in those final months. "Some days, I'm fine, and get around with no problem," he wrote. "Other days, I'm curled in [the] fetal position in bed the whole day (and more often, several days), racked with pain the whole time. Some days I'm on the subway getting the stink-eye from some old or pregnant lady who clearly wants my seat, and can't tell just by looking at me that I'm sitting because I'm on my way home from a doctor's appointment, and if I stand for one more minute, I'm going to fall on the ground."

When grieving friends were packing away Cox's possessions after his death, they found a shelf of unopened medicine bottles and a drawer of unfilled prescriptions. Apparently Cox had stopped taking his hard-won medicine, accounting for his quick demise. Angry speculation about this consumed his friends, but most agreed it signaled a post-trauma syndrome unique to survivors. Many of the five hundred people waiting outside the Cutting Room recognized that they shared the symptoms. In the tradition of the movement, people in line accorded it an irreverent name—AIDS Survivor Syndrome, or ASS—and took it very seriously.

The doors swung open at precisely 2:30. The mood inside was mostly somber and reflective, despite the efforts of a pair of drag queens done up as Joan Crawford and Cox's totem, Bette Davis, greeting the mourn-ers. A video played scenes from the old films that always ran through Cox's mind and frequently spilled from his lips. The camp sensibility was lost on almost nobody except perhaps for Cox's mother, Beverly, who had traveled up from Atlanta. She steadied herself on the arm of Nick Cox, Spencer's only sibling, who was also gay. They took seats in the first row, alongside friends of the family. A mother's grief was a thick wall around them.

When Larry Kramer arrived, one of the organizers took him by the arm. "Follow me, I have a seat for you," he said, leading him through the crowd to the second row. Among the activists, Kramer alone was accorded this special treatment. No individual was more responsible for galvanizing the AIDS movement than Kramer. His plays, books, and essays over the years pushed the gay community to demand that the world take notice. Now seventy-seven, he stayed as busy as ever, though AIDS had slowed him noticeably and he too felt a touch of the survivor's syndrome. That morning he seriously considered not com-ing. What finally motivated him to take a cab uptown was a need to stand with his fellow survivors, for whom his emotions were boundless. "Love was always love, anytime and anyplace," Gabriel Garcia Mar-quez wrote, "but it was more solid the closer it came to death."

Chip Duckett, a professional party planner who had organized the affair, walked to center stage to begin the service. "If there was ever any question that Spencer Cox would stop at absolutely nothing to be at the center of attention"—he broke for over-eager laughter—"this is it."

He passed the microphone to a succession of speakers, eventually introducing Mike Isbell, Cox's partner for more than eight years. After their breakup they had remained friends for many years, but as he had with so many people, Cox pushed Isbell away as his troubles grew. They hadn't spoken in some time. "Spencer often didn't make it easy for people who loved him," Isbell began. "The AIDS epidemic traumatized Spencer, and I imagine this trauma stayed with him until the end. I recall being at dinner parties—some of you were probably there—or out to meals with friends, where someone would talk about 'living with AIDS' and Spencer would immediately reply, 'I'm not *living* with AIDS, I'm *dying* of AIDS!' He'd say this in a tone of defiance, but I knew he was scared to death."

Isbell spoke of how ironic it was that Spencer lost his way after the treatments arrived and the lifesaving mission came to an end. "He desperately wanted another life outside of AIDS," he said, looking around the overflowing room. "It seemed that in the 'treatment era,' he was always in search of something but not finding it."

Peter Staley was the last to speak. He had been unable to sleep the previous few nights, struggling to find the words to make sense of Cox's death and life. Staley was among a small group of people who had raced to Cox's side when they'd learned about the final hospitalization. By the time he arrived, Cox was already in steep decline. He'd gone into cardiac arrest three times, and his kidneys had failed. Staley stood outside the hospital door as medical personnel rushed in and out. He could hear the defibrillator lifting Cox's chest off the table again and again. When Cox was stabilized, Staley and Tim Horn, another activist, were allowed inside briefly. Minutes later came another heart attack and another brutal resuscitation.

From his telephone, Staley posted a note to a private Facebook message group where he'd been coordinating support for Cox. It landed in my phone with a vibration and a jingle as I stood in the cold morning sun on Sixth Avenue, a mile and a half away: *Spencer passed.* I slumped, lightheaded and bereft, against a plate glass window.

The four weeks between then and the memorial service had done little to dim Staley's pain. He placed the pages of his planned eulogy on the small lectern, squinting into the harsh stage lighting to study the faces before him.

He said, "I first met Spencer when he started showing up at ACT UP meetings in the fall of 'eighty-eight. We were all so young. I was younger than most. But he was seven years my junior."

He caught his breath, remembering.

"It was a wonder watching him wow the FDA, and in meetings with the biggest names in AIDS research, like Anthony Fauci. He earned the respect and the love of his fellow science geeks and those of us lower down the learning curve. . . . Eight million on standardized regimens. Eight million lives saved. It's a stunning legacy, and so bittersweet. How could that young gay man, confronted with his own demise, respond with a level of genius that impacted millions of lives but failed to save his own?"

Staley spoke of Cox's last failed burst of activism, and called on the weathered activists to snatch meaning from his death. "He spoke out forcefully about the depression and PTSD that the surviving genera-tion of gay men from the plague years often suffered from, regardless of HIV status. While many of us, through luck or circumstance, have landed on our feet, all of us, in some way, have unprocessed grief, or guilt, or an overwhelming sense of abandonment from a community that turned its back on us and increasingly stigmatized us, all in an attempt to pretend that AIDS wasn't a problem anymore."

He scanned the vacuum-quiet room. "That is Spencer's call to action," he said, "and we should take it on."

PART I

•

When It Rains, It Pours

I

Independence Day

I arrived in New York City for the first time on a college sojourn from Michigan, in September 1978, for an internship at the United Nations and a chance to explore Christopher Street, the mountaintop of gay life. At nineteen, I was not yet comfortable with the longings of my heart. But Manhattan struck me as a city of promise, at once grimy and magical, an enormous, thrilling place where people could hide and be found. I committed to both city and self after collecting my degree in June 1981. My college roommate Brian Gougeon and I took up in a tiny one-room apartment in Midtown, sleeping chastely on opposite edges of a narrow, lumpy bed.

Gougeon had grown up in a large Catholic family in a rural part of Michigan, yet he possessed an innate cosmopolitan sensibility, which I lacked thoroughly, an easiness with being gay, and a strong ambition as an artist. I envied Gougeon's ability to create beauty from nothing, which suited our finances. On our walls he hung his paintings, mostly of faraway places he'd only imagined. One featured pyramids and palm trees, which he titled "Egypt." Another depicted an idealized living room scene. He called this one "Home," though in significant ways he had never truly felt at home, nor had I, not until getting to New York. We were part of the largest influx of gay men and lesbians in New York's history, a vast gay reverse-diaspora; born into exile and separated from our own kind, we were reassembling in a place that had only existed in the imagination, the "new City of Friends" conjured by Walt Whitman a hundred years before. "Home" was an ambition, as fanciful as the pyramids.

Our timing was unfortunate. Just two weeks after unpacking, on the Friday of the long July 4 weekend, *The New York Times* carried the first news of the plague. "Rare Cancer Seen in 41 Homosexuals," ran the headline. The cases were concentrated in Manhattan, with a few in the San Francisco Bay Area as well, and consisted of violet-colored spots appearing somewhere on the body, easily mistaken for bruises though they were sometimes raised and textured. The cancer was not just skin-deep; it killed by spreading to the lung, liver, or spleen. One in five was already dead. The article noted that "most cases had involved homosexual men who have had multiple and frequent sexual encounters with different partners, as many as 10 sexual encounters each night up to four times a week. Many of the patients have also been treated for viral infections such as herpes, cytomegalovirus and hepatitis B as well as parasitic infections such as amebiasis and giardiasis. Many patients also reported that they had used drugs such as amyl nitrite and LSD to heighten sexual pleasure."

I later learned that men who read the paper on the ferries to Fire Island that day, having immediately recognized themselves in those demographics, spent the long weekend examining one another's flesh. They found purple lesions by the dozens. It was possible to stand on those boardwalks and pool decks and beaches that weekend and foretell the whole terrible future. But none of the signs appeared among our new acquaintances in the city. We thought for a while that our economic marginality put us out of reach even from this—what became a disease of the poor began by assaulting the gay bourgeoisie, the "Beautiful People of the Fire Island Pines," as a popular ad described the niche.

Although a doctor in the article called the outbreak "rather devastating," I was more annoyed than alarmed by the news. The story seemed like a new slander on the gay community, which had existed cohesively for barely more than a decade since the Stonewall Riots in 1969. Every advance since then was met by an extreme and paranoiac counterforce. The 1970s produced the fiercest round of anti-gay legislation the nation had ever known, hammered into place in the name of protecting children, of all things, from us. Dozens of states and cities adopted measures preemptively blocking gay rights ordinances. Anita Bryant, a Miss America runner-up and the movement's obstreperous leader, still exercised considerable national influence on the July morning when the "Rare Cancer" story hit. It was impossible to read the news outside of this context; it seemed like just another lie, a call to more hatred, a fiercer backlash. Anyone could see prejudice in what news of us was or was not being covered. On the day in 1980 that the U.S. Senate candidates John Lindsay, Bess Myerson, and Elizabeth Holtzman debated their gay rights planks before a citywide gay Democratic club—a first in history and the suggestion of coming political clout—the *Times* instead ran a story entitled "Rest Room Shut to Foreclose Use by Homosexuals," the toilet in question being in suburban Westchester County. A few months later came one of the most hideous anti-gay crimes in the nation's history, when a madman drove through the Village emptying a submachine gun into crowds of gay men. He killed two and seriously injured seven. For the community, it was a devastating watershed; for the *Times*, it merited a few paragraphs inside, with no mention of other rampages in the weeks and months leading up to it, no quotes from advocates, no elegiac background stories about the victims, and no follow-up coverage in the coming days of the large candlelight vigil for the victims outside St. Vincent's Medical Center or the community's two memorial services that drew thousands and thousands of gay men and lesbians.

I didn't bother to check for spots in the mirror. I had never contracted a venereal disease. Though the potential for unlimited sexual exploration is what drew me to New York in the first place, I had had fewer than a dozen sexual experiences in my life (a number of them women) and I struggled with self-confidence. My childhood had been a difficult one on account of my gayness. I paid a steep price every day for being effeminate and soft-voiced, not just when a pack of young men separated me from my friends behind the auto shop and left me broken on the ground, or buried me in a dozen fists on the basketball court, purpling my cheeks under the supervision of the coach, who locked eyes with me and rejected my pleas for help with a bemused smile—I feared him most, for his authoritative complicity, for closing the official court of appeals to the likes of me. I was seized with fear almost every moment. I felt it at the Marathon gas station, in the 7-Eleven parking lot, outside Woodland Mall, every time the eyes of a stranger flickered with recognition. My innate demeanor betrayed me; I was incapable of getting away with the lie.

By my eighteenth birthday I'd had just two furtive sexual interludes with men: one with a middle-aged Mexican gentleman who gently undressed me one New Year's Eve, and the other with a spirited and "straight" twenty-one-year-old motel clerk from Canada who sprung into my bed to demonstrate the multiple "disgusting things" he had learned from other guests. Those two men were the first hapless evidence that I wasn't alone. Had I been more resourceful, or less isolated, I might have discovered the affirming work of James Baldwin and Gertrude Stein, or the first dozen or so nonfiction books already published from gay social thinkers. Instead, I went to the card catalog in the school library to look up "Homosexuality." My heart pounded with fear of being caught. There, just past "Homogeneous" and "Homo sapiens," was the card that said: "Homosexuality. See 'Sexuality, deviant.'" Moving through the literature I learned that "oral regression" (Edmund Bergler) and "paraphilia" (Sándor Ferenczi) had caused my "sociopathic personality disturbance" (the American Psychiatric Association). I was clearly ill. Mine was a "counterfeit sex," a "third sex," an "intermediate sex" which precluded any expectation for happiness. Dr. Stanley F. Yolles, the director of the National Institute of Mental Health, part of the U.S. Public Health Service, wrote, "With broadened parental understanding and more scientific research, hopefully, the chances that anyone's child will become a victim of homosexuality will eventually decrease." I was a scourge, something to be eradicated. I entered counseling at nineteen and let a psychologist put me through a discredited regimen called Reparative Therapy, alleged to make me straight.

I don't know how, but I eventually dismissed the entire public discussion about my condition as bunk. By the time I relocated to New York, I had rejected every authoritative thing published or said about my kind as malicious calumny. It was into this category that I put the *Times* article about a new disease that could somehow distinguish one's sexual orientation. I crumpled my copy of the paper in disgust. In any case, officials from the Centers for Disease Control doubted it was contagious.

THE AIR that Friday morning was hot and close, sluiced by sheets of rain. Inside a cramped medical office, dog-legged off the dark lobby of an apartment tower on West Twelfth Street in Greenwich Village, Dr. Joe Sonnabend, a specialist in infectious diseases, was swallowing his own anger, a copy of the *Times* in his grip. He had been expecting the "Rare Cancer" story; in fact, he was partly responsible for getting the news out in the first place. He had seen the malignancy in one of his own patients, and in May had discovered that there were eighteen other cases at the NYU Medical Center, all in young gay men. This was astonishing to him. Previously, Kaposi's sarcoma, the cancer in question, was so rare it struck just two Americans out of every three million, almost always very old men of Jewish or Mediterranean background. It was typically so slow to progress and clinically so meaningless in terms of morbidity and mortality that there was no need even for treatment. Sonnabend learned of the other cases from Dr. Joyce Wallace, to whom he had referred his KS patient, and she had learned of them by calling the National Cancer Institute in Bethesda, Maryland. Someone there referred her to the NYU Medical Center's Dr. Alvin Friedman-Kien, an overnight KS expert who was quietly treating the majority of the new patients.

Eighteen KS patients were a significant cluster, a trumpet call that said something remarkable was going around, Sonnabend felt. In his opinion, doctors throughout New York should have been alerted to the outbreak. At a minimum, he believed, the CDC and officials at the NYU Medical Center should have reached out to the doctors with bustling gay practices, like his, telling them what to look for and what to do with suspected KS cases. The oversight disgusted him. Though soft-spoken and remote, Sonnabend was quick to disappointments and muffled rages. He held people to towering, often impossible standards, and he was prone to interior furies against those who disappointed him or systems that failed his moral test. The silence around KS was one such failure. "To me, this is absolutely, absolutely extraordinary," Sonnabend stammered. "By the time you get to number five and number six, you know *something* is under way."

In New York medical circles, Sonnabend was a curious, enigmatic figure. He had studied medicine and infectious diseases in his native South Africa, and for many years worked as a research scientist in the UK, where he held prestigious appointments at the University of Edinburgh and the National Institute for Medical Research. His specialty was interferon, a natural protein produced by white blood cells to fight off infections; he had trained with Alick Isaacs, interferon's discoverer. The field was new and relatively little had come from it so far, but interferon research held the promise of being useful in the war on cancer, as the compound also seemed to show antitumor activity. A temporary professorship at the Mt. Sinai Medical School first lured Sonnabend to New York in 1969, and the offer of a grant to set up his own interferon lab brought him eagerly back in 1977.

He was a changed man in New York City, animated by the promise of personal freedoms that were unthinkable in Johannesburg or even in London at the time. He left behind an untidy private life that included a wife and two sons (by two other women) as well as a history of numerous, mostly fleeting encounters with men. Now middle-aged, lanky, and tank-chested, with a speckled beard and thick eyebrows, he found it possible in New York to uncage his desires for men without shame. He settled on Greenwich Street, emboldened in the neighborhood's restaurants and clubs, especially the anything-goes International Stud, which he visited many evenings before bed; he had only to cross the street. He also developed significant though short-lived love relationships in New York City, including with a male model who lived with him for a year and a half, and with Harley Hackett, a mild-mannered and generous playwright who held him in reverence and awe. He was, finally, a contented man.

Then, in 1979, his research grant was not renewed, leaving him suddenly jobless and panicked. His savings were unlikely to outlast the slow pace of job hunting in academia. So at age forty-four, he borrowed $25,000 and went into private practice, taking along Hackett, now just a good friend, as his office manager. It would be Sonnabend's first turn as a treating physician. He settled on a boutique practice diagnosing and treating gay men with venereal diseases. It was work a good deal beneath his ability and training but it capitalized on his research background in infectious diseases and his independent experience in the field: to supplement his professor's salary, he had moonlighted in the city's Bureau of Venereal Disease Control as director of continuing education. He knew next to nothing about flu and broken bones, but at the darkfield microscope and the anoscope alike he knew he could render a peerless service to patients. Indeed, it was the only field in which he felt he could responsibly practice on his own.

There was no shortage of business. The 1970s saw an explosion of sexual experimentation across America. At a time when the birth control pill freed sex from at least one of its consequences, "swinging" and "free love" flourished among heterosexuals. Feminist literature on sex and power proliferated. Among gay men the sexual revolution was profound and significant. Before the Stonewall Riots, homosexuals were an "unacknowledged minority . . . without a spokesman, without a leader, without a publication, without a philosophy of life, without an accepted justification for its own existence," as a 1951 bestseller put it. The era of Gay Liberation began a process of discovery. To act flauntingly on one's sexual appetence was essentially an act of rebellion, but also of self-affirmation, identity exploration, and community forging. What from the outside might have looked like pure carnal zeal was the rudimentary first pass for this emerging young culture.

A tidal wave of disease followed. In some quarters of the community, lengthy diagnostic profiles became bragging rights. But whether embraced or regretted, VD was suddenly a fact of gay men's lives, and around the gay precincts of New York people knew to see Joe Sonnabend, as much for his discretion and geniality as for his apathetic billing practices. He soon had a patient base of well over one thousand, and even more over at the Gay Men's Health Project, the inexpensive community clinic on Sheridan Square where he volunteered, and where I first met him, as a patient, in 1981. Syphilis, hepatitis, herpes, venereal warts, and gonorrhea were at record highs, and the trend showed no signs of reversing. Unusual cases of protozoan infestations of the gastrointestinal tracts of gay men had risen 7,000 percent in the previous six years and were now so common that a new diagnosis was officially coined, gay bowel syndrome, recognized by the McGraw-Hill manual *Colorectal Surgery,* an industry standard, and the Centers for Disease Control alike. There appeared to be concomitant epidemics of cytomegalovirus and Epstein-Barr virus, and a bizarre incidence rate of lymphadenopathy—knobby and swollen lymph nodes, which one would expect to encounter infrequently. Sonnabend diagnosed lymphadenopathy in 40 percent of his patients, a consequence, he believed, of the body's reaction to various other venereal infections. That same causal link could also have explained the simultaneous preponderance of enlarged spleens, low white blood cell counts, and low blood platelets.

But Kaposi's sarcoma?

When he first heard about Friedman-Kien's cluster, Sonnabend called him immediately. Friedman-Kien, a brash and well-regarded dermatologist about Sonnabend's age, confirmed his unusual caseload. Previously in his long career he had seen only seven or eight cases, in elderly men as expected. He saw his first anomalous KS lesion in January 1981, on the flesh of a young man originally from the Midwest who worked as a decorator in the city. The KS was only part of his troubles. He had been treated for a remarkable constellation of health challenges including fever, weight loss, enlarged spleen and liver, and hardened lymph nodes in his neck and groin. Surgeons had opened his abdomen, removed his spleen, and taken biopsies of his liver and lymph nodes, but nobody had thought to wonder about the lavender splotches covering his legs. The laboratory confirmed Friedman-Kien's suspicion about KS. Within weeks, he diagnosed a second patient, a witty Shakespearean actor with lesions on his face, a disaster in his line of work. Both men were gay, a fact Friedman-Kien, not himself out to his colleagues, found unusual enough to bring up at the hospital's biweekly tumor conference.

Soon another NYU doctor, an oncologist named Linda Laubenstein, told him she had a few KS cases. Like some of Friedman-Kien's patients, hers had collapsing immune systems as well, and all were gay.

Suspecting there might be others, Friedman-Kien queried half a dozen gay and lesbian doctors in the city and contacted a gay dermatologist in San Francisco, Dr. Marcus Conant, to see if the disease cluster had traveled. Conant was unaware of the problem. But the following night, after attending a Bay Area dermatology meeting, he called Friedman-Kien with a quavering voice. Three cases, he said, all gay. Days later he called to raise the total to six.

As Sonnabend listened to Friedman-Kien's history, he itched to return to the laboratory. It would be easy enough to learn if an infectious agent were involved, Sonnabend figured. He would start by looking at interferon, his old métier. Friedman-Kien offered to make room for him in his own lab, and he accepted.

Before ending the call, Sonnabend allowed himself a smoldering rant, decrying the silence around the disease cluster and delivering an emphatic plea for Friedman-Kien to sound the alarm throughout the city. With the authority of the NYU Medical Center behind him, his warnings would reach every area practitioner and, eventually, every gay man with KS lesions, bringing them into immediate care. Friedman-Kien, rankled by the scolding, said he had already alerted the gay doctors he knew and was already preparing a physician warning about the unusual cluster.

That was in May. When no public announcement appeared in June, Sonnabend's mood darkened further. In the first days of July, he leaned over his typewriter to pound out the alert himself. He was not sure how he would disseminate it, but even before he could make copies, Friedman-Kien beckoned him to his NYU office. There, in what seemed to Sonnabend like a kind of performance piece, Friedman-Kien grabbed the phone and dialed Lawrence K. Altman, the *New York Times* science writer and a doctor himself, an acquaintance of Friedman-Kien's from their training days, finally doing what Sonnabend had requested in the spring. He told Altman about the mystery and announced that a letter alerting his fellow physicians would go out with the morning mail.

So Sonnabend wasn't surprised to see Friedman-Kien quoted prominently by Altman in the *Times* on July 3, announcing the gay cancer. What did surprise him was news that the current weekly journal from the CDC, issued that same day, contained a detailed report on the mystery, and one of its lead authors was Friedman-Kien. Sonnabend drew the least generous conclusion from this. The journal piece must have had weeks of pre-publication drafting and review. Had Friedman-Kien delayed going public in order to complete the article, he wondered (and

Friedman-Kien denied), assuring maximum personal exposure for himself? In that time, how many doctors mistook lesions for bruises? And meanwhile, the caseload had grown from eighteen to forty-one.

Greed and personal aggrandizement, Sonnabend fumed, was going to be the soil from which this plague would bloom.

WHEN LARRY KRAMER read the *Times* piece in his large apartment at Two Fifth Avenue, his thoughts were very personal. He had come of age in the furtive 1950s, then left for London and a series of screenwriting jobs that kept him somewhat naïve to the sexual revolution of the American 1960s. He returned stateside after the sexual radicalism had already taken hold, with the resulting conveyor belts of antibiotics, antifungals, and microbicides. He found the sexual Olympics unnerving; when it came to matters of the flesh, he was Jane Austen in Erica Jong's world. For so many in the community now, whether or not someone was bedworthy had eclipsed all other attributes to become the singular measure of a man. Kramer was past forty, balding, and boxy in the waist. He had a steely brow and soft shoulders. His considerable warmth and intelligence sometimes served him well enough, but any luck in dating invited even more frustration, as he tended to fall in love with the people he slept with, leading to unhappy tension on the subjects of monogamy and cohabitation. Breakups and heartbreaks added up, most dramatically involving the bright-eyed and delicately-featured architect David Webster, ten years his junior.

Their nasty separation turned Kramer against the gay world entirely, which he burlesqued in a venomous 1978 novel he called *Faggots*. The book, a thinly veiled roman à clef, took readers through clubs with names like "The Toilet," through sex acts involving fists, bodily waste, and nephews, all of it fueled by more than seventy recreational drugs the totality of which caused impotence and gave rise to dull stretches of sadomasochism to fill the drug-addled hours. In his view, the new world that gay men had built was devoid of evolutionary purpose, its inhabitants no more advanced than randy bonobos.

Condemnation for the work and the author was fierce and widespread. The gay bookstore in New York refused to stock *Faggots*, and the Canadian gay newspaper *Body Politic*, not content with a vituperative review, urged a boycott. His pilloried acquaintances and ex-lovers howled about his caricatures, none more than Webster himself, parodied as a depraved and shallow leather queen called Dinky Adams. It was "a total invasion of my life," Webster protested. "Larry was going through my drawers, piecing together scraps of paper in the waste-basket." Its publication made Kramer into a pariah. That summer, he stayed away from Fire Island and obsessed bitterly over his thorough rejection—personally, socially, sexually, and now literarily.

Then came the *Times* piece about gay cancer. Kramer immediately seized upon it as his vindication: gay men were involved in something that was not just disastrous to the soul, in his view, but incompatible with life. In the previous year, a number of Kramer's friends had come down with ailments that stumped the best medical minds in New York City. Reading the article, he recognized that they had similar venereal disease profiles. So did Kramer, for that matter. He felt the burn of imaginary KS lesions on his legs and arms.

Immediately following the holiday weekend, he called Dr. Friedman-Kien, and a few days later arrived for an appointment on the seventh floor of the NYU Medical Center, overlooking the East River. There in Friedman-Kien's tiny waiting room Kramer bumped into a friend, Donald Krintzman, a marketing director for the Joffrey Ballet. "Yes," Krintzman offered, looking ashen and panicked, "I've got Kaposi's sarcoma."

Friedman-Kien examined Kramer inch by inch and found no signs of cancer. Kramer's feeling of relief was overwhelming, and short-lived. "We're only seeing the tip of the iceberg," the doctor told him. "We don't know what it is. It would appear to be a virus, but we don't have any concrete evidence." Noting that the *Times* had gone silent, he added, "I don't think anybody is going to give a damn, and it's really up to you guys to do something."

Friedman-Kien had joined Sonnabend in the research lab, but he lacked financial support. "We're applying to the NIH for funds, but we won't get money," he told Kramer. "Just to collect specimens and freeze them—a freezer is an expensive item, and nobody will let me put my specimens in their freezer because they think they spread the disease." He had received $1,000 from the philanthropist Lily Auchincloss, who was concerned about her gay brother, but it was barely enough. He implored Kramer, whom he considered "somebody who's known in the community," to do what he could to help.

Kramer had never engaged in any kind of community organizing before. But his mother was once a Red Cross executive in suburban Washington, D.C., where he grew up, so he knew what it took to gather resources in an emergency. He promised to help. It was the right thing to do—and also an opportunity for social rehabilitation.

In August, Kramer submitted a fund-raising appeal for publication in the *New York Native*, a tabloid-sized newspaper aimed at gay men. Though it had only a few thousand readers, there existed no better way to reach the people worried about the new disease. "In the past," Kramer wrote, "we have often been a divided community; I hope we can all get together on this emergency, undivided, cohesively, and with all the numbers we in so many ways possess."

Later that week he hosted a gathering at his apartment. About eighty people attended, including the writer Edmund White, Dr. Sonnabend, and Kramer's unlucky friend with KS, Donald Krintzman. Friedman-Kien addressed the crowd, describing the cases he'd seen and repeating what he'd heard about similar cases in California—mostly in San Francisco but also in Los Angeles now, where doctors had reported a cluster of gay men coming down with *Pneumocystis carinii* pneumonia, or PCP, a disease as relatively uncommon as KS, normally striking only a few hundred Americans a year, typically organ transplant recipients who required strong immune-suppressing medication to prevent rejection. This was more evidence that severe immune suppression was involved. Untreated, PCP resulted in a quick and agonizing death akin to drowning. With timely access to pentamidine, a drug administered intravenously, the death rate could be lowered to 50 percent. But as a sign of how rare PCP was, pentamidine was no longer in production; for emergencies, the CDC kept only a small national reserve. A treating doctor had to call CDC headquarters in Atlanta to request that doses be shipped out on overnight planes. In New York, doctors dispatched messengers to meet incoming shipments at JFK airport, hoping to reach the patients in time.

The way Friedman-Kien explained it, both the pneumonia and the skin cancer indicated the arrival of a never-before-seen disease with an inexplicable predilection for gay men. "We think there might be something about gay sexual activity," he remembered telling them.

Lacking any better data, he advised sexual restraint.

There was an immediate uproar. "It was pandemonium," he recalled. "The reply was, We have fought for this freedom and we're not giving it up." Edmund White remembered it somewhat differently. "Everybody looked at everybody like, Is this guy crazy?" Still, $6,635 was raised for his research efforts that night, and follow-up campaigns were planned, specifically on Fire Island.

Over the next several weeks, Kramer emerged as the de facto leader of the response effort, passing out literature and calling for a community-wide fund-raising drive, but almost no more money materialized. Too many gay men refused to allow his social rehabilitation. As the playwright Robert Chesley wrote in the *Native*, "Now, with Kaposi's sarcoma attacking gay men, Kramer assumes he knows the cause (maybe it's on page 37 of *Faggots?* Or page 237?), and—let's say that it's easy to become frightened that Kramer's *real* emotion is a sense of having been vindicated, though tragically: he told us so, but we didn't listen to him; *nooo—we had to learn the hard way, and now we're dying.* Read anything by Kramer closely. I think you'll find that the subtext is always: the wages of gay sin are death."

To which Kramer parried, also in print, "Why is Bob Chesley not chastising *The New York Times* for ignoring us? Why is he not going after CBS and NBC and ABC for not running any items whatsoever on their programs? . . .

"Why is he not asking every homosexual in this city: Why are we here? What are we here for?"

Early Thinking

Sonnabend had a numbing schedule of work in the summer of 1981. Through the week, his office filled with frightened young men with a confounding array of symptoms. And every Saturday morning he studied their sera under microscopes in his borrowed NYU Medical Center lab. His initial thesis about interferon had proved correct: he identified dozens of his patients who tested positive for extremely high levels of a subset called *alpha* interferon, in response to significant infection, though by what wasn't clear. Rudimentary as it was, this discovery was important. It meant the disease was caused by a pathogen rather than by a chemical, such as recreational drugs, or by homosexuality per se, a macabre suggestion being advanced in certain quarters. "The idea . . . is bizarre to me," Sonnabend told a writer for *Emergency Medicine*. "I don't think anyone is claiming that homosexuals are so biologically different."

On the two coasts, he was joined by a handful of physicians treating the mysterious cases. Most were very young—a decade behind Sonnabend and Friedman-Kien in age and experience—and most were themselves gay, part of the first generation of out-of-the-closet doctors. Perhaps it was a consequence of his dyspeptic personality, but Sonnabend dismissed most of them as timid, unimaginative, and undertrained, and he removed himself from their social circles, though they tended to share common ground in their political views, which leaned far to the left. Sonnabend considered medical care a right, not a commodity. He could easily spend an hour examining patients, unconcerned about the impact on his cash flow or the bottleneck it created in the waiting room. Most patients considered the long delays a small price to pay for his attentiveness, his reassuring telephone reports, his willingness to make house calls, and his heartfelt interest in their journeys through gayness. Even before KS and PCP, he was unusually devoted to his patients. Now the worry consumed him. He began to feel that everything in his life up to this point—his experiences with interferon, venereal disease, virology, gay men, bench research—everything had been part of some cosmic plan to prepare him for this challenge. From his first phone call to Friedman-Kien, he felt the whole weight of the community of gay men upon him.

According to the CDC, by the end of August the official number of sick patients had almost tripled, to 111. Sonnabend feared the problem was much larger than that. In his practice alone, he now had three patients with KS and scores more with swollen lymph nodes. Leaving work late one Saturday, he confided in a colleague that his exhaustive efforts in the laboratory had failed to produce a working hypothesis linking them all to a single syndrome. There was one thing, though: he discovered an overwhelming epidemic of an old infection, cytomegalovirus; almost every one of his patients showed telltale antibodies for CMV, remarkable since only one-third of the general population tested positive. A member of the herpes family, CMV could be passed by way of semen and urine. But it was known to be dangerous only for newborns, resulting in seizures, pneumonia, and enlarged organs. In adults it ordinarily provoked no symptoms whatsoever, certainly not catastrophic immune suppression, and never death. But there was an undeniable flood of CMV in the gay community, as confirmed by a later study of gay men under thirty in San Francisco: 93 percent had been exposed to CMV, and a disquieting 14 percent were actively contagious at the time of testing. Unlike with some other viruses, getting CMV once didn't make a person immune to getting it again. Following the law of probability and a reasonable estimate of the community's sexual appetites, if one in six gay men was contagious, a typical sex life resulted in almost sixty new exposures every year.

It was at least plausible, Sonnabend thought, that an onslaught of CMV re-infections could destroy one's immune system and open the door to conditions that strike the weak—the so-called "opportunistic infections," like PCP. But how to explain the KS cases? No cancer had ever before been thought to be opportunistic. What might CMV and KS have in common? This question weighed heavily on Sonnabend's mind as he drove toward home that evening. He hadn't planned to stop at the baths. When he saw the rugged facade of the century-old Everard Spa Turkish Bathhouse on West Twenty-eighth Street, he spontaneously slid his car into a parking space without giving the detour much thought.

He unsnapped his seat belt and popped a penicillin pill into his mouth.

For his tours through the sexual landscape, Sonnabend swallowed antibiotics to avoid infection. As unconventional as this seemed, it wasn't novel. During World War II, the U.S. Army handed out "chemical prophylactics" to soldiers leaving on furlough (or immediately upon their return). Military medical officers called it "early treatment," though it functioned as a preventative to block syphilis, gonorrhea, and chancroid before the infections could take hold. The evidence for its efficacy was spotty and dated back to the 1940s, but in Sonnabend's personal experience it was solidly reliable. The one time he forgot the pill resulted in his only bout with VD. "Risk reduction," he called the approach. Still, most public health experts discouraged the practice as unwise. The overuse of antibiotics risked creating resistance to the pills and giving rise to super strains impervious to available medicines.

He climbed a flight of stairs, paid five dollars to a distracted attendant, scrawled his name unintelligibly into a ledger, and took a locker key, hoping a relaxing interlude might ease his mind. After undressing, he headed for the showers, the threshold to the dark catacombs that filled two floors. It took a long time beneath the hot water jets for his thoughts to turn to the surrounding scene. A man stood opposite him, also showering. On his legs was an array of purple splotches.

Sonnabend's heart pounded. "I'm a doctor," he blurted out, "and if you don't mind my asking: The stuff on your legs?"

The man smiled politely. "Bruises," he guessed. "We were moving furniture."

"There's something going around," Sonnabend continued, his voice rising with urgency. "You should see your doctor."

"A few minutes later I saw him checking out," Sonnabend told me long afterward, "and I went to him and I said, This is my name, this is my telephone number. And in fact he came and saw me on Monday at my office." They both went directly to see Alvin Friedman-Kien. "Alvin didn't think that they were cancer, but in that climate you never knew. It's a gay guy and he's got purple things. So we did a blood count on him."

"What did it turn out to be?" I asked.

He shook his head. "Bruises. Just bruises. I was hallucinating disease, I was seeing it everywhere."

And this was still only the beginning.

LATE ONE MORNING a few weeks later, Sonnabend pulled a file from the stack of patient records that Harley Hackett had prepared for him.

Next up was Michael Callen, one of Sonnabend's first patients when the practice opened in 1979, and by far his favorite. Twenty-six years old, tall and confident, Callen had flowing hair, satiny skin, and eyes the color of jade. He was, he himself acknowledged, a markedly effeminate young man, skinny and wan. Adding to this overall impression, he possessed a voice that naturally reached falsetto ranges, a voice that brought him as much admiration as a singer as it did grief as a high school student in Ohio, where his father derided him as "a sissy" and boys in his gym class had made a sport of holding him down and soaking him with their urine. He found his way to New York after college, settling down in the "gay ghetto," as the part of Manhattan between Fourteenth Street and Houston Street was known—Greenwich Village, the East Village, and Alphabet City were among the few neighborhoods where it was possible for gay men and lesbians to live without constant fear of being evicted, menaced, or assaulted.

Like many others in the ghetto, he found work in the clerical industry. His job as a legal secretary barely taxed his intelligence but left ample time to pursue songwriting and performing, which he considered his true loves. What he loved even more, though, were the city's bathhouses, bookstores, and sex clubs, which became his abiding distractions through much of his twenties. This made him one of Sonnabend's more frequent patients as well.

Doctor and patient had much in common. As a child in Johannesburg before following his mother into medicine, Sonnabend showed great promise as a musical composer, and he dreamed of scoring for the silver screen, as did Callen. And, of course, they shared a passion for the bathhouses. The doctor was never coy about his own sexual practices. For him, as for Callen, sexual abandon was a means not only of release, but also of liberation, a utopian ideal and a necessary antidote to years of repression.

It was likely that even Sonnabend's most sexually adventuresome patients attached some residual shame to their desires, considering the hostilities experienced by most gay people of that generation. Only a few years earlier, same-sex attraction was classified in the *Diagnostic and Statistical Manual of Mental Disorders* as a sociopathic personality disturbance. Until the mid-seventies electroshock therapy was ordered for recalcitrant cases. Gay sex was still illegal in most of the country, a felony in some states. Suspicion of homosexuality was enough to block applications for security clearance, deny housing, defrock clergy members, fire schoolteachers, and bar foreigners from entering the United

States, even as tourists. It would be nearly impossible to avoid internalizing the stigma. Sonnabend considered it important when speaking to his patients to defend sex generally and anal sex particularly. He could be extraordinarily frank. "The rectum," he would say, "is a sexual organ, and it deserves the respect that a penis gets and a vagina gets."

It took some time, but Sonnabend did come to accept that this liberation strategy had its perils. No patient illustrated the risks more than Michael Callen. In a few short years, Callen had been treated for shigella and other bacteria of the gut, chlamydia, syphilis, gonorrhea, human papilloma virus, herpes simplex I and II, amebiasis including *Giardia lamblia* and *Entamoeba histolytica,* plus mononucleosis, urethritis (nonspecific), and the complete hepatitis suite: A, B, and non-A/non-B, later reclassified as C, D, and E.

What brought Callen back now was another case of gonorrhea, though the new mystery illness was not far from his mind. "What do you think about all of this?" he asked Sonnabend. "You think it's some kind of new virus?"

Sonnabend "moaned like a cow in labor," Callen told a friend later.

Was there something Callen might do to protect himself?

Sonnabend tapped Callen's lymph nodes along his jawline and under his arm. They were hard. He considered Callen's extreme accomplishments in the city's sexual arena and his utter failures as a musician.

"Move," he answered curtly. "Get out of New York."

This seemed an outrageous proposal to Callen, who had finally found sanctuary in New York's gay community. He showed his anger and Sonnabend immediately regretted his flippancy. That night, Sonnabend called him at home to apologize. And he offered an amended answer to Callen's question: what Callen could do, he said, was to give blood for a small study he was undertaking. Four other patients had already agreed to become research subjects. The object of the study was to look at the immune function of gay men who did not have either KS or PCP, but who had similarly long VD histories and swollen lymph glands. Callen was initially reluctant, but Sonnabend prevailed.

When next they saw one another, Sonnabend extracted a quantity of blood to ship to the lab, with instructions to examine a subset of Callen's white blood cells called T-cells (because they're produced in the thymus). T-cells, which coordinate the body's immune response, come in two sorts: CD4s and CD8s. The CD4s are considered "helper" cells. When disease strikes, they manufacture cytokines that serve as field marshals to coordinate and execute the body's immune response. Without CD4 cells, the body is vulnerable to every known infection. The CD8s, known as "killer" cells, then physically destroy the infected cells. On average, a healthy person has anywhere from 600 to 1,100 CD4 cells per cubic millimeter of blood and 400 CD8s. The technology for counting these cells was only a few months old.

The results came back quickly and were as worrisome as Sonnabend suspected. Callen's CD8s had remained stable but his CD4s had plummeted—his immune system was "compromised," as were those of the four other patients he studied. Delivering the news, Sonnabend counseled against dire conclusions. "I don't want to frighten you because we really don't know what this means other than that you're susceptible to disease and you should probably be careful," he said. He added that there was no demonstrated connection between being compromised and getting the new disease.

Still, Callen was inconsolable. That afternoon he called his parents and announced, "I'm going to get cancer—I feel I should tell you."

Recovering from her initial shock, his mother, a schoolteacher, took refuge in midwestern optimism. "You're made from good American Indian and Pennsylvania Dutch stock," she reminded him.

"Mom," he persisted, "I'll probably be dead in six months."

But in the coming weeks the spots didn't come and his lungs didn't fill. By Christmastime he was sometimes able to push his presumed fate out of mind. He still had not met anyone with "it." By year's end, there were 180 cases of KS, PCP, or other unusual infections from at least fifteen states, with New York City hardest hit. Of that number, only one of the victims was a woman. Of the men, 90 percent identified as gay or bisexual and the rest were presumed to have lied.

Half those patients were dead. Some met their ends so quickly they were only diagnosed posthumously. Though she didn't know it initially, Dr. Barbara Starrett saw her first case in mid-November 1981. The young man was anemic and had advanced syphilis, which caused a carpet of pink bumps all over his body. For Starrett, this was nothing unusual. As the director of lesbian and gay medical services at the St. Mark's Community Clinic, a free facility based in the East Village, she had seen a stupefying number of gay men with syphilis. But this case defied treatment. The patient's anemia worsened to the point of grave concern. She told him she wanted him in the hospital for tests. Instead, he headed home to Boston for Thanksgiving with his family. He died before the turkey was served. An autopsy showed PCP.

The pneumonia also soon claimed Donald Krintzman, the friend

Larry Kramer had bumped into at Dr. Friedman-Kien's office. That July afternoon Krintzman was robust and vibrant, a thirty-four-year-old at the peak of his physical prowess. Four months later, on a breathing machine in intensive care, death came on him painfully. In the brief obit published in *The New York Times*, only Krintzman's mother and brother were listed as survivors, but not Paul Rapoport, his devoted partner and the one person at his side throughout. Death and grief were not insults enough. It was the paper's policy to withhold recognition of homosexual relationships.

Krintzman was Kramer's fifth acquaintance to perish, and the one that hit closest to home. At the funeral, he wept. But instead of sharing his grief he found himself surrounded by hostility directed at him, as though he were a death-portending figure, the gay Grim Reaper. *Faggots* had made a lasting impression. So had his *Native* article about the looming crisis. The letters section filled week after week with denunciations of him. He had grown inured to the anger, but never imagined he would be shunned at a funeral.

Unrepentant, Kramer soon published a new piece in the *Native*. "Two new cases of KS are being diagnosed in New York each week," he wrote. "One new case is being diagnosed in the United States *each day*. Nothing is being done by the gay community to insist that the straight community, which controls all the purse strings and attention-getting devices, help us." In his own defense, he concluded, "I'm not glorying in death. I am overwhelmed by it. The death of my friends. The death of whatever community there is here in New York. The death of any visible love. 'Whom do we hate most?' George Steiner has asked. And answered: 'We hate most those who ask of us more than we want to give, who suggest to us that we are far from stretching to the full height of our own ethical possibility.'"

The following week, on January 4, 1982, Kramer opened his spacious apartment once again. The occasion was proposed by Nathan Fain, a young friend of Kramer's. Fain was a writer and editor for the New York nightlife magazine *After Dark*, and a meticulous organizer. He had joined as an enthusiastic participant in the efforts to support Dr. Friedman-Kien's research—the total raised so far was $11,806.55. But he wanted to discuss a more enduring response, perhaps a formal organization to respond to the whole sweep of issues surrounding the disease. He reached out to Lawrence Mass, Edmund White, and two others who had been so helpful in the fund-raising efforts, both motivated by the illness of their lovers: Paul Popham, a publishing executive

and Vietnam veteran; and the grieving Paul Rapoport, a lawyer and philanthropist who was the only one among them with experience working
with gay organizations.

Their meeting started at 6 p.m. Before it ended, they had formed the
first nonprofit in the world to deal with gay-related immune deficiency,
or GRID, as the disease was being called. Various names were proposed,
without gaining traction. Then Rapoport mused about the obvious,
which was that "gay men certainly have a health crisis," and Kramer
shouted, "That's our name!" The founders of Gay Men's Health Crisis
began laying out the work ahead: political advocacy, community self-
help, and fund-raising for research and other needs. As Fain looked
around the room it seemed to him that gay men were emerging for the
first time as a constituency.

THE YEAR 1982 had begun brutally. Biting winds brought some of
the lowest temperatures New York had ever seen. A long East Coast
drought added to the city's discomfort; restaurants were barred from
serving water, and washing grime from windows or sidewalks was made
illegal. Nationally, as President Ronald Reagan put into practice his
trickle-down economic policies, the gap between wealthy and working-
class Americans began to expand sharply. The digital dawn arrived:
Sony would introduce the camcorder, making moving images available
to ordinary people for the first time, and the Commodore personal computer would launch a revolution. But unemployment was at its highest
since the Great Depression, making the electronic revolution a distant
dream for most. Instead, poverty-gripped neighborhoods fell victim to
heroin and cocaine as the most violent scourge of drug violence and
addiction in the nation's history gained devastating momentum.

When the immensely popular Reverend Jerry Falwell sent out his
national funding appeal over the winter, it was infused with grave concern for the country's future. Falwell was not focused on poverty, crime,
nor drugs but on the same thing that mobilized Pat Robertson and a
growing chorus of evangelical Christians and televangelists: the stirrings of the gay movement, spurred by GRID. Falwell and his group,
the Moral Majority, urgently sought funds for a television documentary
he planned to call "Is There a Gay Conspiracy? You Be the Judge." His
own opinion was already fixed. He wrote, "This is a project to investigate, document and expose the gay conspiracy whose goal is to completely legitimize homosexuality in America in the very near future—in
fact, during 1982." He offered an important piece of evidence: "The

gays have gained so much influence in New York that they were allowed
to have a Christmas program in Carnegie Hall this year." He was referring to a concert by the critically acclaimed New York Gay Men's Chorus. This was, he said, "only the beginning."

That spring, Brian Gougeon and I had settled in separate apartments. He moved to a building on Eleventh Avenue, near the warehouse where he found a job as an urban horticulturist. I made my way
to a far corner of the gay ghetto on Avenue C in Alphabet City, the
locus of the city's bohemian culture. Both our new neighborhoods were
profiles of squalor and urban abandonment, but mine was a uniquely
dire landscape of empty buildings, flattened cars, and rat-roiled heaps
of garbage. Along my block, athletic-looking young men occupied the
shadows of doorways, peddling cocaine and heroin. They used baseball
bats to keep order among their frail and impatient customers, who at
times stood fifteen deep outside a dingy mid-block laundromat, creas-
ing small wax-paper envelopes into their palms. Up on the rooftops
were this economy's junior league, teens and preteens whose job it
was to sound the alarm when suspicious strangers approached. They
called down their warnings in a coded language of staccato whistles and
clipped shouts that on some nights could sound as haunting and beautiful as a jungle aviary.

I never once saw a police cruiser turn onto the block.

Awkwardly, the dealers and their customers shared this forsaken
neighborhood with artists, musicians, Puerto Rican families, urban
homesteaders, Ukrainian widows, squatters, writers, and, in increasing
numbers, poor gay men like myself, drawn by cheap housing and the
area's relative proximity to Christopher Street. Allen Ginsberg lived
around one corner, Quentin Crisp was around another. Robert Map-
plethorpe, Cookie Mueller, Madonna, Penny Arcade, Kiki Smith, Jean-
Michel Basquiat, and David Wojnarowicz, all early in their careers,
either lived or played in Alphabet City. I took a first-floor apartment for
$179 a month, the very limit of my budget. I soon learned that the drug
merchants would tolerate me as long as I never stopped on the block,
not even to knot a shoelace. "Keep moving," they'd say firmly, but with
kindness, the only thing they would ever say to me.

For money, I worked nights as a word processor in law firms, driving the fragile transitional technology that was replacing the typewriter, and in addition took a part-time job running the cash register at
Oscar Wilde Memorial Bookshop, the oldest gay-themed bookstore in
the country. As there still were not many gay-themed books, the shop

served as much as a community center as a store. The main action was in the cramped back office, where the owner—a fiercely opinionated Chicago transplant named Craig Rodwell—ran the movement's unofficial headquarters. The first gay pride march in the world was planned there, in 1970. Strategies for getting the Mafia out of gay bars, confronting police violence against transgender sex workers, and supporting gay-friendly candidates for office were revised and enacted around Rodwell's desk. I longed to be in those conversations and one day found the courage to ask Rodwell for a job. He let me stand behind the counter one Saturday a month, and loiter in the office anytime I liked.

There was no simple optimism about gay liberation like existed in the early days of the civil rights struggle, no sense that we would overcome. This was not because of "The Crisis." *The New York Times* and the other influential media outlets had yet to return to the subject. Only the *Native* hammered away at it, with pieces by numerous MDs and PhDs. That spring, Rodwell was among those who believed that the health dangers were entirely overblown, and he held Kramer personally responsible for the overblowing. "First, he was a terrible novelist, and now he's Chicken Little. I don't know why anybody's paying any attention to him at all," he told me. To Rodwell, the most important agenda item was a local gay rights bill, stalled in the city council for almost a decade, which sought to ban discrimination on the basis of sexual orientation in housing, employment, and public accommodations. Mayor Ed Koch—about whose permanent bachelorhood the community always whispered—officially backed gay rights, but with decreasing passion over the years. As a congressman in the early 1970s, he joined Bella Abzug to sponsor the first-ever gay nondiscrimination federal bill, prompting a hail of antipathy, even from fellow New York City Democrats. Abzug, a firebrand, responded with stridency; unmarried Koch, with expiation. After becoming mayor, he spent none of his considerable political capital on gay rights. During more than three years at city hall, he had avoided even appearing before a gay audience. When reelection jitters finally caused him to accept the invitation from gay business leaders, he told them he would never intervene for their rights. "I respect people who are against gays for religious reasons," he said to a silent room. "Prejudice is a matter of conscience."

It was impossible to say exactly how widespread anti-gay discrimination was. No city office kept track of the allegations. The NYPD refused demands to track anti-gay crimes, though there was an undeniable epidemic of violence following news of the plague. Assaults grew so numerous by summer that the *Native* mapped "The 15 Worst Danger Zones" of the city, including all of Greenwich Village and most of the East Village and Alphabet City—the whole of the gay ghetto—plus Chelsea, Central Park, Riverside Park, and parts of the outer boroughs where small clutches of gays and lesbians had put down roots. Not coincidentally, the more the *Native* was dominated by news about the disease, the more frequently articles about gay victims of violence appeared.

"See? This is why Kramer's dangerous," Rodwell said one Saturday afternoon. "The message we need to be getting out there is that we need rights, we deserve rights. Not that we spread disease."

GIVEN THE LACK of anything definitive about GRID, officials at the CDC in Atlanta added Sonnabend's hypothesis—CMV superinfections—to the growing list of official suspects. Though they supposed the answer would prove to be a new virus or bacteria, the public health system would examine all plausible explanations. This was a lesson they had learned a few years before, when 221 members of the American Legion fell ill during a convention in Philadelphia, thirty-four of them fatally. Then, the CDC's list of possible explanations grew several pages long, and included everything from typhoid to sarin gas to seventeen specific poisonous metals. The investigation was massive, the largest in the federal agency's history, involving twenty agents from the epidemiology division, scores more from the state, and millions of dollars. No guess was ignored, not even the suggestion to check the air-conditioning unit serving the banquet room at the Bellevue-Stratford Hotel, which was where the lethal bacteria causing Legionnaires' disease was discovered six months following the first reports.

The parallel between Legionnaires' disease and GRID didn't escape Sonnabend. It was now seven months following the discovery of the KS/gay link. The death toll was already almost four times the total among the Legionnaires, yet not one CDC official had come to see him. There were no million-dollar budget lines, no massive public health campaigns. The agency's apathetic approach was matched by the nation's, as measured by media interest—six brief articles now in *The New York Times*, compared to eighty-six in the first months of Legionnaires' disease. In another comparison, the *Times* also made room for thirty-one stories in 1980 for another national health crisis, when sixty-five women died from toxic shock syndrome linked to a brand of tampons. Homosexuals would not be accorded anything similar.

The silence on GRID added to the burdens Sonnabend carried. Absent any coordinated response, he pursued his research with an energy level bordering on panic. He thought it was far-fetched to suspect a new and deadly microorganism, a mutant Andromeda Strain that had somehow developed a taste for gay men. "We shouldn't jump on the first virus we see," he told Hackett one night, "because we may find a lot." In a letter to a fellow physician, he suggested it was just as likely that semen itself produced the "deleterious responses" they were seeing. This thought first arose after a colleague examining blood samples from Sonnabend's sickest patients discovered that their white blood cells were coated in a bizarre, thick layer of antibodies. He recalled seeing something similar only once before—in chickens exposed to the blood of other chickens, touching off a chaotic immune response.

This fascinated Sonnabend. Gay men weren't consuming one another's blood, but they were exposing themselves to semen, which contained blood cells. Could men be allergic to other men's semen? There were ample studies on the affect of semen exposure on women, but none on men. The lining of a woman's vagina did not react to semen as a dangerous substance and therefore produced no antibodies to fight it. Perhaps the male rectal membrane was an "immunogenic site," that is, a region of the body capable of producing antibodies. When he tested this by exposing the rectums of male rabbits to large quantities of rabbit ejaculate, he managed to trigger the same condition seen in his patients: antibodies attached themselves to their white blood cells in thick carpets. Rabbits exposed to semen from more than one donor had an even more profound immunological response, developing unique antibodies to each overlapping exposure. None of the rabbits took grievously ill. But their peculiar new immune profiles gave strong credence to a theory that male-on-male promiscuity alone was capable of compromising the immune system.

Combined with the stupefying proliferation of communicable diseases in general, and the preponderance of cytomegalovirus in particular, Sonnabend grew convinced, semen exposure could be powerful enough to collapse a healthy immune system in ways no one had ever seen before.

He called this the "immune-overload model," in contrast to the "new germ model" gaining popularity among other researchers who were lured, he suspected, by the glory and renown that would come to the discoverer of a new virus. He also feared that the "new germ" proponents played into the hands of the religious right. If a brand-new killer virus were on the prowl, the thugs preying on the community would multiply and lawmakers might be tempted to throw suspected carriers behind barbed wire. Already, some commentators were openly suggesting quarantining sick gay men in order to protect everyone else.

The Moral Majority had even more draconian ideas. "I agree with capital punishment, and I believe homosexuality is one of those that could be coupled with murder and other sins," said Dean Wycoff, spokesman for the Santa Clara, California, chapter of Reverend Falwell's group. Sonnabend's "immune-overload model" would not inspire such hysteria because it only threatened the wildly promiscuous. The solution to an overtaxed immune system was to let it rest and never overload it again.

Numerous other theories didn't make much sense to Sonnabend. "It could be the bugs out of the pipes in the bathhouses," surmised Dr. Yehudi M. Felman of New York City's Bureau of VD Control, some environment-specific villain as in Legionnaires' disease. Others hypothesized that the suppression was caused by excessive use of Flagyl, a super-powerful antibiotic taken for amebiasis, endemic in the community, but gay people weren't the only ones taking repeat doses of the drug. In fact Flagyl was more often prescribed to women for trichomoniasis, a similar parasite of the bowels, and they weren't dying as a result. Others blamed amyl nitrite, the main ingredient in "poppers," a recreational inhalant that enjoyed a certain popularity among gay men, who found it enhanced their experiences on the dance floor and in bed. But amyl nitrite was much more regularly used by cardiac patients for treating angina, with no link to the mysterious disease. Sonnabend kept all these theories in a single file folder. In a parallel folder he collected academic clips speculating wildly about the social interaction of gay men, a new preoccupation of sociologists. He felt a sudden sympathy with tribesmen from remote corners of the Amazon.

In some aspects, the various theories about cause suggested the same course of action to the sick and the healthy alike: moderation in all things recreational, including drugs and sex. "People who are promiscuous, whether heterosexual or homosexual, are going to be exposed repeatedly to virus infections, some of which in themselves will be immunosuppressive," Sonnabend told a reporter for the *Native*. When his quote appeared in print, hostile feedback from his patients exacerbated Sonnabend's natural persecution complex. Even other gay doctors defended the sexual turf as sacrosanct, the necessary battleground for gay liberation. Feeling the need to defend himself, he asked for and received space in a subsequent issue of the paper to deliver a fuller explanation. "The term 'promiscuous' is used here with the full knowledge that its use may provoke some resentment," he wrote. "In connection with this, it should be stated that gay men have been poorly served by their medical attendants during the past years (and I must include myself in this criticism). For years, no clear and positive message about the dangers of promiscuity has emanated from those in whom gay men have entrusted their well-being."

He knew this salvo would further inflame the other gay doctors, but he could not in good conscience hold his tongue. Just how incensed they were was clear on March 14, when he attended the founding meeting of a citywide group intended to support gay and lesbian clinicians, called New York Physicians for Human Rights. Dr. Barbara Starrett and the group's leaders had been pressing Dr. James Curran, the CDC's point man for the new disease, to come discuss the epidemic with them. He had been in and out of New York forty-four times since the first hours of the epidemic, but had largely avoided the frontline doctors until now. The gathering was in Dr. Starrett's large Chelsea loft. Sonnabend's reception was icy.

More than two hundred gay and lesbian doctors, nurses, and medical students filled the loft to capacity. Also attending was the new health commissioner for the city of New York, Dr. David Sencer, who previously had been Curran's boss at the CDC. Starrett was relieved that he'd accepted her invitation. She hadn't met Sencer yet—almost no one there had—and there was great hope he would assume a proactive role in the epidemic. Sencer had overseen the CDC's nimble Legionnaires' disease investigation and led the successful campaign to eradicate smallpox, his greatest success. The city doctors welcomed his leadership.

When it was his time to speak, Curran—a cheerful and diminutive man of thirty-seven—climbed to a spot halfway up the loft's ornate spiral staircase. What he first noticed from this elevation was how young everyone looked: there were only two or three white heads in the crowd. Then he noticed how ordinary everyone appeared. He had never addressed a specifically homosexual group. There had been no gays in his own medical class at the University of Michigan, and the subject of homosexuality had never come up during his public health studies at Harvard. His experience with the community came from his work in the CDC's VD division, and those patients had struck him as not so different from himself. Now that sense of identification, of oneness, ran throughout the room—he was among professionals like himself, drinking wine and speaking animatedly, ambitious young men and women who just happened to be gay. He wondered how many were already sick.

He began with a repudiation of Sonnabend's hypothesis. The best minds in the country believed this was an infectious agent, he said. "If this is a sexually transmitted disease, it's going to be heterosexually transmitted as well as homosexually transmitted and it's probably going to go in both directions, the receiver and the—uh, the—the inserter." He felt embarrassed talking this way to this audience, yet it hardly fazed them. "It isn't going away," Curran cautioned. "Even if we find a causative virus or other agent, it will be considerable time, probably years, before we can develop a vaccine or some strategy to eradicate it. We are in for a long haul." He fell silent for a time, moved by the hush in the room. But he wanted to end on an optimistic note.

"You're showing great leadership," he said reassuringly. "Epidemics come and epidemics go. Keep calm and don't be too upset."

Almost immediately after he descended the stairway, one of the young physicians touched his arm, introducing himself as chief medical resident at the NYU Medical Center. He spoke in the lyrical cadence of a native Georgian. He hailed from Columbia, a city two hours east of the CDC headquarters. "I've had PCP," he said. Every available statistic counted his life expectancy to be a few months. Curran thought what an idiot he was to tell these people to keep calm.

Before returning to Atlanta the following morning, Curran paid a visit to the office of Dan William, whom he first met in the late 1970s. In contrast to Sonnabend, William was a community insider. Though both volunteered at the free gay clinic, William had been asked to advise the new Gay Men's Health Crisis board and was voted in as the first president of New York Physicians for Human Rights. At Curran's request, he scheduled a number of his lymphadenopathy patients for Curran to examine—to see the disease for himself. This was not difficult to arrange. Among his nearly two thousand patients were some of the most obscure diseases described in medical literature. GRID "needs five or six text books to describe it all in its various and sundry manifestations and complications," William explained. "The tragedy part is, how many people would have to get sick and die as a result? Would it be 30 percent of my patients? Forty percent? Twenty percent? Who knows?"

BY SPRING OF 1982, with the Falklands War dominating the evening news, the caseload across the city built. Dr. Linda Laubenstein turned her attention entirely to KS patients, disregarding warnings from peers about becoming associated with the gay disease. Around NYU, she was well known for her willfulness and defiance, two traits that had roots in her childhood in Rhode Island. Stricken with polio and left a paraplegic at age five, her obstinate self-confidence got her and her battery-powered wheelchair through medical school to where she was today, in the highest ranks at the Medical Center's oncology department, though only thirty-five years old.

There was a curious pattern among her KS patients: two of them reported having had a sexual link to the same third party, a French Canadian flight attendant who, they told her, also had the spots. She noted the man's unusual name in her records.

"Gaëtan Dugas," she told Friedman-Kien. "With Air Canada."

Intrigued, Friedman-Kien wanted to examine Dugas. He called the airline's medical director, who in turn reached the employee. Within weeks Dugas was in Manhattan, introducing his lesions to the New York team with a thick Québécois accent. He was young and strikingly handsome, a magnetic, mustachioed, blue-eyed blond. Friedman-Kien took note of the man's outsized vivacity as he described his conquests along his flight routes. It wasn't until months later that the doctor discovered how many of his own patients had also slept with Dugas. The idea that one man's vast sexual black book included so many of the sick deeply troubled him.

The two NYU Medical Center doctors now had sixty-two KS patients between them, a quarter of the nation's total. In Europe, where the epidemic lagged by more than a year, the number of patients in each country stood in the single digits, and Brazilian officials had recently reported a lone diagnosis, the first in Latin America. In Africa, people had been perishing for a number of years, their deaths sometimes credited to a disease they called "slim," a mysterious wasting syndrome. But no research was under way that would link them to the epidemic. So Friedman-Kien and Laubenstein were responding to their patients in a bubble.

Their approaches were very different. Using the tools of a dermatologist, Friedman-Kien tried freezing the lesions with liquid nitrogen, or cauterizing them, or excising them with a knife. Each technique proved both disfiguring and futile. Spots would reappear elsewhere without pause, usually in symmetrical pairs—one on the left ankle and one on the right—or else clustered on the body's midline, often on the end of the nose. The only remedy Friedman-Kien had for patients with engulfed faces was a new staff cosmetician who gave lessons in the art of pancake makeup. They were lucky if the KS stayed on the skin. If it spread to the mouth or on the tongue, KS made eating intolerable, and in the lung it produced a sensation of suffocation and led to a hasty death.

Laubenstein favored the oncologist's weapon of aggressive chemotherapy. When she first employed the method on a patient who had only two small lesions behind an ear, many of her peers criticized her, concerned that the approach might accelerate immunological decline. She seemed vindicated initially when her patient's lesions shrank in size and softened in color. But his progress quickly reversed. Upon his death he had seventy-five lesions despite her ministrations. Laubenstein started her subsequent patients on higher and higher doses until one day an autopsy report came back with the good news she had been hoping for. She pointed the line out to Friedman-Kien, slapping the desktop with pride.

"No KS!" she declared.

Friedman-Kien studied the autopsy report.

"But Linda," he said, "he died of every opportunistic infection. We bumped him off." The allegation infuriated her, and she found the suggestion preposterous.

It had to be acknowledged, though, that death by chemo only hurried along the inevitable. In Dr. Sonnabend's practice, nothing he did could stem the immunological declines of his patients. They would succumb to fevers, oral thrush, or maddening cases of diarrhea that would strip them of nutrients and body mass. Exacerbating his frustration, in a peculiarity of the New York City hospital system, many doctors, Sonnabend included, could not admit their own patients to hospitals. The authorities at St. Vincent's turned down his application for privileges. He suspected it was because he hadn't had an American-style medical education, with the years-long residencies that mark U.S. training. But many of the city's gay doctors faced similar rejections, and it soon seemed there was a barrier of prejudice at the doors. Whatever the cause, when his patients' health invariably declined, Sonnabend had little choice but to send them to Dr. Friedman-Kien, who could get them into NYU. Too often he would never see them again.

On the day that spring when he bumped into Mathilde Krim, an interferon researcher with whom he had collaborated years earlier, he was wracked with self-doubt and frustration. Nationwide, there were now 335 official cases of the new syndrome; almost half of those patients had already died. Years later, once the causal virus was discovered and

antibody tests developed, researchers would go back to a large bank of
stored blood from 1982 and confirm a huge infection rate among gay
men. In San Francisco, 42.6 percent already carried the virus, and in
New York City, 26.8 percent were likewise doomed. In Sonnabend's
boutique practice, the rate was even higher—hundreds already showed
early signs of the syndrome.

"You know, Mathilde," he lamented, "I am losing my touch as a
physician."

Dr. Krim was not thrilled to see him. Their relations had been stormy
since the late 1970s, when they fell out during the organizing of an
important interferon summit, and for some years they had not spoken.
Like Sonnabend, Krim was frequently impatient and quick to anger,
though she was mostly able to mask her moods behind a courtly, old-
world manner. She too was an immigrant. Born in Italy and raised in
Switzerland, Krim spent her post-graduate years conducting research
in Israel, at the prestigious Weizmann Institute. Sonnabend had also
done some work there—Israel was where they had met—but similarities ended there. In contrast to his constant financial troubles, she led a
storybook life of wealth and glamour courtesy of her second husband,
Arthur Krim, the founder of the Hollywood film company Orion Pictures and a leading figure in Democratic Party circles. The Krims had
played host to President John F. Kennedy's most memorable birthday
party, which famously began with Marilyn Monroe's throaty serenade
and ended at the Krims' grand East Sixty-ninth Street townhouse with
guests including Shirley MacLaine and Jack Benny. That she continued
her work in a research laboratory was testimony to her romance with
science. She now was director of interferon evaluation programs at the
renowned Sloan Kettering Institute for Cancer Research in New York.
As she was setting up that lab, she suspected Sonnabend of undermining her efforts, and the last time they were face-to-face was in the back
of her limo, when she found him so disagreeable she ordered him out
of the car still miles from his destination. The driver hustled him onto
the Park Avenue sidewalk so quickly he never had a chance to offer his
defenses.

And now, having met once again, Krim might have kept walking if
Sonnabend hadn't been so obviously distressed. Instead, she invited
him to lunch at a coffee shop across the street and listened to stories
about his patients and their mysteries, about the KS and the PCP. "And
they're all young men, and they're all gay people who live in the same
area in New York," he said. Krim, who had never knowingly met a

homosexual, found the demographic coincidence bizarre. But she did not doubt Sonnabend; her respect for him as an infectious disease specialist was not diminished by their poor personal chemistry.

Without a moment's hesitation, she offered him a $5,000 check to further his research, and he accepted it gratefully. Her generosity would continue over the coming months. Her envelopes brimmed with large donations, sometimes accompanied by brief words of encouragement laid down in her beautiful penmanship: "Hang in!" The reconciliation they began in the coffee shop that day, and the ensuing collaboration, would change the face of the epidemic.

Krim returned to her lab that afternoon vowing to learn all she could about KS. She called Dr. Bijan Safai, a dermatologist colleague from Memorial Hospital, the in-patient facility attached to her research institute.

"It's rare," he told her. "Over twenty-five years, Sloan Kettering has only seen nine cases. But you are lucky because right now I have twelve cases on my ward." All were young gay men. Krim, fascinated by the mystery, was now committed to trying to help solve it.

3

Compromised

Since getting the frightening news about his inverted T-cell ratio, on his doctor's advice Michael Callen had sworn off sex. There were lapses. As the weather warmed, he tried a distraction, resuming efforts to form a rock band, which he would name Lowlife. He put an ad in the *Native* seeking musicians. He told each candidate arriving for an audition that he had "the disease," whatever it was. He would understand, he said, "if you didn't want to invest time in a group knowing that the lead singer has a life expectancy shorter than that of a garage band." Most retreated in fear. A slow-speaking and thoughtful drummer named Richard Dworkin had a different response.

"I'm a gay man living in New York City," Dworkin replied. "I'm going to have to deal with this disease sooner or later. I may as well begin now." By morning he was not just the Lowlife drummer but also Callen's unexpected lover. No previous relationship had ever lasted more than a few months, and Callen's attempts at monogamy did not go any easier this time. "Once a whore, always a whore," he used to say. But taking himself mostly off the circuit gave him new insights into his character. He began to think about what had propelled him into the corridors and pitch-black rooms of the sex clubs and baths in the first place. The main allure, he now thought, was the darkness itself. Despite his bravado, he was self-conscious about his looks: his skinny chest, his Streisand-like nose, his overall "sissy" appearance. But in the shadows he could overcome those insecurities and blossom into a formidable sexual juggernaut. Dworkin brought him something he hadn't experienced before: a physical self-confidence. He watched with amazement as Dworkin became more and more attached to him, and this helped him find peace with his body.

Unfortunately, his body didn't reciprocate. One humid June day in 1982, Callen collapsed of dehydration and was admitted to St. Vincent's as an emergency patient, with bloody diarrhea and a burning fever. It was days before a diagnosis emerged. Callen wasn't surprised by what the doctor said, just by the way she said it, all plumped up with "the satisfaction of Miss Marple."

"Well," she said, "it's GRID alright."

The news gave him a strange sensation of relief: the waiting that began with Sonnabend's small-scale study was over. No longer merely "compromised," he had gay-related immune deficiency. But the relief was fleeting. "You have cryptosporidiosis," the doctor told him. "Before GRID we didn't think that cryptosporidiosis infected humans. It's a disease previously found only in livestock. I'm afraid there is no known treatment. All we can do is try to keep you hydrated and see what happens. Your body will either handle it or . . ."

She patted him on the leg and smiled. He had six to eighteen months of life left to enjoy, she told him. She pulled a business card out of her lab coat. "Here's the number of Dr. Stuart Nichols. He's starting a support group," she said. "I think you should go—if you beat this bout."

A medical resident followed her into his room and coaxed out of Callen the details of his life to include in a case report for the CDC. In poetry and lyrics, and occasional short stories, Callen had sometimes looked back at his long history of sexual exploration, which began at age seventeen. This was the first time he made that journey with a calculator. He arrived at a figure by estimating the number of men he might have sex with on an average day, times seven average days a week, times fifty-two weeks a year, times the ten-year span of his active sexual life. Conservatively, he'd been with three thousand men. As stunning as that tally was, he had purposely underestimated. "I only counted anal penetration," he admitted to a friend, "on aesthetic grounds." Nonetheless, his statement cast him as almost three times as prolific as the typical man at diagnosis.

Richard Dworkin visited the hospital each of the five days Callen convalesced there and physically steadied him on the short walk home after his discharge. Before they reached Callen's apartment, the driver of a New York sanitation truck, offended by their close proximity to each other, barreled toward them. "Faggots, you're disgusting!" he yelled. The truck swerved away at the very last moment, barely missing them. Not even this rattled Dworkin. In a few months, the two moved in together, sharing a cavernous fourth-floor loft at 129 Duane Street in Tribeca, anticipating a quick and dramatic denouement worthy of Puccini.

After his strength returned, Callen braved the rain one Tuesday to join about a dozen patients in a weekly support group, the first of its kind. Afterward, he made his way to see Sonnabend, waiting three hours before his name was called, such was the chaos in the office. Sonnabend thoroughly examined Callen for more than thirty minutes before being called away for a lengthy phone call. Left alone, Callen grew restless, impatiently pacing the small room in his gown. On the doctor's desk, he noticed the draft of a thirty-page manuscript meant for publication in a scientific journal. The last page was still in the typewriter's platen. Annoyed by Sonnabend's absence, he sat down at the doctor's desk and read the whole paper, which described the doctor's "immune-overload model" for GRID. Callen tripped on some of the vocabulary, but for the first time he saw the unnecessary risks he'd taken with his sex life. It hit him with the force of an explosion: *of course* the body has a limited ability to recover, *of course* VD has a cumulative effect, *of course* he was sick and dying, *of course* he'd brought it upon himself.

But he saw something else in this explanation, a possible course of action for him and people like him. Sonnabend surmised that an over-loaded immune system needed time to recover—no sexual exposure to anyone for a year or more. This made perfect sense to Callen. If GRID was death by a thousand cuts, the sooner one dropped the knife the better chance one had of getting well again. Despite his bloody diarrhea and distended abdomen, Callen now saw his path to improvement. He was *hopeful*.

Sonnabend's telephone call lasted forty-five minutes. When he returned to the examining room, Callen greeted him with a torrent of questions and self-revelations, ticking off his own long cycle of infection and treatment. If he'd have been able to read Sonnabend's essay beforehand, he thought to himself, he might have avoided GRID in the first place.

"You have to publish this in the *Native*," he said. "You've got to let people know there's hope."

"You *read* that?" asked Sonnabend, showing his pride. But the point of the paper was to prompt a discussion within the medical community, he said. A general audience would require a much more accessible draft, which he lacked the wherewithal to produce. What little writing he did was accomplished after midnight, when insomnia allowed.

"Look, I'll help you," Callen said. "I'm pretty sure I can get an article in the *Native*. Anybody who is anybody reads the *Native*." He was referring to the fact that among the paper's small readership were the most influential members of the community; indeed, there was no other way to reach the community. But he knew no one at the paper. In fact, he knew almost nobody in the community. He was quite reclusive, actually; the orgiastic nightlife substituted for social whirl.

Stretched beyond exhaustion, Sonnabend shook his head. "You do it," he said.

Callen didn't have that kind of ambition personally. But Sonnabend had another patient who had professed a desire to warn the community about the wages of promiscuity, a young man Callen's age with a vast network of contacts. Like Callen, he had signs of GRID.

"Maybe you two should meet and together you can pursue this," the doctor said. He slid a scrap of paper across the desk. "Put your name and number here. I'll see if he wants to call you."

One early afternoon toward the end of July, at the start of the second year of the epidemic, Callen received a call at the law firm where he worked from a young man with an excitable voice. Richard Berkowitz spoke with the nonlinear fluidity of a regular marijuana smoker, which he was. To help keep track of life's twists and turns, he had begun recording his phone calls. This was one of those times.

After formalities, they spoke excitedly about Sonnabend's immune-overload model, to which they both wholeheartedly subscribed. "We're in the minority," Berkowitz said. "The general consensus is that there's an infectious virus. Which is—"

"It's just a very romantic notion," Callen agreed. "I just finished reading *Illness as Metaphor,* by Susan—"

"So did I!"

Callen liked Berkowitz instantly. They shared an interest in the writings of feminists in general. "Why aren't you in the group that I'm in? It's a really wonderful group," Callen said, meaning the GRID support group. In fact, he was leaving shortly for a meeting and would have to cut the conversation short. Despite being sleepy after a long writing session, Berkowitz expressed an eagerness to attend; Callen gave him the address.

An hour later, a dozen support group members flowed into a second-floor room at the St. Mark's Community Clinic. Berkowitz chose an inconspicuous seat and spoke to no one, too fearful to make eye contact with the sick men in the room. But they surely noticed the compact and intense twenty-six-year-old with dark eyes, soft black hair and mustache, a leather jacket tight on his shoulders. Berkowitz was accustomed to being stared at by gay men. He loved it, in fact. But the men staring at him now gave him new terrors. This was a coalition of the unmistakably sick. A man in his early twenties with pretty eyes and a timid smile was ashen and bald from chemotherapy; he slumped painfully in a metal chair. A working-class man from Brooklyn named Artie could no longer harness his thoughts, though he was far from elderly. In conversation, the men dwelt on their shared history of excruciating travails. Appearing sick had cost them jobs. Friends had abandoned them and relatives shunned them, barring them from family gatherings, never letting them see their nieces or nephews. One man said he had just returned from Kentucky, on what he expected to be a heartwarming farewell journey home. In one breath he told his family he was gay and dying. He braced for their tears. Instead, his father punched him on the nose and disowned him on the spot.

Berkowitz was by far the most robust man in the room, having remained healthy despite his ominous lab results. Looking around, he prayed he would never decline like them. Somehow, seeing them convinced him he was going to stage a full recovery. He would will it.

When Callen spoke, Berkowitz recognized his voice from the phone. Though he had been out of the hospital for a couple of weeks, Callen still had "a hospital pallor," Berkowitz thought. He spoke of being "bone-tired" and in lasting pain, and confessed the small indulgences, like frosted cake, he allowed himself as a consequence. Berkowitz noted how the others hung on Callen's words. "Every time he spoke, you could see everyone in the group stop," he said later. "Like Gandhi—he spoke, they listened."

Following the meeting, the two retired to Rumbul's, a café on Christopher Street. They sat at a table by the window.

"I have trouble dealing with death," Berkowitz said delicately.

"Who doesn't?" Callen chirped. But he knew how Berkowitz meant it. "I can see that unlike most of the queens there, you're not ready to glamorize or embrace dying, and sick as I am, neither am I." He picked up the menu and added, as if absentmindedly, "I hope when my time comes that I can face it without turning to God or religion, because if I do, that would be a betrayal of everything I fought for and everything I believe in."

This shocked Berkowitz. He was also an atheist, but he feared saying something like that out loud just in case there *was* a God. *He's a queen,* Berkowitz thought, *but he's really got balls.*

When their beverages arrived, Berkowitz described his own credentials. He had earned a degree from Rutgers, where he studied journalism, then spent a semester at NYU's master's degree program in film. The way he made his money and the way he got sick were probably one and the same: Berkowitz, a Jewish boy from New Jersey who spoke to his mother on the phone every day, was a professional sex worker. For his promotional material he adopted the name Vinnie, a "hot Italian" from the boroughs. It began as a lark. While still in college, hustling replaced his part-time job restocking the dairy cases at Krauszer's Food Store, though it soon proved infinitely more profitable. At twenty-two, with money in his pocket, he left graduate school behind and dove into the business without reservation. The specialty he had developed set him apart from his competitors—he practiced sadomasochism, serving as a master to his mostly married and suburban clientele.

Berkowitz used Dr. Sonnabend the way Formula One drivers used a pit crew. Earlier that year, he'd complained about a bump on his neck, just below his earlobe. Sonnabend's hand shot to his neck. "That's a swollen gland," he said. "Lift up your arms so I can check for more." There were many others.

Sonnabend referred him to a lab to have one of them biopsied, but Berkowitz just put them out of his mind. They didn't hurt and barely hindered him, except for one night at a neighborhood bar when the man who had agreed to come home with him noticed the growths and changed his mind. He took to wearing a turtleneck, even in the heat of summer. It wasn't until another hustler died that Berkowitz made the biopsy appointment.

On his way out of New York Hospital after the procedure, a terror overcame him. He ducked into a stairwell and wept violently. When he made it back to his apartment, Berkowitz closed the blinds and climbed into bed. An impulse moved him to reach for the latest *Advocate*, a national gay publication, and turn to his hustler ad in the classifieds section. It was there, as usual, adjacent to an ad the deceased hustler had placed before taking ill. It was three days before Berkowitz rose from his bed, and when he did, he called *The Advocate* to remove his ad from future editions, then dialed the phone company to have his popular telephone lines silenced.

That was a week ago, he told Callen. He was no longer in the business, taking the break his doctor ordered.

Callen listened with great curiosity. Here was an articulate sex worker who shared his recent conversion to sexual sobriety. He told Berkowitz of his own amorous compulsions, the diseases they brought, and his moment of transformation following a diagnosis with cryptosporidiosis.

"Previously found only in livestock," Berkowitz interjected. "I read about that in medical journals."

This impressed Callen. He told Berkowitz how he had stumbled on the doctor's manuscript. "When Joe returned from his call, I was bouncing off the ceiling, frantically telling him we had to get his ideas out to the community. When he said he had another patient who felt the same way, I begged him for your number."

Despite Callen's prissiness and odd formality, Berkowitz felt a kinship developing. He was glad to have support in his new abstemious course. Before parting, they committed to writing an article for the *Native* popularizing Sonnabend's views about the consequences of sexual overconsumption.

"Two major sluts like us," Callen said, "are just the ones to do it."

THE ENERGY Larry Kramer poured into Gay Men's Health Crisis was much more intensive than any of the other cofounders, in part because his financial circumstances freed him from the burdens of a day job. (This was thanks to his older brother, who managed his investments and exercised parent-like control over his finances.) It was a time of great purpose and humanity for Kramer—he felt relieved to be able to share this important work with other gay men. A core group of about a dozen volunteers, meeting in a succession of living rooms around the city, steadily built the organization. Committees were set up to handle fund-raising, a newsletter, and "victim social services." Rodger McFarlane, a towering young southerner Kramer had begun dating, volunteered to advertise his home phone as a GRID hotline. On the first day he received one hundred calls, none of them presenting simple problems. He heard from men in hospitals without staff to clean them; men at home with no strength to shop for groceries; men desperate for help in committing suicide. They were "uniformly thrown out of jobs, uniformly couldn't get benefits, uniformly without legal protection," he discovered. "And these are our friends and lovers and you couldn't just let them lay in shit until you talked the nurses into cleaning them up."

McFarlane was twenty-seven, and his background was in the military, then hospital management, not crisis intervention. But with his quick Alabaman wit, disarming humor, and deftness at managing people, he had an unfailing way of making the horrors appear more endurable while he worked to correct them. "Honey," he would tell the callers, "what they're doing to you is a crime and I'm coming right over there to put an end to it. They will *never* forget having to answer to a 6'7" Alabama queen."

Kramer won appointment to GMHC's newly formed board of directors, but he was shocked when nobody nominated him for leadership.

Instead they recognized Paul Popham, whose dark, square face was off-set by a voluminous mustache, as the ideal leader. Thanks to his steady charisma and extensive connections on Fire Island, GMHC was grow-ing quickly. Kramer thought Popham was the worst possible choice to lead the group. Popham, who by day was a vice president at a major bank, was closeted at work and therefore unable to make public appear-ances on behalf of their organization. In fact, for the first several meet-ings, he tried to remove the word "gay" from the organization's name (the other directors decided "to stick with GAY MEN'S HEALTH CRISIS and say what we mean," as the secretary noted in meeting min-utes). In a goodwill gesture, Popham asked Kramer to recruit a formal advisory board of top researchers and clinicians and Kramer, nursing his bruised ego, accepted.

In the fall, GMHC moved into its first permanent home, a vacant room the size of a large closet in a dilapidated Chelsea welfare hotel. McFarlane had befriended the owner, Mel Cheren, the disco pioneer and founder of West End Records, and convinced him to make the space available free of charge. The arrangement was less than ideal. There were uncomfortable hallway encounters with residents, some of whom were mentally ill. And their tiny room, damp and infested with cockroaches, offered only enough space for two tables and half a dozen chairs. There were just two telephones. When two more rooms opened downstairs, Cheren moved in more tables and helped GMHC keep pace with the expanding needs.

Kramer ensconced himself there, effectively acting as GMHC's office manager, though his workplace style was disastrous. He was a flash flood of emotions, demanding and impatient, a screamer who chafed at the ordinary constraints of collegiality and consensus. No disagreement was too trivial for an explosion. Recognizing the need for change, Popham pressed for hiring a professional to lead the organiza-tion. He had in mind an acquaintance, Mel Rosen, the aggressive and balding vice president of a social service agency called Wildcat. Kramer, sensitive to Popham's motives, argued instead for hiring McFarlane, his lover, who would bolster rather than undermine Kramer's influ-ence. Both McFarlane and Rosen had the requisite background and experience, but Rosen made the winning argument: he had concocted a way to draw unemployment insurance from Wildcat, allowing him to take the position on a purely voluntary basis. The board enthusiastically named him executive director, with Kramer dissenting.

With Rosen at the helm, the group quickly proved adept at institution building and fund-raising. For their first major public event, a disco party at a SoHo nightclub called the Paradise Garage, GMHC netted $32,086 plus a flood of new volunteers, scores of whom showed up at the next regular meeting. Rosen put them to work stuffing envelopes, typing letters, answering phones, and keeping the coffee pot filled, while McFarlane dispatched them to assist his callers across the city. The work was exhausting, overwhelmingly sad, and never ending. "They come in the door and across the telephone, and it's our task to manage the madness, not to be sucked into it," said McFarlane.

Despite Rosen's arrival, Kramer continued to assert himself around the office. He treated Rosen terribly, Popham even worse. He later admitted rather blithely to a crush on Popham, made even more painful by the sudden exit of McFarlane, who left New York City that fall. This didn't go unnoticed by the others. Kramer's confessed inability to keep a man and the role that played in his whipsawing moods was a matter of snide conversation around the office. Still, much of Kramer's ire was aimed at the board of directors' changing priorities. He exploded when the board voted to spread GMHC research funds around to several labs, ending the informal monopoly Kramer had granted Friedman-Kien. They believed that the community's donations should be allocated based on medical priorities, not what they saw as Kramer's personal allegiances. There were more fundamental disagreements. The GMHC board felt that funding research, though a pressing issue, should come second behind patient care and advocacy. At a time when GRID victims were being thrown out of hospitals, ignored by ambulances, and stranded in their apartments, board members felt an urgent responsibility to respond directly to their suffering—and to the suffering of their loved ones. Most hospitals restricted boyfriends to formal visiting hours, if they let them visit at all, and no hospital in New York would allow them to enter the ICU; nationwide, only one hospital had a "significant others" rule acknowledging gay couples. There was much work to be done.

In his unwritten blueprint, Mel Rosen and his team planned to grow GMHC into "a top notch social service organization in the gay community," as he later said. Another board member, a soft-spoken former prosecutor named Richard Failla, advocated for the legal needs of the sick. Employers were firing people diagnosed with the disease, insurance claims were being rejected, and landlords were locking patients out of their homes. Thousands of people urgently needed wills, because without them estates were being swept up by estranged family members who were stripping the surviving partners of everything, even the photographs and cherished ephemera from a shared life. GMHC used volunteer lawyers for estate planning, and to help with living wills and health care proxies. "Every contact with the system is a confrontation," said Robert Cecchi, a volunteer crisis counselor. "As the number of cases grows, it becomes harder to handle the numerous complaints."

The suffering moved Kramer as it did the others, but he felt the Red Cross and the other state and local agencies had a sacred responsibility to handle these matters instead of abdicating the work to the community, and he angrily excoriated his colleagues for letting the homophobia of the social safety net go unchallenged. This was more than a matter of fairness to him; it was the root of all his rage. He tended to see the world as a battle between aloof parent figures and rejected children, a fixation set into motion by his own father, George, an underachieving and vindictively angry presence, who wished out loud that his gay son had never been born. "I should have shot my load in the toilet," was his unfortunate phrase. For thirty-three years, until his father's death, Kramer fought an operatic, losing battle for his kindness, if not his love. In his view, GMHC's clients deserved the same sort of love from the nonprofits aiding "the general population," as the non-gay world was euphemistically called. He felt the same way about city services. He considered Mayor Ed Koch "the father of us all," with all the responsibility that entailed, and condemned him for denying his children empathy. And he held *The New York Times,* the greatest of authority figures—"the newspaper of record!"—to an even higher standard. He wrote letter after letter to its top editors and reporters, pleading in the most personal terms for recognition of the community's pain. He fought stubbornly for GMHC to keep pressure on the paper to report on the crisis—to raise awareness in general, to reach the majority of gay men who never read the *Native,* and to force city hall and the White House to fund research and care. Political pressure and political action were his proposed priorities; he hoped his tantrums would warm frigid hearts.

He also returned time and again to the theme that won him infamy: he wanted GMHC to assume the role of stern father, telling gay men to stop having sex. The other board members opposed this proposal as being without solid merit medically, and toxic politically. Some were more fervent about this than others. Even McFarlane, when he was still involved with GMHC, thought Kramer was going too far. "The rest of us thought, We all have it anyway—we all slept with one another—so it was illogical to think we weren't all infected. What would stopping fucking do?" Instead, GMHC endorsed the advice of the gay doctors' support group to "have fewer partners, who are in good health." Dan William, chairman of the group's medical board, called this "the Elizabeth Taylor model of behavior—serial monogamy."

Under ordinary circumstances, working out these differences might have been a simple matter. But even the smallest deviation from Kramer's wishes could launch angry eruptions. It also seemed to both Popham and Nathan Fain that Kramer was laying an untenable personal claim to the organization and to the disease itself. In public statements and private clashes, he had begun to assert a right to special privileges by virtue of being GMHC's "mother" (and its volunteers and clients his "children"), a claim founded on the relatively inconsequential fact that the first meeting had taken place in his apartment.

Talk of "the problem with Larry" animated telephone calls around the city, further taxing a group of people already crippled by the daily horror of the disease itself. The tensions were especially hard on Lawrence Mass. He had known Kramer for fifteen years, and was his only "old friend" on the board. He too was dismayed by the role Kramer was playing. It was destabilizing and alienating, he felt. Fain was already talking about the need to make changes on the board. But when pressed for his opinions, Mass, constitutionally averse to conflict, sought to acknowledge Kramer's weaknesses *and* strengths. The strategy did little to keep him out of the line of fire.

Mass was already overwhelmed by the crisis. His full-time job at a methadone clinic gave him little time for his writing and reporting on the epidemic, yet he felt the urgent responsibility to provide news to the community—desperate people stopped him on the street seeking it. Sleeplessness and lack of appetite further undermined his writing and inflamed his feelings of guilt. Being drawn into the friction around Kramer pushed him over the edge. His spirits dived. Exhausted and morose, his thoughts began turning to suicide. One evening he admitted to his new lover, Arnie Kantrowitz, that he had taken the elevator to the top of the Empire State Building to investigate what physical contortions would be necessary to clear the lip. Kantrowitz took him straight to the psychiatric ward at St. Vincent's. Mass wouldn't return to GMHC or to his medical writing for another year.

DURING HIS TIME in the hospital, doctors had put Callen on Bactrim as a possible remedy for his cryptosporidiosis. When Sonnabend read this in Callen's chart it triggered a thought. While working in London,

Sonnabend had had some experience with transplant patients, whose suppressed immune systems made them susceptible to *Pneumocystis carinii* pneumonia, the same pneumonia haunting GRID patients. The PCP also plagued patients undergoing chemotherapy for leukemia. In those cases, it was routine to prescribe Bactrim as prophylaxis, the same way he used penicillin before a night at the baths. As early as the mid-1970s, studies confirmed that Bactrim was near 100 percent effective in preventing PCP in at-risk populations. Why, Sonnabend wondered, wouldn't the approach work for GRID patients?

It was now clear that PCP was by far the most common cause of death in the epidemic. A quarter of GRID patients diagnosed with PCP died of it, even with treatment. Statistically, those lucky enough to survive one bout were bound to experience another within a year. Fewer than half survived the second PCP infection, and a third bout did in most of the rest.

To be safe, Sonnabend advised Callen to continue taking one double-strength Bactrim tablet two times a day. He then made the same treatment recommendation for all his patients with advancing disease. He immediately noticed that people with GRID showed more adverse reactions to the drug than expected. Fully half suffered fever, rashes, hives, photosensitivity, and other skin reactions, some so severe they had to discontinue the medicine. But for those who could tolerate Bactrim, the drug appeared to help prevent PCP as expected.

Other doctors made the same leap of faith. In New York, Barbara Starrett put all her patients on Bactrim after their first PCP infection; a handful of GRID doctors in Los Angeles did similarly. Like Sonnabend, they noticed a decrease in PCP as a result. The approach didn't occur to most doctors in the community, though, so Sonnabend began promoting it wherever doctors gathered. Surprisingly, his efforts were met with stern opposition by the research establishment, because there was no published study showing Bactrim helped GRID patients better than a placebo. This infuriated Sonnabend. The main difference between most GRID patients with immune suppression and most of the other populations with immune suppression was sexual orientation. Why would anyone suppose that Bactrim wouldn't work on gay men?

AFTER MATHILDE KRIM'S lunch with Sonnabend, her thoughts frequently returned to the KS clusters. Spending long hours at the laboratory, she struggled to make sense of the disease's sudden explosion. She knew next to nothing about the tapestry of gay sexual life, which she felt undermined her ability to investigate the disease. She confessed this one afternoon to Sonnabend, whom she had always presumed to be heterosexual, and, avoiding an uncomfortable conversation, he sent over Callen and Berkowitz instead, knowing they would tutor her without censorship.

In a succession of meals near her lab, they led their very formal older student on an anthropological survey of their community's way of life, sparing nothing. Though sometimes she nearly went lightheaded at the descriptions, Krim seemed genuinely fascinated, and was riveted especially by Berkowitz's stories from his dungeon. "Oh my," she gasped again and again. Like Sonnabend, she was developing a strong suspicion that GRID selectively attacked the sexually voracious by a thousand blows to the immune system.

She called a number of her colleagues to request KS samples to study, but Memorial Sloan Kettering, she was told, had instituted a formal ban on treating victims of the gay cancer. That the city's preeminent cancer hospital was turning away people with cancer made no sense to her. The hospital administration told her the directive came from the president and CEO, Paul Marks. "It was not to be encouraged for people with GRID to come to Sloan Kettering," she was told. The cold cruelty of her hospital's GRID policy was to her a scandal, and not an isolated one. Forced to look elsewhere for tissue samples to study, she soon discovered that other New York–area hospitals had also begun to refuse GRID patients. Only the NYU Medical Center, where Friedman-Kien and Linda Laubenstein had dived headlong into Kaposi's sarcoma, was openly taking patients. But even there, tensions arose. When Friedman-Kien presented his earliest case at grand rounds, Dr. Saul Farber, the bombastic head of internal medicine, had his retinue of residents and interns wear head-to-foot protective gear, and he himself wore the unnecessary garb. They looked like an expedition of space explorers, and gave the sick patient a fright.

"This," Friedman-Kien said of his patient, "is just the beginning of a disaster. This is going to be a pandemic."

To which Farber replied, still in earshot, "But why does NYU have to be the *Titanic*?"

Farber later adpoted his own anti-GRID policy, ruling that those patients could not be admitted to shared rooms, and consequently had to be held in the ER when the limited number of isolation rooms filled up. He knew that GRID patients posed no risk to roommates. But Farber considered the containment policy necessary because applications for residencies at NYU from top medical schools had lagged, either from fear of GRID or because a hospital overwhelmed with the disease presumably lacked the diversity of illnesses that ambitious physicians sought. The effect was to keep sick patients on temporary gurneys lining the first-floor hallways, held there for days or weeks, sometimes breathing their last breaths without ever having been admitted.

Next Krim reached out to Craig Metroka, a young, unimposing oncologist who was seeing KS patients at another hospital, in a hematology clinic that met one afternoon a week. He agreed to provide her with tissue samples. Through trial-and-error experimentation, he had settled on a treatment protocol with a form of chemotherapy that could be delivered directly into the purple tumor. This inter-lesional approach was much more easily tolerated than systemic infusions. It appeared promising, he said. It turned the purple flesh black and kept it from growing, while managing to avoid the disastrous immune-suppressing consequences of using chemo in the bloodstream. He admitted to wishing he could treat all the patients referred to him, but as the clinic allotted space to him just one day a week, he was forced to turn away many.

Hearing of this newest barricade against KS patients nearly filled Krim's eyes with tears. Krim had a tremendous capacity for empathy, which had sometimes led her into extreme actions. As a teenager growing up in Geneva, she tucked into a movie theater one afternoon just after the Nazis' defeat, and gasped when a newsreel presented the first footage from the liberated camps. The images of haunted men and women reduced to unblinking skeletons caused her to cry for a week, at the end of which she had entirely personalized her identification with the Jewish people. She converted to Judaism, to her parents' lasting dismay, and threw herself into Zionist causes with an unconditional zeal. Before Israeli statehood, she volunteered for the paramilitary organization Irgun, unaware of its involvement in terror campaigns in Brittain's Palestinian territory. She meandered through French villages after the war soliciting arms left behind by the resistance and delivered them to the Israeli underground. ("A pretty girl on a bicycle," she discovered, "can get away with a lot.") In later years, after her economic circumstances improved, she and Arthur Krim played host to Israeli prime minister Menachem Begin when he visited New York.

With all the GRID and suffering around her, intuitively as before, she joined the resistance. She invited Metroka to turn her lab into an underground center for GRID patients. Krim knew they had to carry out this operation without detection or they would be shut down. "Tell your patients to come to my office after six o'clock," she said, and he gratefully agreed to do so.

Thereafter, she convened an informal group of researchers, including scientists in San Francisco and Los Angeles, to begin collecting blood and tissue for future examination. On this, she worked closely with Sonnabend. To avoid contamination, the samples would be stored separately. This required obtaining additional equipment and hiring support staff, which quickly strained her husband's largess, but she made it clear this was now her calling and he knew better than to stand in her way.

Every night, on her way home, she secretly greeted Metroka and his furtive KS patients as they snuck past security. Those young men, wasting away with disease, had the same hollowed gaze she had first seen in that 1945 film clip, some so weak they gripped the wall for support.

AMONG THE 452 cases on the CDC list by July 1982, nearly a fifth of them—79 men—strenuously denied being gay. The obvious explanation was that the non-gay group must be deeply closeted, but many had a history of using intravenous drugs, raising alarms at the Atlanta center. In drug-shooting culture, sharing syringes was commonplace, and a well-documented method for transmitting disease. This was a first suggestion that whatever caused GRID could be transmissible via blood. But it was hardly a foregone conclusion. It was just as likely that drug abuse caused the debilitation, a version of Sonnabend's "immune-overload" theory.

Even more baffling, half of the professed heterosexuals with GRID were recent immigrants from Haiti, having arrived within the previous eight years. By mid-1982, thirty-four Haitians were diagnosed in five American states, eleven in the New York metropolitan area. Their clinical presentations were the familiar ones: PCP, cryptococcal meningitis, toxoplasmosis of the central nervous system, disseminated CMV, lots of herpes, and swollen lymph glands. Most ranged in age from mid-twenties to mid-forties. The CDC hadn't interviewed each one—a few were only diagnosed after death—but the twenty-three men they were able to speak to forcefully denied a history of IV-drug use or same-sex sexual experience. Investigators wondered if cultural strictures kept them from confessing to risk factors, even after Dr. Curran had teams of investigators reinterview each of the twenty-three. The authorities were stumped. There were no alerts in global health circles to a similar disease striking Haitians living inside Haiti. "Is this the same thing that is going on in homosexual men and intravenous drug abusers?" Curran wondered to a reporter. "If so, what does that mean? What is the unifying hypothesis or cause? The answer is, we do not know."

Just before the CDC planned to announce the Haitian conundrum in their weekly journal, a doctor at Mt. Sinai in the Bronx told Curran he had treated a sixty-two-year-old man with a long history of hemophilia A, a disease that keeps blood from clotting. The patient was neither homosexual nor Haitian, and swore he'd never injected drugs, yet after multiple hospitalizations and an immunological collapse, he died of PCP, a disease that had not previously been reported among hemophilia patients. The only thing making him unique was that he had received the standard treatment for hemophilia A, regular injections of a special clotting factor, called factor VIII, derived from fresh plasma donations. Soon, a second hemophilia patient took ill in Denver and a third in northeastern Ohio, raising frightening questions about factor VIII. There were twenty thousand Americans who required factor VIII for their everyday survival. Records were hastily reviewed to determine the manufacturer and lot numbers for the clotting factor each of the three sick patients received. There was no overlap, meaning that if factor VIII were contaminated with GRID, the problem could not be isolated.

Curran knew that the implications were disastrous if GRID was transmissible by blood products. Even without proof, he and batteries of government health officials called emergency meetings with blood bank operators around the country and implored them to adopt a policy to protect the nation's blood supply. Anybody donating blood would have to fill out a questionnaire. If their answers marked them as coming from one of the at-risk communities—the so-called 4-H Club: homosexuals, heroin addicts, Haitians, and now hemophiliacs—their blood would be thrown away.

By now sensitive to the tribal behaviors of gay men, Curran worried about losing the community's trust over the ban on gay blood. He used his strained travel budget to traverse the country, meeting with gay leaders in an effort to ease the sting of it. Gay men, he learned, were extremely avid blood donors. In fact, in recent months an unnoticed and massive blood drive had been under way in LA's gay neighborhoods in response to the mounting GRID crisis there. Week after week long lines of men rolled up their sleeves to donate blood, dutifully offering up pint after pint of harm they never dreamed of.

The blood questionnaire proved an effective tool, though too late to slow the disease. Looking back at saved samples from the time, it was apparent that tens of thousands of blood recipients were already infected, including three-quarters of all those on factor VIII.

THROUGH AUGUST 1982, the *New York Native* publisher Chuck Ortleb had run twenty pieces on the epidemic, far more than any other periodical in the world. He gave them considerable real estate in the paper, promoting many on the cover, and paid writers as much as $400 for a feature, a sum unparalleled in gay publishing. Though the content generated strong objections from some advertisers, particularly the bathhouses and bars that feared scapegoating, the coverage proved a wise business decision. Circulation soared to twenty thousand, such was the hunger for practical, unbiased information.

It was an unexpected new calling for Ortleb. The son of a meat company manager, he earned his degree in poetry from the University of Kansas, then headed for New York in 1972 in search of the gay literati. Blond-haired and lithe, he possessed an enthusiastic mind and a charming curiosity about the city's inner sanctums. Soon he was dating Arthur Bell, whose work as the nightlife columnist with *The Village Voice* put Ortleb in the embrace of gay café society. While he was able to publish some of his work in obscure periodicals, he made a modest living as a typist. His profile changed in 1975, when he managed to borrow enough money to start a gay literary monthly he named *Christopher Street*. It was an immediate cultural bellwether, a gay-themed *New Yorker* publishing new works from Andrew Holleran and Christopher Bram and giving early exposure to a generation of younger writers including David Leavitt and the graphic novelist Alison Bechdel. The magazine was wildly popular, but never profitable. Ortleb launched the *Native* in 1980, convinced that the revenue from advertisers would keep both publications afloat.

He took to newsgathering with remarkable instinct, and personally drove the voluminous GRID coverage. The disease played into his low-level anxiety about dying, something that first seized him in his early twenties, after a relative's sudden death. Once, during a physical exam, he fainted dead away because the doctor said nothing more ominous than, "Lost a little weight lately?" He adopted odd survival tics, like habitually familiarizing himself with emergency exits and washing his hands pink.

By mid-August 1982, at the beginning of the second year of the epidemic, Ortleb penned one of his first strident editorials on the terrible political challenges facing gay men. "It has now been a year since the epidemic surfaced as a serious health crisis, and we are no closer to a cure or an explanation than we were a year ago," he wrote. "[I]f the CDC exists for the purposes of monitoring this—or any—epidemic, who exists for the purposes of monitoring the CDC? . . . Who can assure us that not one ounce of homophobia is affecting the progress of this investigation when we are all too familiar with the medical establishment's formal history of homophobia?"

In fact, as he soon learned, the CDC had been ordered to *reduce* its GRID budget—part of the Reagan administration's war on big government. The disease agency had been able to locate only $2 million for the mushrooming epidemic. And the NIH, with an annual budget of $4 billion, had announced it would be able to set aside just $5 million, one-tenth of the amount already requested by researchers. So it was infuriating to read in the paper that Washington had responded to a deadly flood and landslide in Central America by donating $25 million in foreign aid. Though twice two doesn't equal four in human life, as Dostoevsky wrote, five times as many people had died of GRID as had died in the landslide. Reagan, who had not publicly acknowledged the epidemic, issued a statement: "The American people join me in sending sympathy to those injured, their families and the families of those who lost their lives." Why weren't the American people expressing sympathy to the gays? It was no better in New York. Like Reagan, Ed Koch had not mentioned the disease in public, despite being the mayor of the city at the epicenter of the plague, where one new case was diagnosed every day.

The liberals were as silent as the conservatives. Most just never thought about it, or else mined it for jokes. The scabrous publisher Al Goldstein, a drum major for sexual liberalism, marveled about the new bug that was capable of turning fruits into vegetables.

WITH THEIR DOCTORS' guidance on matters of science (and with Callen's lover, Richard Dworkin, as editor and muse), Callen and Berkowitz began work on a somewhat hectoring, always strident exhortation to the community, imploring people to learn from their mistakes and abandon their promiscuous ways. Neither had much of a literary track record. Berkowitz's output consisted of a few film reviews in his college paper, a stint at a trade journal, and a couple of freelance profiles. Lyrics were the extent of Callen's writing. But they labored through draft after draft, emboldened by Sonnabend's faith in them.

"This isn't a game. People are dying—very real, horrible, and unnecessary deaths," they wrote. "Sure, the baths are fun, but the risks have simply become too great. A year ago, new cases . . . were being reported at the rate of one a day; today the rate is three times that. . . . What ten years ago was viewed as a healthy reaction to a sex-negative culture now threatens to destroy the very fabric of urban gay male life."

If they seemed to be assigning responsibility, that's exactly what they had in mind. "Deep down," they declared, "we know who we are and why we are sick."

They gamely waded into the "cause" debate, listing their reasons for discrediting the belief in a "new, mutant, Andromeda-strain virus" in an averment that went even further than Sonnabend's in describing it as not just improbable but impossible. It was an error of rhetoric they would come to regret. "We veterans of the circuit must accept that we have overloaded our immune systems with *common* viruses and other sexually transmitted infections. Our lifestyle has created the present epidemic. . . . But in the end, whichever theory you choose to believe, the obvious and immediate solution to the present crisis is the end of urban gay male promiscuity as we know it today."

The piece was carefully edited by Ortleb's team, who challenged the writers on context and presentation. Callen had the bristly reaction of a novice: he vehemently resisted the editors' insertions and fought their deletions, both stylistic and substantive. He and Berkowitz loved the title, "We Know Who We Are," but Callen threatened to pull the article over Ortleb's subtitle, "Two Gay Men Declare War on Promiscuity," which missed the delicate point they made about every gay man's sexual prerogative. "Ultimately," their piece flatly stated, "it may be more important to let people die in the pursuit of their own happiness than to limit personal freedom by regulating sex." Despite the storm of unpleasantries, Ortleb's subtitle remained unchanged. He further inflamed them by assigning a companion article arguing the single-virus theory. "Confusing? Contradictory? Of course," the publisher's introduction would read when the two pieces appeared. "But then, so is much of the discussion surrounding the present health crisis. It's a discussion that we feel virtually everyone should be involved in—gay people as well as non-gay, laymen as well as physicians, policy-makers as well as the citizenry—and it is in that spirit that we publish these pieces."

The writing process built a tight bond between Callen and Berkowitz, and despite whatever jealousies may have arisen between Callen and his lover, it also gave rise to a deep and shared admiration between them, fortifying their relationship and cementing their love for one another. The article would run in the *Native* in the early fall. All three knew their lives would be transformed overnight, from anonymous men on the periphery of the gay movement to public figures at a time of crisis. It was Callen's idea to spend the last night of their anonymity revisiting their old life. The three went on a tour of the Mineshaft, the sleaziest of sex holes in Manhattan's legendary Meatpacking District. The entire scene amazed Dworkin, but nothing surprised him more than a spare downstairs room with a bathtub as its centerpiece, where men took turns soaking in urine. "Call me naïve," he declared.

They didn't stay long. As they were collecting their jackets, Callen watched a man pass out, fortuitously landing atop the pool table. Thinking he'd had a heart attack or perhaps a drug overdose, Callen rushed to revive him. When that failed, he ran to get the bartender, but when the two made it back to the pool table, Callen was appalled to find someone attempting to have sex with the unconscious man.

Disgusted, the three men marched out to the street with all the righteousness of Luther. "This is *exactly* what we're talking about," Callen fumed. "We're gonna nail the fucking door *shut*."

In the morning, when the *Native* hit newsstands, the backlash was overwhelming and personal. Callen and Berkowitz were mortified. In subsequent issues of the *Native* they were called "sex-negative" hysterics, self-flagellators, and "religious converts," the cat's paw of Reverend Jerry Falwell and his gay-obsessed Moral Majority. The uproar spilled out of the *Native* pages to gay periodicals across the globe, and even *The Village Voice* published articles denouncing them. The Toronto-based gay paper *Body Politic* ran a stinging editorial titled "The Real Gay Epidemic: Panic and Paranoia" which quoted a gay doctor arguing that Callen, Berkowitz, Sonnabend, and Dworkin were nearly treasonous in their abandonment of the cause. "In the same period that 200 [GRID] cases were diagnosed, more than 400 gay men died in traffic accidents because they chose to go outside," he said. "Lesbians and sexually active gay men are going to have their rights denied and infringed upon—all because 400 cases of a disease have appeared among 20 million of us."

Being so brutally reviled gave Callen recurring nightmares and planted seeds of a budding persecution complex in Berkowitz. They spent hours on the telephone with one another, denouncing their detractors and crafting and recrafting a lengthy written response, which the *Native* repeatedly refused to publish. Ultimately, Callen reluctantly concluded that they had deserved the lashings. "We were arrogant enough to assume that we could use the word *promiscuous* without setting off an absolute furor," he said during one of their calls. "Along comes us, *screaming, yelling,* saying, '*Oh my God there's an epidemic! You've got to cut out [sex] completely, THIS IS A CRISIS!*' And who are we? I mean, really, who *are* we?"

Despite the tensions, Berkowitz recalled this time fondly. "We saw the light, we saw Joe's model, and there was a certain obligation to do something," Berkowitz told Callen. "You and I were on the top of a mountain looking over and seeing something that no one else was aware of, that no one else could see. And that made me feel so incredibly close to you." Callen, despite his public mortification, felt the same. They weren't backing down.

ON A CRISP, fall-like afternoon, Sonnabend found his way to the back booth at Joe Jr.'s, a noisy coffee shop on Sixth Avenue in the Village. Berkowitz could see he was angry. His temper had a tendency to further rumple his appearance and tie his tongue even more than usual. Sonnabend had been watching as the city's weekly health bulletins continued to report PCP deaths. Any trained physician should know how to prevent such a fate, he felt. "These doctors are not delivering, they're just windbags," he said. "Deadheads." He handed the most recent Department of Health briefings to Berkowitz.

Berkowitz thumbed through the papers, not quite understanding.

"NYU has the *distinction*," Sonnabend underscored with sarcasm, "of having the largest number of patients by virtue of their advertising and help by people like GMHC, and they've done *nothing.* . . . By keeping all these patients it means they are keeping them from people who know what to do."

Berkowitz interjected timidly. "Like immunologists?"

"Yes! They haven't proven that they are competent to do this work. Who *is* Dr. Friedman-Kien? He's a society skin doctor as far as I know. He's certainly not equipped to get into this kind of stuff!" Diners from the surrounding booths could make out every word. "These people have lymphadenopathy, and he's not equipped to deal with it. So they're dealing with KS. They grab up all the patients. *They've killed any number of patients.*" He narrowed his eyes. "He's a *skin doctor!*"

He was even more venomous about Dr. Linda Laubenstein. "Laubenstein has got no expertise at all. She's a very young woman, she hasn't been out of medical school that long. Why should you go to a person who has no experience? She's fooling around, fucking with these fucking chemicals. *They're fooling around!* I would never let any patient of mine go near NYU." He shook his head balefully. "The patients I've had there I've taken away. One patient, thank goodness, he went there and he's still alive. He would have been pumped full of chemotherapy and he'd be quite dead by now, there's no question."

These were serious indictments. But rather than challenging the other doctors, Sonnabend let his observations feed a deepening well of resentment against them, Friedman-Kien especially. Their laboratory-sharing experiment had come to an acrimonious end when Friedman-Kien could no longer put up with Sonnabend's disorganization. Such was the communication gap between them that Sonnabend believed he had quit in disgust and Friedman-Kien was certain he had evicted him.

For all his assertiveness while trashing his rivals, Sonnabend was timid in his self-promotion and a terrible advocate for his own ideas. This was partly due to his shyness but also because he saw himself as a perpetual minority of one, a leader incapable of gaining followers. This frustrated Berkowitz and Callen, who often complained that Sonnabend's faulty communication skills kept his disease model from gaining wider traction, and left patients in other practices unaware of his thinking about treatment and prevention. Berkowitz had asked for this meeting to propose a role for himself and Callen as the doctor's mouthpieces, taking his theories public so that doctors and patients could judge for themselves. Despite their public pillorying, they planned another *Native* article, this one telling patients what to demand of their doctors.

Sonnabend enthusiastically agreed to the arrangement. As they ate their lunch, he said he didn't have to be an oncologist to know that people had not done well on traditional chemotherapy. "There are new agents that are not that devastating," he said.

"Interferon?" Berkowitz asked.

Sonnabend shook his head. His experiments had shown it offered little hope. It caused fevers and inhibited development of white blood cells, especially of CD4 cells, the body's elite disease-fighting squadrons. Interferon's massive proliferation in people with GRID appeared to contribute to the course of the disease. Yet numerous well-meaning researchers, including those at the NIH, were injecting even more interferon into immune-deficiency patients, believing its antiviral properties might simultaneously fight whatever was causing illness.

"I wouldn't let anybody of mine even *smell* the stuff," he said. "There's only one treatment that is rational, and that's plasmapheresis."

Plasmapheresis was used for lupus and other autoimmune diseases in which the body produces excessive antibodies, just as GRID seemed to do. The procedure removed those antibodies mechanically, by rerouting blood out one arm, passing it through a centrifuge, then returning the blood through the other arm minus antibodies. He had sent Callen to Boston for the procedure, noting that the patient felt much less fatigued afterward. "It's relatively harmless," Sonnabend said. Still, most other doctors were not offering plasmapheresis and some had openly criticized Sonnabend for championing it.

"In other words, it cleans your blood?"

"Yes!" he snapped impatiently. Then more tentatively, "It might have saved lives."

Berkowitz looked up from his food. "If a person has the immune deficiency, but doesn't have any of the debilitating diseases," he wondered aloud, describing himself, "what do you think the chances are that the immune deficiency could reverse itself?"

Sonnabend answered carefully. "I think if you get plasmapheresed, it might help. *You* would be a candidate, for example. I'd like to get you plasmapheresed to see if we could reverse your parameters."

Berkowitz was numbed by the recommendation. He thought his "parameters," though cockeyed, didn't merit dramatic intervention yet. Since his trauma-provoking gland biopsy, he'd gone totally celibate to protect against any new challenges to his immune system. Consequently, he was also off cocaine—in the world of sex work, they went together like tea and crumpets. Only cigarettes and marijuana remained in his regular routine, though in dramatically reduced quantities. He was eating better, sleeping better, showing his body respect. He had hoped that this alone would allow his body to heal from the dual infections of CMV and hepatitis A, which Sonnabend had diagnosed over the summer. Obviously his doctor was less confident.

There was a plasmapheresis center in New York, Sonnabend said, but the director there had so far refused GRID patients. "I have to call Bruce Gordon and beg him to do you," Sonnabend said, adding another item to his impossibly long agenda. He sighed. "It's being denied people because doctors—*the great experts* . . ." He didn't finish the sentence. Waving for the waiter's attention, he looked exhausted. "I have to get to the office." They sat in silence waiting for the check.

After a time, Sonnabend tilted his head toward a tape recorder that Berkowitz had brought with him. "All this is happening and there really is no one of substance to chronicle this—the tragedy of this. A person who knows how to write, who knows people, where is such a person? This is New York City and nobody is chronicling this?" If he was asking Berkowitz to create that record, he didn't say so directly. Nor did he have to.

THAT FALL, Callen spent $39 on a recorder of his own and joined Berkowitz in taping new Sonnabend disquisitions. By now, researchers had started using a new name for GRID, answering to concerns about naming a disease after the community. There was nothing "gay" about collapsed immunity, as Sonnabend put it. The disease was rebranded as "acquired immune deficiency syndrome"—AIDS. But the new name didn't change perceptions. In the guise of AIDS rage, across the country came wave after wave of anti-gay violence, just as Sonnabend had prophesied.

Callen and Berkowitz taped Sonnabend over lunch, when he met with other researchers, and during late-night phone calls, which had become commonplace. Cassettes piled up in both apartments, where they were reviewed and swapped. They had become Sonnabend's unpaid amanuenses and self-styled acolytes, standing in the spillway of his developing thoughts so that others might benefit. "I've got it on tape," Berkowitz would announce, "if you forget."

Despite their painful experience with the first piece, Berkowitz and Callen had plunged back into the fray. They didn't have time for fighting the attacks. "Let them say what they want," Callen said. "They'll see what's going on and they'll see that they were wrong."

Of the two, Berkowitz had the most to lose by becoming a public figure. Fear that his former occupation would be used against him consumed his thoughts. "I was never ashamed of the work I did," he said later. "I just didn't have any faith that people could get beyond that label and that they'd hear anything that I had to say. To be honest, I didn't want to put myself up for public scrutiny and ridicule." Callen argued for full disclosure, saying, "Gay men are dying and there's no more time for secrets." In that spirit, he had decided to openly discuss his own bathhouse history. When Berkowitz hesitated to do the same, Callen made the matter moot by telling everybody he met that Berkowitz was an ex-prostitute. Though Berkowitz protested mightily, he was quietly relieved to be unburdened of the secret.

Berkowitz and Callen planned to call their second article "A Warning to Gay Men with AIDS," specifically focusing on the dangers of chemotherapy. "We believe that it is crucial for us to begin to share with others like ourselves our personal experiences in getting treatment," they began. They declaimed their advice in nine numbered and foot-noted paragraphs, the first one taking aim at Dr. Laubenstein's zest for chemotherapy, though they did not mention her by name. "Three out of four men with KS die of severe opportunistic infections after two years—and most of these men will have received chemotherapy. Chemotherapy may in fact be destroying what is left of your immune system." They went on to advise against interferon therapy ("NO ONE KNOWS WHAT THE EFFECTS WILL BE!"), too much sunlight ("definitively immunosuppressive"), and allowing doctors to remove an enlarged spleen, which was too often their first plan of action ("this treatment may kill you").

Once they completed the article, they walked it over to the *Native* offices and submitted it for publication. After deliberating for a few days, Ortleb rejected the piece. He told Berkowitz that he had taken a lot of grief from readers after their first article, accusing him of endan-gering gay sexual liberties and confusing the community with mixed messages at a time of crisis. But he accepted that controversy was the price of running a paper, and he was prepared to court it again. What he wasn't willing to do was deal again with such difficult parvenus as Callen and Berkowitz.

Then Ortleb confided his own AIDS theory. "It definitely has some-thing to do with poppers," he said. "They smell of death."

As Berkowitz and Callen saw it, Ortleb's censorial move put his read-ers in grave danger. Frantically, they brainstormed with their doctor about another way to reach the community. One of them offered the off-hand suggestion that they simply buy space in the *Native* to run the story as paid advertising. Assuming Ortleb would not be so craven, they sent in their piece as a two-column ad. Remarkably, he accepted it, along with their check for $240, a sum Sonnabend collected with the help of a few of his patients. The ad appeared around Thanksgiving, set apart in a black box and attributed to a new group, Gay Men with AIDS, listing a post office box for correspondence. Callen and Berkowitz chose this name for themselves to highlight their credentials. Unexpectedly, their box filled with letters from men wanting to join. What began as a front became the first patient advocacy group of its kind in the world.

THOUGH TIMIDLY, the dominant media was beginning to take notice, too; after eleven months of silence, the chief science writer of *The New York Times* returned to the subject with three brief articles in 1982, all deep inside the paper. But it seemed that every minor advance in public attention brought sickening waves of violence. Everybody knew a victim. My friend Andy Mosso was stabbed nine times as he scurried around a clutch of young men in Tompkins Square. Nobody took his wallet; this was no robbery. They left him gasping in his vomit, his pain and death being the whole point. Convalescing in the hospital, he was interviewed once by police, but no arrests were made. It seemed futile even to lodge reports. These crimes were carried out mostly by young white men in their teens and twenties who if caught might say they acted out of self-defense in response to unwanted sexual advances, importunings that disgusted them to the point of temporary madness. Lawyers called it the "gay panic defense," and acquittals were routine.

Ermanno Stingo, whom I met at the Pride March that year, made it his business to attend such trials. A courtly figure in his mid-sixties, with a square head and one crooked front tooth, he took up "court monitoring," as he called it, on his own initiative after retiring as a personnel director. Several mornings a week, he fixed a pink triangle to his suit and planted himself on courthouse benches around the city in silent vigil, hoping to influence judges and jurors. Most nights he called me with his sad dispatches, which he encouraged me to work up for publication in various gay newspapers.

I had done time on my college paper, and I knew something about deadlines and inverted pyramids, so I agreed to help. I had no illusions about the alternative press being able to force the criminal justice system to reform itself. If I needed proof of our impotence, it was provided on the night of September 29, when a friend called about a police raid on a gay bar in Times Square called Blues favored by black and Latino clientele, some of them transgender. When I was allowed inside the next day, the evidence of physical brutality turned my stomach. Chairs were splintered, broken glass covered the floor. The cash register had been twisted open and emptied. Blood pooled on the linoleum in the back, where the patrons had pressed against doors that wouldn't open. A dozen people were reportedly hospitalized, though this couldn't be independently confirmed; the police were offering no comment.

"About a dozen cops came inside and locked the door, and they just started swinging," the bartender told me.

"Did you call anybody?" I asked.

"Who do you call when the police are attacking you?"

No arrests were made in the days that followed. The mayor's office was maddeningly silent. *The New York Times*, whose main entrance stood directly across the street from Blues, never ran a story, not even after gay publications around the country printed the shocking photos. I felt called to do more than impotent community journalism would allow, so I joined a committee to organize a march. I even gave a strident speech at the rally that October. But playing a public role like that did not suit me, and I returned to the idea of journalism more seriously. Pursuing the Blues case, I requested and was granted an interview with the longtime New York County district attorney Robert Morgenthau, his first with an openly gay reporter to anybody's knowledge. I soon became the first reporter from a gay periodical to obtain credentials to city hall, covering Mayor Koch's combative press briefings for the *Native*. The first news conference I attended concerned an aggressive new policy to respond when cab drivers were victims of violent assault. When called upon, I rose nervously to ask if the policy worked both ways—I'd written a story about a driver who clobbered two men he'd caught kissing in his backseat.

"Don't be ridiculous," Koch said, turning quickly to the next questioner. "Cabbies don't attack customers—they *need* customers."

I didn't ask him about the health crisis then; I was still trying to assess for myself the severity of the epidemic. When I read about a community-wide forum to discuss the issue on November 30, I made plans to attend. It took place on a cold night outside the Julia Richman High School auditorium on the Upper East Side, where well over 2,500 people, more than would fit inside, assembled. The crowd was almost all white and male, the majority gay.

Inside, the mood was fragile. Larry Kramer was there, along with the other GMHC men. Dr. Craig Metroka from Roosevelt Hospital and Dr. Jeffrey Laurence of New York Hospital took their places on the stage. When the dermatologist Dr. Bijan Safai of Memorial Sloan Kettering climbed to the lectern, the room fell into an eerie stillness. A slide projector flickered on and threw the title of his talk onto a huge screen behind him: "How to recognize Kaposi's sarcoma." He began by describing the history of KS, and the importance of reporting any suspicious skin lesion to your doctor. Then he switched slides. Now looming large was the enormous image of a man's cancerous arm: misshapen purple blobs, some with deeply colored centers, sprouting against freckled white flesh.

"Oh no," came a cry from the balcony—the terrible outburst of recognition pierced the room, followed by a loud thud as the man hit the floor in a dead faint.

• • •

IN SAN FRANCISCO that November, Dr. Arthur Ammann was feeling frustrated as he studied the results of a bone marrow test he had ordered on a very sick toddler. As an expert in pediatric immunology who traveled regularly throughout Africa, Ammann thought he'd either seen or read about every immune disorder that could plague a child. At the UCSF Medical Center, where he taught and practiced, he was a recognized expert in infantile CMV infections. But this little boy baffled him. He was born prematurely on March 3, 1981, with pronounced jaundice, a problem caused by toxins accumulating in the blood. This was not extraordinary, and the standard course of treatment was followed: every ounce of his contaminated blood was replaced with donated supplies. The process was repeated five times over a four-day period, followed by additional infusions of blood products like packed red blood cells and platelets. When his blood makeup came back to normal, he was sent home with best wishes. But at four months of age his health began to dive. He suffered an enlarged spleen and liver. Jaundice returned, followed by hepatitis of no known origin, then anemia and diarrhea. Now the little boy was twenty months old and in intensive care.

Ammann suspected an infection in the child's bone marrow, which would be highly unusual. Test results were even more surprising than he'd imagined. The child's culture was positive for *Mycobacterium avium-intracellulare,* the dreaded cause of wasting syndrome in adults with AIDS. Recently there had been a number of reports of babies who seemed to inherit the disease at birth from their sick mothers, but that was not the case here. Ammann wrote in his case notes that both parents of his patient were "heterosexual non-Haitians and do not have a history of intravenous drug abuse." He submitted both to extensive testing, and found no signs of immune deficiency.

All he could think was: The blood supply is contaminated.

Pulling the boy's hospital records, he saw that blood donations from twenty-one separate people had been transfused into the child. Their identities were masked. All Dr. Ammann had were coded identifying numbers, corresponding to confidential records maintained by the Irwin Memorial Blood Bank in the Financial District.

In the morning, he headed for the blood bank with his list of numbers. Given the possible public health significance, Dr. Herb Perkins, the blood bank's research director, agreed to break the code and release the donors' identities. That afternoon, he sent twenty-one names over to the city's health department, which, by law, closely monitored each of the city's 125 AIDS cases. There, Dr. Selma Dritz, the specialist in charge, cross-referenced the two lists and easily pinpointed a man in his late forties whose name appeared on both. He had donated blood in early 1981. His health had remained unremarkable until that October, when he complained of fatigue, swollen lymph glands, and clouded vision in one eye—classic AIDS symptoms. Doctors diagnosed PCP in December, and he was dead nine months later.

This was the first irrefutable evidence of transmission through the blood supply. The cases involving hemophiliacs only hinted at the possibility, but this baby was the first AIDS patient to be matched to a specific blood donor with AIDS. The implications for research and prevention were obvious. But from a public health point of view, the discovery was horrific.

Ammann brought the sickening news to his superiors at the UCSF Medical Center. At their suggestion, he closed his office door and called the CDC. Dr. Harold Jaffe came to the phone. Jaffe was the CDC's top VD expert and a member of the agency's new AIDS task force. This was a call Jaffe had feared. He got on the next available flight from Atlanta, and the two doctors sat in Ammann's windowless office at the medical center poring over the boy's records, meticulously confirming transfusion dates and donor numbers. The work took them deep into the night, and produced the same devastating findings.

Ammann and Jaffe silently considered the ramifications. "This has important implications. We should report this," Jaffe said. He suggested that the CDC's *Morbidity and Mortality Weekly Report* would be the ideal outlet, because it was the quickest to publish of any medical journal, and was read regularly by public health authorities. "But I need to warn you," Jaffe added, "if you publish it in the *MMWR* you may not be able to publish it in the other journals, because of the 'Ingelfinger Rule.'"

Jaffe explained: "Ingelfinger is the editor of the *New England Journal of Medicine*. He has a blanket rule that if you publish your findings anywhere, even a letter in *MMWR*, he won't take your study there. We get a lot of researchers who won't give their information to the *MMWR* because they want the prestige that Ingelfinger can give them, even though he might take a year or more in prepublication review."

Ammann had enough experience in academic science to know that publishing in a prestigious journal would be to his advantage in certain circles. But concern for the blood supply outweighed any thoughts of his professional advancement. His *MMWR* letter appeared in early December, and touched off the first round of real interest in the disease. A scrum of journalists burst through the CDC's door for the first time, including correspondents from countless television networks and affiliates. The attention was long overdue. But with images of bouncing toddlers, the reporters warned America that the gay disease was now killing children. It unleashed a torrent of anti-gay violence the likes of which the community had never seen before.

4

Doubt All Things

It was nearly eleven o'clock when Sonnabend finished his work and loaded his bag for the short walk to his dark and messy Village apartment a few blocks away. He had always been as indifferent to décor as to tidiness. In a gesture of pity, an old boyfriend once gave him a vanload of antiques, which now sat behind discarded food cartons and dunes of dust, grime, and cat dander. Mathilde Krim was mortified the first time she saw how he lived. "Joe, you're a doctor," she said. "Forty dollars a week and you can have somebody come in and clean!" She had the same reaction to his office. After one visit she sent over a carpeting crew to replace the threadbare floor covering. But Sonnabend's everyday troubles were out of the reach of cosmetic fixes. Each dollar that came in went toward spiraling research expenses—FedEx bills for shipping blood samples to Nebraska, lengthy phone calls to Europe. By early 1983 he was in arrears to two landlords, who threatened eviction from home and office. The IRS was preparing serious fines for his failure to withhold payroll taxes. Krim continued her cash donations, but had taken to giving the money to Berkowitz instead of Sonnabend, with strict instructions to keep the creditors happy.

It wasn't enough. On his own initiative, Harley Hackett, the office manager, refused his salary and started using his own savings to cover basic office needs, a tremendous sacrifice. Hackett had worked as a stage manager and rising playwright, with the standard privations that entailed. Now he had come into a bequest from the estate of an old friend, $10,000, meant to enable him to write for a year. He poured half of it toward Sonnabend's debts and used the other half to cover his own living expenses. Sonnabend objected, but what could he do? One low afternoon he had to borrow $22 from a patient just so he could buy groceries.

Hackett's stoicism finally broke when, in the middle of a maddening day, Sonnabend appeared from a ninety-minute exam and announced that there would be no charge for the appointment. In mute resentment,

Hackett rose from his desk and left the roiling mess behind. Sonnabend pursued him to the sidewalk, imploring him to return, but Hackett, who admired Sonnabend for his humanitarian—if unreasonable—tendencies, could no longer afford to underwrite the enterprise. He took another job, supervising bookkeepers for a chain of menswear stores. But every evening, and each Saturday and Sunday, he returned to the squalid office on Twelfth Street and continued juggling the books pro bono and helping with laboratory experiments when needed.

As he extinguished the lights for the night, Sonnabend took measure of the epidemic. Nearly nine hundred cases had been reported in thirty-three states, plus sixty-seven cases in thirteen foreign countries; a third of the worldwide cases had resulted in death. Every week brought him more patients for whom he could do so little. He was already exhausted.

Then a ringing telephone called him back to his desk.

It was Berkowitz, who lately had made it his business to see to his doctor's emotional well-being.

"You're losing faith, I know," Berkowitz told him. "I don't blame you."

"Harley paid my phone bill, I discovered, without telling me," Sonnabend said. "Otherwise they would have cut me off today at home. He's got no money to do things like that." The thought of it made him grunt in shame.

"I've got a hundred dollars if you need it! I'm not kidding," Berkowitz said.

Sonnabend was tempted. "I've got to pay Bobby back," he thought out loud, meaning the patient who had lent him grocery money.

"Okay, so I'll get you cash. I have to go to a Citibank. It's there! It's money from Mathilde." He was sorry he let that slip. "I could forward you a hundred or whatever."

Sonnabend cringed. "It's terrible," he said.

"It is, but we just have to deal with it."

A little while later, when he was home with a container of Chinese food, Sonnabend was on the phone with Berkowitz again, rejecting the cash offer. "I'm freaking out," he admitted softly. "I can't look out after all these people, my god. I still haven't been to the hospital to see John Indrasek—and they said he's in intensive care and his condition was critical. I haven't even been there to see him yet, and he's been there for a month."

"I know," Berkowitz said. "It's a full-time job just talking to the patients and explaining things to them."

"I also have to preserve my interest in this, too, my model and the writing," Sonnabend said. He had an offer to publish in a journal put out by the National Cancer Institute, though he would have preferred a more prestigious outlet, like *The Lancet*, "something that really has a wide circulation."

"So spend ten bucks," Berkowitz said, "and Federal Express them your version."

"Oh," Sonnabend said suddenly. "I need some help tomorrow, that's what I wanted to ask you."

"You got me."

In fact, Berkowitz needed money, too. It had been six months since his diagnosis, and six months since he pulled his ad from publications and unplugged the dedicated telephone lines. His savings were gone. He had admitted to a friend he was tempted to go back to his old prac-tice, maybe just part-time so that he could pursue his newer avocations. "If I turned one trick five times a week, at $100—$500 a week—and had a part-time job with Joe [Sonnabend] counseling gay men with AIDS, and kept the support group going, and started working on a book? Wouldn't my life be complete?"

He added, "I'm tired of being poor. I'm really sick of it."

The temptation to resume hustling was made greater by a continual stream of former clients to his doorbell, undeterred by disconnected phones. He turned them away one by one, bending his abstinence rule only once, when a client simply would not be turned away.

"Look, we can't have sex," Berkowitz told him. "People are dying, something terrible is happening. Sex is the furthest thing from my mind!"

The man pleaded and pleaded. "Just put on your boots and let me worship your boots," he begged. "Just do this." Moved as much by pity as anything else, Berkowitz reluctantly laced up the Fryes.

After the client left, the scene replayed over and over in his mind, launching a reevaluation of his theories on promiscuity. Most of the theoretical causes of AIDS required direct exposure to bodily fluids. But most of the things men paid him for—spanking, verbal jousting, bondage, and restraint—didn't involve so much as a drop of sweat. He took a pad and began making a list of the specific acts in his repertoire. Berkowitz soon realized he and Callen had been on the wrong track. It wasn't promiscuity per se causing AIDS, but a certain *type* of pro-miscuity. Sex *could* be safe. Why hadn't this occurred to him so clearly before?

Berkowitz had found the theme of their next article. He got Sonnabend on the phone immediately. We can "come up with some kind of sexual ethic" about risk, he said excitedly, ticking off a litany of S&M maneuvers. "It doesn't have to be negative!"

The doctor had never endorsed the idea of S&M. But he understood immediately what Berkowitz was contemplating. "I think first one has to say that sex is terrific—it's not dangerous, it's an important activity that is—"

"Necessary!" Berkowitz interrupted.

"It should be *fulfilling* and *enjoyed*," Sonnabend corrected him, "and above all it should be healthy."

Next, Berkowitz brought the idea to Michael Callen, who had no interest at all in reassessing his stance against promiscuity. So Berkowitz was left to work on his theory alone, expanding from his own area of expertise to other fluid-free expressions, like hugging and voyeurism. "The advice has to be to have sex in ways where you're not going to kill yourself," he told a friend on the telephone. "Basically it goes through almost every aspect of sexuality you can possibly imagine and explains what's high risk, what's low risk."

In late February he handed a draft to Callen, who read it aloud. Callen was not impressed.

"They're predisposed to hate you," Callen reminded him. "They'll say, If sex has to be this mechanical . . . it's not worth it. Life is full of risks. Some you take, some you don't. *He* shouldn't tell *me* what risks I should take!"

Callen's reaction betrayed a deep uneasiness he had developed about sex in any form; intimacy had merged entirely with disease in his mind. Even in bed with Richard Dworkin, something so simple as a kiss could trigger a panic attack. When they made love, which was not often, his mind spun toward recurring dark montages: a snapshot of his beautiful friend Roger on a respirator; the look on sweet Chip Edgerton's face after he'd fallen into a vegetative state in his final, mute hours. He often claimed an AIDS symptom as an excuse to avoid sex. Memories of his past trysts could cause sudden, pounding anxiety. Recently, when someone he had had sex with showed up at his support group meeting looking near death, Callen flew into a moment of sheer madness: he interrupted the meeting, jabbed a finger at the frail man, and growled, "*You* gave me this. *You had this and you gave me this!*"

The man looked at him emptily and said, by way of apology, "I've had over 30,000 people—I just gave the CDC an interview on it."

Berkowitz's list of safe sex acts initially left Callen nauseated and cold. Over the next few days he began to understand the thinking it was based on. When Sonnabend called him to discuss it, he agreed that they had perhaps been a bit overly didactic in their earlier push against promiscuity. But overtly promoting a pro-sex message made little sense to him.

"Michael, this is part of what we're saying, part of what we're doing," Sonnabend told him. You didn't need to stay on the beach in order to keep from drowning, he reasoned; learning to swim could be just as effective. "You have to get on board with this. Richard is a better writer with you."

Still, Callen declined to help. But when he met an editor at *Mandate*, a popular porn magazine, he was kind enough to promote the Berkowitz project, and the man seemed open to considering it for publication. "Take him a copy," Callen advised Berkowitz. "You need a better introduction, though. Why don't you put it into context by talking about your own personal experience?"

"I'm not telling the whole world I'm a hustler—in a porn magazine," he said, laughing. But he did rework the top of his article to make the piece less like a menu of sex acts. And the next day he was sitting in *Mandate*'s swank SoHo offices, across from George de Stefano, the editor. De Stefano's unusual vision for a gay porn magazine included leftist politic essays and cultural analyses sprinkled among the photos. He loved the idea of addressing the epidemic, and told Berkowitz he would make a place for his treatise in the next issue—which would hit newsstands at about the same time as the first snowfalls of 1983.

"I'm like: I'm going to wait eight months for safe sex to hit gay men? I told him, forget it," Berkowitz reported to Sonnabend. "You got to get Michael to work on this. We have to find another outlet." He didn't have much hope in this regard. Editors in other cities were only slightly more eager than Ortleb to publish the work of "the Callen/Berkowitz/Sonnabend Axis," as they had been branded unsympathetically in the pages of *The Advocate*.

Sonnabend had another thought: they should self-publish the work in the model of left-wing and feminist political tracts. "It's not just an article," he said. "This should be a booklet."

Callen, fresh from a hospital stay with mononucleosis, had a change of heart. He called Berkowitz and offered to help finish the manuscript. The idea that the two "anti-sex heretics" would be producing a sex manual now appealed to him very much.

"We're the Trotskys," he said to Berkowitz. "Let's just hope we don't come to the same end."

. . .

THE WINTER WEATHER only got more brutal, the result of the most powerful El Niño effect in centuries, and in mid-February 1983, it delivered the worst blizzard New York had seen in two generations. Twenty-two inches of snow fell. Taxis and subways froze in their tracks, and the furnace in my building failed. I called my old friend Brian Gougeon and begged for temporary shelter in Hell's Kitchen. He sounded awful. He'd been in bed for almost two weeks, so debilitated that lifting the phone left him panting. "It's like the flu, times a thousand," he whispered. "I've got the strength of Saran Wrap." When he saw a doctor, she diagnosed a shocking multiplicity of infections, most of them sexually transmitted. He also had painfully swollen lymph nodes along his jawline, beneath his arms, and in his groin. But they didn't seem to alarm her. One of his infections was mono, a common cause of lymphadenopathy. She said her nodes would be the size of strawberries too, if she were as sick as he was.

"When it rains, it pours," he said.

I was leaning on his buzzer within the hour. He greeted me at the door in his underwear, almost six feet of slouching and clammy flesh. His fever was still climbing. When he turned weakly and headed back inside, I could see he had lost weight—his shoulders were like a coat hanger. He headed straight to bed and slumped to the mattress we would share that night. Though he parroted his doctor's cheery optimism, I sensed he was afraid, and that scared me. Still, I wanted to believe he was right. I served him some egg-drop soup and administered alcohol rubs. He was comforted and grateful. As I stroked a cloth along his baking flesh I was relieved to find nothing remotely like the KS lesions I had seen on the doctors' presentation slide. But I let my fingers learn the shape of his massive lymph nodes. I had never seen the condition before. Brian's nodes were walnuts, hard and sensitive to the touch. "I think they're shrinking," he winced. "From the antibiotics."

His temperature soared and sank through the night and sweat poured from his body, leaving us both in puddles. We changed the linens twice that night, then wised up and made him a nest of towels to blot the stream. It took two months for his condition to improve enough that he could go back to work. Much later, experts would name this the "seroconversion flu." Most people with AIDS get the same crushing symptoms in the first weeks of infection. We didn't know that then.

And we did something that night that I have not been able to easily explain. In a feat of exquisite timing between Tylenols and linen changes, he reached for me, and with the precautions of a scrub nurse

I made love to him. Such intimacies had never been a subtext between us during our years as college roommates, as we were stretching into adulthood together. Now, as twenty-four-year-olds in a treacherous city, with the shadow of plague stretched over that bed, we felt a need to connect profoundly. Afterward, ironically, I was a little less frightened, and I think he was too.

I ran my thumb over his lip. "I love you, Brian," I said.

"Be careful," he replied.

LARRY KRAMER jumped in to edit the *GMHC Newsletter*, filling a void left by the resignation of Nathan Fain, who also left the board of directors, battle weary as much from nasty internecine politics as from the plague itself. Paul Popham was not happy about the new arrangement, which he correctly predicted would become an occasion for drama. As Kramer put his first issue together, he announced that GMHC had raised $150,000 to date, of which a third went to support research; the rest was earmarked for printing and distributing literature plus a long list of services Kramer for the most part dismissed privately as "candy-striping": responding to the five thousand people who had by now had called the hotline; creating a network of "buddies" to visit the sick at home and help with chores; setting up therapy groups, legal clinics, and financial workshops demystifying the welfare system; arranging multiple "open forums" for keeping community members up-to-date about fast-breaking developments; investigating and exposing improper hospital care; and training and fielding a small army of "crisis intervention counselors" to comfort all patients immediately upon their diagnosis, wherever they might be. "That GMHC has accomplished all of this (and mostly in the last six months), and that so many responsible gay men have stepped forward to accomplish all of this, is one of the most inspirational developments ever to occur in the New York gay community," he wrote.

But then he veered into his own agenda, hijacking the board's collective voice to endorse a message of sexual restraint. In a stroke, he aligned GMHC with the widely detested principles of *Faggots*.

"The gay community itself is not yet united on AIDS," he wrote.

We've been too accustomed to fear, particularly the fear that our sexual freedom, so hard fought for, will be taken away from us. But we must realize that sex is not the fabric holding our community together; that's a very questionable assumption indeed about our commonality. We must realize that we are much, much more, that we have a sense of self and identity and relating such as exists in any religion or philosophy or ethnic background, and in which sex plays no more a role than it does in heterosexual identity. And if it takes an emergency epidemic to teach us this lesson, then let this be one of life's ironies.

That alone would produce a mushroom cloud of outrage among his colleagues. They had never argued that sexual abundance was at the top of a gay agenda. Rather, they supported disseminating information from the best minds in the crisis, and allowing those in the community to make their own decisions.

Kramer continued, "Doctors are telling us to lessen the number of sexual partners we come in contact with, so that, if a transmissible agent is the culprit, we will decrease our chances of getting or giving it. No doctor we know of is trying to make moral judgments with this advice. Quite the contrary. They cannot bear to see one more AIDS diagnosis, and so they are understandably in favor of seeing us live at the expense, perhaps, of our temporarily suspended sexual liberty." He added, begrudgingly, "But GMHC believes that each individual must make his own decision."

Accompanying Kramer's piece was one by Lawrence Mass answering frequently asked questions, one by Roger Enlow advising against donating blood, a list of AIDS-savvy physicians, a call for volunteers, and a piece promoting GMHC's most ambitious fund-raising effort to date: they'd bought out all eighteen thousand tickets at Madison Square Garden for a night at the circus. The newsletter came to sixty-two pages. As a courtesy, Kramer showed a copy to Popham, and Popham circulated it to the board. They held a tense emergency meeting on December 20 to determine how to handle Kramer's essay and "the larger question it poses." They came back to him with demands for changing his text or pulling it altogether. He refused their edits for reasons of timing, revealing that he had already sent the newsletter mechanicals off to the printer. Some fifty thousand copies arrived with the winter snows, provoking the most serious crisis in the agency's short history. The board members had no option but to distribute the newsletter, despite their displeasure—there was no time to produce a replacement before the upcoming Madison Square Garden event.

Kramer had won the day, but the anger he created at GMHC would never subside. He followed the *Newsletter* with another piece for the

Native, again over Popham's objections, amplifying his alarms and calling for an avalanche of rage, the very thing that was splitting GMHC apart. It was a screed of seven thousand words, as seemingly overreaching as it was powerful.

> If this article doesn't scare the shit out of you, you're in real trouble. If this article doesn't rouse you to anger, fury, rage, and action, gay men may have no future on this earth. Our continued existence depends on just how angry you can get.
>
> I am writing this as Larry Kramer, and I am speaking for myself, and my views are not to be attributed to Gay Men's Health Crisis.
>
> I repeat: Our continued existence as gay men upon the face of this earth is at stake. Unless we fight for our lives, we shall die. In all the history of homosexuality we have never before been so close to death and extinction. Many of us are dying or already dead.
>
> Before I tell you what we must do, let me tell you what is happening to us.
>
> There are now 1,112 cases of serious Acquired Immune Deficiency Syndrome. When we first became worried, there were only 41. In only twenty-eight days, from January 13th to February 9th (1983), there were 164 new cases—and 73 more dead. The total death tally is now 418. Twenty percent of all cases were registered this January alone. There have been 195 dead in New York City from among 526 victims. Of all serious AIDS cases, 47.3 percent are in the New York metropolitan area. . . . These numbers do not include the thousands of us walking around with what is also being called AIDS: various forms of swollen lymph glands and fatigues that doctors don't know what to label or what they might portend.
>
> The rise in these numbers is terrifying. Whatever is spreading is now spreading faster as more and more people come down with AIDS. . . . After almost two years of an epidemic, there still are no answers. After almost two years of an epidemic, the cause of AIDS remains unknown. After almost two years of an epidemic, there is no cure. . . . Why isn't every gay man in this city so scared shitless that he is screaming for action? Does every gay man in New York *want* to die?

He then turned his pen on Mayor Koch. "I sometimes think that, like some king who has been so long on his throne he's lost touch with his people, Koch is so protected and isolated by his staff that he is unaware of what fear and pain we're in. No *human* being could otherwise continue to be so useless to his suffering constituents," he wrote. He spoke of the community's frustration with Herb Rickman, a gay man the mayor appointed as our go-between, and the "Inter-Departmental Task Force" he had set up, which hadn't met in months. "With his silence on AIDS, the Mayor of New York is helping to kill us," he wrote, initiating a theme he would return to for many years to come.

Ortleb played the piece big on the cover, and it was picked up by gay papers across the country—syndication by public domain. When they saw it, Popham and the other GMHC board members were beside themselves. For months they had been seeking a meeting with Koch, the first of its kind. They wanted to press for everything from more hospital beds to declaring a formal state of emergency, and worried that Kramer had set back negotiations. But three weeks later, on April 11, the mayor sent word that he would receive ten community representatives.

A board meeting was hastily arranged to select the delegation. Kramer arrived at the GMHC offices late, in time to learn he had not made the cut. His colleagues had chosen Mel Rosen and Paul Popham, with other members coming from groups including the National Gay Task Force and the New York Physicians for Human Rights.

Kramer flew into a fury. Nobody, he believed, had done more to make this meeting happen. The meeting was his idea, and his victory. Kramer threatened to resign from the GMHC board unless he was included, but he saw in Popham's expression that the board would prefer his departure. He quit in a tantrum and spun out the door.

Thereafter, he threw himself into a violent battle of words against the group he helped found, expending at least as much energy attacking GMHC as AIDS itself. He excoriated them in scathing letters to the editor, and crashed their fund-raisers to denounce them. At the same time, he recruited countless intermediaries to cajole the board into asking him back—he wanted them to beg for him to return. When that failed, he announced he was withdrawing his resignation. But it was too late. The GMHC board members wanted nothing to do with him. Retaliating, Kramer slipped into a GMHC event to honor volunteers, barged into the DJ booth, and grabbed the microphone, calling on the rank and file to demand his reappointment. "We need fighters," he screamed. "We need a board of directors that will get confrontational and slug things out!"

It did no good. Kramer conceded defeat and retreated from the fray.

He made plans to spend a year in Europe, telling people he had in mind a new roman à clef that would settle scores.

The prospects of another publishing salvo like *Faggots* led Nathan Fain to write Kramer an acid letter, circulated openly to various leaders in the AIDS fight. "You use the tactics that southern rednecks and the Moral Majority have used for years—and for this you should beg the forgiveness of every gay man who you have caused pain." He reluctantly credited Kramer with raising the visibility of the epidemic like no one else by working to become, "like Goethe, the personification of an era much linked with sadness and death." But the cost was intolerable. "I have never seen such damage as you have wrought, such willful, horrible wreckage."

GAËTAN DUGAS felt as healthy as ever. After rejecting Dr. Laubenstein's suggestion to begin chemotherapy, he simply stopped flying to New York for intrusive examinations and Atlanta for interviews with CDC investigators, who outraged him by suggesting he might have carried AIDS to ten cities across the world—his Air Canada routes. He was done with the American health care system. When he experienced trouble breathing over the winter, he saw his regular doctor in Quebec City. When that cleared up he used his prerogative as a flight attendant to relocate. He chose Vancouver, a city with a vibrant gay community and just six cases of AIDS. He made friends quickly, and they became his support network when a small KS lesion appeared on his porcelain cheek, his first that couldn't be masked by clothing.

He made it his business to study the evolving medical literature on AIDS. That convinced him he didn't meet the clinical definition of the disease. His T-cell count remained high and stable, and beyond the painless purple spots he had no other AIDS symptoms. In his calculus, his cancer could be just that—not good news, of course, but not part of a cataclysmic plague. The fact that he officially remained an "AIDS patient" instilled in him a strong feeling of being persecuted.

The frigid evening of March 12, 1983, gave him another opportunity to state his views, for the first time publicly. Some local doctors had formed a new organization called AIDS Vancouver to convene the city's first emergency meeting for the community, coinciding with a visit by Paul Popham from New York. Shortly after sundown, the hall at the Westend Community Centre quickly filled to overflowing, leaving many of the 250 people standing against a back wall. Dr. Brian Willoughby, a local doctor who had just returned from a gathering of concerned physicians in Hawaii, arranged by the CDC, began by describing the bizarre symptomology.

"Herpes has probably affected [some of] you by causing small little blisters, which last perhaps a week and then go away. A person who suffers from AIDS or has immune deficiency may develop a herpes sore that is eight inches across and takes three months to go away," he said, provoking murmurs of concern throughout the room.

He turned the microphone over to Popham, who, despite his casual jeans and flannel shirt, was an arresting, authoritative figure, a forty-one-year-old former officer in the Fifth Air Cavalry during the Vietnam War. He didn't know it yet, but he was infected, as were a likely preponderance of the men in his audience.

"Most of you know now how devastating this outbreak of AIDS has been, and nowhere more so than in New York," he began, putting aside the few notes he had made. A dead stillness filled the room. "Most of my friends in New York have been touched in some way by this tragedy. Friends have died. The deaths have almost always been long, painful, and unbelievably heartbreaking. I have been through this twice myself, and I think it is fair to say that it's changed my life—just as it's changed the lives of so many others in New York City."

His voice failed him. He took a moment to recompose. Like audiences he had addressed in Boston, Dallas, and Atlanta, he wondered if these men were strong enough for the coming trial.

"This epidemic has challenged us like we've never been challenged before. And we've met the challenge. It's hard—it's *real* hard. But I think we're finding out just what we're made of, just how strong we are. And probably most important we're showing how gay men came through in a crisis," he said. "So far, medical science has not been able to tell us much that is conclusive about what to do and not to do, other than to cut down on the number and variety of sexual contacts. So far, efforts to pressure political groups to help us have been great, but subject to great difficulty. We are left, finally, with ourselves."

These words of self-reliance resonated with Dugas's thinking. Once Popham had concluded his remarks, Dugas approached a microphone stand placed in the middle of the auditorium, a sheath of literature in his hand. He was dressed in a dark V-neck sweater and green collared shirt. Because of his heavy accent, his question was difficult for Popham to understand easily. It pertained to what he saw as the pariah status assigned to AIDS patients, particularly in sexual matters. "You shouldn't fear someone who has AIDS, or [has] symptoms of AIDS, because there's no specific reason why you should get in contact with AIDS—with an infectious agent—like you mentioned. Like, if you have a lover who has AIDS and you don't have AIDS, what is the warning you give these people? It seems like there's kind of a fear toward those people," he said.

Popham replied gently. "My personal feeling about it is, and again it can't be proved, is that some contagious agent *is* probably involved in the transmission of AIDS, and if I were an AIDS patient and were going to continue to have sex with people, I would tell that partner that I was having sex with that I am an AIDS patient, so that they can make that decision. . . . It's what the doctors are telling AIDS patients in New York. And for their own good, they shouldn't be out there exposing themselves to other illnesses, besides, because if they get other infections it's only going to hurt them."

Wasn't it true, Dugas persisted, that it was impossible to really know for sure if you had AIDS? "If you present yourself to your doctor, what kind of test do you ask him to be undertaken in order to confirm if you are possibly a carrier or not?" This touched a nerve with the audience, many of whom had wondered the same thing. And the scientific explanations for risk behavior seemed to change every few months. Was it poppers? Was it sex? Confounding matters further, in the U.S. one of the nation's leading AIDS researcher, Dr. Anthony Fauci, now claimed that AIDS might be transmitted by "routine" household contact. Without any way to know for sure who had it and who didn't, or how to infect others, Dugas objected bitterly to being tagged as infectious.

Dr. Willoughby, while conceding the lack of consensus among experts, attempted an answer, saying it was prudent for every gay man to assume he was sexually infectious, and that anybody he met was also a carrier. Dugas stared back, rocking on his heels, unhappy with this approach. Willoughby attempted to call on another questioner, but Dugas refused to yield. Wasn't it more likely, he asked, that the hepatitis vaccine doctors had been giving to sexually active gay men could be behind this mystery? While Willoughby's fellow panelists corrected Dugas on his misinformation, Willoughby leaned over to the moderator and whispered, "Please, if you don't get him off this microphone he will undo any good we have done in the last hour."

When the meeting drew to a close, Willoughby made a point of introducing himself to Dugas, and when he heard the man's name, it took him only a moment to place it. While Willoughby was in Hawaii, Dr. Harold Jaffe from the CDC had told him about the airline steward whose sexual history had included so many of the sick in New York and Los Angeles. Here he stood, in the flesh. Willoughby saw the KS on his face. He gave Dugas his card. "Come see me," he said.

Dugas never did make an appointment. In a few weeks his health stumbled precipitously, convincing him to move back home to Quebec. There, the purple lesions spread across his body. He died at age thirty-one in the same month that a CDC research paper appeared in the *American Journal of Medicine* linking one non-Californian AIDS patient, called "Patient o" (shorthand for the study's central subject), to other cases in Southern California and New York. Although he wasn't named in the paper, researchers knew that "Patient o" was, in fact, Dugas. Epidemiologists found that 8 of the first 248 gay men who got AIDS had slept with "Patient o"; those men were subsequently linked, directly or not , to another 11 patients. This was a breakthrough study, proving for the first time that AIDS was passed sexually from person to person—the proof that Dugas had demanded.

In death, Dugas's life took on a more sinister interpretation. The writer Randy Shilts, in his book *And the Band Played On,* painted Dugas as a hardened sociopath who did his best to spread the disease far and wide. "With Gaëtan you get a horrible set of circumstances," Shilts once explained. "You get a guy who has got unlimited sexual stamina, who is very attractive so he has unlimited opportunity to act out that sexual stamina, and he's a flight attendant for Air Canada, so he gets these flight passes so he can fly all over and have his fun in any number of cities." In telling this story, Shilts renamed "Patient o" as "Patient Zero," the man not only at the center of a twenty-one-person cluster but at the core of the plague itself. He called Dugas quite possibly "the person who brought AIDS to North America." A frenzy of condemnatory press followed. On *60 Minutes,* a reporter called Dugas the "central victim and victimizer" of the epidemic.

No evidence emerged to support this view. Years later, long after Shilts was also gone, the editor of *And the Band Played On* would admit that the publishing house made a conscious decision to vilify Dugas in the book and publicity campaign in order to spur sales. "Randy didn't want to do it," said the editor, Michael Denneny. "It was my idea. And I regret it."

WHEN APRIL ROLLED around, as most of the world reacted in horror to the deadly terror attack on the U.S. embassy in Beirut, Sonnabend's caseload was double what it had been in the fall. The federal efforts, meanwhile, were going in exactly the wrong direction. After more than a year in the trenches, the CDC had pulled all its Epidemic Intelligence Service officers out of New York. They stopped automatically interviewing every new diagnosed patient. Larry Kramer, who continued serving on the quasi-independent AIDS Scientific Advisory Committee of GMHC, arranged a meeting with Dr. James Curran of the CDC in a fervent effort to get the agency to resume gathering information on the disease—how it might be transmitted, what risk behaviors should be avoided, and the like. He even offered to field an army of volunteers—para-epidemiologists, as it were—to carry out the work if only the CDC were to collate and analyze the data. Curran, his hands tied by red tape, declined.

Sonnabend was powerless to help. What little influence he had mustered in the early days was gone. Colleagues in the medical community had branded him a kook for his increasingly strident jousting against the "killer virus" proponents. GMHC appeared to isolate him further when, in a newsletter article about new findings regarding AIDS, it analyzed two of three articles in *The Lancet* while omitting the one he wrote, an important article with findings about "T-cell ratios in homosexuals." Pettiness seemed the only explanation for ignoring his piece. He now had four published articles on AIDS in the world's most prestigious journals, yet at GMHC his name had been removed from the official list of recommended doctors. Mel Rosen, the executive director, told a caller he wouldn't go to Sonnabend if he were "the last doctor on earth" and labeled Callen as equally unhinged, "a Moonie" in Sonnabend's thrall. Callen wanted to go to war with GMHC, but Sonnabend had no hunger for battle. He took it as a challenge to spend even longer hours in the lab.

His practice was in even more disarray as a result. Including back taxes, his outstanding debts surpassed $50,000, according to the detailed records that Harley Hackett was keeping. His bank accounts were frozen. Lacking options, he found himself once again sitting across from Mathilde Krim at her favorite restaurant. She had seen this moment coming, and had already talked the situation over with her husband. After hearing Sonnabend out, Krim presented a startling proposal. She would like to begin a private research campaign against AIDS, to be called the American Medical Foundation, or AMF. Sonnabend would be medical director, conducting research, attending conferences, and writing policy papers while still seeing patients privately. She, as chairwoman, would see to the financing and positioning of the nonprofit in the world of medical philanthropies.

The proposed undertaking was consciously modeled on the work of Mary Lasker, a groundbreaking philanthropist who turned her husband's fortune—from a career in advertising—into a scientific juggernaut that was credited with promoting the National Institutes of Health into a major world research facility. Mrs. Lasker had already agreed to join the AMF board, as had Dr. David Baltimore, whose study of cancer-causing viruses earned him a Nobel Prize. Through the family foundation, Arthur Krim had committed $100,000.

She proposed a salary for Sonnabend of $52,000, the answer to his dreams. He accepted her invitation on the spot. "Mathilde," he said, "our friendship is a profound one. We have had our falling-outs and will have them again. But the way you have supported me—us—in this crisis. . . . I don't know how to thank you."

Things moved very quickly thereafter. As the Krims were friends of the New York real estate magnates Harry and Leona Helmsley, Mathilde Krim was able to secure prime office space in the iconic Helmsley Building, straddling Park Avenue. She asked Harley Hackett to be AMF's part-time bookkeeper, which he accepted, while still keeping his day job. Within a few weeks of proposing the new foundation, she put Sonnabend on a plane for a week-long science summit in Sardinia, his first foray as AMF's science head.

And the moment his plane lifted off, Krim and Berkowitz, who had a key to Sonnabend's apartment, were inside his home, determined finally to cure the problem of his disheveled inner sanctum. Krim did this out of love and great concern, praying that his generally depressed mood took cues from the apartment, not the other way around. She also felt it would help ready him for the high profile she intended for AMF. She brought in her personal decorator and gave him carte blanche, all paid for by the Krim Family Foundation. Upon his return Sonnabend was floored to find not just a coat of paint, but new wall-to-wall carpeting and built-in bookshelves, with shiny file cabinets and fancy lighting fixtures—and Mathilde Krim herself, standing in the middle of the living room daintily feather-dusting the new furniture. His mouth fell open. He staggered into his bedroom to find a brand-new closet where before had leaned a damaged coatrack, and, behind the brand-new closet door, a rack of new suits as well.

"Too embarrassing for words," he told me later. "I sent the clothes back to Bloomingdale's. That was over the top."

In his disorientation, it took him some time to realize his cat was also gone. Years later, Krim admitted culpability with her usual sentimentality. "When I am asked: How did you start? I say, first, we threw out the cat." Sonnabend was in no position to complain. In a stroke, Krim had put him on sound financial ground for the first time since the bloom of plague.

I DIDN'T HAVE serious concerns for my own health. What I worried about was Brian Gougeon. I checked on him frequently. Neither of us brought up AIDS directly or his health specifically, though I sensed he resented my calls as reminders of that scare. Like characters in a Saramago novel, we talked about anything else. The news was generally good. He resumed the physically taxing work of tending the vast vertical jungle of ficus trees and philodendron bushes that filled high-rises throughout the city. He confided that the East Village gallery scene had been cool to his work, but reported the good news that he was back with his college boyfriend, and had never been happier.

I don't want to overstate our sense of impending doom. The truth was, the storm clouds massed near the horizon, not overhead. Unless you were personally admitted into what Susan Sontag called "the kingdom of the sick," it was not hard to put the growing epidemic out of mind. It took two years and almost six hundred dead before *The New York Times* put a story on the front page. Except in passing, few television news programs made any mention. The progressive *Village Voice* ran a feature that called the danger overblown, and was nearly silent otherwise. You would have to read the *Native* for news on AIDS.

Brian Gougeon avoided the newspapers. I know he saw the first major report in prime time, since we watched it together on my small black-and-white TV. The ABC newsman Geraldo Rivera, flamboyant and hyperbolic though he was, broke the near-complete media blackout with the first network broadcast.

"It is the most frightening medical mystery of our time," Rivera said, leaning toward the camera. "There is an epidemic loose in the land, a so-far incurable disease which kills its victims in stages."

And then appeared the face of a man in grotesque medical distress— the first plague-sickened man either Brian or I had laid eyes on. He was a freelance lighting designer named Ken Ramsauer, age twenty-seven. In an old photograph, he looked as polished and angular as a shampoo model. The difference between then and now was shocking. His head appeared swollen nearly to the brink of popping; his eyes vanished behind swollen muffins of flesh; oblong purple marks covered his skin. Confined to a wheelchair, he hung his head weakly. A friend handed him a glass of water, which was almost too heavy for his trembling arms.

"I thought I was a pretty good-looking guy," he said. "And now, I actually see myself fading away."

Ramsauer said he had just returned from the hospital, where they offered him neither medicine nor hope, and least of all pity. "One night I heard two, I believe, nurse's aides—not the actual nurses—standing outside my door sort of laughing," he said.

"What did they say exactly?" Rivera asked.

He blinked his slivered eyes and looked down at the water glass in his scarlet fists, remembering: "I wonder how long the faggot in 208 is going to last."

Four days later, I opened the paper to discover that Ramsauer was dead. When I read that a public memorial was planned at the Naumburg Bandshell in Central Park, I asked Brian to go with me. But he was taking a different strategy. "I'm just staying out of the whole thing," he said, meaning AIDS. "Worrying isn't good for your health. And it does nasty things to your art."

Instead I went with another friend, a graphic designer named Ian Horst. That evening was unusually still and hot. As we approached the service from the south, beneath a vaulted canopy of American elms and a row of towering statuary, a macabre scene confronted us. The plaza was crowded with 1,500 mourners cupping candles against the darkening sky. As our eyes landed on one young man after another, it became obvious that many of them were seriously ill. A dozen men were in wheelchairs, so wasted they looked like caricatures of starvation. I watched one young man twist in pain that was caused, apparently, by the barest gusts of wind around us. In New York there were just 722 cases reported, half the nation's total. It seemed they were all at the band shell that sweltering evening.

My friend's mouth hung open. "It looks like a horror flick," he said.

I was speechless. We had found the plague.

From there, it was an avalanche. A Friday or two later, a colleague from work ran out the door for a weekend of social commitments. He looked as healthy as a soap opera star, which he aspired to be. We never saw him again. I heard from a mutual friend that he was found dead by neighbors the following week, shrunken and hollow, in a room washed in his own feces. In whispers, we wondered if he had taken his own life—and debated whether it would be more stoic to face the disease or commit suicide.

As the summer of 1983 opened, *The New York Times* finally started covering the plague, but often in bizarre ways. In May, the paper revealed that prisoners on Rikers Island had declared a hunger strike, unwilling to risk using plates or utensils after an inmate dropped dead from AIDS, and a week later reported on a sanitation worker who might have caught AIDS from handling trash. Readers were left more frightened than ever. We read reports of parents who would not go near their infected sons, not even to bid farewell. Many hospital workers felt the same way, abandoning AIDS-sick patients in diarrhea-soaked sheets out of fear and prejudice. Dr. Robert Gallo, head of the Laboratory of Tumor and Cell Biology at the National Cancer Institute, a branch of the National Institutes of Health, was disgusted when he first heard the sick joke that pancakes were the only food fit for an AIDS patient, because they could fit under the door. In this environment, even doctors felt justified to exempt AIDS sufferers from the Hippocratic Oath—in one survey, over half admitted they would refuse them medical attention if given a choice.

The patients' indignities did not end with death. Across New York, the global epicenter of this outbreak, almost every undertaker refused to work with the corpses. Even in the ancient plagues of Europe there were individuals tasked with collecting remains. In *The Betrothed*, the novelist Alessandro Manzoni called them *monatti*, those unflappable Samaritans who, for profit or otherwise, braved the "rags and corrupted bandages, infected straw, or clothes, or sheets" to convey the lifeless flesh to the ditches. In New York at the dawn of AIDS, only Redden's Funeral Home, operating continuously since the Spanish influenza epidemic of 1918–19, would handle the embalming. Yet its owners begged the grateful mourners to keep their kindnesses a secret for fear of boycotts by the aging Catholic community in Greenwich Village and Chelsea, the bulk of their business.

PETER STALEY got to New York City just before the weather turned warm, having completed his coursework at Oberlin College for a double major in political science and economics. A compact and sweet-faced young man with dark eyes and an ornate smile, he began his studies as a piano prodigy at Oberlin's Conservatory of Music before transferring to the main college. He developed an outsized ambition in those four years. His plan was to make a quick fortune on Wall Street then move into politics—specifically the House, having twice interned at the Democratic Congressional Campaign Committee.

It was the year that the bond business defined conspicuous power, the dawn of the Big Swinging Dicks—callow white men who pushed money around the global marketplace by day and cocaine into thick hillocks at night. Following in the footsteps of his brother Jes, a rising star at J. P. Morgan, Staley had been accepted to the firm's exclusive Commercial Banking Training Program for six months of lectures and drills, a high-speed MBA equivalent. He moved into a small studio apartment on Maiden Lane, in the dark canyons of the Financial District. His Yamaha grand piano, a gift from his parents on his twelfth birthday, was the home's steroidal centerpiece, covering a third of the total floor space. With the rigors of the training program consuming his days and nights, he used the place as a bedroom only, and didn't feel at all cramped. Friday and Saturday nights were the exception to his routine, spent playing pool in one of the East Village gay bars or else joining in the show tune singalongs at the Duplex, a piano bar on Grove Street in Greenwich Village where courageous amateur performers put themselves at the mercy of a gladiatorial crowd of gay men.

His plan was to stay in finance just long enough to bank a few million dollars. He was quick-tongued in arguments, with charismatic appeal to women and men alike and an easy and commanding presence when in the limelight. With his slight build, dark hair, and pale skin, he looked the part of a politician, giving off a purposeful, "young Kennedy" vibe, at once boyish and enthralled and self-possessed. His one apparent weakness was a slight lisp—not the sibilance that suggested gayness, but the result of an oversized tongue. To most people, it added appreciably to his appeal.

A much bigger problem was his sexual orientation. He didn't delude himself about what would happen if anyone found out. The sharks at Morgan would surely make his life a living hell and voters would put an end to his political ambitions. He planned to remain in his elaborate and hopefully impenetrable closet. He convinced himself this would entail no great sacrifice. One thing bond trading, public service, and life in the closet have in common: they're all high-wire acts requiring nerves of steel. Staley qualified. This was true of many gay men and women, whether in the closet or out, because nobody who was out hadn't first spent many years in. You hid from the people who knew you best; you were a character actor so convincing your own mother was fooled.

What Staley's mother believed was that he was romantically involved with his closest Oberlin friend, Tracey Tanenbaum, who had followed him to Manhattan, where she had grown up. He brought her home to Philadelphia for holidays and even took her along on vacations. They had pantomimed the sweetheart routine so convincingly that his parents had begun prodding him to set a wedding date. "I don't know," he'd aver. "It's not something she and I ever discussed." Technically, this was not true. They *had* discussed marriage, but only as an accommodation. According to the plan, if by their fortieth birthdays neither found an acceptable man to settle down with, they would ford the rivers of life together as platonic best friends.

When he started at Morgan, the stakes grew exponentially. "I'm going to need a girlfriend for Christmas parties, that sort of thing," he told her.

Tanenbaum loved Staley and would do almost anything he asked, but she was tiring of her role. "Peter, you know I don't like the idea of fooling someone," she objected. She had argued with him the last time she had accompanied him to a Staley family holiday, when his mother made them a single bed to sleep in and they had to wander off hand in hand to their evening's rest, like a scene from *The Blue Lagoon*. "It's plain weird," she said.

"Please? Can you pretend, so they don't ask me questions? You wouldn't believe how homophobic that place is, Trace."

He didn't need to remind her. She had sat cross-legged on the sofa in his apartment as he recounted the language that flew in his training class, and later hung silently on the other end of the phone when he reported what it was like once he graduated to the bond traders' floor. It broke her heart to picture him red-faced and mute in the hail of their hateful opinions.

She relented, with conditions. He was not to think of her as his "fag-hag," a sobriquet she detested. She would tolerate being called his "beard." It would never have occurred to her that this charade would last for years.

Peter thought he could get away with it forever, jockeying through his Wall Street period and on to Capitol Hill with her—or someone like her—standing by his side. The lie would be so frequently told it would even feel accurate to him. He planned to be in the closet forever.

5

A Man Reaps What He Sows

The sex manual Callen and Berkowitz had undertaken to write went through multiple iterations, with the authors challenging every word in lengthy editorial sessions, held either in Sonnabend's office after hours or in Callen's Tribeca loft. They were careful to avoid the mistakes of their two previous articles. Once again they would promote the "immune-overload model" over the "new germ model," but this time they made room for the *remote* possibility of a new virus, the discovery of which was still months away. And they would take greater care with their language choices, which had resulted in more discussions about their "superior tone" than their ideas. Callen excised any hint of arrogance or condescension. For lessons in influencing people and changing culture, he had been reading Hannah Arendt, Alexis de Tocqueville, Barbara Ehrenreich's *For Her Own Good,* and especially Saul Alinsky's *Rules for Radicals.* "Stand up and take a position," Callen told Berkowitz, "and then you say to people, 'Let's talk about this—what's *your* opinion?'"

This was how they invented what they called "safe sex." Their self-assigned mission was outsized, almost radical. In order for safe sex to staunch an epidemic, it had to be embraced by the entire community of gay men—a fundamental and universal change in behavior. If they had consulted social scientists first, their ambitions might have been reined in. But they proceeded as they had before, with naïveté as their guide.

For weeks they parsed the two main models of causation and produced recommended sexual acts that would be safe in each theoretical realm. Their first rule was the only one that entailed an unwavering sacrifice. "Safe sex requires that you be sober. Alcohol, poppers and other recreational drugs can impair your decision-making abilities. Gauge yourself honestly."

After that, the advice was all affirming. In frank and sometimes playful language, they ran through, and measured the risk involved in, mutual masturbation, kissing, and, of course, "leather, bondage, discipline, spanking, titplay, verbal, worship, teasing, affection, humiliation, gadgets, toys, etc." They came to an easy consensus on the risks of sucking ("moderate") and getting sucked ("safer"), but not on anal sex. Callen and Berkowitz instinctively put it in the "never again" column. Sonnabend challenged them. "It's not that simple," he said, adding that anal sex carried different risks for the insertive partner than the receptive one.

"How do I know that?" he asked. "I know who comes in each month and gets a penile STD, I know who comes in each month and gets an oral STD, and I know what guys come in and get into the stirrups and spread their legs because they always have anal STDs. So when I went through my patients, the minute I looked at who was getting sick and who wasn't, it just flew off the page to me: It's the guys who are into getting fucked." This was without doubt the preferred sexual position for Callen, and though Berkowitz's commercial persona was as a "top," during off hours he was a "bottom" as well.

Thinking of his circle of hustler friends, Sonnabend's observation held true for Berkowitz. "It was all the bottoms who were getting sick and all the heavy-duty bottoms who were getting sick the quickest," he said.

"It comes from the semen," Sonnabend surmised. He knew there was a simple way to interrupt the passing of semen: those foil-wrapped sleeves which the French called "English Overcoats" and the English knew as "French Letters." Before that moment, gay men had as much use for condoms as for tampons. "I think most gay men said, Oh thank god, that's *one* thing we don't have to worry about," Sonnabend told me. In 1981, even despite the endemic levels of VD, less than 1 percent of gay men in New York used them, and perhaps fewer in San Francisco. Condoms had fallen into disuse by straights as well, amid the advent of the birth-control pill, the IUD, and the cervical cap. There was universal amnesia about the role they could play against disease, despite knowledge dating back to ancient Egypt. A precise history of condoms can't be fixed, but Norman Himes, the dean of contraception scholarship, gives credit to a slaughterhouse worker in the Middle Ages as the first to stretch an animal membrane over his penis, whether for reasons of prophylaxis or puerile fascination. The earliest known reference in literature came in 1564, when an Italian anatomist named Gabriele Falloppio (of the eponymous tubes) published a study of a medicated linen sheath meant to protect the bearer from syphilis. It was, he wrote, a great success. "I tried the experiment on 1,100 men, and I call immortal God to witness that not one of them was infected."

"If we prevent the transmission of semen—exposure to semen—which is the vehicle by which unknown and known potentially pathogenic things are transmitted, we could interrupt the cause of this disease," Sonnabend said. Benefits would be felt by the healthy and sick alike. Berkowitz testified to the power of that thought. His health had improved steadily in the year or more since his last exposure to semen. "I have become very close to many gay men who may not be able to recover," he told a reporter from *Sexual Medicine Today*. "I have come to believe that the difference between my recovering and their possible death may be that I was warned in time and they were not."

When their piece was typed and copyedited, Richard Dworkin gave it a thorough read and shook his head. "You've written how many pages about sex," he said, "and you haven't mentioned the word 'love' once."

Sonnabend saw the glaring absence instantly. It made him think back on some of his gonorrhea patients who had returned to the baths while still infectious, without care for the people they might be infecting. He had witnessed this himself, as he told Berkowitz over the phone one night. "If people approach their sexual partners with some responsibility, that will be a way to avoid getting sick—not necessarily monogamous relationships, but . . . being able to put love back in lovemaking," he said. "Part of the whole 'promiscuous' business seems to have eliminated all of that. Maybe there are limits to the promiscuity—maybe the body can interact with more people than one's spirit can."

Callen and Berkowitz cared deeply for their vast sexual communities. That love—certainly not the money—was their motivation in assuming the public role they'd assigned themselves. "Temperamentally, we must have been quite alike," Sonnabend recalled later. "Richard particularly, who could find even in his sex work some room for feeling. And I had those same thoughts myself: you could really love somebody even for just four hours. Genuinely."

They drafted an addendum on love. "It has come as quite a shock to us to find that we had written almost forty pages on sex without mentioning the word 'love' once. Truly, we have been revealed as products of the '70s," they wrote. "Men *loving* men was the basis of gay male liberation, but we have now created 'cultural institutions' in which love and even affection can be totally avoided. If you love the person you are fucking with—*even for one night*—you will not want to make them sick. Maybe affection is our best protection."

More than a sexual manifesto for the movement, their manuscript combined feminist critiques of the male ego, an introduction to CMV and other viruses, a frank discussion of sexual ethics, and a detailed primer built around their amended view that exposure to body fluids, not promiscuity, was the risky behavior—in short, a survival guide for the plague years. They called it *How to Have Sex in an Epidemic*. Avoiding any semblance of arrogance, they added a deferential-sounding subtitle: *One Approach*.

Now came the hard part: finding the money for publishing. Berkowitz called a number of his former clients, who all turned him down. Mathilde Krim also declined to help, seeing little value in explicit sex talk in these times. They managed to pull together about a thousand dollars from other Sonnabend patients and rolled in Callen's own tax refund, though given that his annual salary was not quite $10,000, this was a token sum. Just before Memorial Day, they were able to send their forty-six-page monograph to the printer with an order for five thousand copies. The heavy boxes containing the finished product arrived at Sonnabend's office in early June 1983.

The distribution plan was simple: the three of them placed copies on sale at various gay-oriented shops and scattered them among the city's gay social venues, including the Bar on Second Avenue, where the thud of a stack of them landing on a bench pulled me away from a group of friends early one evening. The pamphlet was starkly designed, with no artwork inside and a tombstone-like cover. I read through it in one sitting. I wasn't the only patron absorbed in it. The pool table sat idle as a dozen of us passed around copies, hungry for guidance through the terror that sex was causing.

"Today in most large urban centers, what began as sexual freedom has become a tyranny of sexually transmitted diseases," it read. "Finding ways to have sex and avoid these epidemics might seem impossible, but we believe it's not."

With that, the Callen/Berkowitz/Sonnabend Axis had discharged a self-perceived duty. The three went home to await what Callen called "the gay historical tradition of reducing most controversies to personal polemics." But the letters that began arriving in their post office box came instead from people clamoring for more copies of *How to Have Sex in an Epidemic*. A second printing was ordered just two weeks after the first, then a third, with copies being sent around the world.

And then, to their great surprise, *How to Have Sex in an Epidemic* received a review in the highbrow *New York Review of Books*, which in turn prompted the B. Dalton Bookseller branch in Greenwich Village to create a window display around the work. Fan letters came in from Europe, Asia, and Australia. A television news producer in West Germany traveled to New York just to interview Callen. "It was a lucky accident, because if the *Native* had been less loathsome and if things had happened as we had planned," the audience might have been dramatically smaller, Callen said. "It turns out historically to have been one of the advantages of our status as heretics."

Unbeknownst to Callen, at almost the same moment a San Francisco group produced a different handout to promote condom use. In contrast to the somber stridency of the New York tract, the West Coast effort was the product of radical drag activists called the Sisters of Perpetual Indulgence, known for wearing self-styled habits and wild pancake makeup. Bobbi Campbell was a member of the Sisters, which was founded in 1979 with a mission to "promulgate universal joy and expiate stigmatic guilt." He was also a registered nurse, and the first person in San Francisco to speak openly about his infection (he had a T-shirt made that said "AIDS POSTER BOY"). Their pamphlet, titled *Play Fair!*, was shorter, and illustrated with cartoons. "Wrap it up," the Sisters extolled. "Condoms and other barriers are the best way to prevent the spread of some diseases, especially the nasty ones."

Overnight, in gay neighborhoods around the country, rubbers took off as fast as Madonna's debut album, which was making the charts that summer. They were everywhere. At doctors' offices, they were given out like lollipops. Jars full of them proliferated at every gay bar and bathhouse. One night on Christopher Street, I watched a team of lesbians on a flatbed truck lovingly hurl the things into the air like rose petals over the heads of their gay brothers. Manufacturers caught on to the sudden surge in demand and began producing them in every imaginable color, in flavors and textures, in foils that looked like chocolates or coins or tiny flying saucers. And for the first time they were available in a range of sizes, from snug to jumbo and even a style called "nubs," designed to cover only the organ's head. Condoms weren't the only ingredients in "safe sex"; there were other innovations that made sex safer—a fluid-free Kama Sutra became the sexual norm. But it was the latex prophylactic, more than anything else, which came to dominate the culture. So firmly did condoms take hold that summer along the nighttime "cruising" concourses of the West Side piers that they led to the proliferation in the lapping tides of what came to be called "Hudson River White Fish."

As soon became indisputable, transmission rates for all known sex diseases slowed dramatically. Gonorrhea diagnoses were down 73 percent in San Francisco and more than 50 percent in New York. By igniting a craze for safe sex, the activists on both coasts did more to save lives than anything anybody had done before. Although there was no way to quantify it, perhaps tens of thousands of new infections were averted. It came too late for many, though. By then, more than half of all gay men in New York and San Francisco were infected. For them, safe sex at least offered the possibility of a return to intimacy. Callen hoped *How to Have Sex in an Epidemic* might give hope even to the sickest patients. "Hopelessness kills," he said.

AT ABOUT the same time, scientists in two unrelated labs half a world apart were narrowing in on proof that AIDS was the result of a deadly new virus—the "new germ" that Joe Sonnabend had so thoroughly dismissed was coming into focus. But a vulgar rivalry would keep that fact from the public for years.

The study of viruses was just a century old, but the search for the cause of mysterious illnesses and plagues dated to the time of Hippocrates, when it was thought that "miasmas," or the foul vapors exuded by stagnant swamps and moldering corpses, were the cause of illness. In various permutations, this "bad air" theory continued right into the New World, where doctors warned people to avoid "places where vegetable and animal putrification takes place." Hard evidence of the existence of microorganisms had to await the arrival of Antoni van Leeuwenhoek, a Dutch merchant with an amateur's interest in lens grinding. In 1683, using a microscope of his own design, he dialed bacteria into focus for the first time (also: protozoa and sperm). For the following two hundred years, bacteria were thought to be the only disease-causing microbes.

Then, in 1876, a German scientist named Adolf Mayer first hypothesized the existence of something even smaller than bacteria, though evidence proved elusive. Compact, audacious, and wily, viruses are the tiniest of life forms, though calling them life forms at all is to enter into a debate. On the one hand, they carry genetic material, like all living things. But they are incapable of autonomous life; for survival and reproduction, they must invade the healthy cells of animals or plants. No other organism is so fundamentally dependent upon hosts. Historians have put forth numerous evolutionary explanations for their existence, from simple Darwinian selection of the fittest to the more recent observation that viruses, which are now known to add genetic material to the surviving hosts, might be the secret tool of adaptive evolution. But for most, they engender only disdain. The South African virologist Edward Rybicki disparaged them as "organisms at the edge of life."

It wasn't until 1935, when the American biochemist Wendell Stanley got his hands on one of the world's first electron microscopes, that the first minuscular, rod-shaped culprit was finally identified. The second half of the twentieth century was the golden age of virus discovery, with almost two thousand recognized species charted and named, including a peculiar subset called retroviruses. Unlike ordinary viruses, which are constructed around the DNA helix like ordinary plants and animals, retroviruses carry their genetic materials in RNA. This would seem to make them incapable of causing disease. But retroviruses do something no other life form can: at the moment of infection, they transform their very essence from RNA to DNA, then physically meld with the DNA chromosome strings of healthy cells, permanently corrupting them. This is accomplished through the actions of an enzyme called *reverse transcriptase,* which takes the clockwise RNA helix and re-transcribes it in the reverse direction, making it compatible with DNA.

In the 1960s, retroviruses were first identified in chickens, mice, and cats. Researchers even had evidence that they are transmissible, perhaps even sexually, a puzzling notion. But they tend not to cause disease. Some virologists suggested that humans alone among mammals were immune to retroviruses. That changed in December 1980, when a virologist working at the National Cancer Institute in Bethesda, Maryland, discovered the first human retrovirus, and proved it was responsible for a type of leukemia. Dr. Robert Gallo named his new infectious agent human T-cell leukemia virus, or HTLV. Not only did this retrovirus cause cancer, it was transmittable through transfusions and sex. News of a sexually transmitted cancer captured headlines around the world. The disease was extremely rare—it seemed to strike only in certain parts of southwestern Japan and southern Italy, as well as areas of South America and Africa. But this was a major discovery, earning the prestigious Lasker Prize for Gallo, a joyless figure in his mid-forties with a bent nose and raptorial eyes he kept hidden behind gray-tinted aviator glasses.

Initially, the "gay pneumonia" and "gay cancer" didn't interest Gallo or his lab team. Instead, he stayed busy with his family of retroviruses, which now included a second variant, HTLV-II, found primarily among Native Americans and IV-drug users in the U.S. What turned Gallo's attention to the epidemic was a report showing that AIDS patients had a reduced number of T-cells, particularly CD4 T-cells—the same cells that are chiefly targeted by HTLVs. There could be many causes for a precipitous decline in CD4s, but it was a curious enough anomaly that he resolved to attend a discussion of the subject directed by James Curran, the AIDS point person at the CDC. Gallo left the meeting feeling shaken and intrigued, and he immediately committed part of his lab resources to the mystery—using extreme caution, given the reputation of AIDS for being invariably fatal. He told his laboratory staff to look for any evidence of an HTLV link, and he encouraged heads of other prominent virology labs to do the same.

Many rose to the challenge. Typically, virus hunters were the most flamboyant and brash of scientists. This was not the case with Dr. Luc Montagnier, head of a prestigious laboratory at the Institut Pasteur in Paris. Diffident and prone to error, he directed his career toward laboratory analyses of existing viruses, in search of their secrets. The AIDS conundrum hadn't yet captured his attention. There were just 59 cases in France, and 220 recorded in all of Europe. But when Gallo personally encouraged Montagnier to join the hunt, he agreed to give it a try.

His work began in January 1983, when Frédéric Brugière presented himself to the Pitié-Salpêtrière Hospital with swollen lymph nodes in his neck. Brugière, a gay man employed by one of Paris's leading fashion houses, reported a history of exotic travel, a sex life he claimed included fifty assignations a year, and a recent history of VDs. Suspecting an AIDS link, Françoise Brun-Vézinet, a former student of Montagnier's, hand-delivered tubes containing Brugière's blood and a lymph node biopsy to Montagnier. He minced the lymph tissue himself, separated the fragments into single cells, and a few days later added a nourishment substance to see what he could grow. Every day he examined the culture by microscope. A week passed. On January 15, the culture offered up a preliminary answer. A colleague, Françoise Barré-Sinoussi, positively identified a faint telltale footprint indicating reverse transcriptase. That would mean evidence of a retrovirus, as Gallo had supposed. In early February, when Montagnier and Barré-Sinoussi successfully repeated the experiment to rule out laboratory error, then isolated the retrovirus, Montagnier opened the red-covered notebook where he recorded his experiments. "Enfin," he wrote.

He sent a letter to Gallo, alerting him of their fortuitous discovery, which he'd named lymphadenopathy-associated virus, or LAV. Next, he studied his new retrovirus side by side with Gallo's HTLV-I and

HTLV-II. They appeared to be quite different. The HTLV from the American lab performed as expected: when introduced to a line of healthy blood cells, it readily turned them into leukemia cells. Under identical circumstances, the new LAV had no such affect on the healthy cells. The person in charge of the Institut Pasteur's electron microscope, Charles Dauguet, showed how different they appeared to the eye. LAV presented as a pear-shaped particle with a dense and very black core at its center, entirely unlike anything ever seen. It seemed that LAV was unrelated to HTLV.

To confirm, the lab attempted to replicate the results using samples from other young AIDS patients. This time success eluded them for almost two months, but it finally came in early April. They were sure now that Montagnier had identified a brand-new retrovirus as the culprit behind AIDS.

This was towering news, the stuff of Nobel Prizes. Montagnier knew that every step in his announcement would be scrutinized. The journal article he would prepare was only his fourth in twenty years, so he would need to give it special care. With an invitation to submit to the British journal *Nature*, he labored over his report through the Easter weekend of 1983.

That Sunday, Gallo reached Montagnier by phone with news of his own. He and Dr. Max Essex, a Harvard scientist, had a pair of articles for publication in *Science*, one of America's most important scientific journals. Both focused on preliminary findings, he said. Neither lab had isolated a virus. But they both found strong and early confirmation that AIDS was caused by a relative of the HTLV family.

Montagnier interrupted his caller to tell him what he had discovered in his laboratory, but Gallo was not bothered by this contradiction. It was not unusual for two teams to draw conflicting conclusions. He invited Montagnier to submit his written report to *Science* instead of *Nature*, to produce a richer chorus. Montagnier had no guarantee of publication in *Nature;* he knew that submitting with Gallo and Essex virtually assured publication in *Science*. He agreed. He and Barré-Sinoussi finished their manuscript over the weekend and then passed it to an associate to deliver to Gallo personally, on the assumption that he would be one of the paper's reviewers.

In his haste, Montagnier had neglected to write a summary at the top of his article. With the care he and his team had put into the text, this oversight was inexplicable. But not fatal. Gallo, when the manuscript reached him, offered to write the summary himself, and in the interest of time Montagnier gratefully agreed. Gallo has said that his French counterpart approved the exact wording. However, when the three articles appeared in print on May 20, 1983, Montagnier professed to being stunned to read for the first time what Gallo had appended to his piece. Despite the claims in the article to having discovered a new family of retrovirus, the summary argued that the LAV virus should be included in the family of HTLVs.

In his typical fashion, Montagnier did not trouble Gallo with his disappointment, not even when he arrived at Gallo's home some weeks later with a sample of live LAV for Gallo to examine. But his silence did not end their troubles. "Indeed, we were already engaged, without our knowing it, in a scientific quarrel that would not be settled for a number of years," Montagnier later wrote. And it would slow down AIDS research, lead to countless deaths, and cloud the pursuit of effective treatments in a scrim of political intrigue. It was true what Sonnabend said from the start: greed controlled the field.

THE CONFUSING GROUP of articles in *Science* did not generate much attention; Montagnier's historic discovery was obscured by the theoretical hypotheses presented by Gallo and Essex. What exactly they were announcing wasn't clear to most people. Jim Monroe, a public health adviser working with the New York City Department of Health, read the articles as suggesting the science was in disarray—and ironically strengthened the case against a single viral cause. "We have impressive epidemiologic rather than truly scientific evidence to support the single agent theory," he said. "Many of us remain skeptical."

Sonnabend also persisted in his faith in his own model, so Callen and Berkowitz did as well. They had practical reasons for doing so. "If AIDS was something that was just 'bad luck,' if it's just a virus out there," Callen said then, "if it doesn't matter what you eat, who you fuck with or what other infections you get—if you're just a *ticking time bomb* that's gonna go off whenever it's gonna go off, and nothing you do or don't do matters—then I feel powerless. But if AIDS is not a simple question of having 'a' virus or not having a virus, then maybe there's something I can do about it. There's something I can do to increase my chances of survival—and to increase the quality of however much longer I have to live." At a time when the whole community was confronting "a threat as horrible as the Inquisition and the concentration camps," as the writer John Rechy put it, Callen wanted everybody to have that kind of hope.

Thanks to his newfound prominence, Callen was invited to address the New York congressional delegation that summer. This was the point he planned to make. Congressional testimony was well above his level of experience, but he didn't hesitate. He had until morning to prepare, so he and his lover cleared their schedules to work into the night. According to their invitation, the representatives wanted to know what life in the trenches was like: what victims talked about in their support groups and how they handled uncertainties and frequent hospitalizations. He had no intention of giving them the sad laments of a victim. He sat at his IBM Selectric and hammered out an introduction to the entire tragic affair of AIDS, from the politics to the economics to the dreaded hopelessness to a public opinion that only grew more sour— now even half of all college freshmen felt the country urgently needed laws banning homosexual relations.

Richard Dworkin reviewed the accumulating pages of Callen's speech with the cold blood of an editor. "This is way too specific," he said, slashing line after line. Tempers flared. When they finally headed to bed, Dworkin still worried the speech contained too much of a laundry list and not enough punch, but he held his tongue, knowing that Callen needed at least a few hours' rest before the breakfast meeting. He was confident that the speech clearly made the point they both agreed was most important, and made best use of this opportunity: Congress had to do something it had never done before—it had to stand up for gay men by funding research.

Callen snuck out the door before Dworkin awoke. In a windowless conference room at a Midtown hotel, he found himself seated at a long cloth-covered table between New York representatives Ted Weiss and Geraldine Ferraro. He smoothed a stack of white pages before him and, without a hint of nerves, became the first New Yorker with AIDS—and one of the first openly gay men—to give official congressional testimony, a twenty-eight-year-old man who couldn't expect to see thirty.

"On the whole, I believed in democracy. I believed in America," he said.

I felt it would only be a matter of time before education and the de-stigmatization of gayness would bring me my rights. But now I am fighting for my life. I am facing a life-and-death crisis that only the resources of the federal government can end, and I am shocked to find how naive I've been. Not only is my government unwilling to grant my right to love whom I choose, my right to be free from job discrimination, my right to the housing and public accommodation of my choosing. This same government—my government—does not appear to care whether I live or die.

This was not the testimony expected by the delegation. But Ferraro, the tough-talking Democrat from Queens, listened intently.

"Prejudice and oppression are words often bandied about too freely," Callen continued.

Do not allow the shortsightedness of prejudice to delay us any longer from discovering how the immune system defends us from disease. Whatever you and your colleagues do or don't do, whatever sums are or are not allocated, whatever the future holds in store for me and the hundreds of other men, women and children whose lives will be irrevocably changed—perhaps tragically ended—by this epidemic, the fact that the Congress of the United States did so little for so long will remain a sad and telling commentary on this country and this time.

I do not envy you your role in this matter any more than you must envy mine. Nineteen-eighty-three is a very bad year to be an elected official, just as it is a very bad year to be a gay man, a Haitian entrant, or a child living in poverty. And surely when you first dreamed of holding public office you did not, in the furthest reaches of your imagination, foresee that your duties would include having breakfast on a Monday morning with a homosexual facing a life-threatening illness. You can be sure that ten, five, or even one year ago, I could not have imagined the possibility that I, too, would be up here begging my elected representatives to help me save my life. But there you are. Here I am. And that is exactly what I am doing.

Moved almost to tears by his words, Ferraro returned to Washington and at the first opportunity read them into the *Congressional Record*.

A few weeks later, in June 1983, Callen and Berkowitz flew to Denver with their booklets to attend a conference of lesbian and gay health workers, where AIDS was the top agenda item. The idea to attend wasn't theirs. Perusing an out-of-date copy of one of San Francisco's gay papers, called *The Sentinel*, at Oscar Wilde Memorial Bookshop, Callen learned that a number of West Coast patients had petitioned to attend and urged the major AIDS service organizations to pay their expenses so that patients' voices could be heard. It had not occurred to the New York men to demand inclusion at a medical conference, despite their unusual relationship with Sonnabend. When it came to their care and treatment they had been mostly passive recipients of their doctor's medical judgment, as patients had been from the dawn of medicine. Now it made immediate sense to them to challenge that. Though GMHC declined to help with travel expenses, Callen found underwriting from Alan Long, a well-heeled member of the New York AIDS Network, a new coalition of concerned leaders.

Almost four hundred health professionals attended the conference, a record. The hotel staff was not thrilled to be hosting them. After the first morning's sessions, management removed posters containing the words "gay" or "AIDS" from the hotel lobby and deleted any mention of the gathering in the day's calendar of events. Those attending the conference retaliated by adopting a formal boycott of the hotel's restaurants and bars. Amid these hostilities, conference coordinators hastily arranged a hospitality suite where those with AIDS could take refuge.

When Callen and Berkowitz entered that room it was the first time they had met other patients from around the country. Among them was Dan Turner, a stern-faced playwright and actor who had been personal secretary to Tennessee Williams in his declining years. He was the thirtieth person in San Francisco to be diagnosed with KS. With him was Bobby Reynolds, in his mid-thirties like Turner, who had joined the ranks a few months after. The de facto leader of the San Francisco delegation was Bobbi Campbell, the registered nurse and Sisters of Perpetual Indulgence member who responded to his diagnosis with copious amounts of marijuana, humor, and generosity. Campbell posted Polaroids of the lesions on his feet in the window of Star Pharmacy on Castro Street so the community would know what to look for. He now contributed regularly to *The Sentinel,* in a column he called "Gay Cancer Journal." Callen had been anxious to meet him.

Representatives also came from Los Angeles, Kansas City, and Denver. But the encounter between Campbell's crew and Callen's contingent—including six others from New York City, most of them members of Callen's support group: Phil Lanzaratta, Artie Felson, Bill Burke, Bob Cecchi, Matthew Sarner, and Tom Nasrallah—dominated the gathering.

The West Coast cadre saw the epidemic in starkly political terms. They rejected the phrases "AIDS patient" and "AIDS victim" as being reductive; it diminished the personhood of people with AIDS. When he heard this, Callen thought, "How California." But he was impressed that their self-empowerment group, which they called "People With AIDS San Francisco," had fielded speakers at several AIDS meetings and made themselves available to reporters and doctors. In May, they organized a candlelight AIDS march down Market Street to bring attention to the plight of people with the disease, and to remember those who had already died. Campbell gave a powerful speech there about the need to maintain hope in the face of the epidemic, and had helped make a twenty-foot-long banner to lead the procession. It read, "FIGHTING FOR OUR LIVES." *Fighting* was not something the New Yorkers had begun to do, except to snarl at one another publicly and dodge Larry Kramer's harangues.

There were other differences, mostly cultural. The New Yorkers objected to the way the San Francisco men needed time out for spiritual reflection, and the Bay Area gang found their counterparts' faith in mainstream medicine to be misplaced. They clashed most fiercely over the East Coast theory that promiscuity and VD had caused their immune disorders, a position denounced as homophobic by the San Franciscans. But they all agreed it was time for the sick to assert themselves.

Campbell took charge of the meeting. His vision was an ambitious one—he proposed a national network of groups by and for people with AIDS organized under a single umbrella, the National Association of People With AIDS. Heads nodded in agreement around the room. With an eager show of hands, the men elected themselves to form the founding board of directors. Then they discussed the group's mission. With remarkably little discord, they quickly drafted a manifesto. The "Denver Principles," as this document would come to be known, was the founding declaration of the People With AIDS movement, establishing the rights and responsibilities of the afflicted, most fundamentally the right to speak on their own behalf, to be included in every aspect of their care, and to be consulted on all matters of science, medicine, and public health policy. Callen stressed that their participation had to be significant, not trivial—not "like the dancing bears dragged out on stage at the end of forums before passing the hat."

"We condemn attempts to label us as 'victims,' which implies defeat, and we are only occasionally 'patients,' which implies passivity, helplessness and dependence upon the care of others. We are People with AIDS," their document began. From that day on, the acronym PWA took center stage in the lexicon, not just of the community of PWAs and their doctors, but in the national dialogue as well.

This marked the beginning of a new form of patient advocacy, one that fundamentally rearranged the roles of patients, doctors, researchers, and pharmacists. These people took command of the narrative of their lives and their illnesses, fatal or otherwise. And they planted the first seeds, however small and unpromising they seemed, that would revolutionize global public health care and, ultimately, help forge the drug breakthroughs that would make AIDS survivable. When they typed it up for distribution, they decided to seize the stage from the speaker at the closing session to present their demands in the style of the Lavender Menace feminists who stormed the NOW convention stage.

They unfurled Campbell's banner. One by one, each of the eleven men declaimed one of the eleven points until the whole list of recommendations and responsibilities had been publicly uttered for the first time.

RECOMMENDATIONS FOR ALL PEOPLE

1. Support us in our struggle against those who would fire us from our jobs, evict us from our homes, refuse to touch us or separate us from our loved ones, our community or our peers, since available evidence does not support the view that AIDS can be spread by casual, social contact.
2. Not scapegoat people with AIDS, blame us for the epidemic or generalize about our lifestyles.

RECOMMENDATIONS FOR PEOPLE WITH AIDS

1. Form caucuses to choose their own representatives, to deal with the media, to choose their own agenda and to plan their own strategies.
2. Be involved at every level of decision-making and specifically serve on the boards of directors of provider organizations.
3. Be included in all AIDS forums with equal credibility as other participants, to share their own experiences and knowledge.
4. Substitute low-risk sexual behaviors for those which could endanger themselves or their partners; we feel people with AIDS have an ethical responsibility to inform their potential sexual partners of their health status.

RIGHTS OF PEOPLE WITH AIDS

1. To as full and satisfying sexual and emotional lives as anyone else.
2. To quality medical treatment and quality social service provision without discrimination of any form including sexual orientation, gender, diagnosis, economic status or race.
3. To full explanations of all medical procedures and risks, to choose or refuse their treatment modalities, to refuse to participate in research without jeopardizing their treatment and to make informed decisions about their lives.
4. To privacy, to confidentiality of medical records, to human respect and to choose who their significant others are.
5. To die—and to LIVE—in dignity.

The last line was Callen's to deliver. Looking from the dais he saw that there wasn't a dry eye in the house. For many of the assembled delegates, representing parts of the country not yet touched by AIDS, seeing those doomed young men in that line was devastating. But the presentation rattled those with more experience, as well. Paul Popham, for one, choked back tears. So did Dr. Barbara Starrett, Roger Enlow, and a number of other New York doctors in attendance. They recognized at once the watershed this moment represented, that from now on PWAs would take part in every discussion about themselves, whether medical or political. Virginia Apuzzo, who had been running the plenary as the new head of the only national gay rights group, the National Gay Task Force, stood silently at the microphone for several minutes, fighting to compose herself.

Tears burned down Callen's cheeks as well. For the first time since his diagnosis, he felt the full support and love of his community. That night, the founders of the National Association of People With AIDS celebrated their achievement by taking turns squeezing into Bobbi Campbell's comical habit, posing for photographs, and, amid the general merriment, openly flirting with one another—the stirrings of life.

Unfortunately, the high that Callen felt that day was matched by a deep letdown shortly upon returning home. Early one morning near the end of June, his boss at the law firm told him he was being placed on medical leave of absence, without pay. The firm had learned of his condition through an account in *New York* magazine. Callen complained bitterly, but the decision was not open to appeal. Too many of his colleagues had expressed fear about working with him. He was not allowed to return to his desk, such was the urgency of his removal.

. . .

THAT JULY, a sticky heat wave stalled over the eastern half of the country. By mid-August, the extreme weather had claimed the lives of 183 people in fifteen states. The newspapers and televisions gave lavish coverage to their funeral corteges. Now 891 Americans were dead from AIDS, more in New York City than anywhere else, but their deaths generated no similar coverage. Peter Staley, who never read the *Native*, concerned himself not in the slightest with the plague or the heat. He focused squarely on work. His base salary wasn't much in Wall Street terms—though $26,500 in the middle of a recession was more than most of his Oberlin classmates were making. And he could expect a year-end bonus near $100,000. In two years his total compensation might reach a quarter million dollars; twice that in four years. Within the decade, he would have his congressional war chest in place.

With Tracey Tanenbaum at his side, he traveled the city inside chilly limousines, hurtling between expensive dinners and discoteques or the more intimate piano bars, like Marie's Crisis and the Duplex, where Staley would sometimes take charge of the ivories to accompany off-duty Broadway belters. Later, after dropping Tanenbaum off for the evening, he regularly visited the St. Mark's Baths, a five-story emporium of dark rooms and unpredictable encounters in the East Village. Sometimes, he'd spend an hour or two across the street beforehand, at a packed gay disco called Boy Bar.

That's where I first saw him. A year younger than I was and a few inches shorter, he and I occupied either side of a wrinkle in gay culture. In my long hair and worn shoes, I was typical East Village stock, as short on finances as I was on boldness; I only ever came to the bar with friends, stood or danced in packs, nursing a single drink all night. I can't remember a time I struck up a conversation with a stranger who didn't approach me first. Staley was sparklingly attractive, expensively attired, and as bold as an itinerate preacher. When he came up the stairs to the dance floor, the room turned gyroscopically in his direction. He made an impression.

With New York still locked in the heat wave, I traveled to Vienna—my introduction to Europe—to cover the World Conference of the International Gay Association, a nascent group committed to bringing the various national movements under a single umbrella. Some four hundred people attended. A leader of Austria's Homosexuelle Initiative reported on developing negotiations with the European Parliament to acknowledge gay constituents. A Dutch delegate described getting his government to erect the world's first public monument to commemorate gay

and lesbian victims of the Holocaust. Called *Homomonument*, it consisted of a large granite plaza located in the middle of the city, entirely
funded by the Dutch parliament and local and regional governments.
The delegation from the United States had to admit they couldn't even
get meetings with health officials. The Americans were pressed for
information on AIDS—it wasn't much of an issue anywhere else yet. A
representative from Sweden saw the potential for the epidemic to point
us in a better direction politically. "The discussion now is about health
and community, not about sex, not about crimes," he said. "It's a different way to engage the authorities: doctors, research. This disease could
be a good thing. We should be prepared to use it."

His cold calculus startled me, and contributed to the anxiety I was
experiencing on the trip. I wasn't sleeping well. When I got back home
I developed a weird electrical sensation on my head. In a day or two, a
rash appeared on my forehead and scalp, with painful blisters. A friend
recommended a dermatologist on the Upper East Side, who diagnosed
me with a glance. "You've got shingles," he called out brightly, and sent
me home with ointment for the wounds and tablets for the pain.

During my convalescence, I was relieved to be suffering an ages-old
disease, not the one that was on everyone's mind. AIDS was suddenly
a media phenomenon. It made the cover of *Newsweek* in August, with
an arresting photograph of two men with AIDS staring from the newsstand resolutely—San Francisco's Bobbi Campbell and Bob Hilliard,
described in the story as "friends," though they were in fact lovers. This
was just the second time in history that men identified as gay claimed
the cover of a national newsmagazine (the first came in 1975 with a
story about Leonard Matlovich, a soldier dishonorably discharged after
coming out). I brought the issue back to my un-air-conditioned apartment and read through it obsessively, less hungry for the information
inside—which quoted Reverend Jerry Falwell saying, "A man reaps
what he sows"—than I was for the affirmation the pictures of "avowed
homosexuals" inadvertently provided. We were beginning to see our
lives represented in mainstream media; our faces and names and human
narratives were finally meriting national attention. Maybe the Europeans were right and things *were* about to change. But that meant we
needed to rethink the figurative walls around the gay ghetto, which had
begun to seem as cloistering as the closets we had fled. The magazine
included poll results showing that more than three-quarters of Americans had never knowingly met a lesbian or gay man. It was to them we
needed to make our case. We needed to build a bridge back to America.

The heat barely abated. I spent most of August glued to my fan, too lethargic to socialize. Peter Staley made his rounds undaunted, and successfully performed the riskiest high-wire act of the gay bar scene—he made a play for the bartender one Saturday night at the Duplex. Blond and wiry, Curtis Randall was Staley's opposite, a devoted Communist who abhorred everything about Wall Street. But for two weeks, they worked out their tensions in one apartment or the other, until clashing philosophies forced them apart. The idea that Staley was in the closet about his sexual orientation and out of the closet in terms of his quest for a fortune became insurmountable.

A few weeks later, in the middle of his first summer in New York City, Staley came down with the flu.

LATE IN AUGUST, Joe Sonnabend stuffed his unread office mail in a bag, grabbed a quick bite on his way to the laboratory, and spent hours at the microscope before visiting his patients, who were scattered in hospitals around the city. He now was caring for forty men with full-blown AIDS. Somehow he had managed to publish fifteen important and highly visible journal articles about the crisis.

He didn't have a chance to read his correspondence until very late: journals and lab results, bills, and an envelope from the 49 West 12 Tenants Corporation, the company from whom he rented office space. Thanks to the intercession of Krim, he had resolved his issue with back rent, so he was able to tear open the letter without hesitancy. The news was worse than he could have anticipated. "Please be advised and take notice, that your month-to-month tenancy is being and shall be terminated on September 30, 1983 and you are required to vacate the premises on or before that date. In the event you fail or refuse to quit the premises by that date, we shall commence summary proceedings to recapture the premises."

Sonnabend was being evicted.

When Sonnabend bumped into Dan Foxx, president of the co-op board, in the lobby a few days later, he begged for a reprieve. In the middle of a ballooning crisis, a plague, he had no time for organizing a move. He was busy launching a new peer-reviewed medical journal, *AIDS Research*, set to debut in November with him as editor-in-chief. His patients were dying. They needed stability, and a doctor undistracted by real estate matters.

Those patients, according to Foxx, were in fact the issue. The sight of them coming and going gave apartment owners fear for their own safety and concern for the value of their investments, he said. The shareholders wanted the plague out of their lobby.

Like it or not, Sonnabend was engaged in another battle.

Callen rallied the community. He got the Lambda Legal Defense and Education Fund, the community's largest civil rights litigation firm, interested in bringing a preemptive lawsuit, seeking a restraining order and $60,000 in damages. It was the first AIDS-rights lawsuit in history. He even got the GMHC board and Mel Rosen, the executive director, to overcome their feud with Sonnabend and fully support the lawsuit. This would be a defining case, the groundwork litigation establishing the rights of PWAs. New York State attorney general Robert Abrams saw it as an important precedent, throwing the power of the state behind Sonnabend and against "irrational prejudice."

On Friday, September 30, 1983, the day Sonnabend was to be out of Office 1-C, there would be a press conference. He would be expected to make formal remarks. The last thing on earth Sonnabend wanted was to become a cause célèbre, and the prospect rattled his nerves. Late one night several days before the press conference, he called Richard Berkowitz, at the end of his rope. "I'm just—it's going to be horrible, it's going to be awful, you understand?" he said. "How am I going to go there every day?"

Adrenalin swung him in the other direction as well. "I mean, if this—if I'm told that this can be of value in jobs, housing, all kinds of discrimination on the grounds of AIDS? This would be an important issue," he said. But his stoicism didn't hold, and he whipsawed back to stage fright. "I didn't realize they were going to make such a big publicity out of it!"

"Yep," Berkowitz said. "National."

"I thought all this just simply happened in the courtroom or something, you know? I didn't realize until, like, *yesterday* . . ."

Suddenly Berkowitz heard his doctor gasp and begin to cry. "Oh my god, it's really too much," Sonnabend said finally. "All this data is waiting to be done: the practice, the patients, *everything*. . . . On Friday morning, I'll do whatever they want me to do. And then *that is it*."

Bobbi Campbell spent the last days of summer barnstorming for the cause of PWA empowerment and wringing his peculiar celebrity as the AIDS Poster Boy wherever he could, popularizing condoms and patient rights around the country. He managed this while supporting himself on disability, $1,301 a month, and soliciting donated airfare and lodging. On August 17 he found himself in New York City for a meeting

Michael Callen had won with President Reagan's head of Health and Human Services, Margaret Heckler, her first face-to-face with PWAs. Joined by Richard Berkowitz, Artie Felson, and Dan Turner, they met in a conference room in a blocky building on Worth Street. Campbell found Heckler receptive to suggestions and feedback, but the one issue he personally pushed was out of her realm of influence: PWA claims for Social Security were being held up, including his own. She promised to investigate the matter with her counterpart at the Social Security Administration, which was more of a victory than he'd expected. He was exultant.

"WE DID IT!" he wrote in his journal that afternoon, before celebrating with a hit of acid.

It had been twenty-two months since his diagnosis, and his health was declining. He had just ended a six-month "drug and booze fast," which to his disappointment didn't slow the accumulation of KS lesions, so he returned to a liberal dalliance with mind alteration, sometimes a trip a day. His argument was: *So what?* Being high helped him cope with recurring bouts of depression. And besides, his hallucinogenic sojourns did not slow his work on behalf of PWAs.

In early October, Campbell flew from San Francisco to D.C., wrestling two large posters on his lap. Through relentless advocacy, he had won an invitation for the National Association of PWAs to attend the first Nursing Clinical Conference on AIDS. Campbell demanded a chance to speak at the open plenary as a PWA and a nurse himself; organizers offered a compromise, giving space at the lunch-hour "poster session," where new studies were presented on poster boards arranged on easels in one large hall, usually with researchers standing nearby to answer questions. Campbell accepted, and, with an eye on theatrics, he packed his white pants, white shoes, and clinical lab coat for the occasion.

On October 7, he headed out early in the morning to set up his two posters in the empty hall. One carried the headline "WE ARE PEOPLE WITH AIDS" above snapshots of happy-seeming young men, and the other used the banner "NOT VICTIMS" to introduce some of the literature the activists had produced, including fliers promoting condoms and decrying discrimination and fear, in some instances signed by the Sisters of Perpetual Indulgence themselves.

With the setup complete, he had time to take in one of the formal presentations going on in the conference center. Looking crisp in his hospital whites, he ducked into a talk by an NIH infection control nurse as she discussed what she called the agency's policy of "maximum awareness." She held aloft an electric-green tag with the words "AIDS Precaution" in bold. At the NIH medical center, these tags were hung from the doors of all AIDS patients' rooms, tied to their blood tubes, their laundry, and everything else. It didn't matter that there was no safety reason for distinguishing between AIDS patients and non-AIDS patients. The hospital facility there also generated lists of all AIDS-related admissions and sent them to every department on the agency's campus.

Campbell was horrified to learn this. Shouting from the back of the room, he denounced the policy as "creepy" and entirely inappropriate. The idea that the nation's preeminent research facility was practicing such blatant fear pandering was galling. Artie Felson joined his protest, but, sensing the cause was lost, they retreated bitterly.

They arranged an impromptu NAPWA meeting that afternoon to formulate a response. Campbell remembered their rapport with Heckler. She had ended their historic meeting with an open invitation to her Bethesda office. So "in the spirit of 'Lobby Day,'" as Campbell put it, they marched straight over there. They were not received like old friends, however. For one thing, by the time they knocked on her door it was already ten minutes to five—on the Friday before the long Columbus Day weekend. Heckler, if not already departed, was not available. The best her secretary could arrange was a hasty meeting with Shelley Lengel, who unbeknownst to them was spokeswoman for the new and underfunded national AIDS hotline (it consisted of a small bank of eight phones; some callers reported getting only busy signals for weeks on end). She graciously invited them into her office.

"We want to maintain a spirit of cooperation with the department in continuing information exchange," Campbell began. As Lengel nodded and smiled at the young men sitting across from her, she couldn't help noticing the fluorescent-green "AIDS Precaution" signs hanging from their ties. But she didn't ask about them, and claimed no knowledge of the policy of "maximum awareness." She promised to learn more about the upsetting NIH policy and committed to calling them back on Tuesday. The call never came.

SOON IT WAS New Year's Eve in New York, where entire circles of friends were laid up in hospital beds. Callen and Dworkin had planned to spend the evening with a lesbian couple they had just befriended—Lowlife's bass player, Pam, and her partner, Lindsy. This would be their tradition, new friends for the New Year, a fresh beginning uncoupled from the difficult past. The previous day had been a blur of meetings for Callen that hadn't ended until nearly eleven o'clock, overtaxing his weakened body.

He awoke that morning feeling depleted and feverish. So instead of marking auld lang syne, Callen climbed into bed and sent his lover off without him.

Callen's temperature rose to 102 degrees, causing his thinking to go fuzzy. Every time he closed his eyes, the faces of people he had fought with over the past year—Chuck Ortleb at the *Native* chief among them—returned to haunt him. When his thoughts veered to Dworkin, he was overcome with a feeling of guilt for making his own health their central concern as a couple. Not that Dworkin was all that well himself. In their first months together, Callen talked him into joining a study of healthy gay men and in the course of blood work and physical exams it came out that Dworkin was also compromised. This was life in the '80s, Callen thought.

And now they headed into Orwell's year. There was so much work ahead, urgent work, and so much to remember. Callen took out his tape recorder at about ten o'clock and began a memo to himself, going over it all again in feverish disorientation: the hepatitis B model; autopsy records; risk variances in Toronto, Cincinnati, Des Moines, New York. He needed to write a letter to James D'Eramo at the *New York Native* and to someone named Rick Bebout. Where was that quote from Dr. Thomas Quinn, the NIH researcher who allegedly found AIDS in non-promiscuous men? Quinn, who played right into the hands of the censors? He needed to find that quote for his riposte. His mind reeled. "Now," he said, "I need to put in print my little thesis that . . . my little thesis that amoebas really changed the notion of responsibility for disease." He took a deep, meaningful breath: "I can't sleep. Every time I fall asleep I seem to dream about my enemies."

Then: "I lost my train of thought, but I just—I don't know. Thank god for aspirin and for my sweetest man. AIDS is really getting me down."

PART 2

•

Incurable Romantics

Life, Apparently

I t wasn't until the end of 1983, which I spent back in the shag-carpeted bedroom of my unhappy childhood, that I saw how three years in the city had changed me. I was no longer the man who hid and lied to myself and to others, always alert to the potential for physical violence. Now I walked and talked in a way that was natural for me, in parody neither of masculinity or femininity. Out of the closet, I had found my natural place on the androgyny quadrant of the gender matrix. I wore my hair long and hung a pair of chandelier earrings on my ears. My sexual orientation, which had always been *self-evident*, in the words of Quentin Crisp, was also self-claimed.

But my equilibrium was fragile outside the bubble of the gay ghetto. In my daily rounds through Alphabet City it was possible to go for weeks with only the briefest encounters outside of my kind—the silent Korean woman who pushed a loose cigarette across the deli counter to me, the tiny Ukrainian couple on their daily path to church, the junkie who trembled pleadingly in the hallway outside my apartment door, a needle dangling moistly from his neck. Our ghettos may have occupied the same geography, yet we were all but invisible one to the other.

Being back in the Midwest, I felt as conspicuous and alien as ever. It was destabilizing to feel my gayness so acutely again, to feel myself swelling toward confrontations, to recognize how the fear and the shame had never gone away. I discussed these feelings with my parents, uneasy as they still were with my gayness. The problem, they believed, was self-made, the consequence of having come out of the closet in the first place. "It's like wearing shorts to show off a wooden leg," my father said. I didn't resent him saying this; it was a familiar sentiment, the reason I'd moved away in the first place. It was a relief to return to New York.

That winter, I was in the *Native* offices more frequently. The paper was housed in a dingy two-room suite up a flight of stairs from a

Tribeca pharmacy. Both the larger editorial space and the cramped cloister that housed the advertising and circulation departments were woefully under-appointed. But it hummed with the energy of a gay *His Girl Friday*. Staff writers took turns before the one Selectric, cigarettes clamped in their teeth, and a succession of freelance photographers squeezed into a hallway mop closet to print their black-and-white pictures. Competitiveness and bitchy infighting were inflamed by exhaustion and meager salaries. When tempers crested dangerously, Tom Steele, who oversaw our sister magazine, *Christopher Street*, played the role of peacemaker, walking through the office with colorful paper crowns to bestow upon the Evil Queens of the moment. A crinkled coronet, it seemed, could defuse the dankest turpitudes.

The mayoral election was more than a year off, but Ed Koch was already campaigning for a third term. He had much atoning to do in the community. In the thirty months of plague, a time in which 1,340 New Yorkers were diagnosed and 773 were already gone, Koch had spent just $24,500 on AIDS. In the same time frame, San Francisco had allocated and spent more than $4 million on care and prevention. That gap was even more striking considering that the city by the Bay had just 12 percent of the nation's caseload compared to New York City's 42 percent. Koch's pitiful largesse was allocated to a single program, run by the Salvation Army to provide home attendant care to AIDS patients. But even this contract would soon be canceled when, after fifteen months, Salvation Army officials managed to enroll only seven men. Nobody there had bothered to install phone lines so that patients in need of services could sign up.

It's not that Koch had done absolutely nothing. He issued a proclamation recognizing the "scientists of New York City who are in the vanguard of activities directed toward solving the riddle of AIDS." He made an unannounced appearance at GMHC's circus fund-raiser, which filled Madison Square Garden. He wrote a letter excoriating the New York State Funeral Directors Association for urging its members not to embalm AIDS corpses. But he didn't spend money, he resolutely refused requests for policy meetings, he did nothing to prevent the disease's spread, and he almost never mentioned AIDS on television or to the local papers.

Koch strategically avoided events where gay leaders might appear. In the *Native*, Larry Kramer wrote piece after piece attacking the administration's dereliction and Koch's refusal to meet with community leaders. "How much more manly and humane it would be if the Mayor, as the father of this city, were to wonder just what it is that hurts and frightens and provokes his constituencies so, and try to respond in a helpful, positive, constructive way," he wrote that April. "But no: evidently to question or criticize God only gets you excommunicated."

More than once Kramer crashed Koch's public events to denounce him as a murderer or, even more incendiary, a "closeted homosexual" who, in order to bolster his bona fides, had forsaken the community in its time of suffering. On this campaign, Kramer had no critics in the community. Cause and effect are hard to pinpoint, but it seemed to us that in the wake of Kramer's assaults, Koch was finally prepared to placate the community with real changes. In a first, he created an Office of Gay and Lesbian Health Concerns. Community leaders hoped this prefigured a shift in his AIDS policy. But no change followed. Instead, he took a strong stand against anti-gay workplace discrimination, a move meant to prove he wasn't disenfranchising the entire community—and one, not coincidentally, that required no additional funding. Though unlinked to the crisis, it was not at all frivolous. Despite the city's reputation for progressivism, in respect to gay civil liberties New York was little different than Des Moines and the rest of the country, where 63 percent of the public was "unsympathetic to the homosexual community." According to polls, outside pockets of the city's cultural worlds, almost every gay person had experienced some sort of barriers at work because of their sexual orientation.

Every year since 1971, the city council had rejected a ban on anti-gay bias in employment, housing, and public accommodation. They openly cited personal revulsions and "concerns for the children." Only once did the gay rights bill win the handful of votes needed to get out of committee. That was in the summer of 1973, but the momentum was halted by the full body, which swiftly voted it down. They did this with the complete support of the city's religious leaders and newspapers, none more plain in its view than the *Daily News,* which just a decade before had editorialized that "Fairies, nances, swishes, fags, lezzes—call 'em what you please"—should be barred "from jobs in which their peculiarities would make them security or other risks."

After Koch became mayor in 1978, the bill's prospects faded even more. As a consolation, early on he issued an executive order barring discrimination on the basis of sexual orientation or "affectional preference," bringing New York in line with a number of other progressive cities. But his measure was decidedly limited, covering only the agencies under his direct control, including the police, but specifically barring any affirmative action on the grounds that intentionally reaching out to the community would be, as he tactlessly put it, "insane."

Nonetheless, the executive order was hugely controversial. Anita Bryant's anti-gay religious coalition, which she called Save Our Children, helped foment a frothy backlash across the country. As one letter-to-the-editor writer from Ohio put it, "Someone once said, 'You can be so open-minded that your brains fall out.' I think that the agonizing reappraisal of homosexuality now in vogue is a classic illustration of that." Despite this, the executive order drew no significant organized opposition in New York City.

That changed in the early 1980s, when the administration expanded the executive order to include all civilian agencies entering into contracts with the city. Called Executive Order 50, the policy still didn't apply to private companies but nonetheless doubled the number of covered employees, and drew the first serious challenge to the policy. The Salvation Army refused to cooperate, claiming that it impermissibly impinged upon religious freedoms. Besides the AIDS care contract it wasn't honoring, the Salvation Army had a $5 million deal to provide senior citizen drop-in centers, a foster home, and an adoption service, affecting about 1,100 New Yorkers. At the *Native,* we tried to imagine what religious principle might collapse under the pall of an old lesbian at the pinochle table. We called for a boycott of those ubiquitous Christmas kettles. It was a very small imbroglio.

What suddenly made this an issue in early 1984 was the installation of John O'Connor as archbishop of New York. He declared the Catholic Church's intention to sue, asking a judge to invalidate Executive Order 50. In comparison to the Salvation Army's small role in social services, the church operated enormous city-funded child care and foster programs, homeless shelters, and health care programs. Their contracts totaled $76 million. Church leaders made it clear that if forced to hire gays, they would shut down the whole operation, leaving tens of thousands of at-risk New Yorkers in a lurch. It was a cheerless position for a charitable entity—but not a bigoted one, they argued in court papers. In the courthouse hallway one afternoon, the archbishop's white-haired lawyer told a scrum of reporters that the church never practiced discrimination, period.

He added, however, that it was just "plain common sense" to restrict some sensitive jobs to heterosexuals. "It would be totally inappropriate, in my judgment, to hire a blatant homosexual and put him in as a house parent to a group of young, troubled teenage boys," he said.

With an excess of vinegar in my voice, I asked how he defined a "blatant homosexual," and he sourly surveyed me from my pierced ears to my colorful sneakers in a gesture that said, "Exhibit A." In fairness, the reporters from the *Times* and the city's tabloids gave me the same look. They drowned out my effort to discuss the escalating reports of inhumane treatment of gay patients inside St. Vincent's, the church's flagship hospital.

Such tense confrontations didn't fit my character, but were everyday features of the job. Among my colleagues at the *Native*, I was perhaps the most timid of reporters, constitutionally soft-spoken and still somewhat self-doubting as a result of my formative years. But I was beginning to harden. Confronting the church's lawyer, I realized I was reticent but no longer buckling in fear. I shared the belief that by asking the questions no other journalist was asking—by aggressively covering the affairs of the gay community—we were adding a momentum to the march toward freedom, we were gaining strength, we were becoming citizens.

How many of us would survive to see the Promised Land was the unasked question. The disease had already swept into our tiny operation. Derek Peterson, one-third of our ad department, came down with the classic complications. A freelance writer named Fred Canteloupe was covered in spots. Canteloupe made it to the first week of March, Peterson to the third. One Thursday, sexy Tommy McCarthy from the classifieds department stayed out late at an Yma Sumac concert. Friday he had a fever. Sunday he was hospitalized. Wednesday he was dead.

The trio of tragedies destabilized the staff and weighed especially hard on Ortleb, whose mild hypochondria had grown into fantastic bouts of medical paranoia. He didn't fear catching AIDS himself, at least not through sexual means, given his chaste personal predilections. (He and his lover, Francis, appeared as domesticated as the Cleavers.) But microorganisms and their ghastly consequences consumed his private thoughts. He grew reluctant to shake hands or handle money. He had begun to fear the very air in the newspaper's office. I overheard him on the telephone one day saying, "I'm coming in here every day, an office full of *gay men*, putting my life on the line." He spent more time than usual closed up in his private office, where panic attacks punctuated his days. But as quickly as they came, those bouts would subside, and Ortleb would be hard at work at our side, trying to crack the enigma.

He proved a quick study. As 1984 unfolded, he took to accompanying James D'Eramo, the staff science writer, on his interviews—ostensibly as a second pair of ears, but soon as his journalistic partner: he paired D'Eramo's just-the-facts articles with his own fiery editorials, rich with professions of doom and rage.

Lacking definitive evidence, he was disinclined, like Sonnabend, to accept the hypotheses of Dr. Robert Gallo at the National Cancer Institute or Dr. Luc Montagnier at the Institut Pasteur. He scoured the science journals for alternate theories, making note of each new finding under the rubric "AIDS news," which he allowed to devour page after page of the *Native*. He solicited an article by a California biology professor who believed that chronic parasitic infections were enough to explain the many ailments and deaths. He ran news from a Nebraska researcher amplifying Sonnabend's "overload theory;" from an Australian study suggesting the effects of too much suntanning as a cofactor; and from a French scientist who admitted we were no closer to an answer than we had been six months earlier. Never before had a gay periodical devoted itself so thoroughly to a single news development. He jokingly referred to the paper as the *"New York Native Journal of Medicine,"* and in an editorial bragged that "this paper has provided more diverse and up-to-date information about AIDS than any other non-medical publication in America."

In reality, it was the only periodical of any kind to provide digests of nearly every development in AIDS—the science, the politics, the toll on us and our culture. This was appreciated by the core readers, which included the most engaged and proactive members of the gay community, as well as by the growing network of AIDS doctors, scientists, policymakers, and activists. As we regularly heard from Ray Nocera, the lanky and bearded general manager, subscription cards were coming in from the NIH and Capitol Hill, from Pfizer and Burroughs Wellcome, Harvard and Yale.

ONE PARTICULAR THEORY held Ortleb's attention more than the others. Jane Teas, a young pathobiologist working at Harvard, was the first to notice that the constellation of reported AIDS symptoms bore a striking resemblance to those experienced by ordinary domestic pigs infected with a highly contagious disease called African swine fever virus. Pigs with ASFV became susceptible to opportunistic infections: half died of pneumonia, and some developed skin lesions that looked rather like Kaposi's sarcoma. The condition was almost 100 percent fatal. She had no personal experience with ASFV, and less with AIDS; breast cancer was her expertise. But she found the casual observation significant enough to write a letter to *The Lancet*, which was intrigued enough to publish it on a page featuring educated hunches. She proposed that the virus might have jumped to humans by way of undercooked pork.

What drew Ortleb to Teas's theory was how well it met the test of time and place. In 1978, a plague of ASFV swept Hispaniola, the Caribbean island shared by the Dominican Republic and Haiti. This might finally explain how Haitians became an AIDS risk group. Epidemiologists now believed the earliest cases were in Haiti, in 1978. But how did the disease specifically poison the gay community? This question consumed Ortleb. Almost every night, sitting at the bar across from the office, he and his deputy, Tom Steele, dove deep into conjecture, examining old newspaper articles and new books to test the hypothesis.

For Ortleb, it started to fall together convincingly. Was it a coincidence that Haitian boat people fled to Cuba in 1980, when coincidentally ASFV killed 500,000 Cuban pigs? Was it just coincidence that in that same year a massive exodus of 125,000 Cuban refugees fled by raft and boat to Miami from the beach town of Mariel? Among the "Marielitos" were an estimated twenty thousand Cubans who had escaped prosecution and prison terms for "crimes against the normal development of sexual relations, the family, and children." (It was the largest mass asylum claim by gays, lesbians, and transgender people in history. Unfortunately for them, they washed ashore in a land that formally and categorically excluded gays—or, in the language of the statute, "aliens afflicted with psychopathic personality, or sexual deviation, or mental defect." Their arrival here put Washington in a bind. Keen to score cold war points against Havana, immigration officials wanted the public relations boost of extending citizenship to Castro's huddled masses. So ultimately they pushed the *official* estimated number of Mariel gays down to 276, then bent the rules to allow in any "victims of communism" so long as they didn't make "an unequivocable [sic], unambiguous declaration that he/she is a homosexual.")

Ortleb, who prided himself in his ability to "connect dots very easily," found this new pork connection strangely exhilarating. James D'Eramo, who had a PhD in medical ecology and infectious diseases, felt similarly. He called it "a most uncommon, exciting, and plausible theory." They invited Teas to the office, whiling away an afternoon in consideration of her propoundings and continuing the inquisition over dinner. Teas was invigorated by her avid dinner companions, and preened under their intense interest in her work. Ortleb found her vulnerability refreshing, and told her so. In a field obviously dominated by self-aggrandizers and braggarts, he saw her as among the least self-interested—a scientist with no special interest in AIDS who was willing to share the products of her mind.

Not everybody was so appreciative, she confided in them. A dozen researchers and officials called for more information, which because she was new to AIDS and ASFV she was unable to provide. Her callers dismissed her as naïve. "It was like being queried about an ancient civilization just because I had found an artifact from the site of an old city," she said. Three weeks after her letter appeared, *The Lancet* published a reply from a Belgian group that found no evidence in support of the swine disease after testing Teas's hypothesis in seven AIDS patients from Africa, where the epidemic was spreading wildly.

She found the reply striking on several counts. "How had the Belgians," she wondered, "managed to set up a new experiment with an animal virus, perform the test, write the results, and get them all published in just three weeks? And why were they so certain, when they had only tested seven sera, in a model that used pig antibodies? The first time a test is done, particularly with a novel experimental procedure, there are almost always new problems in working out the test procedure. Why hadn't they done the test at least twice, and with more samples?"

She was left with the unsettling belief that the purpose of the Belgian letter was to shut down interest in her and her virus. But why? "As a veterinarian said to me," Teas reported, "'What if your theory is right? It would destroy our $10 billion pork industry.'"

The implication of a cover-up sent a chill through Ortleb. A headline emerged in his thoughts: AIDSGATE. He would use it often in the future.

THOUGH THEY HAD only been dating for six months, Bobbi Campbell and Bob Hilliard were profoundly in love. It was the first serious relationship for either man. They were complementary characters: whereas Campbell was gregarious and moody, Hilliard was sedate and predictable. Campbell, of the two more romantically inclined, had saved a message from an old fortune cookie that predicted, "You or a close friend will be married within a year," aware that virtually no one he knew would be allowed to marry and besides, despite his weekly chemo, he suspected he wouldn't see another Christmas.

They spent New Year's Eve watching *Gorky Park* through the lens of some mushrooms, then wandered over to Castro Street at near midnight for the annual spectacle of gaiety and cheer. They found a crowd that was glum and subdued, reduced by half from the year before. In a lackluster gesture to anarchic tradition, Campbell grabbed his lover's hand to invade the intersection of Castro and Eighteenth, calling, "Take the streets! Take the streets!" But almost nobody joined them, and cops brushed them back onto the sidewalk with little effort.

In the coming days, Campbell had to admit the gloominess had snagged him too. The chemo sapped his energy and, by mid-January, gave him a wicked case of stomatitis, with painful ulcerations on his tongue and lips. His appetite vanished, leaving him perpetually exhausted. He spent his days watching cartoons on TV, obsessing on his fluctuating CD4 cells, and counting the KS lesions on his arms and trunk. At the insistence of friends in the Order of Perpetual Indulgence, he returned to his psychotherapist after a long absence. This seemed to do some good. On January 28, sun warmed the neighborhood and Campbell turned thirty-two years old, feeling somewhat positive again about life. To celebrate, he and Hilliard blew $115 on groceries and $5 on helium balloons for a large birthday bash. But before the deviled eggs and canapés were eaten, Ronald Reagan announced he would seek reelection, and Campbell's emotional progress was reversed.

The prospect of a second Reagan term also mortified Michael Callen. The president had still not acknowledged the crisis with so much as a word in public. Congress was hardly better, having conducted only a few unproductive hearings. But Callen was focused on more immediate problems. On a dark Friday evening in early February, what consumed his thoughts was a wicked case of thrush. It coated his tongue with white fuzz that, besides looking atrocious, caused pain and bleeding and made food taste so bad he had nearly given it up altogether. His latest CD4 count was more abysmal than it had ever been, which is why the thrush had taken hold in the first place—the fungus exploited the immune suppressed. He was on heavy medication. He knew he needed rest.

Even Sonnabend scolded him for continuing his punishing schedule of community meetings and hospital visits. But in fact he did both mostly at Sonnabend's behest, to defend his scientific theories and to be his emotional brace on his unofficial rounds with patients. It seemed like Sonnabend never entered a hospital room without being preceded by Callen. In contrast to Sonnabend's teary and apologetic bedside manner, his best-friend demeanor, Callen mostly managed these visits with the chirpy detachment of a hospital head resident. He knew how to squeeze the patients' arms without bungling their tubes and needles, how to say positive things when they were least merited.

When he entered those hospital corridors, he walked more quickly than usual, unconsciously, lest anyone mistake him for one of the patients. He had developed a strong ability to put his own health challenges out of mind. There simply was too much to do to indulge in self-pity, even long after everyone else had gone home for the night.

One evening, Callen called Dr. Roger Enlow to resume a conversation about the bathhouses. Enlow was a winsome young physician who wore his hair shorter than prevailing styles. He was one of the gay doctors whose reputations Sonnabend mercilessly impugned. Sonnabend considered him a bumbling rheumatologist who turned to treating AIDS only because he was gay, not because he had the skills to contribute. But a few months back, city hall had tapped Enlow to head Koch's new Gay and Lesbian Health Concerns office. He took heat for accepting. Many people were convinced that the whole enterprise had been created simply as an election-year crumb, a way to deflect criticism without offering anything useful. And it was true that Enlow found himself in a largely ceremonial office, without budget or portfolio, and with little access to the Department of Health or the Health and Hospitals Corporation, where decisions about hospital policy and public health strategy could be made. He was given a staff of two assistants plus an unpaid predoctoral student. He passed his first six months preparing and giving basic testimony before various panels.

But Enlow, adept at realpolitik, was determined to convert his meager office into a kind of official catalyst for the community, to become a cheerleader with an enviable power: the city's imprimatur. So a few weeks earlier, he had convened a meeting of community leaders to discuss the knotty issue of the baths, which were as likely to have long lines now as ever. The Coalition for Sexual Responsibility, as he called it, included GMHC, the gay physicians' organization, Mel Rosen (who had left GMHC to start the AIDS Institute, a state agency), and leaders of the New York PWA group including Callen, Berkowitz, and Sonnabend.

All had agreed that padlocking the bathhouses was off the table, including Callen. "I'd like to see them closed," he said, "but I'd like to see them closed *because people stopped going*." Meanwhile, they were regarded as a ripe opportunity for the prevention squads, logical locations for reaching the community's most at-risk members. In a surprising show of unity, the New York Civil Liberties Union, GMHC, and even the city's department of health militated for keeping them open. The rest of the country saw the situation differently. Epidemiologists at the CDC considered them dangerous "amplification systems" for spreading disease, and entirely indefensible. And public health officials in San Francisco joined with a plurality of gay community leaders to demand closure there.

Enlow's coalition had held three productive meetings to discuss creating an educational poster to be distributed at the bathhouses. At the last meeting, the group agreed that a playfully raunchy poster would be the ideal tool for popularizing safer-sex techniques. But when it came to adding text, consensus collapsed. The draft language that appealed to the majority was silent on the various scientific theories of the day, notably CMV, the villain in Sonnabend's model. Callen strenuously opposed its elimination.

He reached Enlow at home, though Enlow, not eager to rehash the issue at any time, much less after hours, let his frustrations show.

"I can live with the poster," he said impatiently. "I can live with it as it has evolved."

"I understand that consensus makes life *easier,* that people don't have to get conflicting signals," Callen said. But he added that CMV in recently months had moved from a matter of philosophical differences to one of clinical urgency. A rare form of the disease had been entering the eyes of PWAs, creating an unusual type of retinitis and resulting in blindness. The city's AIDS wards were now filling with men hugging walls and scraping the air to find their nurses. Stripping the poster of specifics left the community without the alert Callen believed they needed.

"I know of one case where the person, who was admittedly quite stupid, didn't even know anything about the AIDS epidemic and was continuing to go to the bathhouses. I'm not saying that we should continue to gear absolutely everything to someone that dumb. But I think the fact that in 1984 someone that dumb could go to a bathhouse, of all places—"

"There's probably ten guys who are *that* dumb," Enlow moaned, "who don't know anything about *any* sexually transmitted diseases. But give me a break. This entire lifestyle is dangerous."

Enlow immediately regretted saying those words. For all his years volunteering at the free clinic, he had carefully refrained from judging the lives of gay men, a posture he had intended to maintain. Besides, he knew it wasn't the bathhouses that were dangerous, it was the bodily fluids.

Callen snapped to life. "Why isn't it being said?" he demanded. "*Why isn't that being said clearly?* People look to the public health authorities . . . for some *sign*! They're not reading between the lines. If all [anybody] talks about is 'civil liberties,' then that's all a lot of people will think about!"

He demanded to know why Enlow wasn't backing his proposal to put even these few words on the poster: *We don't recommend that anyone have sex at a bathhouse because a number of sexually transmitted diseases have reached epidemic proportions. However, in terms of civil rights, we are opposed to the closing.*

"We mustn't underestimate people's intelligence," Callen scolded. "People are looking for some sort of guidance and we're giving very mixed signals!"

Enlow saw the difference between the approaches as being one that affirmed safe behavior versus one that condemned unsafe behavior, and strongly felt the positive approach was the best approach. But he had already gone over that with Callen. He drew a breath but found he had nothing new to add. "I've just been told dinner's ready," he said after a polite interval. "To be continued, Mike. I don't talk to you enough."

IN THE END, the poster featured cartoons showing the various sex acts considered medically harmless, and even fun. As disappointed as Callen was with the safe sex literature, he was glad *something* got produced. He went on to help GMHC plan a community forum to further help popularize safer sex, donating his time pro bono because PWA-NY couldn't find independent funding for their work. On February 27, when Albany announced its first round of state AIDS contracts, GMHC got $183,000 for "public information" and Rosen got $150,000 in education money for the AIDS Institute, while PWA-NY, the undisputed public health education trailblazers in the community and the only group with a track record, was awarded only a small travel budget for providing speakers at seminars. Callen complained bitterly. "They put us on at the end to make them cry," he said, "and then pass the hat."

The GMHC forum promised to be the most high-profile public education event in the history of the disease. Gloria Steinem was scheduled to attend, as were Mary Calderone, the famous sexologist and birth control advocate; Congressman Ted Weiss; and Ginny Apuzzo from the National Gay Task Force. But on a panel of ten speakers, there would be no one speaking for the PWA movement. Callen threw in his own name, along with other members of PWA-NY, but GMHC, wanting to suppress Callen's divergent views on the cause of the disease, was not open to suggestions.

For Callen, this was entirely unacceptable. He rallied the other members of PWA-NY, who proposed to picket the affair in protest. But not Richard Berkowitz, who shied from the stage and learned through the controversies they generated in print that he hated public conflict. He worried that anger could destroy their immune systems more surely than AIDS.

When they got together on the night of March 13, Callen tried to rouse him to battle against GMHC. Berkowitz held firm.

"Michael, they're indestructible," he said. Besides, he worried that PWAs faced a far greater threat than being sidelined at a conference. Just the previous Sunday, *60 Minutes* aired a segment on the issue of quarantining AIDS patients. Lawmakers in Connecticut were preparing a bill. "An Act Concerning Quarantine Measures," it was formally called. The Lambda Legal Defense and Education Fund was fighting similar initiatives across the country. Meanwhile, anti-gay violence was surging and the epidemic itself—whatever the cause—was gaining force. The way Berkowitz saw it, the prospect of an escalating intramural squabble was sickening.

"We can't fight them," he said.

"Yeah? Then, so?"

"There's got to be another way to do this," Berkowitz said. Options for averting a showdown ran through his mind. He thought of people who might intervene on their behalf. He thought of ways they could participate from the audience.

"I want to have a serious talk with the guys"—meaning the other group members—"because this could seriously destroy the PWA movement," Callen interrupted. "But maybe it should, Richard. Aren't we a joke?"

Berkowitz was feeling physically sick. "We can't fight them."

"You and I are done in this business—that's what you're wanting me to say?"

That was the opening Berkowitz had been waiting for.

"I'm going to try to move on," he said.

This news, unwelcome though not entirely unexpected, stopped Callen cold. He knew Berkowitz's money troubles were severe. A few weeks earlier, Berkowitz had pestered Sonnabend into hiring him as his filing clerk, a move that only made him more miserable. Sonnabend, unhappy about the manipulative employment campaign, put him on the payroll but was excessively demanding, intentionally making the job impossible. Plus, Berkowitz now had to contend with Sonnabend's financial woes on top of his own—it was a daily struggle to keep the phones connected and placate the IRS agents who showed up unannounced. The waiting room was chaotic, with lawyers for the eviction lawsuit serving papers, reporters running in and out, and the endless stream of dying patients. To Berkowitz, this often meant seeing a friend or former client with thrush, an enlarged spleen, lymphadenopathy, or diseased lungs. The other day, a friend named Ron fell apart in the office after getting his diagnosis. "I don't know how this could have happened," he sobbed on Berkowitz's shoulder. On another day, Berkowitz attempted to console a beautiful young man who nonetheless went directly home and committed suicide; Sonnabend had to identify the body.

Berkowitz came to feel that, for him to make it, if he had any chance at survival, he needed a change—even if that change took him backward. He had begun laying the groundwork for a return to the sex trade. New phone lines were on order. He was back at the gym in search of his faded hustler's physique.

Callen was angrily resigned to this development.

"Keep working out," was his bitchy advice.

But Berkowitz ditched his plans for a resurrected sex career. Instead, he moved to Bal Harbour, Florida, at the invitation of a kind former client. Meanwhile, PWA-NY stopped its regular schedule of meetings. Despondent, Callen abandoned plans to picket the sex conference, which drew five hundred in April, and sank instead into the life of a writer of acidic letters. "How fittingly ironic," Callen complained bitterly in one. "Only in New York was the environment so hostile that the movement could not survive."

Dr. Sonnabend was disappointed in his protégés. But there was no time to dwell on that. Despite his efforts on behalf of his patients, the names of the dead multiplied in his book—Wayne Acott, Tim McCluskey, Robert Melborne (one of the epidemic's first black victims), Bobby Blume, Doug Boyan, Giovanni Siortino, Chip Edgerton, Larry Gueerau. The plague gathered momentum.

Paranoid Fantasies

Chuck Ortleb came to work one morning in March wearing a jacket and tie, which was not his custom, and made his usual perfunctory tour through the editorial office. It was a Wednesday, which meant the newest issue had already spent two days on newsstands across the ghetto, and new typescripts were pouring in for the next one. There were the usual gay-bashing cases Ermanno Stingo was monitoring, and a story on a Minnesota district court judge who had been removed from the bench once his homosexuality was revealed, on the grounds that in a state outlawing sodomy he was a common criminal and therefore no more fit than a safe-cracker for the job.

I was editing a piece on how San Francisco authorities were moving closer to shuttering the bathhouses. Ortleb, glancing over my shoulder, told me to play down the story. "The baths are not our barricade issue," he said. "Close them, I don't care." I took this to be the opinion of a distracted man. Ortleb's investors surely enjoyed the revenues from the full-page ads the sex establishments placed weekly.

"C'mon, we gotta go," he called toward James D'Eramo. A darkly handsome man with spotless skin and a spherical stomach, D'Eramo was always even tempered and impeccably dressed. He grabbed a scarf and the two were off to an extraordinary meeting.

Dr. James Mason, who had just assumed the top job in Atlanta as the CDC director, had requested a private summit with them on the subject of African swine fever virus. To Ortleb, this meant that their strident advocacy for ASFV was paying off. They piled their research into a briefcase and jumped into a cab. At Mason's suggestion, the meeting was hosted by Dr. David Sencer, the city health commissioner.

Despite being new on the job, Mason was already reviled by the gay community. He came to the disease center from a job as Utah's top health director, in a state where not one case of AIDS had been diagnosed. Given Reagan's disregard for the epidemic, this seemed purposeful and offensive. Mason, a bishop in the Mormon Church, had previously served as commissioner of health services for all of Mormonism, where he designed and put into place a strict medical theology against homosexuality in 1973, the same year that the American Psychiatric Association declassified homosexuality as a mental illness. The church's anti-homosexual teaching tightened even further in 1975 and 1978, including the creation of a program to "cure" or expel "belligerent, uncooperative" transgressors. In fact, it was these credentials that helped bring him to the attention of the conservative Utah senator Orrin Hatch, his main champion for the federal job. Mason's arrival in Atlanta in the middle of the gay plague was unfathomable and disastrous.

To his credit, Mason made a point his first week in office to meet with Ginny Apuzzo and other gay leaders to express his commitment to the crisis. But any diplomatic gains were lost when he tripped up almost comically while trying to say the word "gay." He compounded the problem by preposterously asserting that the government was doing everything in the battle against AIDS that could rationally be expected of it.

As obstacles go, even more obstinate was Dr. Sencer, the mayor's appointee, who had responded to the crisis with a policy of formal insouciance, even ignoring questions from the city council on the topic. In defending this stance, he argued that the exponential rate of new infections had reversed, despite overwhelming evidence to the contrary, and he credited his wait-and-see policy for producing the fictional reduction. AIDS, he decreed brightly, was not "an emergency" and didn't require city assistance. This contradicted every available fact and every independent appraisal.

When Ortleb and D'Eramo arrived at 125 Worth Street, they were ushered into a time-worn conference room upstairs. Mason and Sencer, together with another CDC official, greeted them warmly with expressions of appreciation for the *Native*'s extensive coverage. Mason was by far the most elegant. Crisply attired and snowy-headed, his ample eyebrows cascaded over his horn rims like Scottish mist. Sencer was his opposite, the template of a city bureaucrat with a large cubical head fixed to his neck with a bow tie.

Ortleb came prepared with questions about ASFV. Quickly, though, it became clear that Mason's mission was to change the subject. His voice was gentle and disarming when he explained that the disease agency had conducted serology tests looking for ASFV among AIDS patients, finding none. That was almost a year ago. This point was long settled.

Ortleb, feeling the bite of manipulation, wasn't buying it. What strain of ASFV had the agency tested, he asked—was it the one from Haiti? That was the strain Dr. Teas surmised had mutated to become less fatal in pigs and perhaps more likely to make the species leap.

No, Mason said, it was not. With the agency's limited resources, it would not be possible to pursue the matter further, he added. Then he leaned across the table solicitously. He had decided to give the tiny *New York Native* the scoop of a lifetime. He was certain that ASFV had nothing to do with AIDS, he explained, because the agency was getting close to announcing that the true cause of AIDS had been found.

"Work in progress at the CDC on the French retrovirus— lymphadenopathy-associated virus, and related strains—looks very exciting," he said in the slow and overenunciated voice adults reserve for addressing children. Some more questions needed to be answered before confidently declaring LAV the causative agent, he said, but the French had established a correlation between their virus and the disease, the first step in proving causality. Mason said the Institut Pasteur researchers had given a convincing presentation in February at a science summit in Park City, Utah, showing that they had been able to isolate LAV in nearly half of all AIDS patients and most of those who had lymphadenopathy or depleted CD4 cells with no other opportunistic infections, a condition now being called AIDS-related complex, or ARC. They had done so using blood from a variety of AIDS patients— gay men, hemophiliacs, Haitians, and Africans.

Following the Utah meeting, Jean-Claude Chermann, one of Montagnier's two principal collaborators, flew to Atlanta to present additional details in the CDC's auditorium. At the completion of his talk there, the audience of researchers, epidemiologists, and public health experts had broken into applause. It seemed the puzzle was solved. But to be sure, the CDC sent the French dozens of unmarked samples, only half of which were from AIDS and ARC patients. Challenged to identify the healthy donors from the sick, the Pasteur researchers had no trouble. They found LAV in the proper samples, and in none of the controls.

While everyone believed the discovery would hold up to further scrutiny, additional tests were needed, Mason admitted. "This lead is very promising, and so we're going to put all our resources in that direction," he said, adding, "Just because we have an agent doesn't mean we've conquered AIDS. It's simply one step."

Mason's motives may have been unexpectedly generous and heartfelt. But the meeting backfired. When Ortleb and D'Eramo left the Worth Street building, they were more attached to ASFV than before. Hundreds of people must have attended Chermann's Utah presentation, including medical and science journalists, and scores more undoubtedly sat in the open session in Atlanta. If Chermann were so electrifying, why had none of them written or spoken publicly about LAV? Given the stakes—four thousand cases of the mystery killer disease in the U.S. now, with confirmed outbreaks in forty-five states and thirty-three countries, most ferociously in sub-Saharan Africa, largely among heterosexuals—it was safe to assume that a Nobel Prize awaited the genius who could find the cause. If the answer were LAV, why would the CDC be handing the scoop to the *Native*, of all places?

"He was trying to co-opt us," Ortleb said later. "Why else would the government be sending its top guns?"

At our story meeting, the editors decided to give Mason's revelation a single column. It was a landmark story, the firmest news of a virus, halfhearted as it was.

LAWRENCE ALTMAN at the *Times* did not see the *Native* article. He had heard some rumblings about Chermann's presentation in Park City and had exchanged phone calls with Mason in Atlanta, hoping to arrange an interview, although with no particular urgency. Altman was a reluctant chronicler of the epidemic. After his history-making first piece, written with the information provided by Sonnabend via Alvin Friedman-Kien, he had published a body of AIDS writing just a few inches deep. He was impervious to the bitter protestations from Larry Kramer and even Friedman-Kien, who followed their original interview with a year's worth of unanswered phone calls to Altman. When he finally called him back, Friedman-Kien was shaking mad. "You haven't responded to the epidemic for over a year, when we needed the help of somebody like you," he said. Before hanging up on him, Friedman-Kien added, "You're a lightweight."

They finally spoke on the last Friday in April, and he began work on a lengthy story to run on the front page the following Sunday. Beneath the promising headline "Federal Official Says He Believes Cause of AIDS Has Been Found," he quoted Mason as saying the eleven-month silence around LAV baffled him. "There was so little excitement in the scientific community when the French came up with their announce-ment last May," he said, adding his relief that things were now changing.

In the course of his reporting, Altman learned that the NIH—as a matter of fact, all of the U.S. Public Health Service with the exception of Mason and the CDC—considered the French claim about LAV to be a distracting sideshow. They had their money riding on Dr. Robert Gallo, who they believed was on the brink of announcing the true cause of AIDS. So did much of the press corps. For eleven months, many science reporters had been in the thrall of Gallo, who had waged a kind of guerrilla marketing campaign against LAV and in favor of his own *future* discovery. He found time during late-night breaks in his lab to call reporters at home, explaining the research landscape as he saw it, promoting his case in elliptical and often indecipherable detail.

Recently, he had alerted his contacts that he had hit pay dirt. He was calling the responsible virus HTLV-3, linked to his family of leukemia viruses. This was somewhat baffling; there had been no reports of leu-kemia among the AIDS caseload. But Gallo explained this by changing the nomenclature of his entire viral class, from human T-cell leukemia virus to human T-lymphotropic virus, meaning a virus that targets the lymphatic system, where CD4 cells are produced; he managed to keep the "L" by repurposing it. None of this was known to Mason and Cur-ran, and the news only reached Paris on April 3, when Gallo attended a private meeting with Chermann, Montagnier, and Barré-Sinoussi at the Institut Pasteur. He gave few details about his new retrovirus, but bluntly declared he had discovered HTLV-3 not once, but in 48 separate viral isolates—including in 18 patients with ARC, 3 out of 4 mothers of children born with AIDS, 1 apparently healthy homosexual, and, by contrast, in none of the control samples taken from 115 healthy heterosexual subjects.

What's more, Gallo then informed the French that he had identified antibodies produced in response to the new virus, something that he knew had so far confounded them. This would be the foundation for a screening test, the Holy Grail in any epidemic, and a veritable gold mine. Whoever was awarded rights to such a tool would earn royalties for every pint of blood tested, many millions of dollars for whichever institute got there first. Gallo called his findings abundant, and said he planned to publish them in five separate journal articles—it was like slapping a full house on the table.

Montagnier kept his reaction to himself. He was still upset about how Gallo had misrepresented his paper, and relations between the two men had continued to deteriorate since. He behaved politely and held his tongue. So did Francoise Barré-Sinoussi, the ebullient young scientist who led the effort. She masked any disdain behind a pair of oversized tinted glasses, her signature.

Chermann was the only one present who still considered Gallo a friend and valued colleague. He was cordial in his reply. Was there a chance, he wondered, that HTLV-3 was the same virus as LAV? If that were the case, then Gallo's late discovery merely confirmed Montagnier's milestone discovery. Chermann gently reminded Gallo that they had sent him LAV samples almost a year ago. How had the two compared, he wondered?

Gallo had not made the comparison, he admitted. The French team found this fact deeply troubling. Protocol dictated much of how these matters were to be handled. Before declaring a new discovery, Gallo was obliged to disambiguate his virus from Montagnier's and, if that failed and they appeared to be the same pathogen, abandon his attempt to give it a new name. That was the worldwide practice going back a hundred years. Nonetheless, with a handshake, both labs agreed to swap new viral samples and conduct the comparisons in unison. Better late than never.

In the meantime, however, Gallo said his own announcement was going forward, tied to publication dates for his five papers. Gallo left the meeting mistakenly convinced that a bond of collegiality existed among them all.

Altman managed to uncover most of this in preparation for his article, even though Gallo did not return his phone calls. When he reached Mason for comment, the CDC head learned details of the high-stakes catfight for the first time—Gallo had failed to share with him a draft of his submitted articles, which would have been standard procedure. Mason thought the viruses would turn out to be the same. "Logic would lead you to believe that we are dealing with one agent with perhaps some closely related variants," he said.

The day after Altman's article appeared, Margaret Heckler, the Reagan administration's health secretary, gathered her top advisers for a hastily orchestrated press conference, called for the purpose of defending the home team against competitors and detractors alike. Gallo, sweat beading on his brow, stood at her side.

"Today we add another miracle to the long honor roll of American medicine and science," she began in a voice broken up by laryngitis. "Those who have disparaged this scientific search—those who have said we weren't doing enough—have not understood how sound, solid, significant medical research proceeds. From the first day that AIDS was identified in 1981, HHS scientists and their medical allies have never stopped searching for the answers to the AIDS mystery. Without a day of procrastination, the resources of the Public Health Service have been effectively mobilized." She then turned over the stage to "our eminent Dr. Robert Gallo . . . who directed the research that produced this discovery." In doing so, she skipped the paragraph in her speech, added at the insistence of James Mason and over the strenuous objections of Gallo, where she was to acknowledge the work of the French.

The French had no warning about the spectacle of American chauvinism, which came even before the planned comparison of HTLV-3 and LAV. Worse, Gallo told reporters he had not been able to study LAV. "They didn't have enough material to send to us," he lied.

James D'Eramo reached a member of the Pasteur team, Dr. David Klatzmann, by phone. He was unsparing. "We are pleased about the current excitement over LAV and HTLV-3. However, it is unfortunate that this excitement and interest has come only now, nearly a whole year since we first published our findings," he said. "[W]hen we discovered LAV in our lymphadenopathy and AIDS patients, we set out to characterize the biological and immunological properties of the virus which could link the virus to the cause of AIDS. Now, one year later, we have the evidence to say that LAV is the cause, and we believed that initially. I think Dr. Gallo has the same kind of evidence. Undoubtedly HTLV-3 and LAV are the same virus."

It took Chuck Ortleb to find out what else was being masked by this war of words. A slew of competing patent applications had already been filed related to the competing viruses. Gallo applied for a patent for himself and the National Cancer Institute in the car on the way to his press conference with Heckler. Several months before that, Montagnier and the Institut Pasteur had done the same with LAV. A dozen biotech companies were also seeking patents. One, Cambridge Bioscience, listed Gallo as a participant in its prospectus. The battlefronts were multiplying. And still there was not one researcher looking for a treatment.

JOE SONNABEND watched the news conference on television with a hand over his pounding heart. He was acquainted with Gallo and Montagnier equally. He respected their work and their intelligence. And while he was predisposed to doubt the existence of a new killer virus, he accepted that HTLV-3/LAV's pattern of attacking CD4 cells suggested that it contributed to the overall clinical portrait of the disease. Just what role it played was still mere speculation. In a few weeks, researchers fanned out to the "at-risk" communities with the (admittedly imprecise) antibody tests, discovering that 87 percent of junkies in the New York City area were already infected as were 65 percent of sexually active gay men in San Francisco. Surely this virus and this epidemic were intertwined. But how? "It takes much more work than isolation of a microorganism to attribute causation to it," Sonnabend said.

Watching how the news media reported on the Heckler spectacle filled Sonnabend with disgust. Not one reporter remarked on the cravenness of Gallo's conveniently changing his leukemia virus to a lymphotropic virus. "I watch all these things, and intrepid science reporters don't pay any attention," he told me. It seemed farcical to him, and he was far from alone. The prevailing feeling in the gay community was one of suspicion and doubt. A collective paranoia was settling in.

At the *Native,* James D'Eramo gave the staff a lesson in the four criteria that are typically met in order to prove the cause of a new disease. Scientists called these steps "Koch's Postulates," after the nineteenth-century microbiologist who elucidated them. The suspected agent (1) must be present in everyone suffering from the disease but in no one who is healthy; (2) must be isolated from the carrier and must be able to grow in pure culture; (3) when injected into a susceptible and healthy laboratory animal, must be detectable and produce disease; and (4) must be isolated from the newly infected animal and prove to be identical to the original sample. Only the second postulate had been met. Whether owing to the imprecision of the antibody test or not, researchers had only been able to find the virus in most, but not all, of the sick. And to date, no animal proved susceptible to the virus, not mice or palm-sized marmosets.

Without proof that HTLV-3 caused AIDS, it could be equally plausible to say that the virus was just part of another opportunistic infection, a bug that tended to proliferate in people whose immune systems were already impaired—not a cause but a symptom. Or it could be complete coincidence.

"It's a huge stretch to call this settled science," D'Eramo said.

Weeks later, Ortleb blasted into the office waving a book above his head, smiling tightly with rage. "You have to read this," he shouted. "It's all in here. Everything the government is capable of doing, every reason they're doing it."

He turned the jacket to us ostentatiously. The book, *Bad Blood: The Tuskegee Syphilis Experiment,* first published in 1981, was about a perverse Public Health Service experiment to chart the natural course of syphilis by deliberately withholding treatment from hundreds of infected and unwitting sharecroppers, regardless of the human cost to the subjects, their spouses and children, or their communities. Ortleb's eyes shot open and his face reddened. "Some of the same people involved in this are the same people involved in the CDC now. David Sencer *was involved*!" When the study was first revealed internally, Sencer—now the city health commissioner—waged a contorted campaign to continue withholding treatment.

"They did it to the blacks," Ortleb cried. "They let them die in the name of science. And now it's us, it's our turn. *We're the blacks now.*"

Ray Nocera, our business manager, had just finished the book and was equally riled by it. "We're getting all our AIDS information from the government. Well, *thank you very much*, it's the same fucking government who brought us Tuskegee and god knows what else that we don't know about. *Hello? Hello?*"

Tom Steele yanked a cigarette from his teeth and began tearing through a messy tower of papers on his desk. "There was a CIA plot to destabilize Cuba," he said, producing a 1977 article from *The Boston Globe* about an intentional outbreak of ASFV in Havana. Things started falling together in his mind. "A plot to cripple Fidel Castro's economy by killing the pigs. They needed the CDC's help—only it went sideways."

"What do you mean, sideways?" someone asked.

"Crossed species," Ortleb answered. "And then the business with the gay Cuban boat people—the Mariel boat people."

Sweat glistened on Steele's forehead. "They *did* this to us," he said softly. "How do they think they're going to get away with it?"

Whether this grand flourish of speculation was feverish paranoia or a plausible hypothesis, none of us could be sure immediately. Our minds reeled. Could HTLV-3 possibly be part of an elaborate cover-up to draw attention away from the bungled plot in Cuba? We knew how the CIA had covered its footprints in Chile, Zaire, and Vietnam. Could the cold war, of all things, be the reason for the plague? It seemed absurd on its face. But being gay in America, with all we had already witnessed and knew, not one of us could hold the government above suspicion.

Over the coming months, Ortleb tightened his mind around the pig virus to the point of parody. He gave up eating pork. He imagined a backlash after receiving unrelated calls from a USDA staffer, a reporter for a veterinary wire service, and "an 'interested' American," all concerned about his campaign to expose ASFV. He soon banned the use of the phrase "the AIDS virus" as shorthand for the Gallo/Montagnier contenders, convinced beyond reason by his unorthodox theory.

One morning that fall, the staff got to work to find that the place had been looted. Gone were the Selectric and other costly machinery. Ortleb changed locks, and installed hasps on the file cabinets. It seemed like the burglar was interested in things that could be fenced more than things that could be published, but Ortleb was taking no chances. His preoccupations and neuroses grew alarmingly. He hired an armed guard to patrol the two-room office every night. But when the petty cash went missing—a crime of opportunity to which the guard soon confessed—his sense of imperilment only multiplied. He and Tom Steele would leave together at night, evasively varying their routes home, usually through a succession of bars. The staff suspected Ortleb was managing his fears with drink.

One morning that winter his fevers reached a darker depth. He arrived unusually late, in mid-afternoon, having missed many meetings. His face was a brand-new tapestry, sleep deprived and twitchy. His voice jumped on jangled nerves.

"Last night after Francis and I went to bed, the FBI broke into the apartment. We heard them in the living room. We barricaded the bedroom door, but for hours we could hear them out there going through everything, every scrap of paper, whispering—for hours!" He looked at us one by one, silently baptizing each of us with his news. I looked away, embarrassed. "The locksmiths were there all morning," he said, "putting deadbolts on the bedroom door."

It all seemed quite unlikely, though the inconsistencies didn't seem to bother Ortleb. Why would the FBI be interested in him? Why would they break into his apartment—at night, with two men holed up in the other room? He saw these questions in our silence. "I'm about to embarrass the United States government," he said impatiently, "and destroy the $10 billion pork industry."

The paper that had been so pivotal in prosecuting the AIDS war had gone off its tracks. But there was no other outlet for AIDS news, so the staff and the readers stayed put so long as Ortleb permitted the publication of more verifiable stories alongside his obsessions.

SHORTLY AFTER SUNRISE on a glorious morning in New York City, Peter Staley strode off the elevator on the ninth floor of J. P. Morgan's towering headquarters at 15 Broad Street, crossed the company's U.S. bond-trading floor, and dropped into his seat the way a fighter pilot took his cockpit. He clamped a telephone between his chin and shoulder and called the broker he used more than any other, Lou Olivieri, of the firm Garban PLC. Like Staley, Olivieri had little interest in the profession's chaotic social bravado or its temperamental machismo. This morning, as every morning, they spoke only of the overnight markets, the morning papers, the day's strategy.

Staley scanned the room. Acoustically, the trading floor reminded him of the vast casino halls he enjoyed visiting in Atlantic City, though the similarities ended with the din. What animated the flashing machines and felt-covered tables of Resorts International Casino were dreams of fortunes that evaporated one nest egg at a time. Here everyone won, or they wouldn't be here. And while the casino housed a teeming cross-section of American life, this room was no more diverse than any corporate boardroom. All but one of them male, every one of them white. And only a single, closeted gay.

The floor was laid out like a modified gladiators' coliseum, arranged into three tiers of descending rings; on each level was a row of opposing desks. The inward-facing loop was occupied by a swelter of twitchy young men in shirtsleeves: the bond traders, whose brashness drove so much of New York's culture in the 1980s. The bond traders at Salomon Brothers were far more notorious, but the men of Mother Morgan bore the same solemn responsibility with equal unruliness: they chewed up and spit out the debt of the U.S. government. Their workstations put them nose to nose with the company's sales associates, arranged in outward-facing desks. While the traders bought and sold from the other primary banks, it was the sales team's job to ply the secondary market, clients such as Saudi Arabia, Yale University, or the California Pension Fund. Every trader and sales agent was glued to a telephone, and a spikey chorus of calls and responses interlocked each row.

The hierarchy on the floor was vertical. In the center of the room, on the lowest platform, sat the most important men in the room, the high-volume traders, those buying and selling two-year notes and thirty-year Treasury bonds. They were the moguls of the bond market, easily taking home $1 million or more a year. The Pit, as their domain was known, set the tone in the room. When markets lurched in their favor they might leap from their seats with simian roars; when deals went wrong, they'd bray in recriminatorial invective.

Up on the second row sat a no more modest bunch with a slightly more modest portfolio: specialists in the one-year or nine-month Treasury notes, the same securities merchandized by the salesmen sitting across from them. Everything about the medium traders paled slightly in comparison to their counterparts in the Pit, but their power was formidable. Ululations from them were a bellwether of the global economy.

Staley sat on the third and final tier, a position of comparative exile. After completing the training program, he was thrilled to land an assignment in U.S. "govies," which was quite a coup, though he was on the lowest rung: not even short bonds, but something called the "short-shorts." Traders of short-shorts dealt in old notes and bonds, instruments issued long ago that had less than two years remaining to mature—for example, a thirty-year bond that was now twenty-nine years old. There was little action in these vintage instruments, and very little money to be made. Banks didn't regard the business highly. This forced Staley to lower his expectations for a bonus to augment his base pay. At J. P. Morgan, Staley was the only man on the short-shorts. In the entire financial world, just twenty-four traders plied the short-short market. But he knew others had risen—or, more accurately, descended—to bigger portfolios in the past, and he was determined to convert the assignment up in the bleachers into a brief and profitable first chapter.

Coming directly from Oberlin College, that utopia of progressivism, he was unprepared for the barbarism on daily display on the trading floor. Tempers were volcanic. Several times a week, some hideous and costly outcome gave cause for a trader to slam his telephone against his cubicle or a salesman's chair or one of the room's many pillars, with such force that plastic shards shot across several tiers. Almost without variation, the targets of rage were "fags," "pansies," "sissies," "fairies," "cocksuckers," or "queers." Paired with a limited list of approved adjectives, the damning epithets could comprise a major portion of the day's verbiage, the way the names of specialized instruments filled the ear in a dentist's office. Staley never responded, never gave a blink of umbrage. He learned early on that the financial culture was as rarefied as an NFL locker room. Even his older brother Jes, assigned to Mother Morgan's São Paulo headquarters, had developed one of the most homophobic syntaxes Staley had ever encountered. Staley just kept quiet and trained his attention on the three green-hued trading screens on his desktop, shutting out every explosive distraction to give his undivided attention to the life cycles and idiosyncrasies of the short-shorts, with all the intensity of an arachnologist.

Happily, the work fascinated him and the short-shorts began revealing their secrets. Every six months they produced interest payments, called coupons, which were automatically added to the holder's cash balances and invested accordingly. For calculating how the coupons increased the value of the bond, Staley could see on the green screens before him that the industry assumed they earned an arbitrary interest rate, about 6 percent, considerably below the prevailing rate, which was 20 percent or higher. That, in fact, was the number that flashed on his data screens, and the glowing terminals facing each of the twenty-three other short-short primary traders worldwide. Everyone relied upon that number to determine "buy" and "sell" prices. They made their money buying at those published prices and quickly reselling to large corporate investors at tiny markups, an eighth of a percentage point here and there.

He took out a calculator and ran an experiment. Using a formula that took into account true interest rates, he found that the difference between the presumed value of the short-shorts and their actual value to the holder was consistent. If he could buy a million-dollar block of short-shorts that he considered undervalued and hold on to them for a period of months, the difference between the green line on the screen and the actual yield during that period would be pure profit for the bank. Similarly, he could bet against a million-dollar block—shorting it, in Wall Street parlance—and mine a similar return. And if he bet long and short in equal numbers, he could bring his risk down close to zero, a practice known as arbitrage—something no one had done before in the short-shorts. With little fanfare, Staley began accumulating long and short positions in various bundles—amassing a portfolio that at times surpassed $1 billion. Working with such a huge quantity of securities was unheard of among the short-short fraternity, but it allowed him to project between $1 million and $5 million in profits for the bank, significantly higher than anything the other short-short traders were delivering.

The key to succeeding with this approach was to keep the other short-shorters—whether in Tokyo or London, or nearby at Solomon Brothers or Goldman Sachs—unaware of what he was doing. To maintain his stealth, Staley relied on brokerage firms to act as his intermediaries. Their desks were patched to his switchboard: the enormous Cantor Fitzgerald, with headquarters at the World Trade Center; Fundamental Brokers Interdealer, located around the corner; and Garban, whose U.S. offices were at 120 Broadway. Lou Olivieri was Garban's specialist in the short-short market. Of all the brokers, Staley found him among the most nimble and by far the most simpatico. Not once did he profane the gays. (Only years later would Olivieri come out of the closet himself.)

Staley began using Olivieri exclusively, and after a time Olivieri took calls from no one else. Staley got Olivieri on the phone first thing every morning, and typically kept his voice glued to his ear until closing time. It was a relationship of symbiosis. The more money Staley made for J. P. Morgan, the more Olivieri made for Garban—and the more Garban kicked back to Staley in perquisites, the sub-currency of the Street. Staley began enjoying lavish meals courtesy of Olivieri, limousines at his disposal, private helicopter shuttles to free weekends in Atlantic City, even Super Bowl tickets, though those were of little interest to him. In time, he wasn't shy about requesting alternatives, like front-row seats for Madonna's Virgin Tour, and—his most reckless request—tickets for Leontyne Price's farewell performance in *Aida* at the Met, almost a year in the future but impossible to find. (He would sit tenth row center.) He trusted Olivieri to draw no conclusions about his highbrow interests, or at least to keep his thoughts to himself.

This morning was like all others, with one exception. Tommy Kalaris, Morgan's revered head of the government bond department, had chosen today to sit in and do some trading himself—a kind of exhibition event. Kalaris had never shown special interest in Staley. Despite being barely older than thirty himself, he had earned a godly status at Mother Morgan. The room hushed as he took a desk in the Pit. In the moments before trading was to begin he made a Caesar-like gesture to the bleachers and issued a challenge.

"Huey Lewis and the News is playing tonight on the Pier," he called. "Who can get me tickets?" This was the summer "I Want a New Drug" was in heavy rotation on MTV. Scalpers, who had been getting thousands for each ticket, were sold out. Kalaris delivered a baronial laugh. "The first person to get me tickets is gold!"

"You've got to get me these, I need this," Staley barked into the phone to Olivieri, who was renowned for his connections to scalpers. "I know you can do this." Within moments Staley was able to shout down from the rafters. "I got 'em!" When Kalaris looked up at him with a quizzical smile, Staley added a cocky flourish. "How many do you want?"

Kalaris smiled. "One for me and my girlfriend, and if you want to come make it three."

Moments like that made enormous careers.

• • •

THE SUMMER OF 1984 saw a fulcrum of disease in the gay ghetto. At St. Vincent's, the emergency room was visible behind enormous windows on the corner of West Eleventh Street and Seventh Avenue. Before the crisis exploded, how many hundreds of times had I walked past the window oblivious to the small Kabuki dramas enacted there? Now I found myself choked with panic anytime I came near. One sticky afternoon, I slowed to measure the epidemic through the plate glass, praying to see only strangers. Three-quarters of the seats were filled. Scanning the rows I could see that every third or fourth man had "The Look"—sunken cheeks, sparse hair, eyes that showed fear, shoulders that bent in pain. One, all spots and bones, balanced painfully on a pillow he'd brought along from home. Another seemed to be dozing; his head was cocked backward onto a companion's arm, and his mouth and eyes were both wide open. The blind, like horses and snakes, don't need to close their eyes to sleep.

A cab pulled up beside me. A healthy man, first out the door, bent to carefully extract his frail companion from the backseat, an operation as ordered and precise as origami. I held open the hospital door and, blinkered by their mission, they picked past me without a nod. They were no older than I was. I remained on the sidewalk for a long time, watching them navigate the admissions process and settle into bucket seats to await their turn, the healthy partner whispering nonstop into his lover's nodding, sweaty head.

That was my experience with early AIDS. I stood on the sidewalks of the plague, grateful to not enter its tower.

That changed when Tom Ho took ill. Tall and thin and always in white denim jeans, Ho was the assistant art director at the *Native,* and my closest friend there. We were the youngest on the editorial staff, both twenty-five. He swung from health to sickness with disorienting suddenness. I found his room at the elbow of a long hallway inside Lenox Hill Hospital on the Upper East Side. He was propped up in his bed and staring sluggishly out the window, his face still a topography of youthful acne. He was somewhat embarrassed to see me and the box of chocolates I held up in my defense, but nonetheless he welcomed me into his room and his medical journey. His voice expressed amazement, as though he were recounting the events in a film: how he had drenched his bed with sweat, then his own feces, which emptied from him violently; how the pneumonia burned his lungs and robbed his mind of oxygen; how he hadn't told his parents—could never tell his parents. He was born to immigrants, and all that entailed. "I was the kid who grew up in the back of the Chinese restaurant at the strip mall. Doing my homework, folding napkins. They never let me out of their sight, never let me go to another kid's house. I celebrated my birthdays there, all alone with a cake." He straddled three worlds with no overlap: China, America, and gay. And now a fourth: the world of the plague. "They have no idea I'm gay—that alone would kill them."

At the *Native* I had edited and he had pasted up endless horror stories of patients dying in isolation. It was heartbreaking to watch him adjust to the stoicism such loneliness required.

He stared through the window for a long time, ruminating. "The only option I have," he said finally, shaking his head, "is to beat this thing."

He didn't lack an ability to situate his plight in the epidemic's unforgiving time line. "Who do you think will be next?" he asked me. He speculated about Gary in advertising and Bruce in the art department. "Bruce is getting skinny, did you notice? He's got 'The Look.'" That was Bruce's usual appearance; he never did contract AIDS.

"How about Peter?" I asked. "He's been out sick a lot."

He smiled. "If Peter escapes this, it's not contagious."

I would never see Tom Ho again, to my lasting shame. Later, I heard he had left the hospital and returned to his family in the suburbs, having finally told them the truth. I learned that he slid into dementia and it took him more than two years to die. But I mourned his passing that day I left the hospital as if he were already gone, as the old hands in Auschwitz did for those they distastefully called *Muselmänner,* the dead who hadn't died yet, a mere technicality. The look in his eyes seared me, yes, but I was not yet numb from death, just terrified of it to the point of hypochondria and shameful behavior. I lifted my hand out of his with the same cold finality, and let my friend die the death he feared, isolated and alone, pulled back from his gay world through his American world and right back to the China of his parents' home, gone before he was gone.

I went from his bedside and immediately made an appointment to see Dr. Joan Waitkevicz, a lesbian physician in her forties, for a complete physical, and release, hopefully, from fear. She understood my panic and offered comforting words, but there was nothing concrete for me. The antibody tests, far from reliable as they were, were not yet approved for clinical use. Instead, she poked my arm with a four-prong purified protein derivative test, originally developed as a screen for tuberculosis but being used by doctors as an imperfect AIDS test. In patients with no immunity whatsoever, the four pricks would leave no marks. She sent me home to hope my immune system would create bumps. To my relief, marvelous, plump boils appeared on my arm. This gave me no insights into my future, but at least it told me I would not drop dead anytime soon.

THOUGH WE LIVED a couple of dozen blocks apart, I hadn't seen much of Brian Gougeon for several months. He struggled for seclusion from the world of news and doom where I dwelled. The real world distracted him from his art, which he kept producing, though without an audience, and his lack of success frustrated him to the point of isolation. So I was surprised when he called and invited me to a party. "Doug Gould's in town," he said. "It is what it is. So we're having a party."

Doug Gould was Gougeon's boyfriend from college, the one he'd returned to recently. I had known Doug for a long time. He was a shy, pot-adoring theater major, with soft black eyes and a large Afro, a benefit of being half Cherokee (the other half was Scottish). On campus, he kept to a small group of friends. Ironically, we had double-dated once in freshman year, when we were both still seeing women. When he realized his mistake in that regard, in our sophomore year, he came out with little tension and no fanfare, becoming the only out gay person on campus. As I struggled with my own authenticity, he was the first person I reached out to. He amazed me with the list of our classmates he'd had sex with, which is how I learned how many of us there were.

Shortly after he first paired with Gougeon, he came to the conclusion that higher education was not his calling. He had trouble rising for class or mustering interest in the core requirements, and his gradual failure in academe caused a crushing anxiety, which he talked about often until the day he gave himself permission to leave. Landing two hours away in Chicago meant he returned to campus most weekends with news of life outside. He had joined a young Chicago stage troupe called the Steppenwolf Theatre Company, taking responsibility for their light board and appearing occasionally in their productions. During his visits to see us he would produce Polaroids of his new circle of friends, names not yet known outside the local stage: John Malkovich, Glenne Headley, Laurie Metcalf, Gary Sinise, Joan Allen.

And now, his success was turning into acclaim. "He's in New York with a play," Gougeon told me. "He's in *Balm in Gilead* as a drag queen with a big bushy moustache. It's hilarious. Anyway, come to the party. It'll be a scene."

I arrived late with a date, at a packed apartment in Hell's Kitchen. Gougeon looked well, if somewhat underweight. I noticed that the knobs on his neck seemed more pronounced, exaggerated perhaps by his weight loss. But for me the real surprise was Doug Gould, holding court on the fire escape off a living room window. His hair was an enormous black halo tufting in the breeze as he garrulously recounted his experience of sharing an awkward supper with David Bowie, who had treated the entire cast to an evening on the town. Everything about Gould seemed different. Around his neck he wore a knotted cravat, and on his wrist a heavy silver bracelet. His was a marvelous transformation, the look of arrival.

Gougeon snuck up behind me and whispered in my ear, "I'm going back to the Midwest. I've been talking to a guy there about a museum show. Which means I've got a lot of work to do. I need a break from the distractions of New York." He and Gould caught eyes across the smoky room. "And then there's Doug. What can you do? It feels right." Before the summer was over, Gougeon was packed and gone.

BOBBI CAMPBELL and his message of patient empowerment were in great demand, leading to urgent invitations for him to address people with AIDS in New Orleans, Miami, Atlanta, Washington, Seattle, Dallas, and Los Angeles. He appeared on *Nightline,* the late-night ABC news program, and on Phil Donahue's show. On June 28, he was in New York to give one of his inspirational talks and to attend the fifteenth-annual Gay Pride March, reuniting with PWA leaders from around the nation. On that weekend, he fulfilled his biggest dream, formally incorporating the National Association of People With AIDS to further the work begun in Denver the year before.

Campbell returned home in time for the Democratic National Convention, which opened in San Francisco on July 15, 1984. On a gusty afternoon, he stood on a stage across from the Moscone Center with his lover at his side, delivering a well-paced and strident keynote speech to 100,000 protesters demanding a candidate who would respond to the crisis. He looked fragile and tired, but his connection to the crowd was electric and his voice was strong, echoing across the sea of heads.

"I have a message for the nation," he said. "Very often lesbians and gay men are portrayed as isolated, alienated, and alone or else in a pathetic search for desperate sexuality. I don't think that that's true. And I think that it's important for people to understand that lesbians and gay men do not exist outside of a context. We exist in the context of the people we love and those that love us." As the crowd roared, he and Bob Hilliard embraced and kissed.

"I have a message to the person with AIDS who may be in Des Moines or Indianapolis or in Queens or anywhere: Keep the faith baby, I love you!"

Campbell cemented his place as the preeminent infected militant. But his whirlwind efforts took a toll on him. A few days later, a nasty case of shingles engulfed his head, leaving behind a field of deep scars. And in a few weeks he entered the hospital with a brain stem overrun with cryptococcal meningitis, a horrifically painful experience. When the news reached New York City, Michael Callen bought a card to cheer him up, with a photo of the performer Divine in a nurse's uniform menacingly hoisting an enema bag. "How many of this card have you gotten? It's just so you!" he wrote. "Get well! That's an order!"

But Campbell never saw the note. Bob Hilliard, standing at Campbell's side just as he had been on the cover of *Newsweek*, watched helplessly as the blood pressure monitor fell from one hundred to fifty, then forty, then zero. Instinctively he allowed the medical staff space for gently removing all the hoses and pipes and devices from Campbell's spent body. At precisely noon on August 15, 1984, a month to the day after his memorable last address, Campbell ended his battle. He was thirty-two years old.

News of the death spread quickly through San Francisco. It wasn't long before someone at the Badlands bar took the big chalk stick and wrote on the blackboard, "Love After Death for Bobbi." Knowing how devastated the community was, the city shut down Castro Street for his funeral cortege two days later. Mourners filled the intersection Campbell had tried to commandeer on New Year's Eve, the place on the map he used to call "my office." Hundreds of bereaved men and women arrived through the dusky light, followed by hundreds more. Soon a sea of grief stretched down the hill past the famous Castro Theater into the next intersection and beyond—a thousand people standing hushed in Bobbi Campbell's honor. Whether through his work as a nurse or as a tireless AIDS advocate, or through the blessings he bestowed while dressed as "Sister Florence Nightmare, RN," Campbell's gift of courage and leadership had touched the community like nobody else.

The eulogies were touching and stridently political. Holly Near and

Lea DeLaria sang militant tributes. A bit of footage from Campbell's recent speech flickered on a large screen over the stage, momentarily returning him to his beloved people. "I have a message for the lesbian and gay community," he was saying, as if from beyond. "It's important to understand that sex does not cause disease. Homosexuality does not cause disease. Germs do. Learn and practice safe sex."

The throng on Castro Street nodded silently to his manifesto. But then the voice of Campbell added something they had trouble accepting. "It's important for us to learn about AIDS," he said, "but not to panic. There is no reason to become hysterical." At that moment it seemed that there was ample reason for hysteria. The AIDS Poster Boy was gone.

The bad news was piling on. A new study from D.C. in which healthy-appearing gay men were screened for signs of viral infection showed a prevalence rate of 60 to 70 percent, men just like those filling Castro Street. Using conservative estimates of the number of gay men in the country, that meant that eight million were marked for a death just as cutting as Campbell's. A cataclysm awaited the community.

About a week after the massive memorial service, which failed to garner coverage in the East Coast media, a large envelope from Bob Hilliard arrived at the *Native* offices. Inside he'd written a note. "Bobbi Campbell died yesterday, August 15, of AIDS-related meningitis at San Francisco General Hospital." This was how we received the awful news. In the course of my reporting, I had spoken to Campbell on the telephone, but we had never met. I still kept his famous *Newsweek* cover, which had given me such affirmation. Reading Hilliard's note, I wept angrily.

Hilliard went on to say, "The enclosed was found among his papers, stamped and sealed. It seems clear to us that Bobbi intended the letter to be sent. So we are forwarding it to you for publication. Thank you for complying with what was surely among his final wishes."

I carefully smoothed Campbell's last communiqué onto my desktop. It was not a farewell. It carried no hint of the opportunistic infection that would sneak up on him so violently. Instead it was a letter to the editor, addressing the article I ran about the bathhouse battle. In his quiet voice and with gentle optimism, he warned against moral absolutism on either side. "AIDS partisans are not either 'traitors' or 'murderers' or 'heroes,'" he said, levelheaded to the end. My hands trembled as I sat at the enormous photo offset machine and set his last public words into crisp columns of type.

• • •

NATIONALLY, the community's efforts to deal with the bathhouses and backroom clubs never got more in sync. In San Francisco, health officials now required sex venues to make prevention information available to patrons; not so in New York. Most community leaders here stood behind the suggested guidelines drafted by Dr. Roger Enlow's working group, which adopted the name the Coalition for Sexual Responsibility. They included requesting the clubs *voluntarily* to distribute free condoms and safe sex literature, use high levels of chlorine in swimming pools and Jacuzzis, and make water-based lubricants and soap available, in individual packages or pump-top dispensers. From anecdotal reports, only the St. Mark's Baths and the East Side Sauna were in compliance. Management at St. Mark's even went a step beyond, asking patrons to sign a safe sex pledge. Unlike most of the other sex venues, St. Mark's was owned by a gay man. At the dozen or more other bathhouses and sex clubs, most owned by shadowy corporations or suspected mobsters, it was business as usual.

In the months since Richard Berkowitz had left town, Callen had moved inexorably, if temporarily, into the very small camp of leaders who believed the baths should be forcibly shuttered, even if that meant turning over the keys to the city. Short of that he favored making compliance with the Coalition for Sexual Responsibility's campaigns mandatory instead of voluntary. Even that proposal angered the other members. The health department required every restaurant in the city to hang posters illustrating the Heimlich maneuver, he pointed out at a recent forum on the "bathhouse controversy." Why not use the same power to mandate safe sex posters?

"I won't dignify that question with an answer," replied Enlow, the city's official AIDS liaison.

Meanwhile, all the available evidence suggested that the community was clamoring for useful information to govern their behavior. When pressed, GMHC admitted that a third of the 1,500 monthly calls to their AIDS hotline came from men asking about the safety of the baths and sex clubs, among other health issues. But according to their hotline coordinator, they would no more tell a caller not to go than they would reprimand a bathhouse for refusing their posters. In fact, GMHC held its summer fund-raising event at the recalcitrant Mineshaft, a sex club of the least hygienic order. So on a warm summer night, Callen set out on a tour of the baths for an article that might embarrass the community into action. He arrived at the Club Baths on lower First Avenue at about 7:30. He pulled out a small notebook, Sam Spade style, to record his observations.

"Club Baths located next to Ortiz Funeral Home," he noted. "How convenient. Like Sweeney Todd's recycling center."

He paid $17.50, exchanged his street clothing for a towel, and surveyed the scene. There was no risk-reduction information on the bulletin board. In the glass display case there were condoms, but only petroleum-based lubricant, which would dissolve latex and render condoms useless. Wandering through the labyrinth, he counted twenty men: eight blacks, five Latinos, two Asians, and five whites. The racial distribution of the patrons suggested that news of the plague was reaching white men more effectively than minorities, which made sense, given that the *Native* mostly ignored people of color and GMHC's safe sex literature mostly depicted Caucasians. He made a note about the importance of translating brochures and posters into other languages.

But he had to admit he saw no unsafe sex, although what was meant by "safe" was more confusing than ever. From all the intake interviews Callen helped to conduct at Sonnabend's office, it was clear that transmission required anal penetration, with rare exceptions. And yet nobody from the Public Health Service would state this clearly. Making matters worse, the esteemed Dr. Gallo had begun declaring that a peck on the lips was reckless, and a kiss with a tongue was suicide. "I know it's not good news and no one likes the bearer of bad news," he told a colleague at the *Native,* "but I think we will have facts that speak for themselves regarding this, and anyone advocating, go ahead and do a lot of kissing is crazy, in my judgment."

Callen saw a lot of kissing as he circled the hallways, along with mutual masturbation. To the architect of safe sex, it was gratifying at least to see people adopting simple precautions. Still, knowing how many men lost their lives from encounters in those halls, the fact that anyone was there at all, much less in an aroused state, was disturbing to him. Something that Richard Berkowitz once said came back into his mind: going to the baths for sex in 1984 was like returning to Auschwitz for a romantic getaway.

Glancing through a half-closed door, Callen saw a naked black man in his forties sitting alone on a bed in a tiny cubicle. The man kicked the door open and gave a friendly smile. "Smoke a joint?" he called.

Callen declined the smoke but entered the cubicle anyway. The bed gave a heave when he sat on the edge. The nook also held an austere side table and nothing else. The walls were made of thin metal sheets that did not extend as high as the ceiling. The sounds of intimacy spilled overhead from distant corners of the building. Callen let out a dramatic sigh. "I feel weird," he said. "I haven't been to the baths in two and a half years." He looked squarely at his host. "Aren't you worried about AIDS?"

He was not, the man explained, *because he was selective*. He felt confident that he could tell who was infectious and who was not, and he rigorously avoided the former. People with AIDS looked tired, he said.

Callen wanted to blurt out, Can you tell about me? Do I look like someone with AIDS? But he held his tongue. He was there for information, not to correct misimpressions.

"Do you read a lot about AIDS?"

"Too much," the man groaned. In the first years, he had devoured every word of speculation and advice. But he had stopped reading the depressing alerts long ago.

Callen headed toward his locker in a funk. And as he was checking out he looked around the lobby for copies of the new safe sex pamphlet the coalition had recently unveiled with fanfare. If the man had been handed one along with his towel, his dangerous self-deceptions might have fallen away. No pamphlets were in sight. Callen asked the clerk if he had seen any, and the young man pulled open drawers and tore open boxes, rifling his booth until he found a buried supply. He pushed a single copy across the counter to Callen and reinterred the rest.

That Wednesday, Callen continued his stealth investigation with the purchase of a pass to the East Side Sauna, on the fourth floor of a nondescript building on East Fifty-sixth Street. Posters about the Alvin Ailey dance troupe, a running club, and various community groups hung from bulletin boards, but no mention of the epidemic. Here he did see one man penetrating another without a condom, though whether to completion was unclear (and whether that mattered was not yet settled), and he heard moans coming from behind the doors of a few closed cubicles. But the scene here was extremely tame compared to what had existed before.

He got a similar impression the following Saturday at the Everard, the bathhouse with the most notorious reputation for dingy hedonism. Callen had never been there before, so his sense of the place came mostly from Larry Kramer's foul description in *Faggots*. It did not disappoint. In place of literature he found mold and mildew. And plenty of sex. From his station in the steam room, he saw practices that reminded him of earlier days. There was a democratic quality to the lust: men crossing class and age barriers, the good looking with the plain, the light and the dark. He had forgotten that aspect of sexual abandon, and missed it. He thought about his own longings in sex, his gentle contacts with strangers who, stripped of rank and naked of class, might have been doctors or errand boys. How revolutionary it was, how playful, how validating.

And then, remembering the plague, he fled.

Late one night as he worked through his thoughts before writing, he confided his revulsion to Sonnabend. Sonnabend stridently believed that closing the baths was useless and wrong, constituting a war against gay sexuality, not necessarily against AIDS. The problem, he said, was that the *opportunity* of the baths was being squandered. "Look," he said, "at least have other materials out there which we can feel sure will not be—how can I put it?—undermining of a person's homosexuality in the slightest way."

"AIDS," Callen fired back, his voice soaring an octave, "is undermining of a person's homosexuality."

"That's bullshit," Sonnabend snapped. "I suppose one's entitled to hate oneself, and to act on it. But really, I don't think you're entitled to act on hurting other people."

Callen was seething. "What I mean is, the psychological fallout from AIDS—"

"You have to fall over *backwards* to make it positive."

"Let me ask you this hypothetical," Callen said after a beat. "If your choice was between sound medical advice without a gay-positive message or GMHC's slathering about gay positive without any medical advice, which would you chose?"

"I suppose being alive comes first."

"Yes!"

But meanwhile, despite the discord among the AIDS leaders, the community was getting the message. By July, three of the city's twelve bathhouses had closed voluntarily, presumably from lack of customers.

BY OCTOBER, Callen was confined to a bed in room 557 of the Spellman Tower at St. Vincent's Hospital, tethered at the vein to a dripping bag of medicine. At first he had hoped it was flu. Then the tingling began in the leg—like needles pushing out from deep within the tissue. A simple rash gave way to an exquisitely painful knot of blisters—a violent case of shingles. Sonnabend might have taken this as the predictable outcome of a stressful life, which can reawaken the dormant virus that causes chicken pox in children, only now in a more virulent form called herpes zoster. Aging can also trigger the dormant infection. But so can immune deficiency. Callen was fascinated by the development. He allowed a friend to take portrait-studio photographs, and called me with the news, which triggered another of my breathless panics. My own case of shingles had been severe and transient—but was it AIDS related? I ran again to Dr. Waitkevicz for another four-pronged prick test, and failed to find much relief when the raised bumps came.

Sonnabend sent Callen to the hospital. Until recently, except for pain medicine there was no treatment for shingles—or for any virus. But the FDA had just approved a drug called acyclovir for treating various herpes infections, including genital herpes and shingles. An imperfect drug that merely lessened the pain of outbreaks rather than destroy the virus itself, acyclovir nonetheless showed for the first time that the course of a virus's cycle could be interrupted. Millions began taking it at the first sign of genital lesions and as a result were able to resume sexual activity sooner. But in AIDS patients, reactivated herpes zoster promised severe and sometimes life-threatening developments, requiring intravenous administration, which required hospitalization.

Callen was restless and miserable. No one from the nursing staff had seen him since his arrival. He hadn't even been given food or beverage. Now it was late afternoon and although he buzzed and buzzed, no one came. Finally, a middle-aged man threw open the door, giving Callen a view of food trays stacked on the floor outside. Did the staff still fear casual contact in 1984? Then Callen remembered glimpsing the new *Village Voice* on his way to admitting. The cover story unhelpfully declared that Gallo might have found HTLV-3 in saliva. Were they now afraid of spoons and forks that touch the tongue?

The man at the door wore a surgical gown and was further defended by latex gloves and an ear-to-ear surgical mask. Only his eyes were visible, and they looked away with disinterest—a reminder of Callen's own barriers when he accompanied Sonnabend to the AIDS wards. Was this man picking up "the smell," like slightly rotten oranges sprayed over with Lysol—the stench of hopelessness? Callen inhaled deeply. No odors stood out. But then he wondered whether, being the dying one, he couldn't discern his own rot.

The bundled visitor was not there in response to his urgent buzzing. He turned out to be from the hospital's technical staff. Circling the room as far away from Callen's bed as possible, he reached up and adjusted a switch to enable the rental TV. By coincidence, the television came to life just as Archbishop O'Connor announced a new front in the battle against Koch's Executive Order 50. The technician retreated without a word, and without bending to fetch Callen his breakfast or lunch.

Callen didn't speak either. He watched this scene as from another world, then jotted down notes about "the quintessential image of an urban gay man in the Reagan 'eighties: sick, shunned, frightened and frightening; and largely unprotected by either law or popular opinion." He reconsidered the line about "the Reagan 'eighties," and changed its spelling to "the Reagan AIDIES," which gave him a smile, despite the circumstances. "There in the largest gay ghetto on the East Coast," he wrote, "I found myself dependent on the kindness of some very strange strangers."

The acyclovir did its work with amazing quickness. Callen was out of St. Vincent's by the following Saturday, though not well enough for a Lowlife performance at the Pyramid Club scheduled for that Tuesday. Regrettably, he canceled and spent that week giving blood samples to various labs and hospital clinics around the city.

When he was strong enough, Callen returned to his reporting on the literature-free zones of the gay bathhouses. But he was losing his nerve to publish his case for closing them. By early fall, the pendulum swung hard in San Francisco. Public Health Director Dr. Mervyn Silverman had crossed civil libertarians and angry mobs by unilaterally padlocking that city's six bathhouses, four sex clubs, two porno theaters, and two backroom bookstores. There wasn't much dissent in the community there, but the perception among everyday Americans was a big problem. Because the city failed to distinguish between sex that was safe and sex that wasn't, many outside the gay community saw gay men as reckless and foolhardy, driven by self-destructive carnal urges, just as the right wing had always assumed. Naturally, a new round of anti-gay condemnation ensued. Dr. Paul Cameron, chairman of the Nebraska-based Institute for the Scientific Investigation of Sexuality, called gays "worse than murderers" and demanded that, for the safety of the nation, "it should be illegal to be homosexual." In fact, in twenty-three states it already was.

In this environment, and with few allies, Callen felt it was wise to hold his fire. Only a few New Yorkers on the political fringes were joining the calls to padlock. Even Mayor Ed Koch considered closing the establishments a "foolish" public health move, as there was an endless array of other places ripe for sexual exhibition. At the *Native*, Ortleb's position had evolved significantly. Though initially indifferent to the civil rights implications of shutting the bathhouses, his growing hostility to government pushed him to the ramparts. "We sense too clearly that on this roller coaster called AIDS all kinds of well-intentioned evils can be done in the name of public health," he declared in an editorial (having embraced the Royal We through the authority of the epidemic). "In this era of the New Right, we know that there is no such thing as a minor infringement. First there is prayer in school; then there is a state religion. First you shut down the baths; then you shut down the bars. First you impede the sexually active; then you impede the gay couple." Making matters worse, this "first ominous step into your bedroom" was based on a mistaken linkage to a commercial establishment. "Bathhouses don't cause AIDS in Zaire, and they don't cause it in New York or San Francisco."

Callen removed himself from the acrid debate, or at least from the role as provocateur he had created for himself. But in a few weeks, Bishop Paul Moore Jr., the leading figure in the American Episcopal Church, lured him back in.

At a time when most religious leaders evangelized against gay sex, Moore was unusual. Under his liberal stewardship, the Episcopal Diocese of New York unreservedly cared for AIDS sufferers. He never distinguished between gay love and straight love—to the shock of his children many years later, it would be revealed that this policy governed his private life as well. Moore had great clout in the city and the nation, and used his power to become a leading critic of the government's inaction. (And he was having an impact, however minor. In response to his lobbying, Governor Mario Cuomo added $4.1 million for AIDS to the state budget that year, the state's first investment.)

Callen met Moore during a meeting with the governor in Albany, where he bit his tongue and mentioned nothing about the commercial sex venues. Nobody else did either. But on the train ride home, sitting between Moore and Peter Vogel, Cuomo's gay liaison, Callen was surprised when Moore shouted, over the din of the train, "We must talk about the baths."

This was all Callen needed to reawaken his bravado. In the most un-church-like language, he described what he had witnessed at the Everard, St. Mark's, and the East Side Sauna, including the lack of any health awareness campaign.

This had a powerful effect on Moore. "And nobody's telling them about the dangers?"

Vogel jumped in, saying that closing the baths risked "a domino effect" of increasing restrictions on gays and the places they gather. "If you close the baths then you'll close the bars, and then you'll say teachers can't be gay," he said.

"Oh come on, Peter. Now you're just full of bullshit," the bishop said. He proposed that the three of them jointly organize a quiet meeting of concerned individuals to feel out the issue without the pressure of the spotlights. But later, while Moore dozed, Vogel whispered to Callen. "You can't talk about these things to straight people."

"Peter, I really respect you and I know that you think you're helping people," Callen whispered back. "But you're letting people die. You're wrong on this issue. We *can* talk about it, we *have to talk about it*."

Reluctantly, Vogel agreed to convene Moore's quiet meeting.

Callen worried that he and the bishop would need reinforcements if they were to prevail. Though he now spent his days trying to find a dentist willing to examine his decaying teeth—the NYU School of Medicine, Beth Israel Medical Center, and Columbia Presbyterian were all unwilling to work on a PWA's mouth—he sandwiched in attempts to recruit co-conspirators against the baths, with little luck.

Then Callen remembered that nobody had a more anti-sex reputation than Larry Kramer. After a year in self-imposed exile in London, Cape Cod, and a log cabin in the woods outside Washington, D.C., Kramer had quietly returned to New York, resuming his city life, single and lonely after losing Rodger McFarlane's patience along the way. ("I'd had two years of Larry Kramer screaming and I just couldn't take it any longer," McFarlane told friends.)

Callen found Kramer's phone number late one chilly weeknight. "Is it too late to call you? I just wanted to find out what you think about the bathhouse issue—if you feel like talking about it."

"Oh, sure. I think they should close them," Kramer answered sleepily.

"Good," Callen said with exaggerated crispness.

"Actually, I don't think that *they* should close them. I think that *we* should close them," he said.

"Right. The reason I'm asking is, there's this secret meeting tomorrow that Peter Vogel has arranged. People from GMHC are going to be there." He rattled off a few names, including Paul Popham and McFarlane.

Hearing his ex-lover's name gave Kramer a start. "Where is it and what time?" he asked.

"It's at Bishop Moore's. Way the hell up on 110th, I think. But, they're not letting . . ." He was unsure how to put this.

Kramer understood immediately. "I'm going to try to go there," he said, taking down the exact address. "Thank you for telling me."

"Okay, so let me understand your position," Callen said, wanting to be absolutely clear. "It's that you'd like to see them closed and you'd like to see the community close them. But in the event that the community is unwilling, as it seems now, to even consider that possibility, where do you stand?"

"GMHC is against closing?"

"Rabid on the subject."

"Rabid? How dare they. Why?"

Callen nursed a dark theory that the big-budget AIDS organizations were cynically exploiting the baths, relying on them to produce more clients and justifying their salaries. "I don't know," he said cautiously.

"I don't think it should be confined to the baths," Kramer said. "I think it should also include places like the Mineshaft and the Anvil. Where do I stand about the city closing them? I just don't know. . . . I would like to see us picket them or something like that."

"Everybody thinks that education is the answer."

"That would be wonderful," Kramer said. "I think that education would be wonderful, but no one is out there saying there are four new cases a day. I don't hear that from anybody. The media's not doing anything. . . . Why isn't anybody yelling?" He produced a muffled moan upon realizing the yelling would have to come from him—again—when he had turned his life in another direction. The roman à clef he went to Europe to write had turned into a play, a barely fictionalized account of the GMHC battles. "I'm hoping it's going to be done at the Public," he said. "And I have to get new pages over to Mrs. Papp by Friday. I'll know in the vicinity of three tomorrow if I'll be able to come to the meeting or not," he told Callen.

"Anyway," Kramer added, "I feel like I've been a coward in all this."

"Come on, Larry. That's not a word *anybody* would use to describe you."

"Well, I do. I feel like I've let everybody down because the kind of pressure I was putting on, nobody is doing it now. And that was very useful. That's what the media pays attention to, and I was very good at that. . . . That's why I'm doing the play. But if I get sucked back into the community, it'll take away from the writing."

"I know. I'm in a band with my lover." Though the two had shared numerous foxholes over the years, this was the first time Callen had revealed to Kramer anything about his personal life that was unrelated to immune dysfunction.

"So you understand," Kramer said. Then he remembered Callen's very public battle to survive. "How are you feeling?"

"I'm feeling well," he said, reaching for optimism, "but I just got test results back last Friday, and they're the second-lowest ever. So. What can you do?"

"You should be in bed right now," Kramer said, before signing off. "Feel better."

The next afternoon, Kramer did join Callen and Moore at the summit. They held their own but failed to win any converts to their side. As predicted, no consensus developed one way or the other and the bathhouse issue remained unresolved.

3

Testing Limits

It was no surprise that the battle over Mayor Koch's pro-gay Executive Order 50 got nasty. On a muggy August morning, I joined a dozen reporters in Judge Alvin Klein's supreme court chambers for a preliminary hearing. Rather than sending the city's top lawyer to make the case for the anti-discrimination measure, corporation counsel instead fielded a soft-spoken young assistant counsel named Dennis deLeon, who happened to be gay. The lawyer pleaded for a quick resolution, citing the "suffering" the dispute had caused. As a result of the high-profile litigation, deLeon said, young gay men and women were being turned away from important health services by staff members at Catholic Charities and the other litigants. This included AIDS care at St. Vincent's. He submitted affidavits from employees there admitting this. "They are afraid to treat gay and lesbian kids for fear of being labeled themselves gay or lesbian and endangering their job status," he said. Producing another pile of affidavits, he said gay men and women of all ages "do not go to these places because they perceive them as anti-gay."

"Gratuitous insults!" screamed the church's attorney, John Hale, exploding so loudly that spectators jumped in their seats. He stretched his finger toward deLeon like a character from an Ibsen play. "I take *offense* at the city's allegation that we discriminate against *anyone*. My daughter, Elizabeth Mary Hale, treats *victims* of AIDS at St. Vincent's Hospital. Don't say the Catholic Charities isn't *charitable*! *Don't you say that!*"

Dennis deLeon persisted timidly. "There will be a ripple effect," he predicted. "Intolerance will spread from here to affect the entire lesbian and gay community throughout the city."

"Insults," Hale shouted over him. *"Don't you say that!"*

Judge Klein ended the hearing amid the shouting. As the parties spilled into the hallway outside, Hale was pleased with his performance.

The entire case, he told a cluster of reporters, swung on one's definition of "sexual orientation." "The city says that it covers homosexual and bisexual preferences *and practices*," he said. "We cannot condone the *practices* of these people. But if it were just preferences," he continued, turning to look directly at me for the first time, "we could feel sorry for you." Then he did something peculiar. He placed the palm of his hand momentarily on my stomach and smiled—an intended demonstration of his compassion, I supposed. Turning to the CBS News reporter, an apparent heterosexual, he continued, beginning in a near whisper and ending in the timbre of a revivalist preacher, the warmth of my belly still present on his hand: "Did you know, in the homosexual movement there are five organizations of those who prefer sex with children? Does this law mean that if you run a childcare center you have to hire those who prefer children? *Have you been reading about the Bronx?*" Three day care workers there stood accused of sexually abusing children—girls and boys alike.

He turned to address me again. "We have homosexuals in our employ," he barked at me. "We do not discriminate against homosexuals. We are here only to argue legal principles."

In late September, Judge Klein handed the church its victory. Koch had "gone beyond his authority" by attempting to broaden the range of classes protected by existing legislation, Klein determined. Legislation, not executive order, was the way to address this brand-new social policy. I raced down to city hall for a hastily gathered press conference in the mayor's briefing chamber, known as the Blue Room. Few other reporters were present. Koch focused his comments toward me and the *Native*. He intended to appeal the decision, he said, and hoped that Executive Order 50's protections would be back in force by the end of the year. I knew the assurance was laughable; he and his administration had never enforced the provision—discrimination had always been the rule in New York.

Then Koch dropped a bomb. As the ruling called for legislation, he intended to introduce what he called "a limited gay rights bill," covering only agencies contracting with the city. This would supplant the more expansive measure debated and rejected every year since 1971, significantly undermining the aims of the moment. He seemed to think this would please gay New Yorkers. "It will pass quicker than the gay rights bill, because there are people in the council who believe they can't regulate the private sector's right to do business as they please," he said.

"Are you retreating from the gay rights bill?" I asked. "Because the city council has prohibited bias against blacks, religious minorities, or the handicapped in the private sector. Nobody's letting them 'do business as they please' in those areas."

"It's pragmatic," he said. "It's progress."

I told him what I was hearing from gay leaders, who condemned him for failing to throw weight behind the gay rights bill. "Tim Sweeney at Lambda Legal Defense and Education Fund says, 'It's time we had a mayor who used all his power to bring about this protection.' Is he wrong?"

Koch slumped imperiously into a leather chair beside the city's top attorney. He railed against Sweeney in particular and the community generally for insufficient gratitude. Soon his new liaison to the gay community, a sympathetic-seeming lesbian named Lee Hudson, was summoned to his defense. "The mayor wanted E.O. 50 or he wouldn't have issued it," she said. "He has instructed Corporation Counsel to do everything they can in their appeal."

Corporation counsel eventually did file an appeal to Klein's ruling as promised, but not before Koch wrote a sharp letter to the *Native* lashing out at my coverage. Being the typesetter as well as the news section editor, I rendered it for the letters section. "What is outrageous and fundamentally insidious about Mr. France's articles is the allegation that I am backing off from the challenges now faced by my Executive Order and, by extension, all anti-discrimination protection for minorities," he wrote. "I issued Executive Order 50 in April 1980 because I believe in strongly enforced equal employment opportunities for *all* people—including gay and lesbian people. When challenged, I instructed my Corporation Counsel's office to vigorously protect this order *because* I believe in it and my authority to issue it. No one can legitimately term my 'defense of the gay section' of EO 50 as 'apologetic'! I have *never* been apologetic about equal rights protections for the gay and lesbian community."

He concluded,

Ultimately, most unsettling about the unfairness of articles like Mr. France's is the disheartening effect of such frustrating attacks on those, like myself, who are struggling *with* a community for presumably a common goal. After many years of public service, I simply do not expect a community whose rights I fight to protect to turn that struggle into a "rage" and "anger" against me. Such attacks raise a specter of indifference for the community's larger interests and jeopardize the important working relationships with public officials necessary for social change.

Because of people like me, in other words, we were likely to get *even less* from city hall. Though I continued covering him, my working relationship with the mayor never improved.

THAT DECEMBER, Lester Kinsolving, a reporter in his late middle years, took his usual chair at the White House briefing room. Just after noon, he rose with a question. The president's spokesman, an agile, sandy-haired Mississippian named Larry Speakes, eyed him playfully. "Lester's beginning to circle now," he said, as though he were narrating a wildlife show. "He's moving in front."

Kinsolving was more gadfly than journalist, a self-syndicated columnist known for wearing an ecclesiastical collar to briefings (he was ordained in the Episcopal Church) and issuing challenges from Reagan's right-most flank. Sometimes his questions were just plain kooky, like the time, perhaps moved by a tune stuck in his head, he wondered, "What does the president think about muskrat love?" Other reporters christened him "the Mad Monk" and "the price we pay for democracy." Few took him seriously. But for Speakes, Kinsolving's intercessions were occasions for merriment.

"Go ahead," he invited cheerfully.

Kinsolving launched into one of his customary disquisitions. "Since the Center for Disease Control in Atlanta reports that an estimated—"

An explosion of laughter cut him off. The regulars knew what was coming next. So did Speakes. "This is going to be an AIDS question," the spokesman beamed. Kinsolving had raised the subject before, once in October 1982 and once in June 1983. Each time was the same: guffaws and dismissal. These were the only times the subject had arisen in connection to the Reagan administration, which remained silent on the disease.

"You were close," Speakes ribbed him. "You were close!"

"Well, look, could I just ask my question, Larry?"

Kinsolving's poker face never broke. He wanted a serious answer this time. "An estimated 300,000 people have been exposed to AIDS, which can be transmitted through saliva." That last part was never true, despite what Gallo and the *Voice* reported, but his concern was that people with the disease—members of what he called "the sodomy lobby"—were endangering American life. "Will the president, as commander-in-chief, take steps to protect armed forces, food and medical services, from AIDS patients or those who run the risk of spreading AIDS in the same manner that they forbid typhoid fever people from being involved in the health or food services?"

Speakes regarded him warmly. "I don't know," he said. More laughter.

"Is the president concerned about this subject, Larry, that seems to have evoked so much jocular reaction here?"

"I haven't heard him express concern," Speakes winked. Gales now. Everyone knew that only homosexuals concerned themselves with the epidemic. It was beyond the pale to imagine the president talking about it. Chatter flew around the briefing room as the other reporters piped in: "Has he sworn off water faucets?" and "It isn't just jocks, Lester?"

"Lester, I have not heard him express anything on it, sorry," said the twinkle-eyed spokesman, "but I must confess *I* haven't asked him about it."

A year ago he had responded to Kinsolving's question by "acknowledging *your* interest in the subject." A year before that he had parried, "I don't have it. Do you?"

With 7,699 reported cases and 3,665 Americans dead, Kinsolving was no longer satisfied with jokes. "You mean he has no—has expressed no opinion about the epidemic?" he persisted. "Would you ask him, Larry?"

To which Larry Speakes mischievously replied, "Have *you* been checked?"

Reporters fell out of their seats. The press conference was over. That joke always worked.

AS PROMISED, Gallo sent samples of HTLV-3 to Paris and Montagnier reciprocated with his LAV. The French lab immediately undertook a genetic sequencing of both—and in addition, for comparison, another virus more recently isolated at the University of California in San Francisco that was known, for reasons of political neutrality, as ARV, for "AIDS-associated retrovirus." The genomes of the French and Californian viruses showed a variance of about 12 percent. This was as Montagnier had predicted. Owing to ordinary mutations, specific viruses sampled from different patients typically show genetic deviations from 6 to 20 percent. Montagnier concluded that ARV was an additional and confirming isolate of LAV, bolstering his claim to credit for discovering the AIDS virus.

Next, he directly compared LAV and Gallo's HTLV-3. The degree of variation between them was almost nonexistent, less than 1 percent. This was wholly unexpected, and deeply troubling—even Gallo, having made the same observation, had to admit that the genetic similarities were uncanny.

What was the probability of finding two individual patients with AIDS, on opposite sides of the Atlantic, no less, whose virus was so closely matched? Pretty close to zero. Even if they had been lovers and had directly infected one another, the variance would likely have been much greater. Still, such a coincidence was worth considering. Frédéric Brugière, the gay lymphadenopathy patient from whom LAV was isolated, had last traveled to the States in 1979. It was possible that he engaged in sex at that time. But the American isolate had no clear provenance for comparison. The Gallo team admitted that samples had been blended and cross-contaminated during a poorly managed relocation of their laboratory. As a result, their HTLV-3 might have come from any one of a number of people with AIDS: perhaps a gay man in the institute's hospital, or another NCI patient who volunteered bone marrow, or a Haitian being treated at the University of Pennsylvania, or various patients from North Shore Hospital on Long Island. Whether one of them knew Brugière intimately would remain an unsolvable mystery.

Yet unlocking the mystery was more pressing than ever. Nearly two years had elapsed since the Institut Pasteur first discovered LAV, during which time the disease had spread to six continents. The scientific community was as confused as the lay public. This led to gridlock in labs worldwide. Scientists needed consensus on what this new bug was before they could begin work to determine if and how it caused disease, which was the necessary hurdle to clear before one dollar of research money went toward a therapy.

To help clear the fog, Dr. Mathilde Krim joined with Columbia Presbyterian Hospital to organize a meeting of science journalists in New York City. She invited Gallo and Montagnier to make presentations. Anxious for clarity, dozens of reporters filled a public room at the Harley Hotel on a snowy day in early February 1985. Montagnier had arrived from Paris the night before. Gallo, who had only to take a train up from Baltimore, sent his regrets hours before the event was to begin. His boss, Health Secretary Margaret Heckler, also canceled, citing a case of the flu.

Dr. Krim, in her opening remarks, failed to mask her contempt for the American team, telling the assembled journalists that she had made a "deliberate, concerted effort, in absolute good faith, to have you meet face-to-face some of the most authoritative scientists in the world, wherever they come from, in the field of AIDS research. We felt that surely rivalries that can only be considered petty in the face of uncontrolled and spreading *deadly* disease will not stand in the way of a meeting such as ours. For six weeks prior to this meeting we were assured that they wouldn't." Her lips tightened. "I am therefore very deeply . . . *embarrassed,* and I regret very *much,* that Dr. Robert Gallo of the NIH could not be here today and he felt that he could change his plans at the very last minute."

In his lofty manner and through a thick accent, Montagnier described his comparison of the competing viruses and the unlikely findings his study revealed. The reasons for this were inescapable, but it was not his style to spell them out plainly.

Looks of confusion proliferated on the reporters' faces.

Sonnabend lost patience with the whole charade. Leaning to whisper into Michael Callen's ear, he asked, "Why are these journalists so stupid?"

Callen was equally fed up. Just as Montagnier's session drew to a close, Callen grabbed his doctor by the elbow and marched him to a microphone on the center aisle. "He has something to say to you," Callen announced.

Sonnabend's cheeks were crimson. "Well," he said, clearing his throat uncomfortably. The audience settled back into their seats. "What has been generally accepted is that these viruses, that *individual isolates* of these viruses will vary one from another by a small amount." Their faces showed they still didn't get it. "However," he continued, "what we are finding here is that even this expected difference doesn't occur between two prototype isolates. In other words, it would appear that LAV and HTLV are *too* identical."

Still, no signs of understanding arose from the audience.

"They are identical," he tried again, "identical to a degree that would not be anticipated with two independent isolates from the same family."

The hints were just not working. A hum of confusion rose up in the room. Again, Callen interceded from the back row. "Joe, what are you trying to say?"

Sonnabend proceeded carefully. "They appear to be the same actual isolate. Or some strange coincidence."

Montagnier, in his chair, kept his mouth shut. Dr. Krim moved to the front of the room, diplomatically sharpening the message. "Dr. Montagnier felt, I think properly, he was not the person to point this out," she said.

Still missing the point, Lawrence Altman, who had been one of the panelists for the day's event, tried to bring the meeting to a close and move along to the promised cocktails. Then the booming voice of an unfamiliar reporter rang out from the audience: "Are you suggesting that Gallo swiped Montagnier's virus?"

The room went silent. Michael Callen watched one reporter's jaw drop open.

"Or Montagnier swiped Gallo's virus," Sonnabend answered.

This was a story any journalist could understand: laboratory intrigue and low-down thievery. Pandemonium broke out among them. "It was like dominoes, you could see their minds working," Callen reported to Berkowitz later. They finally grasped what had been burning in Montagnier's stomach. It seemed that Gallo had "discovered" his HTLV-3 inside a jar of LAV that Montagnier had hand-carried to his home. There were two ways this might have happened. The most probable explanation was accidental contamination, given what was known about the lab's relocation fiasco. When handling viruses in close proximity, there is always a risk that one will jump from one test tube to another. In fact, this was a problem that had bedeviled Gallo in the past. In a move that nearly sank his career, the journal *Nature* was forced to rescind a paper of his that purported to find a new human virus when it was subsequently determined that the cells it grew in were in fact from an inexplicable mixture of a wooly monkey, a gibbon ape, and a baboon, not human at all.

Contamination would certainly be easier to accept than the alternative: that Gallo had made a fraudulent claim out of hunger for personal fame and riches. Somehow he managed to receive a patent for the antibody screen though he had filed months after Montagnier, whose own application languished without a ruling. Meanwhile, the global research effort was tied in knots. Krim pointed out that Gallo's HTLV-3 claims had already affected research priorities at the NIH, where scientists were being encouraged to commit their resources to take another look at HTLV-1 and HTLV-2, hoping to find a key in the battle against AIDS. If the new virus was unrelated to the HTLV family, as seemed increasingly likely, time and money were being recklessly misdirected. The shenanigans infuriated Krim. As she made clear at the opening of the afternoon's discussion, she held Gallo personally responsible for derailing the global effort. "This rivalry stands in the way of the truth and understanding," she said in her characteristically blunt fashion. "Dr. Gallo has slapped all of us in the face and apparently does not have the courage to face this group."

The whole matter continued to make Montagnier queasy. He declined requests for interviews on the subject that day. What he wanted to discuss instead were exciting new findings about an experimental therapy called HPA-23, which he and his colleague Jean-Claude Chermann found had potential to curb reverse transcription, the process by which retroviruses bind to the DNA of healthy cells. In test tubes, the Pasteur team watched it halt the AIDS virus in its tracks. Buoyed by those results, they enrolled four AIDS patients in a fifteen-day trial. The drug appeared to successfully hinder viral replication.

This was a thrilling finding—the first pharmaceutical agent ever to have an impact against a human retrovirus. Chermann and Montagnier immediately planned a larger study, hoping to enlist the NIH in running an American trial. Given the absence of Gallo and Heckler from the meeting, there was little chance of that happening.

Rumors about HPA-23's hopeful performance rocketed through the patient community. Dozens—then hundreds—of AIDS patients flew to Paris and begged for the pills at local hospitals and the Institut Pasteur headquarters. Only a fraction were lucky enough to be enrolled at Pasteur. Those who were put on a waiting list feared relinquishing their place in line, so they stayed put in Paris indefinitely. Some of Sonnabend's patients were among them.

Sonnabend personally pressed the NIH to undertake its own study of HPA-23, without success. Dr. Sam Broder, the head of the clinical oncology branch at the National Cancer Institute, turned down the request. Although AIDS was now more than likely to be an infectious disease, and therefore might fall under the purview of the National Institute of Allergy and Infectious Diseases at the NIH's sprawling wooded campus, from the beginning it was instead channeled to Broder's division at the NCI. This made sense logically, because of the prevalence of Kaposi's sarcoma. But another advantage of the NCI was that it was the only branch of the country's Public Health Service with deep experience developing and testing pharmaceutical compounds, thanks to the heavily financed "War on Cancer" declared by Richard Nixon. Clinical trials began there in 1971.

The epidemic found a fierce foe in Dr. Broder, a wiry-haired and affable scientist with a comically big moustache who joined the NCI in 1972. When the first AIDS patient was admitted to the ward on campus in 1981, Broder squeezed into the young man's hospital room with other NCI staffers, palpably thrilled at a chance to confront a fascinating and confounding new malady. In his years of training as a scientist and clinician—Broder's specialty was the relationship between immunodeficiency diseases and cancers—he'd never seen anything like it. The fact that the patient was gay seemed more novel than noteworthy at the time. Broder won permission to set up an AIDS drugs initiative at the NCI, with a tiny staff and tinier budget.

Many respected figures in the field thought it would not be remotely possible to treat a retrovirus because of the way it integrates its RNA directly into human DNA—literally becoming part of a patient's genetic makeup. No one yet had put forward a theory for reversing that process without the likelihood of killing the patient in the process. Seeing certain failure, they did not rush to join Broder's initiative. But Broder's tiny "SWAT team," as he called his recruits, shared his view that AIDS offered "a once-in-a-lifetime opportunity" to them as researchers and clinicians. Robert Yarchoan, a veteran of immunology research and cancer, plus a post doc from Japan, Hiroaki Mitsuya, nicknamed Mitch, a gifted virologist known for his preternatural skills in the laboratory, came on board.

Rather than looking for ways to kill infected cells, they hypothesized ways to block viral replication, hoping at least to slow the course of the disease. They guessed that the virus infected CD4 cells selectively, and was probably reproducing within the infected cell and breaking free to infect new, healthy cells. This might explain why CD4s continued dying through the course of infection. Broder gathered his team, inviting them to suggest pharmaceutical compounds that might interrupt this cycle. Thymidine and rifampin were mentioned as strong candidates, and it was agreed to try them both in test tubes. The results weren't good. Unhindered, the virus was able to destroy all cell samples within a few days. They tried a number of other compounds in the same way, and all gave disappointing results. But late in the summer they struck gold. Working in their labs with a drug called suramin, they noted that it seemed to keep the cells alive past the five-day watershed. That meant it was doing something to slow the virus. Suramin was known to be safe. It was already prescribed to treat onchocerciasis, or river blindness, in Africa.

Excited by the results, Broder pushed suramin into human trials in record time, beginning August 6, 1984. Twelve patients raced to sign up as trial subjects, submitting to six weekly injections. The most noteworthy effect of the treatment was that it now took longer to culture the virus from their blood. This suggested a decrease in viral load, for which no measuring tools existed. But there was never a correlated increase in CD4 cells, and therefore no clinical improvement. More to the point, patients felt no better. When the study was replicated in two other groups of patients, the results were similarly meager. Interest in suramin petered out. Broder had to admit that early efforts to find a treatment were dispiriting. Unfortunately, his SWAT team was already out of ideas.

Turning to the pharmaceutical industry for assistance proved no more profitable. Throughout that fall and winter, Broder traveled across the country meeting with industry giants and start-ups alike, but AIDS did not interest them. They talked about it in terms of money, not human suffering. They couldn't justify the necessary R&D cost for a disease affecting so few people, they told Broder. To them, there simply wasn't a market worth chasing.

The only firm willing to break rank was Burroughs Wellcome, the North Carolina–based drugmaker. Wellcome was the company that produced the anti-herpes medication acyclovir, so they were not averse to commodifying sexually transmitted diseases. In a visit to their headquarters that October, Broder enticed them with a highly unusual proposal. If the company agreed to conduct the test-tube work to identify promising compounds, Broder's NCI team would then put them into human trials, taking on all the associated costs. In exchange, the company would, if warranted, rush the agent into production. Burroughs Wellcome liked the arrangement. But there was a catch. Citing fear of contagion, the company refused to accept live retrovirus samples from the NCI. This meant that Broder's people would have to do the initial screening as well as the human trials. In other words, every aspect of this collaboration, beyond the provision of various candidate agents, would be the responsibility of Broder's lab and paid for by taxpayers. What choice did he have? He agreed.

His colleagues were no less frightened than the people in private industry, so, bowing to fears from others at the NCI, his small team scheduled the AIDS research at night, after everyone else had gone home, in a remote office on the thirteenth floor. Mitch Mitsuya was the logical candidate to do the meticulous and dangerous work. He had cultivated a line of healthy human cells, capable of living continuously outside of the body except when exposed to the AIDS virus, which invariably killed them within five days. As with suramin, his task was to combine the drug sample with the healthy cells, then infect them with the lethal virus to see if it made a difference. For the next several months, he received a pharmacopeia from Burroughs Wellcome, each candidate given a code name (soon, a smattering of samples came in from other companies as well, also with the same arm's-length proviso). For Mitsuya, it was tedious work. He put every contender to the test. "Everybody and their brother is saying, 'Try this tincture, try some extract of some flower,'" Dr. Broder complained. But "until we have something better, how do we know?"

If after five days the cells were dead, he knew he had a failure. And in instance after instance, week after week, the cell line was killed on schedule by the pitiless virus.

JOE SONNABEND kept up with these frustrating developments less through the medical literature, where a peer-review process could delay publication for months, than through the grapevine. He considered the possibility that he was wrong to doubt the new retrovirus. Suppose it was nasty enough to collapse a healthy immune system all by itself, without help from other known pathogens or precursors. So what? Every doctor treating AIDS knew that what was killing their patients, what actually tore at their organs and stopped their breath, wasn't a retrovirus, no matter how wily. What killed people were the opportunistic infections, or OIs. There now were twenty-four known deadly infections responsible for nearly all of the AIDS death toll (suicide claimed most of the rest). This was uncontested fact. Many of the OIs lacked any proven therapies. The widespread use of chemotherapy was failing to stop Kaposi's sarcoma, now the second-leading cause of death in the community, behind pneumonia. Coming in third and fourth place were AIDS-related lymphoma and toxoplasmosis, which combined accounted for another 24 percent of deaths, followed by the fiendish wasting disease caused by *Mycobacterium avium-intracellulare*.

While NIH money poured into anti-retrovirals, none of these diseases were even being studied.

The AIDS-related pneumonia revealed an even more catastrophic dereliction. There was no disagreement about how to treat PCP, but once a patient came down with the disease it was often too late. A small number of doctors were following Sonnabend's lead, using Bactrim to prevent the deadly infection from taking hold in the first place. The drug seemed highly effective for those who could tolerate it, though in half the patients Bactrim could trigger painful skin rashes, including a cataclysmic condition in which skin boils up and sloughs off, as if burned crisp in a fire. Some doctors had discovered a way to avoid these problems by starting patients on small doses and gradually increasing them over a number of weeks. These practices were conveyed in a brief letter published in medical journals in 1981, and another, by Dr. Michael Gottlieb of Los Angeles, in 1984, but outside small circles of specialists it was largely unknown. The branches of the Public Health Service—whether the CDC or the NIH—might have been expected to send out an alert, but they did nothing, citing a lack of research. Studies proved Bactrim's power against PCP in various groups of immune-compromised patients, but in the middle of a health emergency nobody had done a formal study to establish that people with AIDS would respond the same. Absent that evidence, a largely preventable disease remained the number one cause of AIDS death.

Had Sonnabend been in a stronger position, he might have been able to influence the research agenda. But he was trapped in the legal tangle around his eviction case. Depositions were taken and retaken. There were dueling press conferences, fund-raising appearances, and confessional sit-downs with reporters. The story went national, casting his tormentors as heartlessly cruel. Meantime, Sonnabend scurried in and out of his office, fearful of making eye contact with the building's other tenants. "I'm their enemy and they hate me," he told Berkowitz one night. "I'm getting a little bit *scared*." Finally, lawyers for the 49 West 12 Tenants Corporation threw in the towel. Conceding that their motives were discriminatory, they agreed to offer Sonnabend a new lease at a fair rate and wrote a check for $10,000 in restitution, plus legal costs. Sonnabend was naturally relieved to have the dreadful matter behind him, but it left him deeper in debt than ever.

"I haven't been able to manage things," he confided to Callen.

"Oh, my," was all the compassion Callen could muster. He had deep money troubles of his own stemming from the lawsuit. Press and other obligations cut into his temp work earnings, pushing up the balances on his credit cards and forcing him to take a secretarial job at the small law firm representing their side in the suit. The pay was insufficient. He borrowed thousands from Krim, but remained $10,000 in the credit card hole, he said. In his twenty-ninth year on earth, he didn't see many good options. Someone had suggested law school—a Hail Mary!—as if he had the $350 to take the LSATs.

"What's going on for me," he said to Sonnabend, "which you can hear, is that I am at present surveying the wreckage."

Sonnabend commiserated. "Unfortunately, like everyone else, you will spend your life working to pay a few bank loans."

"I'm also feeling a little like a fool. I'm the only one who has made no money out of this whole venture."

"Really? Oh, my," Sonnabend stammered. Making money off AIDS was an idea that repulsed him. "That's not really the measure of the quality of anything! That's presumably not the reason one does it."

"No, but when one is in serious financial trouble and feeling the pinch . . . it just makes it a little more painful," Callen said. "You must know that."

Sonnabend rattled off a few undeveloped suggestions for getting AIDS-education grants for Callen, but his protégé was no longer interested.

"I've made the decision," Callen said. "I'm at that juncture about, what the fuck am I going to do with my life?" He had made up his mind to go back to music, full-time for once. If poverty was his inescapable fate, he would endure it as an artist. "I moved to New York to be a singer, and of course I took another path. And I really need to know whether I have what it takes to do that. For me, it's now or never."

He added, "I think I gave this AIDS thing quite the old college try."

THROUGH THE WINTER, Dr. Mitsuya pressed on with his methodical after-hours lab work. Over 180 candidate drugs came his way, all submitted with coded names to keep from influencing technicians. They were increasingly more exotic. Some focused on "antisense molecules," a highly theoretical approach, or on "messenger RNA," unlikely for many reasons to be useful in the long run.

One morning in mid-February, Mitsuya pulled yet another jar from the storeroom, this one codenamed "Compound S." He introduced it as usual to the brew of living cells and retrovirus. On day five, the cells were still alive and behaving normally, a first. They were also still alive on day six, and day ten. It was as if they'd never been infected.

Rumors scattered through the NCI building and right into the panicky gay grapevine. Patients began asking their doctors for the compound before anyone knew its name.

Officials at Burroughs Wellcome, armed with Broder's findings, revealed that Compound S was an old anti-cancer compound called azidothymidine, or AZT. It had been developed in 1964 by Jerome P. Horwitz, a young academic researcher in Detroit on contract to the NCI, using cells isolated from the sperm of herrings. Horwitz had observed that cancer cells used raw materials called nucleosides to make new DNA necessary for rapid cell divisions. Horwitz borrowed an idea from Wile E. Coyote, who lured the Road Runner into traps by painting false vistas on the sides of buildings. To foil the nucleosides, he designed the pharmaceutical equivalent, which he called "fraudulent nucleosides," biologically useless compounds that would appear so similar to the real thing that they would connect to the DNA chain and prevent actual nucleosides from aiding in cell division. With the chain ended, the rapid cell division would stop and the cancerous tumor would cease to grow—in theory.

Unfortunately, it worked no better for Horwitz than it did for Coyote (in a scientific principle known as "cartoon physics," Road Runner could speed right through the trompe l'oeil scenes while Coyote crashed against them). The cancer cells ignored the nucleoside analogues and multiplied unchecked, while the drug itself proved unacceptably toxic to healthy cells and bone marrow. Disappointed, Horwitz threw away his lab notes and did not even seek a patent. "We dumped it on the junk pile," he admitted later.

But apparently AZT was a drug awaiting a mission. In Mitsuya's lab, it performed just as Horwitz had originally imagined. When introduced to HTLV-3/LAV in the cell culture, AZT stopped the virus cold. The mechanism was slightly different than in Horwitz's plan. Rather than impacting cell division as a fraudulent nucleoside, it appeared to interrupt the reverse transcriptase process that was transforming the virus's RNA chain into DNA and allowing it to infect healthy human cells. One of the enzymes involved in that process is called thymidine, and AZT was a dead ringer for thymidine—fraudulently taking its place in the genetic chain and rendering the chain useless.

Dr. Broder was as elated as Mitsuya about the findings. Failure in the drug discovery process would have been catastrophic for him professionally. Broder called Burroughs Wellcome to report the good news on February 20, 1985. At that time, there were 8,597 cases of AIDS, half of them dead.

The pharmaceutical giant had had the foresight to apply for an American patent a few weeks earlier, naming five top Burroughs Wellcome scientists as inventors not of AZT, but of the idea to use it against AIDS. After Broder's call, the company's legal department filed another application to the UK patent office. The applications made no mention of Horwitz in Detroit, nor of Mitsuya and Broder, whose painstaking process discovered its efficacy.

In the summer of 1985, the NCI team began preparing for a small Phase I trial, to study the toxicity in people with AIDS. For this, Broder turned to his other SWAT team member, Dr. Robert Yarchoan, a colleague with considerable experience running clinical trials. Yarchoan enrolled nineteen patients—eleven of them on the ward at the NIH's Clinical Center and eight who were being treated at Duke—in a protocol that included intravenous infusions of AZT three times daily, for two weeks. The first patient came to the lab on July 3, 1985, four years to the day since that first *New York Times* story about the new homosexual disease. He was a furniture salesman from Boston named Joseph Rafuse, and had been treated for an early bout of PCP that left him with roughly forty CD4 cells. Yarchoan and Broder watched as the syringe emptied AZT into Rafuse's arm, worried he might have an immediate and negative reaction. He did not. That evening on the ward, he developed a slight fever. Neither doctor could determine if his temperature was due to drug toxicity or the disease itself; they continued injecting him with AZT three times daily, and the fever soon subsided. The drug seemed tolerable. This suggested it would pass the Phase I test for safety.

Something else was quickly apparent. At the end of the two-week trial, the patient's CD4 count had rebounded from forty to a remarkable two hundred, still a third of the normal count but heading in the proper direction. Usually researchers waited for Phase II trials to measure efficacy. But this turnaround was so dramatic that they changed the protocol, giving the patient another two weeks of medicine, then changed it again to allow for a total of eight weeks, moving from injected drug to oral. Over that time, his CD4 count fluctuated and began descending again, but he reported feeling better—a lot better. This was not simply subjective. As a test of his immune response, doctors were giving him regular skin tests—the four-pronged TB screening test my doctor used on me. They produced no response when he first arrived. After eight weeks of AZT, his skin tests were producing raised bumps—the reaction of a functional immune system. "Not only were the *number* of CD4 cells going up, but they were *working*," Dr. Yarchoan said. "This is something real."

The second patient also showed positive responses, though not as dramatic. He began the study with severe Kaposi's sarcoma, and additional lesions appeared during the course of the study, though he did

RARE CANCER SEEN IN 41 HOMOSEXUALS

Outbreak Occurs Among Men in New York and California —8 Died Inside 2 Years

The New York Times significantly downplayed the first article alerting the world to the coming plague. Appearing beneath this headline on page 20, on July 3, 1981, before the long holiday weekend, the news caused no public health alarm.

Anti-gay protesters in New York City, ca. 1982, were expressing a common American sentiment against gay, lesbian, bisexual, and transgender people, a trend that worsened as the epidemic deepened.

Amid the largest influx of gays in city history, I (below, in beard, June 1983) migrated to New York to become part of what epidemiologists call an "amplification system" for disease.

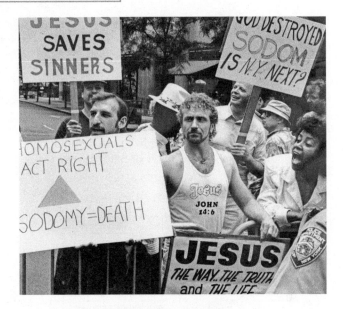

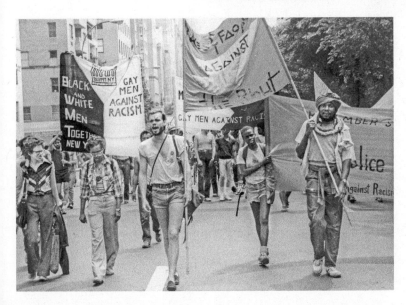

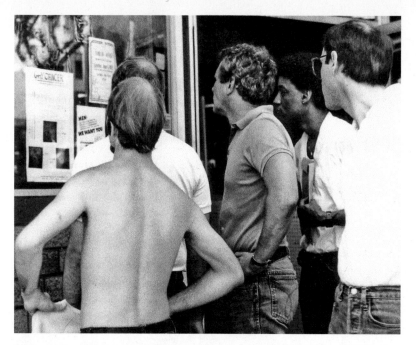

To spread awareness about the new "gay cancer," self-declared "AIDS Poster Boy" Bobbi Campbell posted photographs of his own lesions in the Castro Street window of Star Pharmacy, San Francisco, in 1981.

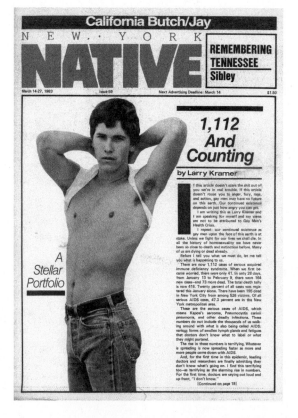

The powerful polemics of Larry Kramer, then a lesser-known playwright and novelist, helped mobilize the affected community and cemented his role as the galvanizing, if sometimes unpredictable, voice of the embattled community.

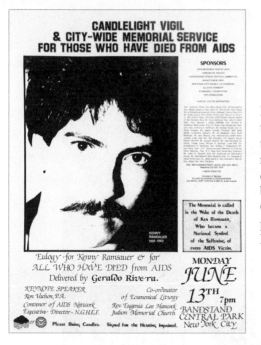

Kenny Ramsauer became the first person with AIDS to be the subject of a national news special. He died days after the *20/20* broadcast, and newsman Geraldo Rivera organized a public memorial service in New York's Central Park.

Some 1,500 people attended Ramsauer's memorial on June 13, 1983, the first large gathering in the plague's wake and a sobering acknowledgment of the horrors to come.

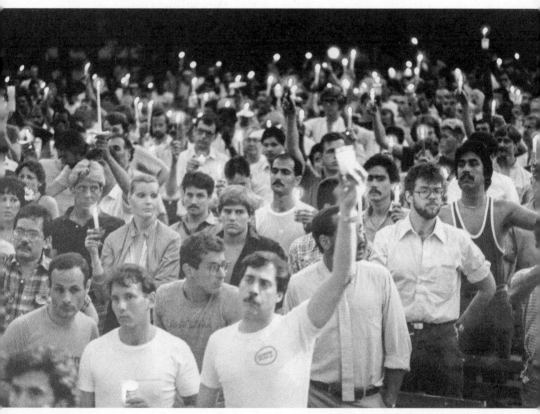

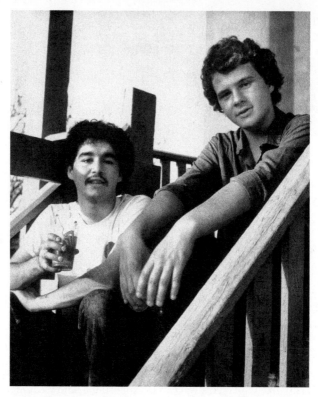

Brian Gougeon (right) was my college roommate and fellow migrant to New York City. He is pictured here, ca. 1980, with Doug Gould, his longtime lover and my future partner.

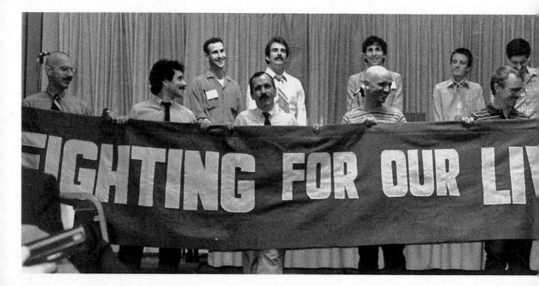

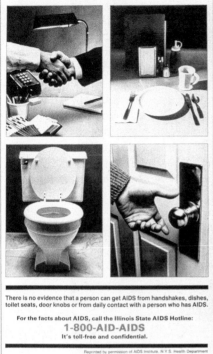

None of these will give you AIDS.

There is no evidence that a person can get AIDS from handshakes, dishes, toilet seats, door knobs or from daily contact with a person who has AIDS.

For the facts about AIDS, call the Illinois State AIDS Hotline:

1-800-AID-AIDS

It's toll-free and confidential.

Reprinted by permission of AIDS Institute, N.Y.S. Health Department
Printed by Authority of State of Illinois
November 86, 30M 50321

By 1987, though it was clear how HIV was transmitted and how it wasn't, workplace discrimination against suspected carriers peaked. Public health campaigns around the country sought to reassure and destigmatize.

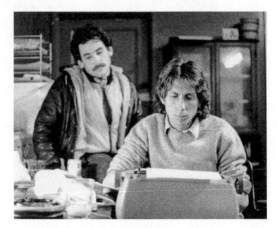

Richard Berkowitz (left) and Michael Callen (right) at work on "How to Have Sex in an Epidemic: One Approach," credited with changing gay sexual practices and preventing untold thousands of infections. The booklet, Berkowitz's brainchild, was written by the two immunocompromised men under the supervision of their doctor, Joseph Sonnabend.

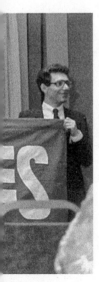

In 1983, AIDS patients from across the country gathering for the first time drafted the Denver Principles, so-named because of the city where the attendees met. The participants were in part insisting on their direct involvement in all matters affecting their lives.

MEDICAL AND SCIENTIFIC CONSULTANT:
JOSEPH SONNABEND, M.D.

Chairman, Scientific Committee,
AIDS MEDICAL FOUNDATION

How to Have Sex in an Epidemic: One Approach

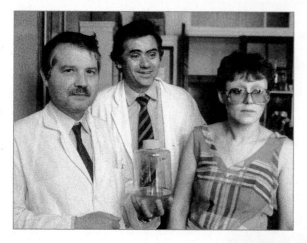

When Drs. Luc Montagnier, Jean-Claude Chermann, and Françoise Barré-Sinoussi of Institut Pasteur isolated a virus they linked to AIDS in 1983, they met strong resistance and obfuscation from the American research establishment.

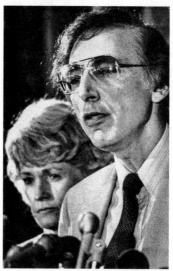

On April 23, 1984, Health and Human Services Secretary Margaret Heckler and Dr. Robert Gallo of the National Cancer Institute touched off a decades-long scientific quarrel with the Pasteur team that misdirected research and slowed progress.

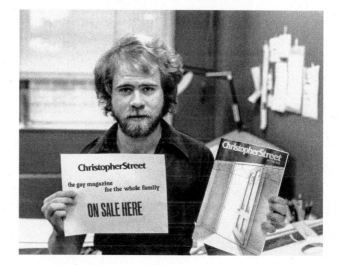

Early in the plague, Chuck Ortleb (photographed on May 26, 1976), my boss at *Christopher Street* and the *New York Native,* published the most authoritative AIDS news available. Subscribers included the world's top researchers.

1515, Wednesday August 17, '83 – Board Rm NYC
Dept of Health

(Waiting for a meeting with Margaret Heckler.
Rich Berkowitz, Artie Felson, Dan Turner,
Michael Callen & I.)

Intraleuken-2; CDC/NIH working hard; has
spoken to President; hopeful for future; And PR
session with PWA at NY hospital; we won't give
up until its done; spirit of PWA is strong.
Will offer to meet č PWAs later in Wash DC,
though a long interview should be č Brandt.
Small meeting.
Asking Congress for 22 million transferring
from other depts transferred to AIDS
to 39.5 million.
Sent letter to Soc. Security requiring to
process AIDS claim.
United Airlines/Columbia U firings
Snapshot photo.
WE DID IT !!

Bobbi Campbell, the San Francisco leader, kept a plague journal throughout his battle. After his death, his family destroyed all but one volume, which documents the first political advances of the national People With AIDS movement.

A panel for Brian Gougeon on the AIDS Memorial Quilt, a vast virtual graveyard that today honors over 94,000 of the dead and weighs 54 tons.

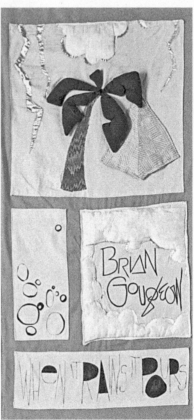

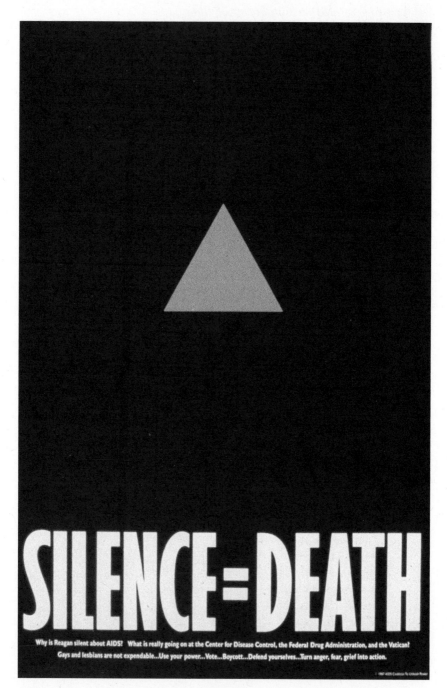

This poster, anonymously produced and pasted on walls in late 1986, touched a nerve in New York City's gay community, presaged the founding of ACT UP, and launched the era of direct action in AIDS activism.

have a minor increase in his CD4 count. A third patient also had an increase, and so did a fourth, though his CD4 cells jumped from five to ten, then sank back to five again. But time and again, by using skin tests they were able to see reliable increases in immunologic activity. To Yarchoan, it was like steering a ship through a soupy fog—he didn't know if what they were seeing was another ship in the distance or just misty apparitions. But he was excited nonetheless.

The drug proved quite toxic, unfortunately. It was brutal to bone marrow, resulting both in anemia, a depletion of red blood cells, and leukopenia, a depletion of white ones. Both were potentially life threatening, but a better alternative than AIDS.

Broder called Burroughs Wellcome with the good news on July 23, 1985, reaching a very excited young scientist named Sandra Lehrman. They both agreed there was ample reason to rush the drug into formal Phase II trials before the end of the year. Broder set it up through his clinical trials network.

But it soon became clear at the NIH that the National Cancer Institute was probably not as strongly equipped as the National Institute of Allergy and Infectious Diseases—NIAID—to study treatments for AIDS. The AZT research would continue in Broder's institute, while future work would be done at NIAID, whose young head was an aggressive immunologist from Brooklyn named Dr. Tony Fauci. Fauci's institute had a smaller budget than the NCI, and no system in place for conducting clinical trials, but that would change. Soon Fauci would become the most powerful man in the epidemic. Just how bad that proved to be depended on whom you asked.

A FRENZY OF anticipation preceded the opening of Larry Kramer's play at the Public Theater. The legendary producer Joseph Papp devilishly hinted to reporters that Kramer took vicious aim at Ed Koch, *The New York Times*, and every other powerful institution in the city. Papp refused requests to release the script to reviewers, and engaged in other buzz-generating maneuvers. Kramer named the work *The Normal Heart*, from the foreboding Auden poem about another "low dishonest decade," so seemingly predictive as it was of the present circumstances, and, of course, of Kramer's quest.

Opening night drew the usual array of patrons. Many were gay, but the AIDS establishment was not in attendance and no one from GMHC planned to see the play, with the exception of Dr. Lawrence Mass, who attended with his lover, Arnie Kantrowitz.

Stage lights came up on a doctor's waiting room, modeled after Alvin Friedman-Kien's office, where panicky Kramer had his flesh examined in August 1981. A doctor arrived onstage shortly, via motorized wheelchair—inspired by Linda Laubenstein.

"Who are you?" she demands of a beautiful young man.

"I'm Ned Weeks. I spoke with you after the *Times* article."

"You're the writer fellow who's scared. I'm scared too. I hear you've got a big mouth."

"Is big mouth a symptom?"

"No," she says, spinning toward the examining room. "A cure. Come in and take your clothes off."

It was clear to anyone who knew the history that Ned Weeks was Kramer's alter ego, and that what was about to unfold in stage makeup was a vengeful rendition of the founding of GMHC, including his own estrangement for, as the script depicts, being furiously impatient in a world of men passively collaborating with their own death. Kramer may have stopped yelling. He may have left the world of activism for the world of art. But he had invented someone to take up the megaphone, someone who could say what Kramer was thinking a touch more eloquently, if even more rudely. Ned Weeks denounced Bruce Niles (a caricature of Paul Popham) as a raging closet case and "an awful sissy," as responsible for AIDS as the virus itself. The GMHC stalwarts were "cowards" and "murderers" in cahoots with the bloodless mayor, whom he dared to call—or Weeks dared to call—a "cocksucker."

By act 2, there was no question in Dr. Mass's mind that the character Mickey Marcus, a health department employee and writer for the *Native,* was modeled after him. Marcus was compassionate and mild, a conciliator, a good friend of Kramer's character. There he was, inside the GMHC stage set, answering desperate hotline callers and trying with diminishing success to ignore the Ned Weeks chaos around him. The screaming and the dying and the towering plague wore on Mickey Marcus. And then the character began in stages to become unhinged.

Mass, seated near the aisle, could not imagine that Kramer would expose his mental breakdown, about which he had been so ashamed. On the stage, Marcus shouted incoherently, "The *Native* received an anonymous letter describing top-secret Defense Department experiments at Fort Detrick, Maryland, that have produced a virus that can destroy the immune system." And, "They are going to persecute us! Cancel our health insurance. Test our blood to see if we're pure. Lock us up. Stone us in the streets. And *you*," he said, turning to Ned Weeks, "think I am killing people?"

Another actor tenderly gripped Marcus by the elbow. "Come on," he said. "I'm taking you home now."

"Ned, I'm not a murderer," Marcus bellowed. "All my life I've been hated. For one reason or another. For being short. For being Jewish. Jerry Falwell mails out millions of pictures of two men kissing as if that was the most awful sight you could see." Lawrence Mass recognized these as his own actual words. The portrayal stole his breath. He held his chest. He rose conspicuously to his feet as the action continued onstage.

"You're just a little tired, that's all," said the other actor, "a little bit yelled out. We've got a lot of different styles that don't quite mesh. We've got ourselves a lot of bereavement overload. Tommy's taking you home."

"No," the madman cried. "I'm afraid I might do something. Take me to St. Vincent's."

Astonished, Mass turned to his lover. Pain filled his eyes. He staggered from the theater. Never before had he been so betrayed. Kramer had done what Nathan Fain had warned him against, he had exposed a friend's private demons to aggrandize himself—unnecessarily, as Mass kept saying to Kantrowitz, who joined him in the lobby. It took him many minutes to stop shaking. Eventually, he followed Kantrowitz back into the theater to witness what other boundaries were being bridged.

Audience members who knew nothing of Kramer's betrayal sat breathless as Ned Weeks fought valiantly to save the life of the lover Kramer conjured for himself, a tall and witty journalist named Felix Turner. The KS treatments weakened him, and we saw them both slowly give up hope. It was not the first representation of the plague onstage, but it was the most brutal—a traumatizing portrait of agonizing death. Projected on the stage set were dense columns of names, actual names of the dead. Donald Krintzman. John Indrasek. David Norton. John Russo. Kenny Ramsauer. It gave the powerful impression of a monument to those we'd lost, as for those who'd gone to war. I knew so many of them. Bobbi Campbell and Gaëtan Dugas. Fred Canteloupe and Tommy McCarthy. I was not the only one gasping for breath.

The set was a hospital room now. In the final and most powerful scene, Felix Turner embraced his death, for what else could he do? "Please learn to fight again," Turner begged Weeks—or Kramer begged Kramer. "Don't lose that anger. Just have a little more patience and forgiveness. For yourself as well."

As a piece of art, the play got mixed reviews, with some critics dismissing it as little more than messy polemics. But it certainly grabbed the attention of New Yorkers, and opened up for conversation subjects that hadn't been dealt with in public before. Emboldened by Kramer's characterization of the mayor, I followed Koch to an appearance at the city's gay synagogue weeks later, and asked him whether he was gay, as the play alleged. He was prepared for the question. "My sexuality is my business. It's not Larry Kramer's business or anybody else's business," he snapped. "I'm proud of the fact that it never deterred me, because I do not believe that, if you say that someone is homosexual, you are slandering them. That is why it is despicable for someone like Kramer to attack me substantively." He narrowed his eyes. "Try," he challenged.

The point in the play, another reporter averred, was to suggest that as mayor Koch was not doing enough to protect gays, not just in public accommodation but from the epidemic, for fear of being revealed as gay.

"Okay, we're not doing enough?" Koch said briskly. "Then we'll do more."

That was his trick—to reform on the spot. A moment later he added, "It seems to me that when we come before God, God is not going to ask whether we are Jews or Protestants or Catholics or non-believers, or whether we are homosexual or heterosexual. God is going to say, 'What did you do on Earth? Should your actions on Earth entitle you to come into heaven?' And if God decides not, then you're going to go to hell."

In the synagogue that night there was broad agreement on this point.

BY SUMMER, an affordable blood test for HTLV-3/LAV was widely available, put immediately to use at blood banks for screening donors and at "anonymous testing sights," set up in part out of fear that gay men would flock to blood donation centers to learn if they were infected. The two-step procedure looked for antibodies to the virus with a method called ELISA and another called Western Blot. Public health officials promoted testing as a breakthrough for protecting the blood supply and offering important information for the afflicted. But the new test engendered universal and unwavering condemnation. Handbills were passed out in the Village and banner headlines darkened the *Native:* the test was wildly inaccurate; it produced a high number of "false positives" and "false negatives," as demonstrated in the scientific journals. A study in California found that live virus could be cultured from the blood of more than 10 percent of AIDS patients testing negative on the antibody test. Their blood could then erroneously be accepted into the nation's blood supply, to be parceled out by health care workers lulled into a false sense of security. Even more people might become infected as a result of the unreliable test.

Equally troubling, Abbott Laboratories, makers of the kit, warned that .02 percent of positive test results in clinical trials were false, as demonstrated by follow-up viral culturing. Based on this percentage, the Conference of State and Territorial Epidemiologists calculated that blood banks would be destroying 200,000 perfectly good units of blood a year for falsely testing positive. Considering that to date only 113 AIDS cases had been linked to transfusions or blood products, this was an ethically troubling waste of precious resources. "Statistically," according to a succinct *Newsweek* article, "you're much more likely to get run over on your way to the hospital" than to contract AIDS through blood products.

Clinically, the test was just as useless for the infected. For one thing, HTLV-3/LAV had not yet satisfied Koch's Postulates—until it could be intentionally transmitted to another animal and cause disease, it was far from certain what it meant to be infected. This wasn't fringe thinking by Dr. Sonnabend and his ilk. The New York State health commissioner refused to call HTLV-3/LAV "the AIDS virus" until it could satisfy all of Koch's Postulates. There still were numerous patients who had every telltale AIDS symptom yet the test failed time and again to find the retroviruses in their bloodstreams. Further, multiple journal articles reported on gay men who were undeniably infected but who showed no signs of disease (at least not yet). Neither a positive test result nor a negative one meant anything useful to the sick. Besides, there was no approved drug to treat HTLV-3/LAV. "To put it simply, this test helps no one," said Dr. Stephen S. Caiazza, president of New York Physicians for Human Rights, the gay doctors' group. "The test is so primitive that we cannot know who is who."

Some public health experts suggested that even a flawed test would make gay men behave more responsibly, and therefore help stem the spread of disease, but frankly it was not possible to further personalize the scare. The community of gay men had already carried out one of history's most remarkable cultural shifts, broadly investing the community in safe sex practices, as proven by a plunging incidence rate of other sexually transmitted diseases. Eighty percent of gay men in surveys showed detailed familiarity with safe sex guidelines. They cut the average number of sexual encounters per person by half. In the months since Callen's survey of the sex establishments in the city, the sex venues had begun setting up voluntary systems of monitors. Gay men knew how many of us were likely carriers already, and behaved with great care in the face of that knowledge, even if it was unrecognized by public health authorities. Across the board, the community had, as the Callen/Berkowitz/Sonnabend Axis reminded us, consciously championed love in its lovemaking. Unreliable tests were hardly necessary as a prevention gambit. Nobody who knew how well the community had already adapted would make such a proposal.

The test had another major drawback. It would potentially allow the selective identification of gay men, putting the eight million believed to be exposed at immediate risk for losing employment, health insurance, housing, and basic freedoms, including the freedom from quarantine. For this reason, the test was, in Dr. Caiazza's emphatic estimation, "extremely dangerous." Police officers in some cities were taking suspected carriers to hospitals in handcuffs demanding tests. Proposals for detention camps were gaining adherents across the country and the culture war against gay sex—still illegal in many states—had whipped into a frenzy. Atlanta's Metropolitan Vice Squad marched into the Club Baths, a wholly legal establishment, and arrested dozens of men there on charges of sodomy, a criminal act in Georgia. In Gainesville, Florida, sick AIDS patients were being deported to San Francisco, no matter the cost. State health officials in California were talking about making results from blood bank tests reportable, converting a voluntary act of civic altruism into an anti-gay dragnet.

In fact, quarantine orders had already been issued by the CDC for any foreign homosexual attempting to enter the country—supplementing the statute that barred gay people generally, even as tourists. This surprising news was only revealed when a reporter from *The Bay Area Reporter,* the *Native*'s sober counterpart in San Francisco, stumbled upon it. The memorandum of quarantine instructed medical officers from the Public Health Service to ask suspected aliens if they were homosexual, and to hold those answering yes in special detention facilities until they could be deported. The CDC claimed it opposed the order but was forced to issue it by the Reagan administration. Gay papers across the country reprinted the *BAR* story, but the news was ignored by the non-gay press. Nobody in America knew the perils we faced. Heterosexual friends and relatives discounted our concerns as overblown. If the perils were credible, surely they would know about it from Mike Wallace or Harry Reasoner. According to the *Native*'s Washington correspondent, the assistant secretary of health, Edward Brandt Jr., said that "such extreme measures as quarantine and mass firings of gays and other high-risk individuals from schools and hospitals have been seriously discussed within administration councils." The draconian political solutions seemed almost as serious as the epidemic itself.

In enormous type on the front page of the *Native*, we warned readers away from the test and from any research trial in which blood would be screened for evidence of viral infection. The National Gay Task Force and most AIDS service organizations strongly advised the community to stay away from blood donation centers as well. We were incensed that so much federal money was being ploughed into the testing campaign, $72 million, which FDA commissioner Frank Young estimated would avert between 50 and 150 transmissions annually. For the eight million already infected, Reagan's new budget offered just $85 million in AIDS research funding, more than $10 million less than was under-allocated the year before.

"This is a pernicious test which will inevitably cause incredibly personal and social pain and damage. *Stay away from it*," Dr. Caiazza, head of the gay physicians group, wrote in a piece he submitted to the *Native*. "Unfortunately there are times when the information collected can hurt the individual. This is, at present, the case with AIDS. The solution is to be informed, to be cautious, and to be careful."

In my circle, we supported the boycott unreservedly. As far as disease control was concerned, we behaved as if we were already infected, as if everyone were already infected. We would take precautions. We would eat well, sleep thoroughly, and conduct our romantic lives with great care. This policy did little to offset our cycles of panic. There was no agreement on the latency period between exposure and symptoms, so perhaps safe sex would have come too late to save us. Privately, I focused neurotically on my own health, fanatically examining my skin for marks and my forehead for fever and my scale for signs of wasting.

Then one morning, I found what I feared. A mark appeared on my ankle, purple in its center with a halo of yellow and blue. I went deaf from fear. I raced to my doctor that afternoon. "It's a bruise," Dr. Waitkevicz told me, patting my leg. "Let's do a workup." She palpated my lymph glands, swabbed me from every angle for gonorrhea, and drew multiple vials of blood.

"I don't want the AIDS test," I told her.

"Good. I don't offer it," she said. "But it's important to know if your immune system is strong. If it's not, if you're compromised, we'd want to start preventative measures for the OIs—the opportunistic infections." One crimson tube would be sent to a special lab for counting my CD4s and CD8, she said. She also shot me in the arm with the four-pronged TB test again. This gave me something to obsess on while awaiting the other blood results. I trilled my fingers over the location for days until the gorgeous red lumps came. In a week I returned to learn I enjoyed a multitude of CD4 cells, 680 of them, in ideal harmony with my CD8s. I was apparently healthy, a member of the "worried well" fraternity who carried the emotional burden of the epidemic without any apparent clinical reason.

The shelf life of good news was incredibly short. A rattling cough a few weeks later undid me once again. I raced back to Dr. Waitkevicz in the middle of a driving rainstorm with the newest evidence of my seroconversion. In the waiting room, I watched as a nurse escorted an unsteady old African American man past reception and toward an ambulance, blinking its lights outside the door. He took each step with a grimace, planting his cane after a few painful yards in order to heave his glasses up his nose. With his eyewear repositioned, a realization shot through me: I knew this man. We had dated sporadically, and with casual vigor, earlier that year. Only a few months had passed since we drifted apart. He seemed to have aged decades. He was, like me, in his twenties, but his hair had thinned, his skin had shrunk around his eyes, his chalky knuckle trembled atop the cane. I reviewed our history frantically. We had used the safe sex rules with precision. Remembering that did little to assuage my fears. I was doomed. A gentle man, a veteran of my bed, stood before me as proof.

Our eyes met. I don't know what look crossed my face, but his became an abstraction of shame, as though humiliated by his own victimhood. He looked away. "Let's go," he begged the nurse, and fixating on my own fate I let him pick his way into the storm without a word of condolence.

NAUSEATED AND PANIC-STRICKEN, I wandered back to the *Native* with a prescription for antibiotics for the cough. It was a July afternoon, humid and close even after the rain passed. In the triangular park across from the office, a crowd pushed around a squat newspaper vending box. The afternoon *New York Post* had just been delivered and on its front page was a pair of pictures of the movie star Rock Hudson, dreamy in his thirties but now looking hideously frail. I knew he had been sick. After appearing ashen and hollow cheeked at a press conference with Doris Day, his well-being was the subject of open and wild speculation. He did little to assuage this by explaining it away unconvincingly as either a liver disorder, a flu, or some intestinal bug he picked up in Israel. Earlier in the week on the local news, the irrepressible television anchor Sue Simmons openly wondered, "Just what *is* wrong with Rock Hudson?" He had raced to the American Hospital in Paris for secret treatment for "fatigue and malaise," she told us, and while there he took a phone call from his old friend Ronald Reagan, wishing him well.

At the office we wondered if he was chasing Montagnier's experimental AIDS drug HPA-23. Of *course* we wished it was AIDS. We wished the worst for poor Rock Hudson. We had also wished catastrophe for Pope John Paul II and Ronald Reagan, both of whom had received blood transfusions after foiled assassination attempts recently. We prayed for a day when the disease struck someone who mattered, prayed for a weaponizing of AIDS, and when I finally saw the *Post* headline I knew our terrible wishes had come true: "ROCK HAS AIDS—And He's Known for a Year."

A friend of Elizabeth Taylor and Carol Burnett, Ronald Reagan's guest in the White House, like a brother to the first lady: Rock Hudson stepped forward to tell the world he had the gay plague. What the article didn't say was that becoming the face of AIDS hadn't been his idea. The crush of reporters on the American Hospital's doorstep in Paris had grown so overwhelming that officials entered his room with an ultimatum: either Hudson would announce his diagnosis, or the hospital would do it for him. After a pause, Hudson waved a hand, and with a thin voice said, "Who cares? Go ahead. We've hidden it for over a year. What's the point."

His team produced a press release. As Hudson stared stonily at his publicist, she sat at the foot of his bed and read him a draft. "Mr. Rock Hudson has Acquired Immune Deficiency Syndrome," she recited nervously. "He came to Paris to consult with a specialist in this disease. Prior to meeting the specialist, he became very ill at the Ritz Hotel, and his business manager Mark Miller advised him from California to enter the American Hospital immediately. The physicians discovered abnormalities in the liver which, without knowledge of an AIDS diagnosis, were suspected to be caused either by infections or were consistent with metastatic liver disease. These abnormalities are currently being evaluated."

Hudson listened silently. "Okay," he said. "Go out and give it to the dogs."

The news tore around the globe, igniting gossip in most known languages, and sending printing presses into overdrive. The *New York*

Post's commuter edition was on sale within hours. I brought the paper to the newsroom, and our collective feeling was clear: At last.

Patrick Merla, the *Native*'s editor, imagined the influence that Hudson's notoriety could bring to funding and to public awareness. It took only a few days to see the evidence of that. In my *Native* column on the revelation, I wrote about the massive number of developments on the AIDS front, from a broken dam of media coverage to sudden voices of urgency at the research bench. Television anchors expressed amazement that an American citizen—tax-paying, upstanding, and beloved—was forced to go to France to receive a medical treatment that his own government was unable or unwilling to offer him at home. Reporters flew to Paris to discover that four hundred Americans were pleading for health care there. In the limelight, Margaret Heckler's chief of staff was dispatched to the morning shows to announce that HPA-23 would be available in the U.S. in under three weeks on a "compassionate use" basis. Even Reagan was prodded into action. Without breaking his public embargo on mentioning AIDS, he spontaneously increased his AIDS budget request by 47 percent, and Congress, not to be outdone, threw in $70 million more, bringing AIDS spending up to $190 million for the coming year—still insufficient, but a sign that the disease was finally on the public agenda.

As the days passed and Hudson failed to drop his other shoe, keeping his homosexuality a secret even in the face of death, Merla's celebration of Hudson's candor turned to anger. He assigned me the story. I called the writer Armistead Maupin, a friend of Hudson's, and asked, "Will he be coming out? Does he intend to reveal his sexual orientation?"

"We discussed it," he said, "but he won't do it. He says Hollywood is not ready for an openly gay movie star."

Despite assuming he would not likely survive to act again, I wasn't about to criticize. "Associating his name with the disease is activism enough to do what thousands before him could not," I wrote in the *Native*. "Rock Hudson is the human face of the disease. Rock Hudson is the sacrificial lamb."

To honor her friend's bravery, Elizabeth Taylor hastily organized Hollywood's first star-studded AIDS fund-raiser. Burt Reynolds, Rod Stewart, Bette Midler, and Sammy Davis Jr. attended, as did former president Gerald R. Ford and his wife, Betty. "Three of my close friends have died," Shirley MacLaine told the crowd that night. "The image is that Hollywood is panicky. Tonight shows most of us have made the choice of love rather than fear." Another of the organizers, the philanthropist Wallis Annenberg—her father was the publishing magnate Walter H. Annenberg—said, "I felt it was time to make AIDS everyone's business. I remember the polio scares of years ago. Friends of mine would disappear from summer camp. We were told old wives' tales, not to let flies bite us because they might have bitten children with polio. I saw the same kind of thing happening again—*don't eat the onions because homosexuals are in the kitchen and their tears carry the AIDS virus.* Rock Hudson deserves an Academy Award because his illness has made AIDS respectable."

Respectable was a bit too optimistic. But his disclosure meant that everyone in America now knew someone with the disease.

On September 17, after more than six thousand young Americans had died of AIDS, after the disease had eclipsed all other causes of death for New York men in their twenties and thirties, Ronald Reagan finally discussed the epidemic in public. It came during a regularly scheduled press briefing, Reagan's thirtieth since the first AIDS death was reported by the CDC. Helen Thomas, the UPI bureau chief already esteemed as the dean of the White House press corps, broke the logjam. "Mr. President," she began, "the nation's best-known AIDS scientist says the time has come now to boost existing research into what he called a minor moon-shot program to attack this AIDS epidemic that has struck fear into the nation's health workers and even in schoolchildren. Would you support a massive government research program against AIDS like the one that President Nixon launched against cancer?"

Reagan wiggled his head genially. "I have been supporting it for more than four years now," he said. "It's been one of the top priorities with us, and over the last four years and including what we have in the budget for 'eighty-six, it will amount to over a half a billion dollars that we have provided for research on AIDS, in addition to what I'm sure other medical groups are doing." He smiled as reporters jotted down his specious dollar figure. "So this is a top priority with us. Yes, there's no question about the seriousness of this, and the need to find an answer."

Reagan's small and defensive comment bridged the void between our tragedy and the American people. His acknowledgment of the plague's "seriousness" was monumental, and long overdue. Rock Hudson's fight for life had moved the mountain.

The screen idol never appeared in public again. After his condition stabilized in Paris, he chartered a 747 and returned to Los Angeles on a stretcher, accompanied by a retinue of medical experts. He spent the next twenty-six days at the UCLA Medical Center fighting various infections. Thereafter, he retired to "the Castle," his home in Beverly Hills, to be among friends. He prepared a statement that Burt Lancaster read on his behalf.

"I am not happy that I have AIDS, but if that is helping others, I can, at least, know that my own misfortune has had some positive worth," he said. "I have also been told that the media coverage of my own situation has brought enormous international attention to the gravity of this disease in all areas of humanity, and is leading to more research, more contribution of funds, and a better understanding of this disease than ever before."

Only a few weeks later, weighing barely 120 pounds and easily confused, Rock Hudson was propped up in bed in his blue pajamas and alone in his room when the life slid out of him.

ON A HUMID summer day in Bethesda, Dr. Tony Fauci strode briskly into the library attached to his office on the seventh floor of Building 31 on the NIH campus for a meeting he knew would produce fireworks. Wearing his trademark crisp white shirt and a look of mischief on his face, he opened the meeting with a promise to his senior staff. "I'm going to surprise you," he said. Mike Goldrich was the executive officer for Fauci's institute, the chief administrator responsible for NIAID's budgets and operations. Though he was not a scientist, he held considerable power over the institute's direction. Sitting beside him was Dr. James Hill, Fauci's special assistant responsible for maintaining NIAID's good relations with Congress and "Downtown," which is what everybody called HHS and the White House.

Hill looked the part of a scientist, with an expansive forehead and straw-like hair, but he was also a natural diplomat, soft-spoken and guileless. He provided Fauci with thorough briefings before every Downtown trip. But there was something else noteworthy about Hill. He was one of the highest-ranking gay men in the research firmament. Before the responsibility for AIDS fell to NIAID, Fauci had already surmised as much. They were close and comfortable in one another's company. They had plenty in common—a sense of humor, a bemusement about the politics of science, and a gourmand's admiration of fine food and wine. Hill was an exceptional amateur cook. Fauci and his wife, Christine, were regular dinner guests at his Capitol Hill townhouse, and frequently reciprocated the hospitality. When Fauci was put in charge, Hill was his first hire. "You need to know that I am a somewhat closeted gay man," Hill confessed then, adding that he didn't want to "embarrass the Institute." To which Fauci replied, "Jim, I knew that you were gay from the moment I met you. So cut the shit and say yes to my offer."

Goldrich and Hill had come to the meeting with their own deputies, junior staff members who had arrayed before them stacks of documents, spreadsheets, and notepads. They knew the subject of the meeting was the 1986 supplemental budget. Reagan and Congress had already augmented AIDS funding following Hudson's revelation. More than $130 million, roughly 70 percent of the new total, was earmarked for NIAID. This presented an opportunity to finally undertake meaningful research. The question that Goldrich and Hill had been debating was how to prioritize the spending. They had produced reports and projections for Fauci, which he had now reviewed.

To their surprise, he called their proposals inadequate. "I'm going out on a limb," Fauci told them. He had decided to make clear to the administration the magnitude of the problem, how aggressive NIAID had to be in trying to solve it, and the cost involved. "I'm going to ask for a budget that will make your hair stand on end."

Lowering his brow, Fauci announced that his budget request would be for $300 million, more than double the current allocation.

Goldrich shifted in his chair. "Tony, be careful," he said. "If you go out and ask for it, they may tell you to do the research but they might not give you the money for it."

"What could happen," Hill warned, "the administration might say, 'Tell us what you need to do AIDS research.' We might provide a dollar amount, and they might say, 'That's very important, it has high priority. Take it out of your other areas.'" If they did that this time, Hill admitted it would shut down all other work in the NIAID's infectious disease portfolio to focus solely on AIDS, an outcome nobody wanted.

Fauci had considered the problem of the "unfunded mandate." He had experienced this response in the past, on a much smaller scale. But he was firm. "I do not think we have any choice. We have to get it through," he said. "I think we would be negligent if we did not stand up and be counted and say we must have major growth in our effort on AIDS."

The plans Fauci had in mind were unprecedented. From scratch, he intended to create a national system for coordinating, funding, directing, and evaluating research on every promising AIDS treatment. At his request, Hill mapped out its structure, modeled after existing but much smaller vaccine evaluation units for other diseases. The system would entail establishing formal trial sites in a dozen cities across the country, engaging top retrovirologists and immunologists from the major universities, and together developing an enormous engine for clinical trials. He called it the AIDS Clinical Trials Group.

Some of the younger people present expressed the concern held by the classical infectious disease specialists at the institute, which was that Fauci was making too much of the disease. That was not Hill's concern, nor even Goldrich's. Goldrich had no objection other than the practical: "Do you think we will be able to get it through?"

Fauci had the face of a poker master. He admitted he had discussed the prospects with his boss at NIH, Dr. James Wyngaarden, and with Wyngaarden's approval he had approached Edward Brandt, the assistant health secretary. "Brandt was very sympathetic to it," Fauci said. "I knew if I could get the budget past the administration and have the Director of NIH and the Assistant Secretary go along with my request, that the Congress would come in and help out even more."

The NIAID division was not run as a democracy, but Fauci was pleased that his deputies endorsed his plan. In the coming days he reached out to his counterparts at the other NIH institutes doing AIDS research to encourage them also to think big while crafting their supplemental budgets. They all sat down for a summit on the epidemic in the spacious conference room in Building 1, the stately flagship structure on campus. The National Cancer Institute head, Dr. Vince DeVita, was there; the National Institute on Drug Abuse sent representatives, as did other institutes. Fauci pushed his counterparts to raise the AIDS alarms with him in the budget process. But after much debate, the others were too concerned about the possibility of an "unfunded mandate."

"We're not backing down," Fauci told them. "We'll take this by ourselves if we have to."

Fauci got his money from Congress. It was the single biggest NIH increase ever approved, and gave Fauci a major domain and daunting responsibility. It meant that for the first time in the epidemic, coordinated and targeted research would be undertaken. Fauci would now centralize all authority in his office, which left the other NIH institutes to do their AIDS work with *de minimis* budgets and a shrinking mandate.

Fauci wanted to focus only on the Gallo/Montagnier virus—not novel theories about co-infections, not a new discipline called immune modulation, and certainly not the old-world opportunistic infections that were blinding patients, scrambling their minds, or colonizing their skin, lungs, and bowels.

ON WALL STREET Peter Staley had attracted the unflattering sobriquet Pencil Neck. The year since developing his special formula for projecting the real yield of the short-shorts had been an extremely profitable one for all parties. He programmed his formula into a bulky IBM computer the tech guys had set up at his desk—the only so-called "personal computer" on the trading floor. It was big and boxy and came in three heavy segments, like something from NASA. Its faint green glow gave his face a comical Gumby-like hue as he bent over it, slapping at the keyboard with the same energy he used on his Yamaha piano at home. He was indeed a geek. He was accustomed to being teased for his faith in the computer. When he was searching for his first job, he made the reckless prediction during an interview at Goldman Sachs that buyers and sellers would eventually be matched by computers—a remark that cost him a job offer. "It's much more efficient," he said in his own losing defense.

Now his IBM was viewed as something to be visited by the curious. Only his boss, Tommy Kalaris—and, of course, his main broker, Lou Olivieri—seemed to recognize what it was able to produce. Staley's bonus rose to a quarter million dollars on the strength of his computer program. His career was on track.

To celebrate, he plotted a vacation to Amsterdam and Copenhagen that August. He invited Tracey Tanenbaum to join him, not as a beard this time but as a friend. He wouldn't need to sneak around in Europe. In fact he reserved a room at a gay hotel he found in the *Spartacus International Gay Guide*. Tanenbaum jumped at the invitation. They had grown extremely close; she often spent evenings at his apartment, serving as his sober guide, for example, during his first trip on Ecstasy, which initially caused him to sprawl naked on the floor of his apartment and talk and talk and talk, then propelled him out the door to dance till dawn at CBGB. Both were grateful that no sexual tensions had ever arisen. Tanenbaum enjoyed hearing Staley's tales of conquest at the baths. And he let her and her boyfriend use his apartment when passions demanded (she still lived with her parents). They were "sisters."

But things changed in Amsterdam. They both felt it. Tanenbaum was miserable from the start. As Staley's hotel was for men only, she let a room in an older woman's home, which turned out to be located on the distant outskirts of town. Worse, the host had strict rules for comings and goings. "I'm like a nun under house arrest," Tanenbaum complained. She was miserable when he bid her farewell in the early evening to head off alone toward the gay discos, saunas, and clubs, cruising the bicycle-choked streets until the first blinks of dawn. What a place, what a time, to be gay! At that moment, Amsterdam was the most tolerant city in the world. Homosexuality had been legal since 1811, and the oldest gay bar dated to 1927, operating almost continuously—there was the matter of the Nazi occupation—ever since. In broad daylight, gay couples walked hand in hand without a care.

On one of his first nights out, Staley met a magnetic, dark-haired man named Peter Launy, from a small town in rural Holland. He was a year older than Staley, charming, excitable, and adventuresome. Staley's infatuation was quickly reciprocated, and for just the second time in his life he was in love. They were inseparable. It took Staley many days to recognize what this was doing to Tanenbaum, who commuted sullenly from her convent every day, seeing the city in the company of a guidebook despite the plans they had made together. On the plane to Copenhagen, their second destination, they had argued. Staley knew she was right. He had been totally selfish, but he didn't care. When they landed, he called Launy from the hotel phone. "I want to come back to Amsterdam," he said. "Do you want anything from Copenhagen?"

Launy, equally heartsick, had prayed for this call. "Cigarettes," he replied. Within twenty-four hours, the two Peters were reunited. For another week they sat in cafés and sparred about politics, both leaning toward center-left thinking. Like Staley, Launy saw a political life in his future. He planned to enter law school in a year. Without measuring the consequences, Staley extended a spontaneous invitation to New York, and Launy accepted, delighted to spend the year before law school with his new lover in a new city. His flight took Launy across the Atlantic a few weeks later, in the cooler half of September, and their courtship continued at the Museum of Modern Art and in Central Park, at Fire Island and the National Zoological Park in Washington, D.C.

They lived literally around the corner from Staley's office. To make sure no colleague saw them together, Staley would arrange to meet Launy in remote neighborhoods, or they would arrive at the apartment at separate times. The closet required great attention and planning. This was a cause of mounting frustration to Launy, accustomed to his European liberties, but as far as Staley was concerned it was very manageable—and, in any case, a small price to pay for happiness.

His behavior didn't go unnoticed on the trading floor. Coworkers noted his later arrival in the mornings and earlier departure, his absence from the rollicking nightlife of the Street. Was he seeing someone new? Staley admitted that he was indeed in love, and he told a story of the beautiful girl he had met in Amsterdam and brought home for an extended stay. This was an easy slide—every fact was true but the gender. He had practiced the deception in his head. What he hadn't anticipated was being pressed for his girlfriend's name. It should be a Dutch girl's name to pair with Launy's surname. But on the spot he could think of only one other resident of that fabled canal-crossed city, not the famous spy Mata or the kindly queen Beatrix, but the unfortunate young Frank girl. "Her name's Anne," he said below a nervous cough.

When Staley told his lover the story that night after work, Launy folded over in laughter. An appropriate choice, he said, for he felt similarly locked away in the attic, an inconvenient being. From then on, in notes to Staley or in answering machine messages, he referred to himself only as Anne.

THE NEWS COVERAGE of AIDS had remained voluminous, in part because of a new tolerance in newsrooms toward openly gay reporters—itself a result of the visibility the community was enjoying, by way of the obituary pages. In San Francisco, *The Chronicle* hired the thirty-four-year-old *Advocate* veteran Randy Shilts, the first time in the known history of journalism that an openly gay reporter made the jump to the mainstream. Later, a *Los Angeles Times* writer named Victor Zonana also came out. Both took the AIDS beat. The first openly gay journalist for a major daily, however, was in New York, not at the *Times* or the *Daily News*, both of which were known to tolerate suspected (but closeted) gays in the features or arts departments, but at the *New York Post*, the American toehold for the Australian media mogul Rupert Murdoch.

Joe Nicholson was a pugnacious former Navy lieutenant with a mouth to match. But because he had never married and didn't engage in macho banter during his twenty-three years at the *Post*, various editors had had their suspicions, and once or twice someone had asked him outright if he were gay. He reversed the challenge in a stroke, rasping, "Give me a kiss and we'll find out." He finally answered the question honestly in an article we ran in the *Native* that generated not one word of comment in his newsroom. His superiors might not have been happy, but the Newspaper Guild made him untouchable. Once he left the closet, Nicholson—an Irish Catholic who graduated Holy Cross College—turned his Cagney-like persona to the gay struggle. He was my role model and a new kind of journalist, the abrupt reporter of legend who melded the role of witness with perspective. He once joined a pickup basketball game with a group of young men who had violently attacked the Olympic medalist Dick Button in a gay cruising area, coaxing out their boastful confessions. For an article about Executive Order 50, I overheard him grilling a Catholic Church spokesman in his piercing tough-guy voice: "Tell me, Father, when you were in seminary and you were in the showers, you never once got turned on, even just a little bit, looking at the other boys' legs and rear ends?" (He told me later that he had been provoked.)

Shilts, Zonana, and Nicholson—coincidentally, Nicholson was his paper's medicine-science editor—produced the most aggressive mainstream AIDS coverage, often stretching the boundaries of their editors' comfort. Nicholson had the more difficult challenge. His editors patrolled his work for ideological deviation and transgressions of language (even the word "condom" was banned), and the photo desk routinely refused to assign camera people to snap sources, citing contagion fears. But by campaigning ruthlessly for space in the paper, he won considerable real estate, assuring that the *Post*, of all places, produced far more useful information than the venerable *Times*—but also some of the worst. To counter Nicholson, editors transplanted Ray Kerrison, a conservative columnist assigned to the arcana of horse racing, to the front of the paper for a regular column devoted to condemning what he called "the gay deathstyle." His invective went over so well with readers that in the summer he anchored a daily series under the banner "AIDS Timebomb," which hammered away at, among other things, the disaster of letting kids with AIDS go to school or men with the disease work in restaurants.

Kerrison's *Post* persona was an aberration in volume, but not in sentiment. Papers across the spectrum were portraying gay men as public health menaces—"walking Three Mile Islands," in Nathan Fain's joyless phrase. In 1985, twenty states debated legislation for quarantining or otherwise controlling people with AIDS and suspected carriers. The dialogue was particularly coarse in Texas, which ranked fifth among states in the number of AIDS cases. San Antonio's health director mailed letters to all AIDS patients threatening a ten-year prison term if they engaged in sexual intercourse, safe or not. The mayoral race in Houston tightened when Louie Welch, who had been trailing in polls, suggested that a better way to block the disease was to "shoot the queers."

By fall, the first reactionary federal legislation was introduced when the conservative Republican congressman William Dannemeyer of Orange County, California, presented a suite of bills proposing "common sense" approaches aimed at "protecting the integrity and the health and the public at large." One measure sought to bar people with AIDS from practicing in the health care industry, even as X-ray technicians; others would pull federal funds from any city where gay bathhouses remained open and bar sick kids from public schools. Finally, he proposed lengthy prison terms for any gay person who attempted to donate blood, whether moved by civic virtue or otherwise. "Strange and weird as it may sound," he said on the House floor, "my office has received unconfirmed reports, which are difficult to check out, that certain male homosexuals in this country are so incensed and frustrated that America has not found a solution to the AIDS crisis to cure them of this disease that they have, in a spirit of spite, threatened to donate blood—those with AIDS—in order to contaminate the blood supply, hoping to reach the heterosexual world so as to increase the level of attention that we of the heterosexual world, the 95 percent of us in this country, may be willing to devote to this tragic disease." It had become perfectly normal to attribute venal motives to the sick and superpowers to the virus, creating what one observer called "the darkest public portrayal of homosexuality since the McCarthy era."

Dannemeyer's bills didn't pass, but they had an impact nonetheless. An otherwise ordinary community in Kokomo, Indiana, went to the barricades when it was revealed that a thirteen-year-old hemophiliac named Ryan White had come down with the virus via blood products and hoped to continue his education regardless. Terror-stricken students and their parents forced him out of seventh grade, demanding that he take his lessons through a telephone hookup. They shunned the rest of the family as well. When his uninfected mother, Jeanne White, went to the grocery store, cashiers would throw down her change to avoid touching her hands. Vandals broke the windows of the family's house, slashed their car tires, and sent a bullet into the living room when the Whites sought relief in court.

To Ray Kerrison, Ryan White was an "innocent" victim "whose suffering is agonizing and whose plight deserves every consideration and resource at our disposal." But he condemned the boy's parents for not just keeping him at home. Feeling beleaguered, Joe Nicholson asked me to join him in the *Post* newsroom, the beast's own belly. There were two other gay men and a lesbian on the payroll, all in the closet, some deeper than others. He needed reinforcements. But there would be a catch. "They won't hire you if they know you're gay," he said. "They'll think you're biased. If you make it ninety days you're covered by the union and you can be open." Lasting three months would be difficult under ordinary circumstances: for budgetary reasons, management liked terminating tryouts before the vesting period was completed. "There's a long history of eighty-nine-day wonders," Nicholson warned me.

On his recommendation, I cut my hair, retired my earrings, and swapped my Chuck Taylors for simple Thom McAns. He counseled me to produce a false work history in which my only qualification for the job was the ability to type. That half-page résumé won me a tryout as an assistant to the investigations editor, charged with keying his discoveries into the mainframe computer.

Life in the closet was more awkward the second time around. At Nicholson's strong suggestion, I showed no professional interest in our stymied community, leaving him to fight that battle alone against a tidal wave of column inches from the right wing. From a distance, I spotted Kerrison as he hand-delivered his columns on colored paper to the news editors for markup. He wasn't what I'd expected. A slight man with unclean hair who favored shiny brown suits, he appeared shy and private in person, not the foaming firebrand that his columns conjured. Kerrison's standing at the paper improved with every gay-themed column he filed. This was not lost on other aspiring reporters and tryouts, who clamored for a corner of the "faggot" beat. The tidal force of it all weighed terribly on Nicholson, but he fought back with journalism, producing strong articles that sank deeper into the paper, eclipsed by every adjective of revilement his colleagues could muster. One brash young reporter went undercover into one of the "AIDS Dens." He buckled on a towel like medieval armor and burst harrowingly into the bathhouse hallways, denouncing what he found there, or thought he found there, or wanted to find there, as the "Skid Row of gay sex." "[W]alk in and go through a turnstile and you see desperate men—men without families, men without lovers, many without real friends."

For me, it required a peculiar kind of psychological contortion to remain silent. More than any other institution in the city, the *Post* was shaping the conversation on AIDS. When the weather cooled, it fomented an ugly riot of parents in Queens when the school board refused to bar a child who tested positive, causing a citywide school walkout. Next the paper forced Mayor Koch to abandon a pilot program giving nursing home beds to ten homeless AIDS patients over community objections. "There is only one certainty about AIDS," the *Post*'s editorial board wrote. "No one knows enough about it to make general statements of any sort." Faring worse than the infected homeless and the children were gay men and, ironically, lesbians, who had the lowest infection rates of any subgroup. A national poll that fall found that more than a third of Americans had changed their opinions about the community for the worse since the onset of AIDS. The *Los Angeles Times* reported that the community's political heyday was over, when in truth what the community tumbled from was already the bottom rung.

A FEW WRITERS from the *Native* joined a number of veteran activists and intellectuals on October 30 to craft a response to the escalating hostility from mainstream media, which Gregory Kolovakos, a boyish translator of Mario Vargas Llosa, said posed "the greatest threat to our freedoms and civil liberties that we've faced since Stonewall." They didn't know how to stop it, but were prepared to stage direct action in the streets after what had been years of post-Stonewall docility.

"The silence only connotes complacency within our community," Kolovakos said. "But I know that there is a lot of anger, fear, and a real sense that we can't be beaten down anymore over fake issues and misrepresentations." To make their goals plain, the group called itself the Gay and Lesbian Anti-Defamation League and crafted a mission statement similar to the one that B'nai B'rith had used to guide *their* Anti-Defamation League since 1913. They would secure justice and fair treatment toward lesbians and gays, and respond wherever untruths about gay lives were being trafficked.

But almost as soon as they put out a call for a town hall meeting to announce their formation came cease-and-desist warnings from, of all places, the very Jewish group they so admired. The Anti-Defamation League felt defamed by association with the gays. They threatened legal action, forcing the new group to change its name to the Gay and Lesbian Alliance Against Defamation, or GLAAD.

The town hall meeting was held on November 14, an unusually warm late-autumn night. A fluorescent sliver of moon hung in the sky. More than seven hundred people descended on the Metropolitan-Duane United Methodist Church on West Thirteenth Street in Greenwich Village. They filled the pews, then the choir lofts; bodies choked the aisles and vestries and snaked out the door. It was the most people inside the sanctuary that the church's administrator had ever seen, even counting Easter and Christmas. It may have been the largest political summit of gay men and lesbians in the city's history. The energy was as electrifying as the night's sky. Most in attendance were middle-class liberals who had never taken a public stand for their rights, but a few were familiar faces in the movement—the street transgender activist Marsha P. Johnson and the feminist author Jewelle Gomez, both African American—who brought a breadth of experience and class consciousness to this still leaderless assemblage.

I arrived late, but in time to hear the speakers call for the formation of a massive street protest at the doorstep of my new employer. "Bring your old rags," someone shouted, "to throw at that old rag." The restless crowd whistled and clapped.

A man few people recognized moved to the front of the church's nave. Darrell Yates Rist, in his mid-thirties, was a darkly handsome man and a fine dresser, favoring three-piece suits to complement a lavish moustache and, usually, a downturned face. I knew him from the *Native*, where he submitted occasional pieces remarkable for their gravity. I had not known him to be a rousing speaker, but these times had called him to eloquence and rage. He glowered over the room, then jabbed the air with a finger.

"Many of us had to live a lie too long," he began. "We spent agonizing years believing lies about ourselves, hideous lies that fed self-hate, that ate away at us until we feared that any minute we would be destroyed. These lies sneered that we are sinful, we are moral blights, we are sick, we are desperate, we're violent, and, more than 'normal people,' prone to heinous crimes. *Lies* that we recruit young children—and 'innocent adults'; that we cannot love; that we're unlovable; we're sexually obsessed; that we're all promiscuous; that our relationships don't last; that we spread disease, emotional and physical; that good, clean folks can catch perversion or a deadly germ by simply being near us in a room. *Lies.* That we cannot control our genitals, as heterosexuals can. That therefore straight folks must control us"—a furious ovation interrupted him—"otherwise, we won't stop copulating as we wish, without a conscience, without precaution, without responsibility, until we've killed ourselves—for we are suicidal—*and* killed others—for we are homicidal, too. All of these are lies and *we are sick of lies*."

The audience responded as to a Dust Bowl revivalist, hands in the air. Their sense of having been mischaracterized was universal. Rist delved into history, his own and our collective stories, through the 1950s and our "stymied puberties," past the fires of Stonewall and the "anarchy of passion" that followed alongside gay liberation. "Not that all the vulgar lies about us ceased. But they *seemed* at times to be contained," he said. "Things appeared to change—slowly, haltingly—and then our progress, more and more, took on a steady pace. Those were heady days—gay and lesbian pride from San Francisco to New York and countless places, we thought, in between. . . . *It seemed sometimes that we were free.*"

He looked around the room at the many young faces. Their faces showed portent, surely, and frustration. And fear. Not defiance.

"Then, AIDS," he said.

How soon the bigots made the issue theirs, manipulating tragedy with hate. "GRID," they jumped to call it—*Gay* Related Immune Deficiency—as though just what they'd always said was true, that we were not like other human beings and this was proof—our very own disease. Or, more spiteful still, that we were damned—because of who we are—to suffer tortured, early deaths, a godly retribution. And from the very time this illness was identified, the air has swarmed with lies—in the street, in the press, and in the legislative halls.

Listen to the lies: *AIDS is a gay disease,* when in the worldwide epidemic, it is straight, striking men and women equally whenever it occurs in Africa and, as *The New York Times* wrote just last week, spread through "conventional sexual intercourse" (that offensive adjective!). *AIDS is not now gay, nor has it ever been.*

Listen to the lies: *Gays, getting buggered by infected boys in Haiti, brought AIDS here.* But, as the Centers for Disease Control too quietly announced, the first AIDS case was not a gay man in 1979—the mythic epidemic's starting point—but a San Francisco woman in 1976—heterosexual, an IV-drug abuser, three years before a case of "homosexual" AIDS was diagnosed. But addicts often die in slums or in the street, their deaths conveniently and callously ascribed to overdose, whether that's *really* it or not. And, as some epidemiologists, even some inside the CDC, confess, if there was one IV-drug related case in 1976, when no one had yet pinned a name on AIDS, there were many others, maybe hundreds, before one gay man got sick. *However AIDS arrived, gay men didn't start it in their rectums.*

Listen to the lies: *AIDS-infected gay men poisoned the U.S. blood supply.* But it was American pharmaceutical companies which in the seventies were buying plasma from the destitute in Africa, the

Caribbean, and Central America—from some of the very countries where AIDS is killing rampantly. And, as late as 1982, some of these companies purchased plasma from U.S. prisoners who, according to investigators, had tracks of needle marks running up their arms from recent drug abuse. This was plasma which became the clotting factors used by hemophiliacs, whose AIDS infections, and whose deaths, were wholly blamed on homosexuals. But *gay men will not submit to lies and bear the wretched burden of this guilt.*

Listen to the lies: *That this country cares about our lives.* That it is looking for a cure for AIDS as feverishly as it would if the victims of this horror were all straight.

Listen to the lies: That the U.S. government, the CDC, the medical establishment *grieve* that some 10,000 of us have been stricken; mourn our dead—now more than 5,000; pray that not one more of us will die. Listen to the lies: *That our sorrow has torn this nation, wrenched it just as horribly as it would if the epidemic were destroying, not gay men, but husbands and their wives.*

His audience rose angrily to pound out applause, denouncing the nation whose cavalry never came. Rist waited for them to settle into their pews before he continued. "We have not forgotten that *The New York Times* cared very little, very late. We do not forget that the *Daily News* still likes to paint gay sex as scandal. . . . And the *New York Post:* We will not be satisfied until this nasty piece of lunacy has folded. There is no place for journalistic filth like that in any sane society."

The room now sparked with the energy of an angry mob. The community had found its rage, given to them by a largely unknown man with his unexpected, powerful speech. For that moment at least, Darrell Yates Rist became the leader the community had been looking for. The look of burden was gone from the faces in the audience. Their voices were a roar of excitement. They spilled out into the city with a purpose and a plan: the "rags protest" at the *New York Post* would mark a new beginning.

When the frigid morning came, I knew I couldn't cross their picket line. Nor could I join them openly without forfeiting my job. So I called in sick and headed over to join the protesters in disguise, fully encased in a balaclava and heavy topcoat, my woolen closet. A sign on my lapel read, "I would lose my job if seen here." Inside the paper's newsroom, I heard later, editors debated hilariously over which young reporter they would punish with the job of covering the protest. They settled on "poor Margie Feinberg," a rookie who emerged from the lobby door as if entering a cage of rabid dogs. She kept a great distance from the chanting protestors, perhaps as many as one thousand before a sleeting rain cleaved the ranks. I was relieved that she did not see through my disguise. Not even my old colleagues at the *Native* did. They unknowingly used a photograph of me on the cover of *Christopher Street*, taking me for the emblem of closet life.

In the wake of the protest, with a few weeks remaining in my trial period, the investigations editor called me into his office. "Found out you're gay," he said through the grin of a poor winner. I looked away. On his desk I saw clippings of my work in the *Native*. "We don't need infiltrators here, bloke, not homosexuals in the investigations department."

I dreamed of being the person who confronted bigotry, who overturned tables and spray-painted bright red truths on walls. I fanaticized about having the last word. But I left the building in silence, not as an eighty-nine-day wonder but as a homosexual flushed safely from the bushes.

RICHARD BERKOWITZ returned to New York in the fall, ending his Florida retirement a few days ahead of his thirtieth birthday. His time in Bal Harbour had been restorative, thanks to the beneficence of a former client, a doctor who not only saw to Berkowitz's comfort for a year but also kept his New York rent current while personally looking after his medical needs. The pampered life helped Berkowitz push the epidemic's clashing personalities out of mind. He kept to a routine of strenuous exercise and mindful consumption—no more drugs, and even less politics. But he failed to find meaningful employment. He offered lectures on safe sex and even landed a gig promoting it in South Florida bathhouses, but a true income never materialized. He conceded defeat after more than a year, returning to New York in top physical form with reluctant plans to reenter the sex trade.

Michael Callen's political retirement was also a success. He thought of himself as a modern-day Cincinnatus, a mere farmer called away from his plow to lead the Roman army at a time of urgent need who returned to the countryside when his work was done. Callen threw himself into his band, Lowlife. Billed as a "dance-oriented, kickass, rock 'n' roll party band," it featured Callen on keyboards and Richard Dworkin on drums, along with two guitar-pounding lesbians, Pam

Brandt and Janet Cleary. Gender parity was Callen's idea, and a radical one at a time when lesbians and gay men inhabited parallel cultural spaces. Femaleness was a source of deep inspiration for Callen. He devoured books on women's history and feminism. If his AIDS work had dragged him into a mostly male world, his music would bring him back—and the audience along with him. As Dworkin put it, "Maybe the men are watching me and Michael, and the women are watching Janet and Pam, but inevitably they have to look at the whole band, and at everyone else in the room."

The group was a marvel, enjoying strong reviews and a growing number of bookings, most recently on October 17 at the Pyramid Club on Avenue A in the East Village, followed by a stretch in the recording studio. Callen was the star, praised for his "screamingly high falsetto" and hilarious country and western yodel.

Finally taking his musical life seriously was, for Callen, a recommitment to life itself. But as with all matters Callen, it was also deeply influenced by politics. He interspersed their sets with queer banter touching on everything from AIDS to homophobic cops to sexual autonomy, themes echoed in songs like "Vigilantes," a rebel call in the AIDS war to "look out for our own," and "We Did It Anyway," about finding love in the clubs that promise only sex. But where Lowlife connected with audiences was with their poignant reinterpretations of oldies. Their rendition of "Secret Agent Man," in the context of their repertoire, was a powerful invocation of bathhouse culture in a time of plague.

> *There's a man who leads a life of danger*
> *Everyone he meets he stays a stranger*
> *With every move he makes*
> *Another chance he takes*
> *The odds are he won't live to see tomorrow.*

Their reputation spread outside the city as well, with invitations to tour. He had dreams that success would carry him to a new life in California, or even Europe.

But as fiercely as he tried, he couldn't leave the battlements altogether. He bowed to peer pressure and retained his board seats with countless organizations, including the governor's Interagency Task Force on AIDS, the New York State AIDS Advisory Council, the National Gay Task Force, and the Bathhouse Subcommittee of the state's AIDS Institute. In addition, his home phone was the unofficial hotline for every one of Dr. Sonnabend's patients, with their onslaughts of fear and need. As long as he was alive and in the city, he knew, this would be his lot.

He saw little of Berkowitz after he'd returned. He was not aware that his old collaborator had resumed his work with the flesh, albeit with a twist. His somewhat unexpected ads in the *Native* and *The Advocate* were attuned to the times—his innovation was to offer "bondage & discipline" as a "safe-sex master." So many New Yorkers had such fond memories of the legendary "Very gdlkg, straight-type Italian" that he did not lack for business.

Still, it proved impossible to cast the plague into the past. Berkowitz began discovering spots on his clients, KS lesions they had overlooked. In a few months he noticed more clients with KS than without, a higher ratio of "gay cancer" than in Sonnabend's practice. He didn't have Callen's ease with patients. He agonized over how to suggest they go for a checkup. Stress built up. He soon reacquainted himself with cocaine, despite his vows. When a client offered him crack, which was sweeping the city, he found a better analgesic. He loved its fast, jagged high, how it reoriented the hideous world. But crack paralyzed him as surely as it did anyone else, and launched him on the darkest journey of his life, one that would alienate him from Michael Callen and, more important, Dr. Sonnabend, at the time he needed them the most.

AT THE END of a long and chilly Veterans Day weekend, 1985, Peter Staley and Peter Launy were in front of the television. With an emotional slurry of obligation and dread, they were watching *An Early Frost*, the first film to deal with AIDS. It seemed as though the entire country felt similarly compelled. Some 34 million Americans turned to NBC to watch the show, far outpolling *Cagney & Lacey* on CBS and ABC's highly anticipated San Francisco 49ers–Denver Broncos football game. In sweeps month, such an audience would normally mean a large fortune for the network, except on this subject. The network lost a half-million dollars in advertising revenue as corporation after corporation fled the time slot, as though AIDS could be borne on airwaves.

This was the first time Americans saw a sympathetic portrayal of a gay couple on television. They watched the actor Aidan Quinn coughing and wheezing, begging for an ambulance driver who refused to take him, making his own way to a hospital where rooms were fumigated after AIDS did its work. They saw the ravages, both biomedical and political, and the cost to the patient in the lost love of family. And there was D. W. Moffett, playing the faithful partner. A sensation of pride coursed through Staley and his lover. On the screen was a couple just like them, two men in love, and one of them coughing. Staley's lungs had been rattling for weeks, accompanied by a low-grade fever. It had become a kind of joke for Launy to say, "You're sweating again." Cough drops, menthol rubs, and Echinacea had all let him down. But Staley had put it out of his thoughts, and so had Launy until this minute, in front of this television movie.

"There's something going on, Peter. Something serious."

"It's a cold," Staley said. "A bad cold."

As the film progressed, Quinn's character confronted death in the experience of his hospital roommate, who perished in a gnarl of opportunistic infections. Launy and Staley wept. And when the film was over Staley agreed to see Dr. Dan William about the cold. A week-long vacation to Disney World and Cape Canaveral would start for the couple on Friday. It would be good to begin the antibiotics before heading south.

Staley had not been to his doctor's office since his case of the flu turned out to be herpes. Not even *An Early Frost* prepared him for how much the waiting room scene had changed in the two years since. The office was jammed with sick patients, men in wheelchairs, men so thin they looked like death camp victims. William labored with the dazed concentration of a war zone surgeon. He extracted Staley's blood samples swiftly. Late Friday morning, Staley called for results.

The doctor's receptionist, Bob, answered. "You've got a low white blood count," he reported. "You need to come in for more tests."

"What are the possibilities?" Staley demanded.

Bob ran down a list of things that cause a drop in white blood cells. And the end of the list, after a pause, he added, "Well, and it could be a sign of AIDS. *But we need more tests.*"

Even this did not yet faze Staley. Thirty minutes later, he stood in the doctor's examining room, leaving more blood behind, this time for CD4 blood counts, then he raced to the airport with Launy. Coincidentally, among the women's magazines and decorating books at the newsstand in the terminal, Staley found the newest issue of *Discover* magazine, which was given over entirely to the "seemingly hopeless" epidemic; "AIDS: The Latest Scientific Facts," read the cover line. That evening and the following morning at the Days Inn in Orlando, Staley devoured page after page, dismayed by how much was still unsettled about the epidemic. The magazine didn't play down the odds. If Staley had this disease, he was in deep trouble. "AIDS is incurable and believed to be always fatal," it said. His death was a dirigible appearing on the horizon. A numbing terror seized him. Sitting on the king-sized hotel bed, Staley wept helplessly.

Then his self-pity lifted as quickly as it had fallen on him. If he had a limited future, he would not spend the time shaking his fist at God. Rather, he would live the life of his dreams, which was the life he now had—in the company of a handsome and devoted lover, his own thick-accented D. W. Moffett.

The following Tuesday morning, standing at a pay phone outside Cape Canaveral, Staley's uncertainty came to an end. Dr. William explained that Staley's CD4 count was a worrisome 351, well below a normal count of at least 600, and his ratio was inverted. It would be weeks before his HTLV-3/LAV antibody test results would cement a diagnosis, but William had no doubt. Four years after the first cases were described, Staley was part of a new generation of infections, a statistical surge of young men who had not experienced the community's adolescent hedonism in the 1970s and felt somehow immune as a result.

How long did he have to live? Staley demanded the cold truth. In an epidemic that remained so mysterious, this was one question for which the answer was definitive. William wouldn't give a prognosis, but he didn't have to—the *Discover* magazine article had made it plain: two years, at best.

That Thanksgiving, Staley returned to Philadelphia to break the news that, as he joked wanly, "I have AIDS, and I'm not Haitian," borrowing a line from *An Early Frost*. He met with siblings one at a time, ordered from least homophobic to most. First up was his brother Chris, a ceramicist, then Janet, the youngest, a college student. The last sibling he told was his older brother, Jes, whose casual anti-gay diatribes had so often offended him. (Jes apologized profusely.)

Staley told them what he told his parents: "I think I probably have a couple of years, but I want to keep doing what I'm doing. I don't want to change my life drastically." He added, "I have a boyfriend. His name is Peter. I want you to accept him as a member of our family."

It was a drama playing out at countless family gatherings that Thanksgiving. There now were 15,053 cases; the number was doubling every year. Stunned as the Staleys were, they powered through the holiday stoically.

IT WAS NOW settled scientific fact. The virus Gallo "discovered" was indeed the virus Montagnier had sent him. Gallo shrugged it off as a common cross-contamination, and no big deal. He had since successfully found his own isolate. More importantly, he retained the patent rights for a so-called AIDS blood test. Within the year sales would surpass $34 million, with up to $4 million going back to the NCI in royalties. Government policy kept individuals from profiting—until 1987, when Gallo and his two main team members were each awarded $100,000 annually off the top. Neither Montagnier nor the Institut Pasteur saw a penny.

As a result, the Gallo group in Bethesda found itself even more at odds with the Parisian brain trust. Over the summer, a friend of Gallo's, a University of Paris researcher named Daniel Zagury, brokered a series of tense dinner meetings between Gallo and Pasteur's top officials. The second of these, at the home of *Le Monde*'s science editor, Dr. Claudine Escoffier-Lambiotte, brought to the table one of Pasteur's directors, Dr. François Gros, and Dr. François Jacob, a Nobel laureate and one of France's best-known scientists.

"The dinner was light and delicious," Gallo reported some time later, "the conversation less so."

Jacob, speaking on behalf of the institute, was unusually frank, characterizing Gallo's behavior as both unfair and shockingly unethical. He contended that the Institut Pasteur, a nonprofit center, was rightfully entitled to royalties as the discoverer of the virus. He proposed that the NIH—and Gallo personally, since the application bore his signature—voluntarily agree to share the revenue equally. It was a compromise, a painful one for the Institut Pasteur, and the least they could accept. Lawyers stood in the wings if Gallo rejected it, Jacob added. If the matter landed in the courts, Jacob said, Gallo would not fare well.

For Gallo, this was a matter of pride, not gain. He felt that his patent application was granted because it was the better one. Of little consequence to Gallo was the fact that his test proved to be wildly inaccurate, while Montagnier's team had improved theirs so dramatically that it was now far superior, according to trials in England and Australia and even by the American Red Cross. He held his ground, and the evening did not end on a higher note.

Gallo returned home to consult with his immediate superior at the NCI and with the director of the NIH, James Wyngaarden, who backed Gallo's hard line.

Jacob had no choice but to carry out his threat and pursue legal and diplomatic action. In August, the Institut Pasteur dispatched a formal delegation to Washington with an official protest. Heading the dramatic mission was Pasteur director Raymond Dedonder, who issued a chilling ultimatum. "I must impress on you that, if a satisfactory agreement is not attained [by] September, the Pasteur Institute is prepared, and determined, and even compelled to utilize all the available procedures to obtain complete recognition of its rights," he said.

September came and went. In December, legal papers were filed as promised, and for much of the next year Gallo was repeatedly distracted from his laboratory work by a bolt of nasty articles in the *New Scientist* and the European newspapers, accusing him of countless perfidies.

4

Warfare

In the aftermath of the promising Phase I trial showing AZT's relative safety, Drs. Broder and Yarchoan felt they had ample evidence
to suggest that the pills were not just tolerable, but dramatically effective. One patient in particular was their polestar, a New York City
nurse who contracted AIDS through a transfusion. Her symptoms
included a nasty fungal infection under her fingernails and severe oral
canker sores. With AZT, both cleared up completely and the nucleus
of a normal nail began to take shape. To Yarchoan, this seemed near
miraculous. But after the trial ended and the AZT was withdrawn, the
clinical progress reversed. Monitoring the patient's blood, he saw new
CD_4 cells collapsing, ratios re-inverting, and opportunistic infections
multiplying once again. "It was something like *Flowers for Algernon*,"
Yarchoan said.

To see if the health gains could be maintained, they wanted to put
the Phase I patients back on AZT and follow their progress for a longer
period of time, but to do so they needed special permission from the
FDA, which was not easily won. The regulatory agency didn't have
a simple procedure for allowing experimental medication to be used
therapeutically. But after initial intransigence, regulators agreed that
it would be inhumane to refuse AZT to these nineteen patients. Even
while answers to significant questions about the compound's efficacy
were still unknown, the FDA instituted an informal agreement allowing
for very limited "compassionate use" of the unapproved drug.

By January 1986, Yarchoan was ready for the Phase II trial, the true
test of a new drug's efficacy. The design of the clinical trial called for
a multicenter, double-blind placebo-controlled protocol, long considered the gold standard. It meant that neither the researchers nor the
patients would know who was on the placebo and who was not—both
blind, in other words—and only half of the patients enrolled around
the country would be receiving AZT while the rest would take a use-

less substitute made from cornstarch or saltwater. The significant end-point of the trial, the key variable in outcomes, would be death. If more people died on the placebo than on AZT, the drug would be considered beneficial. A final Phase III study would go on to determine exactly *how* efficacious the drug was, by measuring how much it extended life.

Throughout January and February, the final details of the trial were worked out. Two hundred and fifty patients would be recruited through a dozen medical centers in San Diego, San Francisco, Los Angeles, Boston, Chicago, New York City, and elsewhere. A center connected to the University of Miami, Jackson Memorial Hospital, would take the lead. The point person there was Dr. Margaret Fischl, a timid general practitioner with a fierce intelligence and towering ambition, though she was just thirty-six. What brought her to the attention of Burroughs Wellcome was not immediately clear. She had authored three AIDS papers to date, one a case report on brain lesions, but had never taken on such a daunting responsibility. Her training was as an internist, not as a research scientist.

The timetable was ambitious. Enrollment would begin immediately, and the study would be completed by Christmas 1986. For patients to be eligible, they were required to discontinue any other medication during the course of the twenty-four-week trial, including lifesaving prophylaxis for PCP. For the trial to produce unambiguous answers, Burroughs Wellcome deemed it essential to test AZT without the interference of other pharmaceuticals. Samuel Broder at the NCI concurred, knowing it condemned people to preventable deaths. "God have mercy, you don't want to do that more than once," he told me.

To Sonnabend, who had been following the trial's development closely, this was tantamount to premeditated murder, no more ethical than denying patients food. His arguments were amplified by Dr. Mathilde Krim and others who testified that summer before congressional hearings about the immorality of these "death trials." Many argued for a more humane study allowing everyone participating to take prophylactics in addition to either placebo or AZT, and most thoroughly objected to the use of placebos. Instead, they advocated for making the drug available to everyone in the study, no matter what else they were taking, then comparing their health to what was already known about the natural course of an AIDS diagnosis. Dr. Krim went even further, advocating for making AZT broadly available to anyone who wanted it, even without solid data showing that it worked. "Do we have the right to refuse a dying person a small measure of hope?" she asked.

"Or the dignity to fight to the end?" But neither Burroughs Wellcome nor the government was receptive.

The last variable for the trial was dosing. This was the trial-and-error area of drug testing. The Burroughs Wellcome team pushed for a very high dose, arguing that bombarding the patient would make it easier to read whether the drug worked or not. Damage to bone marrow, it was agreed, was an unfortunate but acceptable price to pay for certainty. The FDA agreed, approving a dose of 1,500 milligrams per day, administered every four hours even through the night. This was the high end of the doses given in the safety trial. As an additional protection, throughout the trial the patients would be monitored by a data and safety monitoring board whose independent members had access to all test results for each patient, secretly examining them weekly, ready to intervene if circumstances required.

Early research was also under way on a host of other drugs. Ribavirin was being evaluated in a study group of about fifty patients; according to the rumor mill, its power against the virus was not promising. It had many fans on the underground nevertheless. The same was true for HPA-23, the drug that had drawn Rock Hudson to Paris and for which patients were still clamoring. The belated U.S. trials, involving just forty-two patients, found that HPA-23 gave patients a vague and fleeting sense of improvement, with no clinical benefits. Early studies were in preparation or under way on naltrexone, isoprinosine, and cyclosporine A, whose manufacturers seemed to announce price hikes every time the gay papers published upbeat stories. In fact, the drugs seemed to be mostly inert against the virus. It was AZT that gave hope to the community for the first time. The *Native,* keeping track of the original nineteen patients, reported that almost all the Phase I trial subjects were "alive and stable . . . four to eight months after entry to the study." This struck a chord with a dying population, where people would give anything for an extra four to eight months.

FIVE YEARS INTO the plague, a formal nomenclature committee of eminent scientists from around the world took up the task of settling the dispute over the virus's name, if not its paternity. It was an American representative from the University of California, San Francisco, who proposed the inelegant descriptor "human immunodeficiency virus," or HIV, and the people in charge of such things at the Human Retrovirus Subcommittee of the International Committee on the Taxonomy of Viruses found this acceptable. Montagnier and the

French supported the change and quickly sought acceptance from the World Health Organization of the French translation, VIH, for *virus de l'immunodéficience humaine*. Though he had no vote in the matter, Gallo rejected the proposal outright, still fighting for the name he and his NIH colleagues had registered with the U.S. Patent Office, or, at the very least, HTLV-3/LAV. He argued his case obsessively. As the body count surpassed sixteen thousand, his noxious squabble showed no signs of abating.

In his own defense, Gallo made a point of asserting that none of the binational maneuvering had any negative affect on patient care, prevention, or ongoing scientific discovery. This claim was hard to defend. Under constant pressure, whether from him (which he denies) or his supporters, the FDA stymied the HIV antibody test developed by the Institut Pasteur, despite its superiority to the version registered by Gallo and the NIH and approved in 1985. Finally, in February 1986, a year after the French had submitted an application, the FDA gave its limited blessing. But the distributors were specifically prohibited from mentioning studies showing the superior accuracy of their product, on the apparent grounds of national pride.

There was no way to know how many units of tainted blood slipped past the faulty screening test, or how many people got sick as a result. The CDC would soon report one confirmed case of HIV transmission through blood that had been screened with Gallo's test, and shortly announced transmission to seven patients who received vital organs from a donor who had been screened twice, producing two false negatives. These transmissions could be blamed squarely on monopolistic intransigence. (For their part, the French refused to adopt Gallo's screen even when theirs lagged in production. Arrogance was a deadly vice.)

The matter of false positives was equally devastating, though harder to quantify in terms of lost lives. Whether a positive test result was true or false, the stigma was crushing just the same. Kids were removed from schools that year based on rumors alone. In August, an hour after a Manhattan man named Terry Dangelo was told he was positive, he leaped seven floors to his death. If even one of these cases stemmed from the unreliable test while a better one was kept off the American market, the leaders of the American Public Health Service had to carry the heavy burden for those lives as well.

His other assertion, that intensive scientific work had continued meantime, did seem true in important regards. Between 1984 and

1986—the "period of discovery," as it would be called in retrospect—huge strides were made in the understanding of retroviruses and the immune system generally, and in the Solomonicly disputed retrovirus in particular. Its peculiar physical structure was now established, as was its mechanism for infection and reproduction, and its life cycle. It was a typical retrovirus, with a fairly high molecular weight. But genetically it was way more complex than other known retroviruses, able to use a sequence of genes for a wide range of adaptation—in essence, it could modify itself to accommodate each cell it infected. Remarkably, it managed these changes a "millionfold" faster than most other organisms, as Gallo reported. Nothing like this had ever been seen before.

As this exploratory work progressed, it became apparent that Gallo, not Montagnier, was the field's driving scientific mind. He had the idea to test for a retrovirus, he created the first continuous culture in which it would grow, and he showed its relationship to causing AIDS. In his memoir years later, Gallo said that debating whether or not he was the first person to physically lay eyes on the virus missed the point, "the arguments stale and of little relevance to the scientists on either side." The discovery was hypothesized by him, made possible by him, and spearheaded by him. After all that groundbreaking work was laid out, Montagnier's group of "crappy scientists" (as Gallo told a colleague) simply lucked upon the thing, like a bum tripping over a dropped wallet. This point of view had many adherents, even among some in Montagnier's universe. "Around here we say, he stumbled onto the virus and he's stumbling still," admitted a colleague at Pasteur.

Gallo, despite his obsessions and unseemly competitiveness, was the acknowledged genius of AIDS research. His annual lab meetings, attended by the world's top virologists and AIDS investigators, proved he was one of the world's most formidable scientists, a researcher with the star power of Einstein or Freud. Dr. Broder, who openly compared Gallo to both titans, considered him "one of the paradigmatic figures of the twentieth century."

By contrast, Montagnier's lab was stymied. Whether this was caused by the challenging science or because resources were depleted by the battle for credit, as he contended, he and the Pasteur team encountered roadblock after roadblock, with one standout exception. They identified a second strain of HIV in blood from West Africa, where HIV-2 was creating a heterosexual epidemic. Unlike HIV-1, as he called the Western virus, HIV-2 seemed as easily passed from woman to man as the other way around. Developing a clear picture of the catastrophe that this posed for the continent was hindered by Africa's weak health infrastructure and limited resources. Only time would tell.

In the fifth year of the epidemic, the surge of media attention that followed Rock Hudson's death receded and the Reagan administration called for a 22 percent *reduction* in the fiscal year's AIDS budget, including $29 million cut in treatment and related spending. In case anybody contemplated targeting a prevention campaign to the gay community, Sen. Jesse Helms, Republican of North Carolina, attached an amendment making it a federal crime to use any language or images that might be "offensive . . . to a majority of adults." His anti-gay Helms Amendments would proliferate in appropriations bills year after year.

In the East Village, where I shared a rundown apartment on Avenue C with Jim Hubbard, an experimental filmmaker, the scene was grim; every building was a microcosm of the plague. Two floors above our apartment, a slender redhead from Georgia in his early twenties fell into a drunken tailspin following his diagnosis. For the several weeks before his family came to collect him, he lamented his fate operatically in our living room, incapable of steeling himself for the coming battle. At a time when examples of surprising grace and fortitude dominated, his reaction, however understandable, stood out. His sobbing was a tropical squall. We never heard from him again. Across the hall, Evelyn exiled her husband after a bout of pneumonia won him a month in the hospital and a discharge slip that said AIDS. When he tried to return home, she met him in the hallway with a scorching rage over his admitted drug use and, as their two young daughters screamed in confusion, she issued final banishment orders. Day after day he returned seeking forgiveness she was too panicked about her own future to grant. One morning I found that he had made a nest for himself in the hallway between our doors, heartbroken and desiccated, as close to his girls as he was allowed.

"Are you all right, Juan?" I asked. "Can I get you anything?"

I had to lean in close to hear his reply.

"My bones hurt," he whispered, shifting painfully from one emaciated hip to the other. He pinched at his yellow bedroll, unable to turn it into the cushion he longed for. His voice was hollow and raspy, the unmistakable sound of PCP.

"Do you have a doctor? Anyone I can call?"

He shook his head. "At the VA, they told me to go home to Puerto Rico to die. But how?" He stared at the door keeping him from all his resources.

A sudden pain contorted his face. He gripped his abdomen and gave a look of terrified foreknowledge. But there was no time—his bowels emptied with a terrible force, painting a mandala of excrement on the floor where he sat.

"Let me get you some help," I said. Reaching around him, I pounded urgently on the door of his old apartment.

"No, no, no," he cried out in embarrassment. He whispered an incantation in Spanish meant to spare his daughters the sight of their befouled father. He managed to get to his feet, stroking the hallway clean with his bedding, and on fragile legs carried his shame down to the street. He need not have fled. His wife never came to the door.

THE ANTI-DEFAMATION WORK undertaken by GLAAD was beginning to make an impression, if not a difference. The collective slanders against the community still continued from the highest levels, but now the perpetrators had to contend with the response of GLAAD's nettlesome foot soldiers. When William F. Buckley published an article in the *National Review* referring to AIDS as an "avenging angel" and "retribution for a repulsive vice," and demanding that its sufferers have their flesh branded as warnings to the world, the committee erected an impromptu concentration camp tableau on the sidewalk in front of the magazine's office. Though not contrite, Buckley did feel compelled to argue the differences, as he saw them, between his policies and those of Hitler. "It becomes a little harder to callously hurt a population when they're in your face saying, *No,*" said Bill Bahlman, a GLAAD stalwart.

And in significant ways, a modicum of optimism was taking hold for the first time in the American gay civil rights movement. Now fifty cities had adopted gay rights ordinances. Even New York's legislators seemed more disposed than ever to bring the measure to a vote. Sensing this change, religious opponents in the city began a full-court press in the spring. Though admitting that he hadn't read the measure, Cardinal O'Connor warned that the bill promoted "man-boy love" and child molestation. Jewish and Protestant leaders joined in, as did the assistant director of the CDC's AIDS Task Force, of all people, who feared gay rights would prohibit public officials from declaring that "a Christian lifestyle" was the best prevention against HIV. (Thereafter, the *Native* referred to the federal agency as "The Christian Disease Center.") But the pendulum had swung perceptively, and that spring, for only the second time in twelve years of debate, the General Welfare Committee of the New York City Council voted to allow the gay rights bill out of committee for an up-or-down vote.

When the momentous day arrived, I took a seat in the press box in the front of the chambers wearing *Village Voice* credentials. Being inside the august council chamber was a revelation for me. It was a cavernous hall whose soaring ceiling was adorned with enormous murals depicting the "civic virtues." The paint was peeling badly. Whole sections of plaster were missing. Around the room's perimeters, banged-up doors and trim and cheap metal folding chairs reflected the city's lengthy decline. A statue of Thomas Jefferson in mid-stride towered incongruously over the shabby scene.

The first fifty people to arrive grabbed the limited spectator tickets and crammed through the door amid multiple bomb threats. At precisely 1:45, the oratorical combat began. When the leading opponent, Councilman Noach Dear of Brooklyn, rose to speak, gays and their supporters in the gallery stood and turned their backs in silent protest. Calling the initiative "perfidious," Dear offered a dozen amendments meant to neutralize the bill, then drew ferocious shouts of agreement when he stated, "I am opposed to this bill. I am opposed to my own amendments. We must destroy this legislation before it destroys our own family units."

After three hours of debate it seemed that the vote just might go our way. It was left to the Manhattan councilwoman Ruth Messinger to end the cliffhanger. "Nothing makes me prouder than to cast the eighteenth and decisive vote," she said. The longest-debated piece of legislation in city history was law.

I was one of the first people out the chamber doors, making my way quickly to the Broadway location where a crowd of some four thousand lesbians and gay men were held behind police barricades. I pointed skyward and gave a shout. A chorus of cheers rose up. I pulled myself up onto the pediment of an ornate stone column to look for the man I had been recently dating. When we united, we kissed before the crowd and the reporters, unconsciously creating one of those dramatic embraces that mark profound victories in history. Victory, limned with exhaustion.

THAT SATURDAY, I rose early and packed my bags in the dark for a week with my family back in Michigan. At the airport, I picked up a copy of the *New York Post*. The cover held an I-told-you-so piece on the new law. "Soon after the gay rights bill sailed through City Council, living rooms everywhere lit up with . . . pictures of male homosexuals celebrating with embraces and kisses. Forget the closet. They've taken over the whole house." I turned the pages quickly to see if they'd been talking about me, but they didn't print the picture itself—being a "family newspaper," they had censured the offensive display. If that was victory in New York, I didn't expect a celebration in the heartland.

Almost nobody there was out of the closet. Social scientists now estimated there were eighty thousand gays and lesbians still living in western Michigan, but they had no public spokesperson, advocate, newspaper, organization, or meeting center. With notepad in hand, I visited gay bars there for seven consecutive days. I spoke to scores of men and women, and only one—the dandy bartender at the Carousel— would tell me his real name: Tony Denkins. "But if you call me 'the Queen,'" he added, "they'll know who you mean in any bar in town."

One evening before happy hour Denkins talked to me about AIDS. "For the longest time it didn't mean anything to people. Then Abby Roads died in February and things have been different. Abby—that was his drag name—was well known all over. He was crowned Miss Carousel a couple of years ago and did a lot of shows here. When he died, people knew it could happen to them. It hit us pretty hard." He pointed to a sign over the bar announcing a drag extravaganza to raise money for AIDS research "In Memory of Abby Roads."

"People are much more careful," he said. "This place has a reputation of being the cruise bar in town, and that's still going on. We get the carefree types, the more careless ones. But on the whole, people are being careful. Of course, what they do once they go back through that door is your guess. And you don't hear many people sitting around here talking about it." He kissed me on the cheek and spun off his stool to return to work. "When you're out for cocktails," he called over his shoulder, "you don't want to discuss the plague."

I knew some of the statistics. With the caseload surpassing 19,000 nationally, Michigan had 140 AIDS cases in the state, ranking it eighteenth in the nation. Presumably most of those people resided in the more liberal eastern precincts around Detroit and Ann Arbor; there were only three dozen reported cases in Grand Rapids. There was an opportunity to contain it there—an opportunity like the one that had been squandered in New York. Many of the infections were presumably among people who had left town and returned only for end-of-life care. Without a large-scale testing program, there was no way to know for sure how many other people were carriers, but among the first 150 tested at the county clinic, 10 percent were positive.

When I learned that the county's medical epidemiologist was speaking at the local community college, I attended. Dr. Richard Tooker was a well-meaning and progressive public health official. He had authorized the creation of "Play Safe" literature and had a budget line for distributing condoms. But he bemoaned the lack of an organized gay community to partner with. "This gay community is pretty much still behind the times," he said. The reasons for that were obvious to anybody who made his or her way across the campus to attend the talk. On the bulletin board in the lobby was an announcement for a student group that stated, for no apparent reason, that none of its members were gay. Above the urinal in the men's room, in thick marker, someone had written, "Kill a homo a day and keep the AIDS doctor away." Out of curiosity, I entered the adjacent stall to scan the graffiti there. "If I find a homo in the bathroom, I'll cut his balls off and stuff them in the faggot's mouth," one said. This was still a very dangerous place.

Consequently, it was nearly impossible for me to meet the local PWAs to know what their lives were like. Through members of a support group for parents of gays, I was introduced to a mother who had a sick son at home. Even talking to me over the telephone terrified her. I only knew her by a pseudonym, Edith. Her son had come to live with her after being diagnosed, she told me. "We can't afford to have anybody know about this or we'll lose the apartment. Then where would we go?" With great courage, she gave me her address. "And if you see anybody in the driveway, don't come right in. Drive around the block, anything."

A light snow fell on the morning of our appointment. Edith pulled me through the door quickly. "There are young people living in the building," she said, pinching open a curtain to patrol the front sidewalk. She turned to me. "Okay, young man," she said. "First show me identification." I did. "Now," she said, "I want you to sit down right over here, before anything else, and write on this paper that nobody will know who we are. Nobody." A pad and pen sat on the kitchenette counter, past the cloistered living room. I walked past her son, half in shadows on the old family sofa, and did as requested. Only then could I introduce myself.

He was emaciated, maybe under one hundred pounds. He balanced his cadaverous frame on two feather pillows to reduce the pain. "I thought about what name you should use for me," he said in a hollow voice. The effort caused him to grimace. "Jim," he said. I took his hand and sat at his side.

His mother settled into a recliner, protectively. "Only family members know what he's got. It'll remain that way," she said. "And his friends from church. They call him and come to visit. But nobody else. You just don't know how they'd react."

"Metropolitan Community Church," Jim specified. He attended the gay congregation, no longer submitting to the steely Christian Reformed Church in which he was raised, and which since 1973 enforced a policy stating that "explicit homosexual practice must be condemned." He added, "I have no animosity."

Jim had traveled to California some years before and had enjoyed himself there. So when the symptoms came and sent him to the local hospital, he had almost been expecting them. The doctor gave the news to him and his mother at once. The first thing Edith did was to have the phone in his hospital room disconnected so that no one would find them there. They had been in hiding in their small apartment for almost a year now, and planned to remain in hiding until there was no longer a need. "When we write his obituary, it's not going to say anything about AIDS—it's not going to request donations to any AIDS group," Edith said.

"But I'll be dead already," Jim protested in a weak and angry voice.

"I grew up in this town," she said with forceful midwestern determination. "I went to school here. No, it will say 'Give donations to the Christian Reformed Church.'"

Again, he didn't object—why bother? "I think about what it's like to die. I think about my funeral. Who's going to be there, things like that. I've asked people to sing . . ." He paused and let out a gasp, remembering how painful it was to extend the invitations. "I've asked people to sing at my funeral, in the church, and that's hard."

"Tell him what music you've chosen," his mother called from the kitchen.

"I've picked out one song. The Lord's Prayer."

"Tell him the other."

He shook his head. "I've changed my mind," he told me, whispering now. "I was going to have 'Amazing Grace,' but now I don't know."

I wish I had asked him why. Because he wasn't once lost, was not now found? And so many other questions. Did he regret his journey to California or embrace it? Through AIDS, did he know himself more or less? I was too timid to ask, choked up as I already was by his story. I was not yet inured to seeing someone so close to death's ledge and was not ready for the wisdom he had access to. Still, on my flight back to

New York, I vowed to keep that song out of my funeral, too, in honor of "Jim," whatever his rationale.

Over the subsequent weeks, I wrote in my journal of my lucky escape from America. There in the Midwest, the real America, gay life was untenable—consigned either to oppression, hatred, forbearance, or death. I couldn't stop thinking about death. I wasn't sleeping well. My relationship suffered and finally faltered. But in the bigger picture of gay New York, the rhythms of death and life went unchanged after my trip. I didn't attempt to use my new rights to return to the *New York Post* or land anywhere else. Instead, that Easter I expatriated to Nicaragua. The decision to go was impulsive. After five years of daily combat, I chose to experience someone else's war for a time. Nicaragua was cast at the moment into bloody civil war by secret U.S. foreign policy—not a viral plague but something more conventionally cruel, a distraction in saturated colors from my own foredoom.

For the year I was a more traditional war correspondent, covering the conflict for the Religion News Service, and reporting on peace negotiations, such as they were, for *USA Today*. I took stupid risks while embedded with the Sandinista army. I crept so deeply into the jungle at the Honduran border that I could hear the sound of guitars in enemy camps. I crouched in mud ravines as bullets passed above me, handing my fate to an army made up mostly of teenagers in ill-fitting fatigues. I snuck into off-limits military installations to interview prisoners, fixed a tourniquet to the leg of a Canadian aid worker who had taken shrapnel, and floated down the intensely contested Rio Escondido with an AK-47 across my lap, and all the while I felt safer there than in America.

PETER STALEY and Peter Launy were living a dream. Vacations in Tahiti and Bora Bora. Broadway theater openings. The best Japanese, Thai, and Indian food New York had to offer. The fact was, Staley's health weighed more heavily on Launy's mind than on his own. The more Launy read about it, the more he was able to see the landscape of AIDS all around the city—not just in the doctor's waiting room where he accompanied Staley, but at the dance clubs and bars where they went after work. In the context of mass death, he decided he needed to take the test, to know if his fate and Staley's were bound together. He wanted the option of doing things differently if he were positive, though exactly what he would do or how he would do it, he had no idea.

To his relief, his test was negative, and when he repeated it there was no change. He thought the good news would make their sex life less fraught, that it would prove safe sex worked. Unfortunately, it had the opposite effect. Learning he was healthy made him feel unreasonably lucky, like a man still standing after five rounds of Russian roulette. He withdrew physically, sometimes too afraid even to kiss. Staley's drives were similarly knotted up. The idea of sexual love was bound with death—with suicide and with murder.

Their love deepened despite these troubles. As Launy's New York year drew to a close and he looked toward law school, they discussed the future ebulliently. Staley thought they should move back to Amsterdam together—buy a house, take advantage of the health care system. This made Launy very happy. They flew to Europe together so he could introduce Staley to his relatives, who were besotted with the handsome and direct young Wall Streeter.

Back at J. P. Morgan, Staley told his boss that he and "Anne Launy," his fictive Dutch girlfriend, had become engaged. He requested and was given a transfer to the Amsterdam office. Launy went ahead as Staley made all necessary arrangements.

He was surprised by how Amsterdam had changed in one year. When he left, there wasn't a cloud of plague in the sky. Now it was inescapable there, too. He saw the disease in his countrymen's faces, the hollowness in their eyes. He could see it in people who didn't yet know themselves. As he waited for Staley, he submitted himself almost obsessively to HIV antibody tests, each one negative, but the relief would only last for a matter of days before the panic returned.

Finally, in late April, Staley packed up and headed over the Atlantic, stopping first in London for a month of training in the European markets. Then an unpredictable disaster befell their plans. J. P. Morgan announced an international reorganization, including layoffs in Amsterdam. Staley was given the option of Paris, London, or Frankfurt. He loved the UK, but if Launy earned his law degree there he would not be able to practice in either the Netherlands or the United States. Germany and France were likewise unsuited to Launy's planned future. Flummoxed and increasingly desperate, Staley returned to his old job in New York and begged Launy to study American law. The thought of losing Launy was excruciating. Their relationship had become part of his survival plan—a marriage of sorts seemed essential now.

For Launy, this would be an unmanageable expense. His parents had offered to pay his tuition in Amsterdam. They certainly could not afford NYU's $15,000-a-year price tag. He said no.

"I'm going to pay for it," Staley insisted.

"But, Peter, what if halfway in my studies either one of us decides it's over? If you do it, I'm fucked; if I do it, I might think I still have one and a half years to go and so then I can't say goodbye. That's not healthy." What he meant to add, but didn't, was the fact that Staley would almost certainly be dead long before the bar exam.

Staley was inconsolable. His father, who had been monitoring these events, had an idea. He called Amsterdam early one morning. "I can give you a loan," he said to Launy, "nothing to do with Peter. Pay if you have a job. If you don't, you don't have to."

The gesture was exceedingly generous and kindly extended. But it had the unexpected consequence of making Launy feel trapped. Reluctantly, he filled out applications for NYU and one or two other schools. Apartment hunting in Manhattan took the two through June and July, masking their troubles with industriousness. Launy never stopped loving Staley, but every day made him more and more afraid of him. As ashamed as that made him feel, he was obsessed with the danger Staley posed for him. He wondered stupid things. Were the dishes really safe? Someone told him toothbrushes carried the virus. Was safe sex nullified by the toothpaste tube?

In August, when he flew to Amsterdam to sit for the NYU admissions exams there, as the school required, he knew what he had to do. He broke up with Staley over the phone.

For only the second time since his diagnosis, Staley despaired and sobbed.

When he got ten days off a few weeks later, he flew to Holland in an effort to change Launy's mind, but he left Europe after only four days, knowing it was unsalvageable.

DR. ROBERT GALLO also left for Europe. On a Monday in June he flew to Paris to attend the international AIDS conference, the second global gathering of researchers, scientists, and clinicians. He had a number of important papers to present and hoped to focus the attention of his fellow scientists on them. But the increasingly cantankerous lawsuit with Montagnier and the Institut Pasteur made that impossible. On one of the first days of the summit, Danielle Berneman, the patents chief at the institute, organized an off-the-record luncheon for Gallo and his team with the Pasteur delegation. Gallo arrived late to the restaurant, near the Porte Maillot metro station. Montagnier was already there, stony-faced and sullen. So was Lowell Harmison, the American deputy assistant secretary for health and human services. Harmison had brought an official offer from the U.S. government that the Reagan administration hoped would end the legal wrangling. There at the table, he offered Luc Montagnier $1 million. All he had to do in exchange was to publicly declare that LAV and HTLV-3 came from blood isolated in two different AIDS patients, on its face a ludicrous request. It was now settled that both samples came from Frédéric Brugière. Everyone working in AIDS knew the truth. Even if Montagnier took the money and did as requested, which he never contemplated, it would not change the facts around Gallo's HTLV-3.

Another lunch guest had a better proposal. Dr. Jonas Salk sympathized with both sides. In the early 1950s, Salk became the first to develop a vaccine against polio, an enormous accomplishment that engendered the same kind of dismissals from the scientific establishment that were vexing Montagnier, and embroiled him in a bitter thirty-year rivalry with Dr. Albert Sabin, a Polish American who claimed to have crossed the finish line first. Salk, now in his seventies, was a friend and close confidante of Gallo's. He saw an opportunity to use his negative experiences for the good of science, and offered himself as a statesman to broker an end to the feud. These were grave times of global urgency, he said, in which the appearance of self-serving disputes risked great harm to the scientific community as well as to the sick; history would accord all involved with plaudits or damnation, depending on how they behaved today.

Both sides welcomed his mediation. Over time, Salk arrived at a detailed proposal. He suggested that the royalties be split in thirds—a cut for each institute, and another for AIDS research in the developing world, where cases were multiplying at a frightening pace. As for the fundamental dispute over credit for discovering HIV, Salk suggested a method for clearing the air that was as ingenious as it was infantilizing. He invited Montagnier and Gallo to coauthor an official history of HIV's search and discovery, according one another the credit they deserved. Being empiricists, facing the blank page, they were bound to find the truth themselves.

Numerous Nobel Prize winners endorsed the plan, which Salk forwarded to President Reagan, imploring him to "bring the power of your office, your wisdom, and your humanity to bear in helping to achieve a solution." It did little good. Montagnier and Gallo did attempt to craft a consensus narrative, but the process was derailed by disputes over trivial matters like who deserved more citations, as well as by essential ones: now Gallo claimed he had discovered the virus three months *before* Montagnier, but had failed to tell anyone until now. Privately, Salk called the whole affair "insanity afloat." In the following year, the Institut Pasteur would press its suit against the NIH, an imbroglio that reverberated at the highest political levels in both nations. It was finally put to rest in a solemn joint appearance at the White House. Like weary parents, President Reagan and French prime minister Jacques Chirac declared that the lucrative patent rights would be shared equally and that both men would be considered "co-discoverers" of HIV, whether they liked it or not. They didn't. Their unseemly squabble simmered on for another two decades, occasionally revived by angry memoirs, and would only be put to rest by the Nobel Prize committee, which in 2008 deemed the French, and not the Americans, worthy of their award. Montagnier, a gentleman, called Gallo equally deserving.

NEW YORK'S Gay Pride March took place that year on June 29, seventeen summers after the Stonewall Riots. There was much to celebrate in 1986. The hard-won gay rights law, called Intro 2, was the most tangible accomplishment of the local movement to date. Koch signed it immediately and was begrudgingly named the grand marshal of the march as a result, though he only made a brief appearance, in protest of the fact that organizers had named the portable toilets after city leaders who opposed the measure ("Cardinal O'Connor Throne Room," for example). To mark the victory, organizers adopted a rainbow motif—a symbol both of gay people finally joining the diverse landscape of civic life, and of the promise, made by young Dorothy Gale of Kansas, that beyond the rainbow dreams really could come true. Every few blocks along Fifth Avenue, rainbow-colored arches of balloons looped high overhead.

Despite the kitsch and ostentation, which included a lighthearted new gay pride logo donated by Keith Haring, there was little jubilation among the 200,000 people who proceeded down Fifth Avenue under a baking sun, led by people in wheelchairs and walkers. Up in front, Michael Callen helped carry the PWA Coalition banner and Richard Dworkin played a snare drum. Dworkin considered himself an honorary coalition member. He now knew he was infected with HIV, something he learned through a casual reference on a lab report, but he had never been sick. Every test of his immune system showed it was fully intact, giving further credence to Sonnabend's theory that HIV might be at best a co-conspirator in AIDS.

Immediately following the PWA Coalition's contingent came the

New York City Gay Men's Chorus, performing their traditional repertoire of classics and re-gendered show tunes. Then, beneath signs for the GMHC buddy program, came hundreds of caregivers, followed by hundreds more volunteers who were getting fresh meals to the ailing via God's Love We Deliver, or offering counseling through a proliferation of bereavement groups, or there to walk dogs or fetch prescriptions or rub burning feet.

Dworkin and Callen had a Lowlife gig that night at Limelight, for which they needed to conserve energy. At 2 p.m., as prearranged, the drumming stopped and the music faded, in homage to the dead. For several minutes, the length of Fifth Avenue from Central Park to Washington Square fell eerily silent. Thousands of balloons, released by organizers, floated through the canyons and disappeared into the bright sky. When whistles signaled a resumption of the march, people clutched one another, moved to tears. It took some time for the chanting to resume. Even near St. Patrick's Cathedral, where followers of Jerry Falwell carried signs reading "Quarantine Manhattan Island . . . The A.I.D.S. Capital of the World," few in the ranks had enough fight left in them to do more than raise a middle finger.

The rare exception to this collective depression was a mile or so uptown, in the section of the march where political organizations were congregated. The centerpiece of the militant contingent was GLAAD, whose message was to fight homophobia through direct action. The anti-defamation group had divided into various committees since the "rags" protest at the *Post* and the anti-Buckley demonstration at the *National Review*. One of them strategized colorful demonstrations and "zaps"—office takeovers, street-theater actions, and the like—against any offending outpost. They called this subgroup the Swift & Terrible Retribution Committee. In the past six months it had zapped the state's Republican senator Alfonse D'Amato by staging a sit-in in his office to demand more AIDS funding. Bill Bahlman, a Swift & Terrible member, created "The Dirty Dozen Contingent" for the Gay Pride March, listing the thirteen most dangerous homophobes of the day. Tall and angular, with a mop of blond hair crossing his forehead, Bahlman worked as a club DJ and was something of a celebrity in the world of New Wave music. But he had also been a fixture in gay politics since Stonewall. He played a role in the campaign against the American Psychiatric Association, which for a century had classified homosexuality as a mental illness. In one memorable skirmish, at the APA's 1972 convention, he interrupted a session by screaming, "How dare you call us disordered and sick!" Afterward, many mental health professionals approached him with genuine perplexity—the idea that some homosexuals felt normal was anathema back then.

He proved especially adept at working the crowds into chants and applause. He personally handed out thousands of copies of the "Dirty Dozen" leaflets. Included were the pastors Pat Robertson and Jerry Falwell, the publisher Rupert Murdoch, and myriad health officials—leaders in the campaign of "criminal indifference" that threatened the community with annihilation. "It doesn't matter whether you're homeless on the streets or Rock Hudson, if we don't have effective treatments, we all are going to die," Bahlman explained as he pushed through the full sidewalks. "We're taking action," he called out. "We are on the move!"

But back home that night, he couldn't have felt much evidence to support that claim. The march barely merited attention in the evening news, and only a few inches in the next morning's *Times,* which reduced the turnout to "thousands" and the demands to "what they called 'the crisis of AIDS.'"

The affair was overshadowed by plans in the city for an enormous event in the coming days, a global rededication ceremony for the Statue of Liberty to be attended by heads of state, Hollywood idols, and a projected million-plus tourists. Some thirty thousand tall sailing vessels were en route toward the harbor, including ceremonial warships from fourteen nations. The Reagans were coming for the whole July 4 weekend.

But just as those events were about to begin, in timing that added another layer of cruelty to the painful summer, there was news from the Supreme Court in a case followed in the gay press very closely. Police officers in Atlanta, mistakenly believing that an attractive twenty-nine-year-old bartender named Michael Hardwick had failed to pay a fine, had knocked on his door one hot summer day to deliver a warrant. A roommate directed the police to Hardwick's room, where the officers pushed open the door. At that moment, in his own bedroom, Hardwick and a lover were committing an act known in the Georgia penal code as a "crime against nature." Police took both men into custody on charges that carried a jail term of up to twenty years. As the case bounced through the legal system all the way to the Supreme Court, Georgia officials argued that upholding the law against homosexuality was even more essential in light of AIDS.

The cover of the morning's *Daily News* brought the Court's ruling:

"Top Court Okays Gay Sex Ban." On the very weekend the world had come to New York to celebrate the symbol of freedom, the fundamental rights of gay men and lesbians were explicitly excluded.

The opinion, signed by a five-to-four majority, cited good taste and public health as motivating the decision, and dismissed Hardwick's claim to equal protection with pure contempt. The justices noted without commentary that ancient Rome considered such couplings to be a capital offense and to eighteenth-century English jurists it was worse than rape, "a heinous act 'the very mention of which is a disgrace to human nature.'" The opinion concluded, "To hold that the act of homosexual sodomy is somehow protected as a fundamental right would be to cast aside millennia of moral teaching."

Bill Bahlman, an optimist, made a new leaflet, fashioned from the *Daily News* headline. It called for a protest that night at Sheridan Square, the tiny park across from the Stonewall Inn. A friend with a car drove him through the gay neighborhoods as he blasted the announcements out the window through a bullhorn.

"Sheridan Square. Tonight. Seven o'clock. Meeting in Sheridan Square. Tonight. Seven o'clock."

Well over a thousand people showed up that night, including Michael Callen and Richard Dworkin. When Bahlman's fellow Swift & Terrible activist Buddy Noro exhorted the crowds off the sidewalk and onto Seventh Avenue, there was no hesitation. Callen, who wore a favorite shirt with a Dairy Queen logo, sat down on the pavement to block traffic. The police, perhaps under instructions from city hall, did nothing. The sit-in lasted for several hours, and moved to Sixth Avenue as well, blocking both major arteries until near midnight.

Bahlman felt a change in mood in the community, sensing that people were ready to fight back.

"We gotta do another demonstration on July 4," he shouted into his bullhorn, and when the day came, 3,500 people showed up in the Village and marched toward Battery Park at the southern tip of Manhattan Island. At Wall Street, they hit a barrier. A four-deep cordon of riot police had set up a perimeter, stopping the march cold. But Marty Robinson, a veteran of the Gay Activists Alliance, noticed that they were allowing just about anybody else to proceed.

"If we look like tourists they can't stop us," he called out. He advised everybody to split up, make their way down to Battery Park, and reconnoiter there at the monument honoring soldiers killed in World War II.

"Look like Americans," he said, "if you can."

Callen and Dworkin put their signs in the trash and turned down the unfamiliar crooked streets of old New Amsterdam. They were able to walk right past the thick police line. More than a thousand of them reconvened at the war memorial, pushing for a spot on the crowded promenade and erupting into chants. Tourists pushed back. "What are you doing?" one cried out. "You're in the way!"

"We're protesting the *Hardwick* decision," Callen said, discovering on their faces that nobody had a clue what the *Hardwick* decision was. "That's appalling," he snapped. "Here you are celebrating liberty! And this major thing happened, negating our very existence, basically, and you don't even know about it?"

Once again, the protest didn't make the news. Ronald Reagan never heard their chants. Nor did François Mitterrand, the French president, on hand to help commemorate the hundredth year of France's gift of the statue to America. Both men and their wives were instead sitting at a formal state luncheon, with the comedian Bob Hope as their ribald emcee.

"Did you hear that Lady Liberty has AIDS?" the comedian cracked to the three hundred guests. "Nobody knows if she got it from the mouth of the Hudson or the Staten Island Ferry."

There was a scattering of groans. Mitterrand and his wife looked appalled. But not the Reagans. The first lady, a year after the death of her friend Rock Hudson, the brunt of this joke, smiled affectionately. The president threw his head back and roared.

THE REST OF 1986 was a numbing blur of bad news. After the first snow of the winter, a thin but buoyant forty-year-old man climbed to the second-floor offices of the *Native* to share a story he considered miraculous about a simple food supplement. He had written an essay describing how the substance, known as AL721, had reversed his descent into the grave. Ortleb agreed to rush the piece into the holiday issue, beneath the headline, "What We All Want for Christmas." The author preferred to remain anonymous.

I noticed a difficulty with my health during the summer of 1985. I had a painful separation from my job. My energy dropped. I attributed it to mental depression.

During the fall, I suffered with strange illnesses: an ear infection that wouldn't respond to antibiotics; athlete's foot; frequent colds. In January of 1986, I had the worst "flu" of my life, and it wouldn't go away. Toward the end of the month, I developed a tightness in my chest and a bad cough. Then I went to the doctor. The ELISA test, a T-Lymphocyte Subset, and a viral culture confirmed what I did not want to hear. AIDS.

I was given Bactrim for the PCP, and the cough abated. But my strength was gone. I could no longer work. During February and March, I developed painful sores. A fungus spread to my legs and arms. My skin was scaly, with red blotches. I had fits of perspiration at night; I had fevers. I couldn't eat; I became thin. Worst of all was the generalized feeling throughout my body that I was dying. Indeed, I *was* dying.

At this time a good friend of mine—an Israeli citizen—was doing some investigation on my behalf. She discovered a treatment developed at the Weizmann Institute of Science in Rehovot, Israel. By Express Mail she sent me a most remarkable document—a letter full of promise. As I read it, my condition had deteriorated to the point where I had hardly the strength to breathe. I knew my death was imminent.

So I took a leap of faith—I had nothing to lose anyway. After writing goodbye letters to my friends and loved ones, I was taken, in a wheelchair, to the El Al plane, along with my mother and my closest friend. I don't know how I endured that long flight. My Israeli friend met the plane, and took us to our hotel.

The next day I began treatment with AL721, a potent form of lecithin which makes your cell membranes resistant to viral attacks. It is derived from egg yolks. AL721 looks and tastes like butter; you spread it on your bread and eat it morning and evening. My Israeli doctor said to me, "The Americans don't like our treatment. It's too simple for them."

During the first week of treatment, there was no change in my condition. The three of us were planning how to deal with a corpse so far from home. But after two weeks of treatment, lo and behold! I did feel stronger. My diarrhea was less severe. I began to eat. During the first month I gained some weight.

I consumed these Active Lipids through April, May and part of June. When I came back to the U.S.A., I walked off the plane—no more wheelchair. I continued my treatment by taking a heaping tablespoon of granulated lecithin mixed with a raw egg yolk daily. During June, my CD4 count continued to rise, even without the Active Lipids. My sores and skin rashes disappeared.

By the end of August, however, the CD4 numbers were heading down again. Since AL721 is not available in the United States, I once again flew to Israel. Another month of treatment lifted my CD4 number significantly.

In February and March, my moribund condition forced me to let go of my plans, my hopes, my loves, my career, my possessions, and life itself. The pain was unspeakable. When it came over me that some unfathomable hand of fate had determined that I would not die but live, I became semi-hysterical. I remained that way through most of the summer. Why should I have been allowed to receive this miraculous treatment when it had been denied to so many others?

As I write this I have no more physical symptoms. The infections have gone; the night sweats have stopped; I have no more fevers. I am able to eat again, and my weight is close to normal. The last symptoms to disappear were the red blotches and scaling on my face. In October, those too went away.

I am trying to make sense of all this. I tell my story in hopes that it may help someone. I remain easily excitable. When you have been to Auschwitz and survived, I think you never get over it.

The article and the buzz it activated sent the community into a frenzy. For weeks, all anyone talked about was "the egg-based cure." Men wrote to the Israeli researchers begging for samples; a lobbying campaign took aim at the FDA demanding immediate approval. Those who could afford it didn't wait, but flew immediately to Israel or else to South Africa, where quantities were reportedly available. American doctors scrambled for information. Dr. Joe Sonnabend was one of the few people in the world with clinical knowledge of AL721. The *Native*'s anonymous letter writer was a patient of his: Michael May, a chorus and orchestra conductor originally from Morristown, New Jersey. Sonnabend became the fulcrum of pleas in New York, but, lacking any access of his own, all he could do was share information.

The compound was first developed in 1979 under the guidance of a specialist in cell membrane biochemistry, Dr. Meir Shinitzky. His interest was in staving off the effects of aging, particularly memory loss, thought to be caused in part by cell-wall hardening. Shinitzky and his team produced AL721—the AL stood for "active lipid"—by blending the neutral fats extracted from common egg yolks with two other egg lipids, phosphatidylcholine and phosphatidylethanolamine, in a ratio of seven to two to one. The crude substance was all natural, and meant for ingestion. It smelled ghastly and tasted worse. But in vitro, the oily substance effectively removed cholesterol from cell membranes, returning them to a more fluid, youthful state. Tested in sixteen people age seventy-five or older who shared the ordinary complaints associated with age, all showed significant improvement in cellular activity. The benefits to CD4 cells were especially strong. This led one of the collaborators, a lab assistant named David Heron, to surmise that the magical youth potion described in Kabbalist literature had been discovered.

That was in the early 1980s and little had been heard about the stuff since, in part because it fell into the hands of a small startup company under the control of a Hollywood film family unfamiliar with the ways of pharmaceutical research. Their idea was to market it through health food stores, but they made little progress. Meanwhile, fearful of FDA opprobrium, they made it impossible for patients to get access and nearly as difficult for scientists. The Israelis acquired enough for the very small trial involving Michael May, and Gallo, when he learned of their optimism, put some samples to the test. He noted positive results in test tubes, but was unable to secure additional deliveries. That's where the research trail went cold.

Then Michael May put AL721 on everybody's holiday wish list. His story was picked up in the New York *Daily News* and in a San Francisco newsletter, *AIDS Treatment News,* read widely by AIDS patients. Demand was extreme. Callen found a New York phone number for the tiny drug company that produced the substance, Praxis Pharmaceuticals, and begged them to release stores of it for Sonnabend's patients. Martin Delaney did the same from the West Coast. The company refused. But they did allow two doctors at St. Luke's–Roosevelt Medical Center in New York, Dr. Michael Grieco and Dr. Michael Lange, to push forward with the first human trials of AL721 in the United States. Scores of patients rushed to sign up, but Praxis restricted supply so severely that only seven subjects were able to enroll in the trial, a statistically insignificant sample. The doctors went forward anyway. After eight weeks, five of the seven patients showed a reduction in virus levels. They gained weight and said they felt better, though their CD4 counts remained unchanged. There were no side effects, and after being taken off the drug, the patients' conditions reversed. Sonnabend and Callen were watching the study closely. Then Michael May began to decline again.

• • •

TRACEY TANENBAUM had been spending her free time at Peter Staley's apartment. His diagnosis put her into a state of high alert, magnifying the protective instinct she had always felt for him. When fevers caused him to shake and moan, she wrapped him in a blanket; when the cough returned, she sat on his back massaging his lungs. She felt a need to be as close to him as possible. But she reluctantly headed to graduate school in Philadelphia in the fall. She managed to return to the city often, but her departure added to Staley's fear of dying alone. When he heard about a support group for the afflicted, he signed up, hoping to find peace. After work one Tuesday night he made his way to an unmarked storefront on Perry Street in Greenwich Village. The setting was as he had imagined. Fifteen men sat in a circle, most wearing jeans and sweatshirts; Staley was the only one in a suit. A pot of coffee brewed in the corner. He slid into a folding chair desperate to be inspired, but the night's dominant topics were repentance, guilt, and preparing for death.

Far from easing Staley's mind, sitting there made him feel even worse. Then, the moderator called on a man who looked like a Hell's Angel gang member dressed half in drag. Griffin Gold was covered head to toe in black, including a black leather biker jacket. He wore his hair in a bright orange pompadour and filled his earlobes with costume jewelry. Scores of rubber and leather gaskets encased his wrists like shackles.

Gold was as frustrated as Staley by the darkness in the men's voices. He rebuked them in a high-pitched voice, not womanly so much as defiantly gay. "I'm not ashamed at all," he said. "It's just a *virus!*" He declared his right to a robust though safe sex life, and didn't care one bit what others thought about him. His life would go on. "If folks freak out about my HIV status, that's their problem."

Staley was mesmerized by this dramatic creature and his lively manifesto. In Gold, he saw a person refusing to be a victim of AIDS, someone, he said later, "who was in action mode." After the meeting, he introduced himself and invited Gold for a cup of coffee.

"Everybody in the room was about to die," Staley said to Gold. "This isn't going to change my life. I won't let it."

Gold crinkled his deep green eyes into a smile. He told Staley about Michael Callen and the People With AIDS Coalition, of which he was a board member, and their commitment not just to live with dignity, but to advocate publicly for the rights of the infected. They lobbied the government for drugs, the media for accountability, and the hospitals for humane treatment. Staley was deeply impressed. He had never heard of the PWA empowerment movement and though he was closeted and in no position to join them openly, he pledged to help in the way he could.

"I've got money," he said. "I want to start funding stuff." He pulled out his checkbook and made a sizable donation, which Gold folded into his pocket with a brisk "Thank you, darlin'."

Within a week, Staley took Gold to bed. He was as flamboyant as any gay man Staley had ever seen, whose force of personality made him laugh, restored his sex life, and gave him true hope. They never had sex again, but they became inseparable. It took Gold only a matter of days to coax Staley into his first drag costume, an incongruous outfit that paired a tasteful floor-length sequined gown—spaghetti-strapped with a deep décolleté—with black evening gloves, simple pearls, and a towering nylon wig, one half Holly Golightly and the other half Cher. He was comically unstable in the pumps, but as he wobbled out onto Christopher Street and off to the drag affair, Staley had a sense that his disease was going to take him places he had never imagined.

Soon, he opened *The Wall Street Journal* to read about a new group of AIDS activists called the Lavender Hill Mob that had disrupted a meeting at the Centers for Disease Control. A spinoff of GLAAD's Swift & Terrible Retribution Committee, the Lavender Hill Mob was committed to radical forms of patient advocacy. One day in November, ten Mobsters staged a sit-in at the office of New York senator Alfonse D'Amato, presenting him with a fake arrest warrant accusing him of "mass murder by indifference," then zapped an academic forum at the New School for Social Research debating the biases of *The New York Times*. None of the panelists mentioned the paper's AIDS coverage, which recently had included an editorial that advised, "Don't panic, yet, over AIDS," obliviously blind to the tragedy in the ghetto.

"Well over fifteen thousand people have died of AIDS and you say, 'Don't worry, it's only faggots.' How dare you?" one of the Mobsters demanded from the sideline.

A *Times* editor on the panel, William Borders Jr., tried to answer the heckler. "I myself found the editorial reprehensible, but what can I do?" he said.

"Retract it!" the movement veteran Marty Robinson bellowed from the back of the room. "Our lives are at stake!"

The CDC protest was equally confrontational. The agency had arranged a national hearing on public health proposals to require HIV testing for members of all risk groups. The Mob, seeing this as a first step to quarantine, seized the dais and ended the summit with chants of "Test Drugs, not People."

Gold, who knew the activists, arranged for Staley to meet Bill Bahlman. Over dinner Staley underwrote the Lavender Hill Mob's endeavors with a $1,000 check. "Think of me as your bank," he said. There was no turning back.

THE AZT PHASE II trial was enrolled quickly as patients clamored to be chosen for the 282 spots. Most were turned away because their CD4 count was still above five hundred, the cutoff. Others were excluded because they had Kaposi's sarcoma, an arbitrary criterion, or because they refused to discontinue their anti-PCP drugs. In order to be monitored closely, each study participant would spend the first few weeks of the trial living at the NIH hospital grounds in Bethesda, and thereafter would be in the care of the doctors running the study in one of the dozen participating cities. Slightly more than half the patients were randomly assigned to the group receiving 1,500 milligrams of AZT daily, while the rest were put on capsules that looked identical to the AZT but were placebos. The medical conditions across both groups were similar. Most had recovered from a PCP infection within the previous three months, putting them at imminent risk of a recurrence.

One of the first to arrive at the NIH's hospital compound was Roy Cohn, referred by a doctor at Memorial Sloan Kettering in New York. What strings the legendary lawyer pulled for a chance to become one of the first patients to get treatment was unknown. His clinical picture was bleak. He was extremely thin and severely demented. Cohn didn't know where he was or who was president. At times he couldn't even recall his own name. He was sporadically delusional, convinced that one of the nurses was trying to kill him by withholding his medication. As luck would have it, Cohn was assigned to the arm of the trial receiving AZT. Within a few weeks, his mind cleared like the sky after a summer storm. This was wholly unexpected—AIDS dementia complex was thought to be irreversible. His transformation was remarkable. "There's nothing more dramatic than a neurological awakening," Dr. Broder told me. "To see that firsthand is a unique privilege."

Cohn, no longer confined to bed, celebrated his return to discernment by taking lunch at a power restaurant in nearby D.C. He made sure that news of the jaunt was in the columns, along with the fiction that his health problems were attributable to liver cancer. "I'm recovering faster and better than anyone anticipated," he reported. "Those people who have had me at death's door may be surprised to see Roy Cohn leaving his deathbed to have lunch at the posh Madison Hotel."

Some of Broder's colleagues at the NCI, holding to their doubts that any drug could impact any retrovirus, questioned the role of AZT in Cohn's dramatic rebound. Even when five other trial subjects went from neurological impairment to near normal as determined by psychometric tests and positron emission tomography scans, they initially refused to credit AZT.

Toxicity became a problem almost immediately. Nearly half the people taking AZT showed signs of serious bone marrow suppression, and anemia occurred in the majority. One in five required multiple blood transfusions. The problem was so dramatic that a number of the researchers proposed pulling the plug on the study altogether, but Dr. Margaret Fischl, the Miami internist who led the trial, argued strongly to persevere. If the patients' health became seriously compromised, the data and safety monitoring board would take note during its periodic appraisal of the records; in early August, they saw nothing they considered life-threatening. Fischl's view prevailed.

Patients on AZT also complained of crushing headaches and intractable nausea, and had elevated incidents of muscle ache, fever, and abdominal pain. A handful withdrew from the study because of these side effects. Two patients were dead, but both had been on the placebo arm of the study so their demise was anticipated. By the end of the month, the death toll had risen to seven, all from the placebo group.

It went like this week after week: nine dead on placebo by September 5, eleven dead on placebo by September 10 plus one fatality on the AZT arm, the first. The spread between the two groups was beginning to look statistically significant. This gave the monitoring board members reason to hope that AZT was performing up to expectation. But it also gave them cause for concern for the people not on AZT. When they checked in again on September 18, there were now sixteen dead on placebo and still just one on AZT. That day, the monitoring board held a series of secret meetings to weigh the ethics of continuing the study. By evening the placebo deaths had risen to seventeen, and out of mounting concern for the patients on placebo, they voted to halt the study. Two more died overnight, bringing the total on placebo to nineteen by the time their recommendation reached Dr. Sam Broder's office the following morning.

Their proposal presented a difficult problem, as the trial had only been under way for a few weeks and fewer than 10 percent of the subjects had completed it. Would the apparent benefits be lasting? Would toxicity accumulate? Nobody knew. Only a long-term study could tell. Still, Broder was eager to pull the plug. To do so he needed the approval of his boss, Vince DeVita, who coincidentally had just undergone emergency surgery. Broder raced to the hospital with the trial data, which they reviewed together. DeVita inhaled deeply.

"We must stop the study," he said.

They placed urgent calls to each of the trial sites, instructing those responsible to substitute AZT for the placebo without delay. It took a full week to complete the transition. By then the outcome disparity was even more stark. The death toll for the first weeks of the aborted trial now came to twenty-three patients taking the placebo, compared to just three on AZT.

The drug was no magic bullet. Blood tests showed the virus was still present in those taking AZT, and they still developed opportunistic infections. The data showed peak benefit at about four months of AZT use, with most patients beginning to decline again afterward. But even adding four months to the life-span of a patient was a major breakthrough, and of great interest to those with the disease. News of the success tore through the community. In San Francisco, people danced in the middle of Castro Street. "There really is hope now," Dr. Mathilde Krim told a reporter.

Before anyone could get the drug, however, it needed to clear the approval hurdles at the Food and Drug Administration. Responsibility there fell to Dr. Ellen Cooper, a careful young medical officer. She took the restraints of her position very exactingly, always mindful of one of the worst pharmaceutical disasters in history, when thalidomide, developed to help pregnant women overcome nausea, caused ten thousand children worldwide to be born with missing or misshapen limbs. Cooper's predecessor, the trailblazing Dr. Frances Kelsey, limited the disaster in the United States by correctly identifying the drug's toxicities and withholding FDA approval. For a year, the German manufacturer sidestepped her by leaving free samples at doctor's offices, but the number of American victims paled compared with Europe, where thalidomide had won easy clearance. Kelsey went on to author the three-phase clinical trial model that became the standard route for drug approval and led to the modern gatekeeping role of the FDA.

Burroughs Wellcome had not done a Phase III trial yet, and only had spotty efficacy data from the aborted Phase II study. But on December 3, 1986, the company filed paperwork with Cooper seeking formal approval, at the same time submitting a request for special clearance immediately to release AZT on a compassionate basis while approval hearings were arranged. By its own estimate, the company currently had enough AZT to treat a few thousand patients. They were willing to distribute it for free if the FDA would allow.

Ordinarily, the time required for an FDA ruling was at least a year. Concerned that lives depended on her swift action, it took Cooper only a few weeks to set a policy allowing the pre-approval distribution. The news touched off a flood of desperate requests to Wellcome, where over fifty calls an hour jammed the company's hotline. On the first weekend alone, hotline workers registered more than 3,500 names. Soon, thousands of PWAs were popping the little white-and-blue capsules every four hours. To keep to their schedule, many began setting alarms on electronic wristwatches, a new technology. Now it was not possible to go to a movie theater or restaurant in the country's gay ghettos without hearing the chorus of tinny beeps at the top of the hour.

Still, there were many more people needing AZT than could be accommodated by the compassionate-distribution program. Cooper still had to pull together an advisory committee meeting to determine if the drug should get commercial release. It would be months before the company would be able to supply enough pills to meet the wild demand.

LETTERS FROM FRIENDS reached me in the war zones of Central America, sometimes weeks in transit, undermining my efforts to escape the epidemic. JT, Roger, Michael E., and Richard had dropped dead. I started keeping a book with each name and bits of our last conversations or intimacies, attaching a few sentences like buoys to the memories of them. JT, young and charmingly irresponsible, was sleeping on friends' couches to the very end. Roger, a filmmaker, dead at forty, at the cusp of a powerful career. Richard was the husband of Susan, our building's super—a bisexual, it turned out. Michael E. had climbed from poverty to medical school, and had only begun to practice when he became a patient instead. Remembering his heartbreaking thirtieth birthday turned my stomach. His mother, fulfilling an old promise, had come north for the first time, to cook him his favorite southern fare. But before the guests arrived he told her he was gay. This gave her more of a shock than she could handle. Already unsteady at the beginning of the evening, her wobble grow more pronounced each time she returned from the corner in the kitchen where a bar was set up. Before the meal was fully plated, she slid to the floor, unconscious. I helped Michael lift her into bed. "Are you one too?" she asked me before beginning to snore.

"And that was the easy part," Michael said. "In the morning we'll talk about AIDS."

I heard once from Brian Gougeon, my old college roommate. His letter was full of exciting updates—about his art, about life in Chicago, about his lover, Doug Gould, whom he nicknamed Buster. He seemed in good spirits despite the frank last paragraph. "My Frankenstein knobs are bigger—big hard buttons—but at least they don't hurt," he wrote. "I've had a couple of other weird health things. Thrush, which was like a gross blanket in my throat, and shingles, which hurt like hell. Obviously something's gone haywire, but the doctor doesn't know what." He wasn't letting it get him down. "I mean, it's been three years and I'm basically fine," he insisted. He didn't mention whether he'd been tested, and he seemed content—determined, actually—to exist in a state of unknowing. I didn't address the subject in my return note, concentrating instead on lavish descriptions of life in the jungle. In our contortions we were as purposeful as Tolstoy's amputee, who told a judge how he coped with the pain: "The main thing, your honour, is not to spend too much time thinking about it; if you don't think about it, it doesn't seem much."

When the thinking could not be vanquished, it drowned out all else. Sitting on the curb outside my Managua hotel room one night, sharing a beer with a friend, I traced a finger absent-mindedly above the waistband of my jeans and on my hip I came upon a spot, raised and leathery. Quickly excusing myself and returning to my room, I tore off my clothes and stood before a bare bulb staring at the dreaded stigmata. It made sense. I had had the bout with shingles all those years ago. Countless nights in the jungle I awoke drenched in sweat and convinced myself it was from the tropical heat.

The KS got me.

I never mentioned my lesion to anyone. But I immediately began planning a return to New York to face this new reality. For a number of frustrating reasons, this took many weeks. Before departing, I was overtaken by dysentery of a dreadfully familiar kind. The cramping, the inability to control my bowels. I had no appetite. Weight slid off me. It could be anything, of course, in this country of non-potable water, mosquito clouds, and casual hygiene. During the time I was embedded with the soldiers, we had no ready rolls of paper for cleaning ourselves, no barracks for washing ourselves. We had no kitchens for scouring the pots and no silverware at all, just shallow plastic bowls we rotated in a complex choreography, scooping gruel to our mouths with hands as dark as dirt.

In Managua, I consulted a succession of well-meaning doctors who admitted they had no drugs to prescribe and little in the way of diagnostic tools, given the tight embargoes of the Reagan administration. Nobody suspected HIV. There wasn't a diagnosed case in the country yet, and since gays there were rounded up and thrown into a special prison, out of caution I didn't bring it up. Finally I presented myself to a private hospital; I had heard rumors that inpatients were given priority access to the armamentarium. There I received a presumptive diagnosis of *Entamoeba histolytica* infection, a rampant amoebic assault requiring daily shots of a viscous remedy into my buttock. After two weeks they sent me back to my hotel with a supply of loaded needles to finish the course. I proved an unskilled self-administrator. A friend visiting from New York didn't mind helping out, though he proved even less adept. On his first effort, he discharged the needle too shallowly, creating a painful blister in the epidermis that slowly receded into a permanent purple scar that took the shape, eerily, of a crucifix.

This all did little to slow my symptoms. When I stepped on a scale I found I'd lost thirty pounds since leaving New York. Luckily, my ticket soon came through and I returned to the city and to modern medicine, such as it was.

It was winter. After a year away, I was astounded to see the stark visual presence of plague on the sidewalks below Fourteenth Street. Having the same harrowed, trembly appearance, I fitted right in. Dr. Waitkevicz squeezed me into her packed schedule. I stood before her naked as she drew her warm hands along my body to look for knobs on my lymph nodes. She found none. She studied the lesion on my hip with a hurried smile: it was a type of mole, she said, nothing to worry about.

But my bony appearance and abdominal distress stumped her. She sent me to a clinic specializing in tropical diseases, where they diagnosed a spectrum of bacterial and protozoan infections. They prescribed Flagyl, a powerful antibiotic so punishing it put blood in my stool, numbed my fingers, and seemed to compress my brain. Officially, the National Toxicology Program "reasonably anticipated" that Flagyl was carcinogenic, but it served its purpose and put me on the mend.

Despite the fact that I had begun gaining weight, Waitkevicz wanted to see me for a follow-up appointment. She ran down a list of questions about possible exposures and indicators of infection. My answers all fell in the safe column until she asked about shingles. I hadn't thought to tell her before. It hadn't left any scars, and never returned.

"It can mean a compromised immune system," she said, which I knew, but she hastily added, "*sometimes*—not always. Simple stress can bring it on. Sometimes there's no trigger at all," she said. "But I'd like you to consider an HIV test."

With the wildly positive news about the AZT trial hanging in the air, she had reversed her thinking about testing. Her colleagues had referred a number of her patients to Burroughs Wellcome, where they received the experimental drug at no charge. If I were infected, she would consider the same for me.

Reluctantly I agreed, reasoning that a positive diagnosis would do no more harm to me psychologically than not knowing, which was consuming me.

It was by now possible to send blood to commercial labs for testing. But the risk was still too great. Insurance companies were dropping patients who tested positive. Labs were reporting positive results to the Department of Health. The potential for serious ramifications was real. So Waitkevicz recommended using the network of "alternative confidential testing sites" set up by the CDC. After drawing my blood, she filled out a form assigning an untraceable code number to the sample, referenced only inside her medical files. Then she handed me the form, and the deep-red tube.

"Carry this to the Health Department on First Avenue," she said. "There's a drop-off in the lobby—don't sign the visitors' log; just tell them you're dropping a blood sample."

I did as she said. At 455 First Avenue, I passed through a set of glass doors fogged by neglect. The lobby was grimy and nearly empty but for an old gray metal desk on which a uniformed guard rested a lazy elbow. I showed the red of my vial, and without a word he pointed to an alcove beside the elevator bank. Standing there was a simple white refrigerator, the kind you'd expect to see in a suburban kitchen. Opening the door suspiciously, I found nothing inside but a cardboard basket holding more of what I had brought: tubes of blood with confidential identifier forms rubber-banded to them. I placed mine on top of the pile, praying that the next person to open the cooler didn't perversely scramble the vials and the forms, giving me someone else's diagnosis.

Then I waited two sleepless weeks for the results.

The mood in New York had begun to change in my absence. I was impressed to learn of the Lavender Hill Mob. One morning in December, bus shelters and bank windows in a large part of Manhattan were covered with ominous large posters, featuring a pink triangle floating against a black background. This was a potent reminder, not at all an obscure one, of how gays were marked by the Nazis in the camps. The movement had long ago reclaimed the pink triangle to signify liberty. Pins with pink triangles were best sellers at Oscar Wilde Memorial Bookshop. It was the symbol used for gay pride marches, on the covers of gay magazines, on T-shirts from gay cruises. But on the mysterious poster, the triangle had been inverted—no longer pointing downward like a yield sign, it was depicted there as a pyramid, invoking cosmic power and strength. Beneath this image was an arresting message in blocky white letters: SILENCE=DEATH.

Three thousand of these posters went up, from the East River to the Hudson and stretching north from the Village through Chelsea to Hell's Kitchen and the Upper West Side, and as far south as SoHo— not just in the gay ghetto but in the outposts of the arts communities where allies might find meaning in the message. For a full month it was all anybody talked about. Who had made them? What did they mean? It was obvious that the posters were addressing those of us living inside the plague. Part of the message was easily discerned: on the current course, we were surely doomed. Less clear was what these posters were asking us to do. The slogan suggested a corollary. We knew what the opposite of death was. But what kind of non-silence was being called for?

When it was time, I returned to the doctor's office for my results. They were negative. I was so relieved I nearly collapsed. "But don't live your life any differently," the doctor said. "This could be a false negative. Or there could be an incubation period. We don't know. And anyway," she said, gesturing to the fishbowl of condoms on the receptionist's counter, "everybody else is positive, so the rules still apply."

PART 3

•

An Ounce of Prevention

The Barricades, 1987

Larry Kramer lived and worked in a spacious two-bedroom apartment on the corner where Fifth Avenue terminates at Washington Square Park. A small balcony off his living room offered a bird's-eye view of the grand Washington Arch, modeled after the Arc de Triomphe, and the long-dry fountain where NYU students intermingled with breakdancers from uptown and soft-spoken marijuana peddlers, usually with Jamaican accents. He did not spend much time gazing down at the sights, a consequence of a growing struggle with acrophobia. On those afternoons when the beauty of the park drew his attention, he would grab his dog's leash and walk its perimeter beneath the dense awning of London planetrees, Norway maples, and American sycamores.

He enjoyed the attention he regularly received during these circumnavigations. His stage play had been a huge success—it went on to open in Europe and began a long life as college repertory material—and had made him quite famous. The play had even gotten the attention of Hollywood, where Barbra Streisand snapped up an option. She planned to direct a screen version; he planned to adapt the script. Through 1986, Kramer was a regular guest in her Malibu home, dreaming up casting options—of course, she would play the wheelchair-bound physician— and sketching out new scenes. But as quickly as she came into his life, Streisand retreated, dropping *The Normal Heart* to do *Nuts* instead.

He was back in New York at the start of the year, in a venomous mood. He turned his ire back toward Gay Men's Health Crisis. It had been five years since the group was founded in his living room, and four years since his painful resignation and the messy, failed campaign to be invited back. Every one of his cofounders had since moved on. Edmund White now lived and wrote in Paris, and Dr. Lawrence Mass had claimed a more private life since his recovery from depression. His writing now focused less on AIDS science than on the opera, a gentler beat. The other three had traded their public war on AIDS with very personal ones. Paul Popham, the handsome first board president, was now weakened with AIDS and five months from death. Paul Rapoport, another founder, had only seven months to live. The journalist Nathan Fain, who had excoriated Kramer so publicly, had since retreated to East Texas for his last excruciating days.

The organization's budget had grown to $6 million. It attracted some of the most well-connected New Yorkers as supporters, volunteers, and board members, even drawing socialites (Judy Peabody and Joan Tisch) and celebrities (Madonna and Mikhail Baryshnikov). The volunteer army now stood at 1,600 people, personally seeing to the needs of more than 5,000 clients. The agency drew praise around the world and served as a model for city after city.

But Kramer detested what "Auntie GMHC" had become: a service agency and not an advocacy group. One might expect Kramer to align himself with the Lavender Hill Mob, operating in what he considered a "separate and individual cocoon." He appreciated the group's intemperance, but he ultimately dismissed the Mob for carrying on the failed traditions of the movement to date—in his view, having "the great unwashed radicals" of the gay counterculture at the helm was off-putting to America and the majority of gays alike, or at least those in Kramer's Ivy League–educated, Fire Island–going, wallet-heavy circles. It was the baby, not the bathwater, he wished to throw out. So he resuscitated his campaign to goad GMHC into radicalism with boundless stinging invective.

"I think it must now come as a big surprise to you and your board of directors that Gay Men's Health Crisis was not founded to help those who are ill. It was founded to protect the living, to help the living go on living, to help those who are still healthy to stay healthy, to help gay men stay alive," he wrote in an open letter, making a distinction most in the community rejected. "Get off your fucking self-satisfied asses and fight! That is what you were put there for! That is what people give you money for!"

Larry Kramer was back, and he was stirring up trouble.

It was natural, then, for his name to come to mind at the Gay and Lesbian Community Center. Organizers of a monthly speaking series there had booked Nora Ephron for March 10. Her hilarious novel *Heartburn* was a bestselling success. But with barely a week's notice, she called in sick—the flu had felled her. Organizers tapped Kramer as a last-minute replacement.

For Kramer, the invitation sparked an idea to shift tactics. Instead of goading GMHC toward radicalism or the Lavender Hill Mob toward respectability, he dreamed of mobilizing the mainstream community into a sort of asylum uprising. On a recent evening news broadcast he had seen a group of agitated nuns descending on Albany with placards and handbills to show their displeasure over something or other. Why was no gay group up there demanding action? If he chose his words carefully, he thought, he might spark a new middle-class militancy.

In the few days he had for planning, he called and visited key people in the city. One was Michael Petrelis, a leading member of the Mob—its youngest and perhaps its most shrill. A boxy man with curly hair sliced into a mullet, Petrelis had a voice that was as powerful as it was grating, and an outsized personality that made him easy to admire but hard to love. The *New York Native* had taken to calling him "an adamant and abrasive young man." I first saw Petrelis in the audience for a panel discussion where he attacked a *New York Times* editor for the paper's editorial ban on the words "gay" and "lesbian." When the editor began to speak, Petrelis started bellowing, "Call us gay! Call us gay!" over and over, until the event could no longer proceed. Kramer needed him on his side.

Petrelis had fallen on hard times since his AIDS diagnosis in 1985. He was now at Bailey House, a residence at the far end of the West Village where Christopher Street met the Hudson River, conceived as a place for homeless PWAs to live out their last days. Turnover was painfully quick. (Proving there were no bounds Petrelis would not transgress, he referred to the place as "Auschwitz on the Hudson," keeping a grisly tally of his neighbors who left in body bags.) Kramer came to his top-floor room with a Balducci's bag of bagels, cream cheese, and lox, enough for everyone in the building. It was intended as an enticement. "Bring people," he said. "Bring as many people as you can." Petrelis enthusiastically agreed.

Next, Kramer reached out to another AIDS patient, Eric Sawyer, as handsome and cerebral as Petrelis was brash. Sawyer had recently lost his lover, Scott Bernard, who stopped breathing on a flight back home to bid his mother farewell. "I'm going to try to organize a civil disobedience group," Kramer told him. "I'm putting friends in the audience as plants. When I call for people to help me organize a demonstration, I need you to stand up and join in—rabble-rouse." He added, "There are people like Rodger who are going to join," meaning Rodger McFarlane, his former lover. "But if some of the younger guys from the Fire Island scene would step up that would be helpful, especially young, pretty people . . ."

Sawyer was angry enough to give anything a try, even civil disobedience. He promised to spread the word.

In this way, anticipation for Kramer's speech spread through the community. Someone placed a twelve-word notice in *The Village Voice*'s Community Bulletin Board, the equivalent of circling the ghetto in a sky-writing plane. Waves of people filed into the new Lesbian and Gay Community Center, a crumbling former high school that the city had recently made available to accommodate the wild proliferation of AIDS support groups. The main assembly hall on the first floor had peeling paint and a linoleum floor made of a patchwork of discolored tiles. The ceiling was a gnarl of exposed electrical cables and wobbling overhead fans. With no stage, Kramer stood at a music stand facing a semicircle of metal folding chairs. Before him were 250 men and a few women, most in their twenties and early thirties, almost all uncommonly handsome.

I learned of the lecture from a friend and though I planned to attend, it was a symptom of my feelings of impotence that I arrived only as the crowd was spilling out the door onto West Thirteenth Street. The scene on the sidewalk was electrifying. For a March evening, the weather was unusually hospitable; no one was in a hurry to leave. A sampling of celebrities milled among them, exotic specimens in Kramer's growing menagerie. Joel Grey had done time as the lead in Kramer's play at the Public. Martin Sheen, who had joined the London production, emerged from the center's derelict doorway with tears in his eyes. I later learned that his dearest friend, John Douglas Crane—the best man at his wedding—had died that day. Sheen had been at his side throughout his last week. I recognized a few other people on the sidewalk, including my former *Native* colleague James D'Eramo, who had moved to GMHC, but most were newcomers to the scene.

It was plain from their faces that something important had taken place inside. "He had two-thirds of the room stand," a man told me, illustrating the gesture with an unfolding arm. Crammed into his back pocket was a paperback of *The Wretched of the Earth* in the original French. "And he said, 'You will be dead in five years. Two-thirds of you will die. What are you going to do to save yourselves?'"

Kramer's savage oratory power, honed over his years of screed writing, swelled as he read his prepared remarks. "If my speech tonight doesn't scare the shit out of you, we're in trouble," he told them. "I sometimes think we have a death wish. I think we must want to die. I have never been able to understand why we have sat back and let ourselves literally be knocked off man by man without fighting back. I have heard of denial, but this is more than denial—it is a death wish."

He glared at the crowd and locked his large jaw. "It's our fault, boys and girls. It's our fault."

The presentation morphed into a Capraesque town hall meeting. Someone had risen to propose massive street protests, and someone else called for an organizing meeting. The current executive director of GMHC, a fair-haired Montana transplant named Tim Sweeney, offered institutional support, a welcome surprise to Kramer. Sweeney implored everyone in the room to work together and end the vocal antagonism between the political groups and the service agencies. Earlier in the month, when he attended a meeting at the Centers for Disease Control, he said he was shocked when the Lavender Hill Mob turned on him, of all people. Dressed as Nazi camp prisoners, Michael Petrelis and his band had cast the gay and AIDS establishment as deadly kapos in a tense showdown that forced the conference to adjourn prematurely. Attacking one another made no sense to Sweeney. As conservative as it was, GMHC's single-minded focus on care teams, hospital visits, and funerals did not make it traitorous any more than Red Cross tourniquets and stretchers served the enemy, in his view. In the plague war, GMHC was at the battlements, its battalions of volunteers confronting hospitals and undertakers, its flanks of lawyers fighting to keep surviving boyfriends in their apartments, a vast and heartbroken bureaucracy tasked with wrestling dignity and justice from the teeth of inevitable death.

After Sweeney's moving exhortation, a surprising thing happened: Michael Petrelis stood up and on behalf of the Mob apologized. It was neither wise nor productive to be fighting within the community with such towering adversaries on the prowl, he now agreed. The community was pulling together.

Next, the film historian Vito Russo took to his feet. The author of *The Celluloid Closet,* a seminal text on Hollywood's depiction of gays, had just watched the epic documentary about the civil rights movement, *Eyes on the Prize.* He spoke of the parallel strategies, the complementary and sometimes mistaken leadership, and the role of civil disobedience and nonviolence in a coordinated, triumphal movement. The community needed to show its anger, he said; the community needed to take to the streets.

Eric Sawyer shouted his promised endorsement, and the fuse caught fire. Consensus formed around a plan to reconvene two nights hence. Kramer's strategy had worked. Something brand new was afoot.

When the meeting was over and Kramer moved through the room, men called out to thank him for making the truth so plain. Hands touched his sleeve. After years of being a lightning rod, he now was the leader he felt called to be—Kramer the writer had written into formation a militant response to the plague. From that moment on, his words would drive the movement.

Almost 350 people attended the next meeting, held in the glass-walled dining hall of Bailey House with a spectacular view of the sun setting across the Hudson. Besides Petrelis, only one other resident of the facility attended, a man thoroughly ravaged by AIDS who sat quietly for a short while before returning to his room. Chuck Ortleb was there, too, taking notes for his *Native* editorials. So were Andy Humm from the Coalition for Lesbian and Gay Rights, Darryl Yates Rist from GLAAD, and representatives of the PWA Coalition, Gay Cable Network, and the Silence=Death Project. Avram Finkelstein, a top stylist for Vidal Sassoon with a long history of leftist organizing, broke the anonymity surrounding the stark posters with the large pink triangle that had appeared so mysteriously around Manhattan in recent months. He revealed that he and five others had spent the winter planning the poster and its dissemination, with the goal of fomenting the current atmosphere of action into which Larry Kramer's hand grenade had dropped.

A tremor of lingering hostility existed among the veterans, but the majority of people on hand were unaffiliated with existing groups, fresh recruits to the idea of political activism. GMHC's Tim Sweeney, crisp and proper, volunteered to moderate the meeting. Though barely thirty himself, he represented the old movement. In the interest of bridging the gaps, it was decided that a newer face would join him as co-facilitator: Vivian Shapiro, a fixture in the lesbian community. Kramer, as he had in GMHC's early days, jockeyed for leadership, claiming the group as his own, but he was quickly rebuked by Marty Robinson, one of the Lavender Hill Mobsters, who said, "It's not about making you famous, Larry. It's not about making *me* famous. It's about mercy." Stung, Kramer sunk into his chair, content for the time being to be one voice among many.

The first item on the agenda was a discussion of the value of marches and sit-ins generally, and how they might work. Specific actions were suggested and weighed, measured by a show of hands: picket on the doorstep of Memorial Sloan Kettering (thirty-one hands), protest the United Nations or *The New York Times* (thirteen each), block bridges and tunnels (two), shut down Wall Street (forty-three). It was Shapiro who proposed the Financial District. She was maddened by the indifference Big Pharma was showing the community and by the unseemly international tussle over royalties for the AIDS antibody test. But for her the last straw had come just that month. After huddling over the AZT data for weeks, Dr. Ellen Cooper at the FDA gave Burroughs Wellcome the go-ahead to bring the drug to market. It was the fastest journey to approval in FDA history, thanks largely to the unusual collaboration with Sam Broder at the National Cancer Institute. But on the same day the FDA cleared AZT for commercial production, Burroughs Wellcome announced it would charge $10,000 a year for it—more than any other drug in history. Few people without insurance could ever hope to swallow an AZT capsule. And the insured were not always better off. Many policies had annual or lifetime caps well below that figure.

As Vivian Shapiro put it, AIDS, which desperately needed an emergency medical response, was instead mired in spasms of ineptitude, opportunism, and greed. She proposed an informational picket line on the corner of Wall Street and Broadway. By acclamation, the assembly adopted her proposal, and conversation pivoted to making plans for the demonstration later that month.

"Drugs into bodies" would be the rallying cry.

But the group also called for a comprehensive and coordinated national policy on AIDS, overseen by a single independent agency, to eliminate redundancies and oversights among FDA, NIH, and CDC programs; increased funding for studying newer experimental drugs; an open and accessible register for patients wishing to enroll in trials; the permanent elimination of placebos in AIDS trials; and an end to discrimination against PWAs, especially within hospitals and other institutions where nightmare experiences were still common and unchecked.

I missed that meeting, and the next one, at which the assembled group adopted the name: ACT UP, for AIDS Coalition to Unleash Power. By the time I made my first appearance, ACT UP had slimmed down to a working nucleus of about seventy-five members, mostly gay men, mostly white, and, except for a few notable exceptions, mostly new to community organizing. They were young, privileged, and driven to a degree we hadn't seen much in the movement to this point. The plague had given them a mandate to act, to join voices and respond to Camus's edict: "When abstraction sets to killing you, you've got to get busy with it." Their energy and defiance was an invitation to optimism.

Six hundred people followed them to Wall Street for the first protest, assembling at sunrise one chilly morning in March. Larry Kramer arrived along with an effigy of the FDA commissioner, Frank Young, which he had convinced Joseph Papp, the legendary founder of the Public Theater, to produce in the set shop. The posters were handsomely lettered by Avram Finkelstein, but a degree too clever for conveying their desired message: "THE NAZIS HAD MENGELE . . . WE HAVE NIH," and "FDA, YOU SLAY ME." The picketers drew curious stares from passersby.

As he made his way to work, Peter Staley came upon the demonstration unexpectedly. He took one of the flyers being handed out but did not stay to see the protest's dramatic conclusion when, at precisely 7:55 a.m., a phalanx of protesters seized the intersection of Wall Street and Broadway, the service providers alongside the political activists, sprawling their bodies on the ground before oncoming traffic. Banks of cameras chronicled the police effort to roll protesters onto stretchers and cart them off to jail—seventeen in all. It was a story that played widely and sympathetically, in outlets ranging from *The Economist* to the Cleveland *Plain Dealer*. These weren't hardened activists dressed as Nazi camp prisoners. These were fresh-faced, scared-looking young people who could not afford the one drug on offer. Kramer's art direction had had an impact.

Sitting at his trading desk, Staley marveled at the scene he had encountered, filled with gratitude for the efforts. As he prepared to consult his complex trading algorithms, his attention was fixed by the flyer on his desk and its banner headline, "Why We Are Angry."

"Why is the FDA in bed with Burroughs Wellcome?" it demanded to know. "Why does it *IGNORE AT LEAST 8 OTHER DRUGS* considered just as promising and safe as AZT? Who's getting the kickback?" On the reverse side was a reprint of a *New York Times* op-ed published the day before, written by Kramer. "There is no question on the part of anyone fighting AIDS that the FDA constitutes the single most incomprehensible bottleneck in American bureaucratic history— one that is actually prolonging this roll call of death. This has been only further compounded by President Reagan, who has yet to utter publicly the word 'AIDS' or put anyone in charge of the fight against it."

Many others from the bond-trading floor had taken copies of the handout. It sparked an unexpected conversation in the Pit until one of Staley's mentors, a young lead trader named Mark Werner, shut it down with a grunt. "Well, if you ask me, they all deserve to die," he said. "They took it up the butt!"

Nobody denounced Werner. A few traders even laughed. Staley felt his face go red. He leaned deeply into the green glare of his computer screens, fuming silently, and discreetly folded the flyer into his brief-case. Back at his apartment that night, he watched Dan Rather lead his hour-long newscast with reports from the demonstration, which had forced the FDA's Frank Young into making a vaguely conciliatory state-ment. *I've got to be part of this*, Staley thought.

WITH THE GROWING availability of AZT, there was no clear consen-sus among doctors on whom it might help—anyone showing immune suppression, or only the very sick?—or if it would be effective against Kaposi's sarcoma, toxoplasmosis, cytomegalovirus, or the other oppor-tunistic infections. Sonnabend studied the published literature and decided not to prescribe it at all. Although he could see how it worked to kill HIV-infected cells, he believed that the same mechanism made it just as deadly to uninfected cells. It was a blunt-force instrument—"a thermonuclear warhead," in Callen's phrase. The list of debilitating side effects sounded as bad as the disease itself. He called it "incompat-ible with life."

What Sonnabend wanted his patients to take was AL721, which was even more out of reach than AZT. Through the winter, he hammered away at Praxis Pharmaceuticals, appealing to their sense of humanity for a supply of the compound. He had the health of Michael May to worry about—May couldn't afford to make another trip to Israel, and with supply exhausted, his health was precarious. But he had dozens of other patients who might benefit. Praxis officials said there was little they could do. While they did have a sizable quantity of AL721 in a warehouse, it was all earmarked for the FDA trials they hoped to begin shortly. Being a cash-poor startup, they could not afford to produce more at this time. Frustrated, Sonnabend turned to his contacts in Israel, but they were equally unable to meet his demands.

Sonnabend wasn't the only one on the AL721 trail. Larry Kramer also tried and failed to gain community access to the Praxis cache. Mathilde Krim put pressure on Dr. Tony Fauci, the government's top AIDS researcher, to break the bottleneck, without success. Callen put his own doggedness to the task, adding the gravitas of the People With AIDS Coalition. He personally called the Praxis CEO and begged him to do the "moral thing." The answer was no different. Once he had full marketing clearance, which he honestly believed was imminent, the company executive promised that raising money would be simple and the drug would soon flow.

With one PWA dying every hour, Callen lost his cool. "If you don't make it available, *we will*," he shouted into the phone. "We will get it bootlegged!" He hated making hollow threats, but it did make him feel a little better thinking the man might actually believe him.

Then one frigid afternoon, Sonnabend entered his examining room to greet a new patient, a Columbia University graduate student in chemistry named Stephen Roach, who had tested positive but had few other symptoms. Roach had come to Sonnabend in search of AL721 for himself and for his lover, whose AIDS was considerably more advanced. Sonnabend shared the long and frustrating history, encouraging Roach to join the quixotic campaign. So on a snowy morning, he and his lover—a short and charismatic song-and-dance man named Tom Hannan—showed up unannounced at Praxis's Manhattan headquarters.

They spoke to one official after another, before landing in the laboratory of Claire Klepner, head of the company's research efforts. She heard them out, knowing there would be no way to comply with their request. Like Callen before them, they said to her, "If you can't make it available to us, let us try to make it ourselves." She quizzed Stephen Roach about his abilities in a chemistry lab and, when she was satisfied by his competence, she did something extraordinary: she showed him how to make AL721. Klepner did this with the approval of the company's president, who had been moved by the community's pleas. The formula came without conditions, as the company held patents not on AL721 but on the process to upscale production for commercial quantities. But she warned him that the procedure was a volatile one involving explosive acetones; a false step could have serious repercussions. Roach was not deterred. He took detailed notes.

Over the coming weeks, he and Hannan—with Sonnabend's supervision—followed the instructions, using acetones they purchased on Canal Street and eggs from the corner store. But it was even more difficult to accomplish than Klepner had warned, and twice as dangerous. Their failures were numerous. In frustration, they sought out an independent lab capable of the challenge. If they could find a suitable compounder, they could bypass the gatekeepers altogether and actually do what Michael Callen had so flippantly threatened—put bootlegged AL721 into production.

Sonnabend saw this as a thrilling opportunity, one that in his estimation held far more promise than AZT. He tried to get Callen involved, but his protégé wasn't keen to become embroiled in a criminal undertaking. Even if he were, he lacked the time and energy. Besides struggling to finish his first studio album, he was battling yet another opportunistic infection while maintaining a packed portfolio of AIDS work. Between his duties at the People With AIDS Coalition, he had launched the *PWA Coalition Newsline,* a monthly compendium of useful research findings, and served as its editor and publisher. Callen was also beginning work on the anthology *Surviving and Thriving with AIDS,* attending the weekly AIDS Network meetings, singing at AIDS benefits, and serving as a delegate to the New York State AIDS Advisory Council. In between, he was attending memorials, visiting Sonnabend's sick patients, and making regular appearances in housing court to battle his landlord, who was trying to evict him and Dworkin in a loft-conversion dispute.

And then there was the elusive matter of gainful employment, which included sporadic temping assignments and joining the Musicians' Union to work as a "walker," a peculiar theater-world perk in which ordinary people were paid to fill the orchestra pits of Broadway shows that didn't meet the minimum number of musicians required by union contracts. Someone at the union had decided these benefits should go to PWAs. Callen earned scale for eight no-shows a week.

Another leadership role was out of the question. But as a favor to Sonnabend, he agreed to attend an AL721 planning meeting at the doctor's apartment. Hannan arrived alone; Stephen Roach had just been admitted to the hospital with PCP, casting a pall of urgency on the agenda.

With his rapid-talking demeanor and quick mind, Hannan reminded Callen of Richard Berkowitz, though he was considerably more naïve. The plan he spelled out was balanced unstably, it seemed to Callen, on impossible assumptions: Praxis wouldn't sue; the FDA wouldn't intervene; the community would be totally behind them; the drug would work miracles.

To Callen, AL721's potential seemed questionable. It was more likely that Hannan's plan would simply flood the community with a useless concoction. But as Hannan spoke Callen became convinced that, regardless of AL721's efficacy, it offered the community something it hadn't had in years: hope. He came to the conclusion that it was worth the risk and begrudgingly agreed to help.

He volunteered to bring the initiative under the umbrella of the PWA Coalition, although that never happened. Fearing lawsuits from Praxis, the coalition's board of directors rejected the idea after an emergency meeting. They would lend office space and phone service, but Callen, Sonnabend, and Hannan were forced to incorporate a new group. They chose the name "People With AIDS Health Group," on Callen's suggestion. "Who could sue a group with that kind of name?" he reasoned. Its only purpose was to manufacture enough AL721 to create a media storm ferocious enough to force Praxis to open its spigots. Thereafter, they might serve as a kind of consumer advocacy group, mediating disputes between patients and pharmaceutical companies.

No formal announcement of their endeavor was necessary. Word spread quickly and within days preorders flooded their mailbox. People from Texas, California, and Hawaii mailed in $200 checks for a three-month supply. Checks came from Denmark, West Germany, Canada, and Belgium as well. More than five hundred orders were from New Yorkers. Demand was so high that the PWA Health Group had to close the list in a matter of days, when they already had $20,000 in the bank.

They signed a contract with the American Roland Company to produce and deliver the product—and made a decision to keep their contacts at Praxis informed at every step. Callen promised to pull the plug on their illicit operation if the company agreed to start producing the drug. "Please do this," he offered, "there is a big demand." But the weeks progressed and Praxis remained inert.

As spring approached, the PWA Health Group began planning for the day distribution would begin, set for the third week in April. Still wary, the PWA Coalition's board wouldn't allow them to use their offices for this. The Lesbian and Gay Community Center likewise refused, afraid of Praxis lawyers and FDA enforcers. Callen and Hannan then made a presentation to the Judson Memorial Church, one of the most liberal religious institutions in the city. Not only did the board of directors agree to host the distribution efforts, but their pastor, Reverend Howard Moody, a colorful veteran of battles for prostitute safety and free speech, volunteered to attend the launch press conference. It promised to be a circus.

The substance arrived from American Roland several days early in a large refrigerated truck. Contained in thousands of plastic tubs was a thick, oily, orange goo, as dense as fudge and as malodorous as a baby's diaper. Out of abundant caution, Sonnabend sent a sample of it to a local lab to gauge its purity. Late on the afternoon of the day before showtime, the lab called with bad news. The three lipid components were indeed correct, but the ratio between them was off considerably—nowhere near seven to two to one. Over strenuous objections from Callen and Hannan, Sonnabend called off the distribution unilaterally and ordered a brand new batch. The time for hope was delayed by weeks.

But at lunchtime the following day, as the spring weather turned bright and warm, almost a thousand people lined up at Judson's doorstep anyway, only to learn the disappointing news. Some wept, unsure they could survive the delay. The press conference went on as planned. Callen and Hannan took their places before a bank of television cameras and a scrum of radio reporters. The papers and wire services were represented. Photographers took aim. Callen managed an impassioned speech, ending with the unfortunate news about the postponement. Reporters shot looks of confusion at one another and demanded clarification, but without an actual distribution, they had no story. The next morning, no mention of AL721 appeared in the media. A friendly *New York Times* reporter suggested a feature story in the Styles section, to the disgust of everyone at PWA Health Group, but even that never materialized.

It was two more Mondays before acceptable material arrived from the compounder. Two registered customers had died in the interim. A distribution was scheduled for noon on May 4. The line outside Judson was even longer—there now were $100,000 in orders—but the reporters stayed away this time. This was Callen's nightmare: without creating a media spectacle to shame Praxis, all they had accomplished was a bootlegging operation, the last thing in the world he wanted. But as he scanned the faces of the men in line, people like him "with their backs against the wall," as he wrote later, he knew that making AL721 available was the right thing to do.

A feeling of thrilled expectation filled the air. Laughter and shouts rose from the line of people looping across Washington Street and bending south at Thompson.

Peter Staley took his place in the queue, having come directly from work, a briefcase dangling at his side. The esprit de corps surprised him and lightened his mood. It had been eighteen months since he'd been given twenty-four months to live. He had stayed remarkably healthy. His cough was gone, fevers were no longer an issue, and his CD4 numbers were holding steady. If what he had read was true, AL721 might extend his lucky streak. He too felt like rejoicing. In the face of almost total disregard from the pharmaceutical world, the gay community had managed to accomplish the seemingly impossible.

He recognized some of the men ahead of him in line, faces from the support group or the doctor's waiting room, or men he had met through Griffin Gold. Inside the church's great hall, each customer was greeted at a succession of stations: one to confirm orders; one where advisers explained what was known and unknown about egg lipids and lecithins; one where recipients learned how to prepare and administer doses. This last station featured a video looped on a television monitor. It featured Michael Callen, standing in his own kitchen, warbling like Julia Child. At his elbow was a large jug of the orange sludge everyone was there to collect. As a succession of men huddled around the television screen, he proceeded methodically to show how to handle AL721, how to measure it and freeze it into ice cube-sized bricks, and how to blend it up in a large glassful of orange juice. But not before offering a bit of plague-era advice.

"I will digress, but briefly," he singsonged. "The well-stocked kitchen for someone with AIDS has Bactrim or Septra, if you can tolerate it." Rattling his own bottle of pills, he made it his mission to extoll the benefits of PCP prophylaxis, even if the public health establishment was still silent on the subject. He plucked another jar with a coy smile. "Acyclovir, for those troubling outbreaks of herpes, which we are all so frequently plagued with. And of course aspirin or Tylenol for those cyclical fevers that we all get." He reached below the countertop to retrieve two red cans of another elixir in his daily survival regimen. "I know my macrobiotic friends will cringe," he said, "but Classic Coke is my reason for living."

The afternoon and evening filled with an organized bedlam. At 9 p.m., the refrigerator truck empty, Callen slumped into Richard Dworkin's arms, more exhausted than he ever recalled being. With the exception of the media blackout, their event had gone off without a hitch. Like it or not, they were in the distribution business now. Several more times over the next year, they would presell and then hand out truckloads of orange goop. Soon, they branched out to other drugs, importing ribavirin from Mexico and dextran sulfate from Japan, both legally available in most of the world but not the U.S. Groups like theirs quickly formed in as many as nineteen other American cities as a movement of AIDS buyers clubs took hold, serving a long menu of options to tens of thousands of patients. Among them no drug was more in demand than AL721. To everyone's surprise, Praxis never pursued the PWA Health Group.

Nor did they ever go into commercial production. Following the first Judson Church event, the Praxis CEO managed to convince the NIH to do an efficacy trial. Responsibility for the trial fell to Tony Fauci, who didn't hold AL721 in high esteem. The burgeoning underground marketplace worried him, though, so he ordered a quick four-week test at his infectious disease institute involving some forty people and a range of doses. Results were positive in terms of weight gain, but he found "no indication of an immunorestorative or anti-viral effect." With that, Fauci moved on from AL721, convinced it was fool's gold, a waste of time for scientists and patients alike, and as dangerous a form of quackery as the apricot-derived laetrile that had been a distracting and costly craze among cancer patients in the 1960s.

This development did nothing to diminish the community's faith in egg lipids, and only reinforced its suspicions of governmental neglect. Nobody believed that what Fauci learned in four weeks was enough to counter the years-long experience of patients and their doctors. But with a stroke, Fauci delivered a fatal blow to Praxis and assured that no other researcher would return to AL721, condemning Hannan and Callen to delivering a drug with no sure profile of efficacy, a role they refused to accept. Callen spent many months phoning Fauci's secretary trying to get a meeting. Reluctantly, Fauci finally agreed to see Callen in his office, thanks to the forceful intervention of Tim Westmoreland, a legislative aide to Representative Henry Waxman and a gay man himself.

Waxman, who represented Los Angeles and West Hollywood, the region's gay ghetto, was in a unique position to do something about the epidemic, as the chairman of the health subcommittee. He called his first hearing when there were just three hundred cases, and he had chaired several hearings since then, with Westmoreland serving as his fill-time AIDS investigator, instructed to "look for research undone, surveys not conducted." That's how Westmoreland came to know Callen. He pressed Fauci to set a meeting in May 1987—the first time that the putative leaders in the fight against AIDS would sit down with representatives of the population the plague was stalking.

When the morning came, Callen headed to the NIH campus with Westmoreland, Larry Kramer, Dr. Barry Gingell from GMHC, and GMHC's new board president, Nathan Kolodner, by profession an art dealer. They were ushered into a sunny conference room inside Building 31. Tony Fauci joined them momentarily, along with a battery of fifteen colleagues wearing suits, lab coats, and steely expressions. They crowded on one side of the table, an intimidating battalion of scientists squared off against the New Yorkers, whose long-haired leader introduced himself in his most silken voice.

If Callen was intimidated, he didn't show it. He seized the initiative, describing the insatiable demand for lipids not just in New York City but in every American city with infected people. He laid out the anecdotal reports of stronger, healthier, more robust patients, and described how AL721 was being used prophylactically by the uninfected population on a hunch that it might confer protection. All of this was happening despite Fauci's summary dismissal of the drug. People with AIDS—*Americans* with AIDS—deserved a thoroughgoing drug trial and, if merited, a legitimate marketplace for buying it, he said.

Fauci cut him off. "It's useless," he said. "Our committee considered it. There's absolutely no evidence that it works—*whatsoever*."

Callen shifted into his aggressor mode. He was taller than Fauci by a foot, and bitchier by a factor of ten. "What about the anecdotal reports?" he demanded. "What about the Weizmann Institute data? What about the Gallo letter? Are you saying that Gallo is publishing shit?"

Fauci smiled the patronizing smile of a bureaucrat. "Look," he said, "if I take a tube of blood from a person with AIDS and I put oregano in it, it would probably kill the virus."

"Dr. Fauci," Callen interrupted. "If you had this disease, would *you* take AL721?"

A flash of anger lit Fauci's face. Of *course* he would take AL721, he said. Fauci's admission gave Callen the strategic opportunity he was looking for. He planned to take every advantage of it, whether in future issues of the *PWA Coalition Newsline* or during his next congressional testimony. He felt certain that the people at Praxis would be able to turn Fauci's "endorsement" into a full-scale trial. For his part, Fauci said his statement was "irrelevant"; it wouldn't make AL721 any more powerful against HIV.

In fact, Praxis never pushed Fauci again. Instead, with the road to FDA approval blocked, the company unilaterally reclassified AL721 as a food supplement, packaged it in handsome aluminum envelopes, and began placing the product in select pharmacies in AIDS-ridden neighborhoods on both coasts. The experiment ended quickly when the FDA wrote a warning and pledged to seize their materials—once a drug, always a drug, was the agency's apparent philosophy. Claire Klepner, the Praxis research chief, despaired that high-quality AL721 might be destroyed by the federal government. In a caper worthy of a Hollywood movie, she raced to the warehouse on a Friday night, loaded up multiple refrigerator trucks with the remaining doses, and sent them to a friend of the company's president in LA, who because he was a florist had the needed cooler space; he agreed to hand out doses free of charge to anyone who asked. "It was so important that the supplies not be destroyed," Klepner said later. "People were dying. We were all very upset about AIDS, we didn't sleep at night." Dumping the product on the underground market was the last financial blow to the struggling company, inflaming internal battles. A power play later in the year toppled its leadership and sent Praxis permanently adrift. The company still had a death grip on its patents, but absolutely no ability to do a thing with it.

For the next year or more, various underground groups across the country produced versions of AL721, most far inferior to PWA Health Group's product in terms of reliable lipid ratios. Some individuals were making facsimiles in their own bathtubs. My local pharmacy began offering lecithin pellets made from soy instead of egg, with instructions for mixing them in a blender with ordinary stick butter and a powdered egg extract. Countless people were taking one version or another, on the assumption that it couldn't hurt even if the formula were badly mangled. As a preventative, I began buying the local mix and preparing large batches for myself, divvied out in precise amounts and spooned into ice cube trays for freezing. Every morning I thawed a dose and choked it down. Eating that much butter packed a huge amount of weight on me very quickly. My waist swelled from twenty-nine inches to thirty-four. I developed jowls. A friend walked right past me on the street without recognizing me. I was mortified. There was no way of knowing if it had improved the defenses of my cell membranes, but my *Village Voice* editor saw some currency in it as an AIDS-prevention modality. "Makes you a lot less likely to get laid," he said. Reconsidering his put-down, he added, "With AIDS turning everybody into skeletons, maybe chubby is the new chic."

CALLEN'S AGENDA for the Fauci meeting went well beyond AL721 and included his leading concern for saving lives. He told Fauci and his colleagues of his own successful use of Bactrim for preventing PCP.

Since up to 75 percent of people with AIDS eventually succumbed to PCP, there was no more pressing issue. On this day, to the best of Callen's ability to calculate, nearly ten thousand Americans had died unnecessarily from PCP, a disease that was entirely preventable.

Callen, who had been waiting for this meeting since 1982, didn't mince words.

"Look, Dr. Fauci, I have a proposition to make," he said. "I'd like you to just issue guidelines to doctors to consider using PCP prophylaxis." Certainly, the number of lives saved would merit the small expense of mailing an alert to every doctor in America. "I am here to ask you—no, to *beg* you—to issue interim guidelines urging physicians to prophylax those patients deemed at high risk for PCP."

"There isn't a doctor in New York who doesn't prescribe prophylaxis now," Dr. Gingell, from GMHC, added enthusiastically.

Fauci gave Callen a steady look. "I can't do that," he said. "I can't issue these kinds of guidelines."

"Why not?" Callen's voice was steely and sharp.

"There's no data."

Callen knew the data. There were published studies showing that Bactrim prevented PCP in cancer and transplant patients, both infants and adults. There was no evidence suggesting that gay people were biologically different from straight people, or that immune suppression caused by a retrovirus was different from immune suppression caused by chemotherapy. While anecdotal evidence was not data per se, it suggested that using prophylaxis was just as safe and effective. Because the practice was commonplace among New York doctors, death rates from PCP were the lowest of any city in the plague-riddled country.

Fauci did not budge. If Bactrim were rolled out throughout the community, he said, you risked creating an untreatable mutant strain of PCP.

Hypothetical mass deaths, Callen countered, might be the potential outcome of overprescribing, but *certain* mass death was assured by the present policy—every data set pointed to it. The main determinant of whether a person survived or died, he said, was PCP prevention.

Fauci countered. Bactrim itself could be deadly, he said. At the NIH Medical Center he had witnessed the horror of a patient dying from an excruciating side effect called Stevens-Johnson syndrome, which caused every inch of flesh to bubble up and slide off in sheets, blackened as if by fire. *Primum non nocere,* he said: First, do no harm.

"Please, I *beg* you," Callen said. "In wartime, in the trenches, there is a need for emergency medicine. You don't have the luxury of time. The main task is to keep people alive and work out the fine details of science later."

"I can't do that," Fauci said in a voice suggesting he hadn't heard Callen at all. "I need the data."

The plague was six years old, and still there was not one person at the helm of the Public Health Service demonstrating simple human compassion for the victims. Callen looked around the room. Everyone on the other side of the table regarded him sadly, as though they considered him delusional.

I WAS BACK from Central America for just a few weeks when Gary Petkanis, a friend from the *Native*'s circulation department, called to say he had been diagnosed. Petkanis had been my confidante at the paper, and my occasional companion on the town—he was the person who carefully scoured the day's mail for club invitations, and pocketed them for the two of us. He delivered his news in a tone that seemed strangely ebullient. When I responded gravely, his gentle laugh interrupted me. "It's not that bad," he said. "I just wanted you to know how much I admire you, and would like you in my life at this weird time."

I made a vow to him—and to myself, more tentatively—to be his "weird-time" partner, not to withdraw the way I had from Tom Ho. We spoke nightly on the telephone and saw each other several times each week. After movie nights or concerts in Central Park, we sometimes went back to his apartment on the Upper West Side for *Jeopardy* or crossword puzzles, or for reading aloud the increasingly bizarre headlines from the *Native* through fits of laughter. We talked about the movement and our leaders, such as they were, and reviewed and critiqued the evolving liberation agenda. His politics were driven by wise intuition, and always mediated by self-deprecation about the place of "party boys" like him in the cause. We talked so late into the evening on a few occasions that he threw a fresh towel at me and invited me to stay.

On those nights, lying beside him, I never for a moment stopped thinking about death. I awoke each of those mornings in a bolt of terror.

I didn't accompany Petkanis on his medical rounds. His parents and brother, who lived nearby, were the major presence in that part of his life. Following one particularly tiring round of radiation treatments, he spent a week convalescing in his childhood bedroom, waiting for the pain and nausea to subside. He called me from there one afternoon, overcome with emotion. He said he had glimpsed a file folder with his name on it among his father's papers. Inside were notes taken from consultations with the Hemlock Society, the publisher of a backyard guide to home euthanasia called *Final Exit*. His father had copied the necessary formulas.

"If for whatever reason I'm in agony, he knows what to do," he told me. "That's taken care of. I knew I could count on him."

The night he returned to the city, I stayed over at his apartment, the two of us lying in his bed like kids having a sleepover. In the dim wash of the city lights, I could see how frail he had become, but he was not frightened. He said he was counting on me for continued distraction, that when talking with me about politics he sometimes forgot about death.

Luckily, there was much to talk about that winter. The fallout from the Iran-Contra hearings dominated the news. When President Reagan gave his stunning address to the nation maintaining that his absent-mindedness had given birth to the whole affair, I called Gary. When he didn't return my call after a week I grew concerned. Not knowing how to reach his family, I left increasingly frantic daily phone messages on his answering machine. Eventually, a recorded message told me the number was no longer in service. I thought of his dad's file folder and prayed that the end was as gentle and loving as Gary had imagined.

But I waited for many months before penning his name into my book, tenaciously holding on to hope that a call from him might come.

ACT UP had entered a frustrating period of fruitless outreach to the non-gay community after its first burst of energy. Organizers moved the meetings out of the Village to the Midtown headquarters of the Health and Hospital Workers' Union, but quickly returned downtown when "allies" failed to materialize. ACT UP settled into a steady hum at the Lesbian and Gay Community Center, where the weekly head count at meetings hovered between fifty and seventy-five. The few women in attendance had significant influence over the group, owing to their greater experience in political organizing—some from the feminist health movement, others with antiwar and civil rights activism. At their suggestion, weekly meetings were led by one male and one female, elected by the floor.

I was often the only reporter in attendance, challenged from time to time about my intentions. From the start I elected to keep the relationship formal and distant, telling myself that was the way to remain objective. A more honest explanation was that I was intimidated as much by the disease as by their response to it. In sharp contrast to the ACT UP ethos, which turned "anger into action," AIDS terrified me into torpidity. Compared to the confrontational strategies ACT UP was planning, my journalistic quarrel with the epidemic felt cowardly.

Peter Staley entered the center for his first Monday-night meeting a week after the Wall Street demonstration. He was hard to ignore in his suit and tie, a handsome young Wall Streeter among artists and Village types. Something happened to him in that instant, he told me later. The fear that had been his constant companion since getting diagnosed suddenly lifted. For the first time in two years, he was not afraid.

Right away he signed up for the fund-raising committee, a natural fit, taking a low-profile position that would not require him to leave the closet. The committee, which was run by an elegant and arch nursing student named Michael Nesline, was less functional than it was aspirational; it didn't even have a bank account. The first demonstration had been made possible by ACT UP members appropriating photocopies and postage stamps from their employers. With plans in the works for a tax-day picket at the main post office branch, an anti-Reagan protest in D.C., a round-the-clock rally in front of Memorial Sloan Kettering, and a major presence—replete with a stark concentration camp–themed float addressing the quarantine threats—at the annual Gay Pride March in June, a more robust source of finances would be needed.

Staley wrote a check for $1,000, the group's first asset. At his third or fourth meeting, he and Nesline addressed the ranks with a proposal to merchandise T-shirts bearing the same SILENCE=DEATH logo that had appeared around town over the winter. Their presentation inadvertently revealed ACT UP's main weakness. From its inception, all decisions were made by a majority vote of those in attendance. As a result of this unwieldy democracy, decisions were painfully elusive. On the T-shirt issue, sharp discord erupted among art directors, fashion designers, and marketing experts in the room.

An unseemly back-and-forth continued until Larry Kramer could stand it no more. "You sissies!" he shouted from the back of the room. "What a bunch of sissies! People are dying and you're talking about T-shirts!"

Reaching consensus never got easier. Attending meetings could be a painful exercise in endurance. But Monday after Monday, more people arrived, and a momentum built steadily, though toward what wasn't yet evident, at least not to me. At the minimum, ACT UP served as a weekly town hall meeting, the place you went for information about the crisis, a squabbling, teeming, ill-defined entity replacing the void left by the *Native*'s derailment. I missed very few of the meetings, believing that if anyone anywhere in the globe was doing something promising about the epidemic, the members of ACT UP would know it first and I might learn it from them.

2

Things Fall Apart

On June 5, 1987, Joe Sonnabend sank into an armchair in his apartment and turned his television to the news on PBS. To his surprise, Dr. Mathilde Krim's face appeared. In the past eighteen months, he and Krim had mostly parted ways. Sonnabend had been an unbending and difficult partner in the American Medical Foundation, the research organization they founded together, more so once Krim recruited Elizabeth Taylor and changed the name to the American Foundation for AIDS Research, or AmFAR, increasing its ambition and standing. Ultimately he resigned in protest after learning that a *Life* magazine article he considered dangerously alarmist—the cover line was "Now No One Is Safe from AIDS"—had been planted by Krim and her PR staff. The article made the case that heterosexuals were now at equal risk for the disease, which the data didn't support.

He could see the brilliance of her gambit. It made AIDS everybody's problem and it put AmFAR on the national stage. But at what cost? The dangerous conclusion, plainly stated in the piece, was that homosexuals now "posed . . . [a] threat to other Americans." They had barely spoken since.

Krim, who gave off a grandmotherly presence onscreen, was joined by a Columbia University sociologist, Dr. Ronald Bayer, and by Tony Fauci. The purpose of the segment was to discuss the Third International Conference on AIDS, which had just concluded. "The Washington meeting drew 6,000 scientists and other experts from throughout the world, and it attracted much attention to the scope of the tragedy [the] disease has brought, and will continue to bring, to millions of people throughout the world," the anchor, Jim Lehrer, was saying.

"Did anything come up at the conference from a medical point of view that was news to you—that would say, Oh, my goodness, this is new and significant?" he asked his panelists.

Krim was silent. "Well, not really," Fauci said.

Sonnabend stared at the television in disbelief. He had attended that conference, where one very important study had been presented. Dr. Craig Metroka, the oncologist who had collaborated with Krim years before, presented data from a trial in which various drugs were tested to prevent AIDS-related pneumonia. One, a drug with few side effects called dapsone, reduced the number of patients coming down with PCP to just 0.7 percent, compared to 74 percent on a case-matched control. This was the missing data Fauci sought while rejecting Callen's pleas for a national campaign to prevent PCP. This was proof it worked, which everyone already knew anyway, and the formal foundation for issuing emergency guidelines to doctors everywhere.

This meant finally slowing the dying. And to Fauci it was an irrelevance.

Lehrer pivoted. "From a medical point of view, somebody that's diagnosed in this country—or any other country—as having AIDS, what happens to that person?" he asked. "What is the life expectancy after catching AIDS?"

"If you present with an opportunistic infection like *Pneumocystis carinii* pneumonia," said Fauci, "the mean survival is about thirty-six to forty weeks."

Sonnabend shot out of his seat, cranked a sheet of paper into his typewriter, and pounded out a dense two-page rebuttal. "[T]he reality for many community physicians and their patients is much more optimistic," he wrote. "Nobody should be deprived of an intervention that will in all likelihood prevent this pneumonia."

In typical fashion, Sonnabend did not send the letter to Fauci, PBS, or the *Times*. Instead, he submitted it to the *PWA Coalition Newsline* and Michael Callen rushed it into print. The *Newsline* had a small but targeted circulation, reaching most New York and San Francisco doctors with large AIDS practices. At least they would be reminded about proper practice standards. A copy also went to Fauci's office, though he did not reply.

WHILE TRAVELING, Larry Kramer got word from a mutual friend that Paul Popham had died, at the age of forty-five. In recent weeks, Kramer had visited Popham twice to offer deathbed comforts and to seek a final reconciliation, which proved elusive after years of estrangement. Popham was unable to forgive his GMHC cofounder for his vindictive cruelties to other GMHC stalwarts and for parodying Popham in *The Normal Heart* as a man gifted with nothing besides good looks. The *Times* ran a brief and admiring obituary. Under intense pressure from the AIDS community, the paper had recently changed its policy of not acknowledging "intimates other than blood relatives and spouses" in death notices. In Popham's case, it named Richard Dulong, calling him a "longtime companion," a spongy phrase that called to mind Lemmon and Matthau in *The Odd Couple* and helped make gay relationships seem unusual and strange. Both GMHC and the PWA Coalition continued protesting the *Times* obituary policy as demeaning, and the editorial board quietly began an internal review that would go on for many more years, long after Dulong himself was dead.

Popham's death cast Kramer into a deep funk. He spoke of little else for weeks. He described their deathbed conversations as a rapprochement, perhaps assuaging some of his guilt with a bit of wishful thinking. He asserted that Popham had used some of his last earthly energy to exalt him to "keep fighting, keep fighting," something Popham's friends doubted seriously (not coincidentally, Kramer's fictional lover in *The Normal Heart* had the same dying words). Kramer soon turned his grief to anger when he addressed a stone-faced crowd in Fanueil Hall coinciding with Boston's pride week events.

"I don't think you are going to like what I am going to say. It is the last time I am going to say it. I'm making a farewell appearance," he told them dramatically.

I am not overly tired. I am certainly not suffering from burnout. I have a lot of piss and vinegar left in me—too much in fact. No, I'm not tired. Not physically tired, at any rate. I am, of course, as are you, very tired of many things. I am tired of what *they* are doing to us. I am tired of what *they* aren't doing *for* us. I am tired of seeing so many of my friends die—I'm exceptionally tired of that, as I know you are too.

I'm also tired of people coming up to me on the street and saying, "Thank you for what you're doing and saying." They mean it as a compliment, I know. But now I scream back, "Why aren't you doing it and saying it, too? Why are there so few people out there screaming and yelling? *You're dying too!*" I'm telling you, they are killing us. We are being picked off one by one, and half the men [hearing] this could be dead in five years, and you are all still sitting on your asses like weaklings, and therefore we, the gay community, are not strong enough and our organizations are not strong enough and *we are going to die for it*!

Yes, most of all, I'm tired of you.

Kramer received $1,000 for the speech, which he called the angriest of his life. It was received tepidly by an audience that seemed equally tired of its speaker. In peculiar contrast, Kramer had delivered a very different farewell message to the ACT UP ranks the night before. From the back of the room he praised the group's creativity, tenacity, and three months of demonstrations, predicting that they would force new drugs from the sluggish system. "I think each and every one of us can be very proud of what we have been doing with such success," he told them. "I am particularly pleased that everything is going so well because I must say goodbye, and it is easier for me to do so when I know that ACT UP is on a high and is in such good hands."

To that crowd, he described his planned departure as a restorative retreat, a hedge against burnout. But it was also a preemptive strike. He did not say so, but he may have feared that ACT UP would turn against him if he stayed, as GMHC had. In fact, the young men and women of ACT UP venerated Kramer, and tolerated his moodiness and unpredictability. Unlike GMHC, ACT UP owed its creation and its success to him. His flourishes on national television generated letters of gratitude and support from the younger generation. "My children," he called them. He couldn't risk losing that. That's what Paul Popham's death had taught him.

He told ACT UP he was called to write another play. "I would much rather be with all of you out there in the streets than at my computer. But it is to my computer that I must go," he said.

Three weeks later, Ronald Reagan finally exercised leadership in the battle against AIDS. His few comments up to this point, as 19,938 Americans perished, had been defensive and unhelpful; in April he had said, "When it comes to preventing AIDS, don't medicine and morality teach the same lessons?" Now, under mounting pressure from inside his administration, including from his surgeon general, Reagan announced the establishment of the Presidential Commission on the HIV Epidemic, vowing to send the plague "the way of smallpox and polio." He charged the commission with analyzing research priorities, suggesting care standards, and recommending steps for federal, state, and local officials to take in trying to stem the spread of AIDS. A final report would come in twelve months.

If anyone imagined that this would be the turning point in the epidemic, their hopes died when details were made public. To chair the commission, Reagan selected Dr. W. Eugene Mayberry, a man who, despite being a respected physician and the CEO of the prestigious

Mayo Clinic, freely admitted he had no clinical experience with AIDS and knew little about it. Nobody in the public health community could imagine why he was chosen. To fill out the commission, Reagan ignored every name put forward by HHS and the NIH, settling instead on a roster of figures whose lack of experience was matched by their reckless beliefs. Reagan introduced them at a carefully orchestrated unveiling at the White House. One "expert" was New York's Cardinal John O'Connor, whose only involvement with AIDS had been to inveigh against condom use and gay civil rights. O'Connor was joined by Penny Pullen, an obscure Illinois lawmaker who came to the attention of the administration when she warned, without evidence, that a subset of homosexuals were engaged in "blood terrorism" by deliberately donating infected blood. Next was Dr. Woodrow Myers, who as Indiana's health commissioner had supported a quarantine law for "recalcitrant carriers" of the disease. Theresa Crenshaw, a San Diego sex therapist who considered it probable that AIDS was spread by toilet seats, was introduced, as were a bevy of important Republican donors with their own odd theories about the epidemic: the editor of *The Saturday Evening Post,* the president of Amway, an executive with the Metropolitan Life Insurance Company, a Navy admiral, and the uncle of Education Secretary William J. Bennett. It was as bizarre a group of "independent thinkers" as anything filling the pages of the *New York Native.*

The nation's most distinguished scientists blasted the composition as downright irresponsible. The ACLU prepared to sue, on the grounds that the composition violated the Federal Advisory Committee Act, mandating that such groups be "fairly balanced." But the crush of reporters who gathered at the White House didn't challenge Reagan or his policy development adviser Gary L. Bauer to defend any of the ideologues who stood at their sides. Instead, they rushed the stage to confront a single appointee, Dr. Frank Lilly, the chairman of the department of genetics at the Albert Einstein Medical Center and an expert in immunology, making him the most suited for a position on the commission. The press had been alerted by operatives inside the administration who were offended by his inclusion. Lilly, it turned out, was gay.

Anticipating a media storm, Lilly had prepared a statement acknowledging his homosexuality and pledging "to forcefully represent the gay community as well as the biomedical community as a member of this Commission." He added a note about the historical significance of the moment. "As far as I know I am probably among the first openly gay persons to have been appointed to a significant position in any U.S. administration." A dozen reporters pummeled Lilly with questions, asking him to respond to critics who, like Senator Gordon Humphrey, alleged his very presence on the public stage endangered "impressionable youth."

IN NEW YORK that afternoon, Michael Callen discovered that the CDC had quietly compiled a list of people who had defied their death sentences by living with AIDS as long as he had. Including him, the CDC counted twenty-six living patients who were diagnosed in the first wave of the plague. That didn't include people like Richard Dworkin, who apparently had been HIV infected since the late 1970s, but was still so healthy he hadn't developed any AIDS complications.

To Callen, this seemed like more than a small wrinkle in the epidemiology. Those surviving with AIDS might be further evidence in support of Sonnabend's multifactorial model—perhaps it took additional exposures to other pathogens to produce AIDS, a thought thoroughly rejected by scientific consensus. But the tiny band of survivors was significant even if Sonnabend's theories were wrong. Thanks to improved testing technology, the HIV antibody tests were now reliably accurate. It was clear now that everyone with AIDS had contracted HIV, a key element in Koch's Postulates, suggesting a strong causal relationship between the virus and the disease. In that case, the existence of people like Callen who were able to resist HIV's crushing power suggested that they had something, or were doing something, that made the difference between death and life.

Determined to find out more, Callen undertook a major project researching the lives of "long-term survivors," in his phrase. He placed an ad in the *Newsline* seeking anybody alive at least three years post-infection. Dozens of people called—by far more than the CDC had first counted. Talking to them buoyed Callen's spirits. The first thing he learned was that people whose only opportunistic infection was Kaposi's sarcoma were living quite normal lives. Most were taking PCP prophylaxis; having a clued-in doctor made a huge difference. So did individual choices. Only one man he interviewed was taking AZT, a fact Callen, a vocal detractor of the drug, considered paramount. When it came to other health care strategies, they were all over the map. Several swore by macrobiotics, some credited love, while others believed they fared well by avoiding the stress of a relationship. All of them exhibited what Callen called "grit."

The Village Voice ran his interim findings in a surprising front-page piece titled "Not Everyone Dies of AIDS." It was a powerful revelation to the patient community as well as to public health officials at all levels. He wrote,

> Now that published reports prove we long-term survivors offi-cially exist, it's almost amusing to watch those who knew, or ought to have known, that we existed race to excuse their silence. City Health Commissioner Stephen Joseph said recently that the pro-portion of patients surviving five years was "greater than I would have intuitively expected it to be." What the hell does that mean? In New York City, fifteen percent of all people with AIDS have survived five or more years. Shouldn't the Health Commissioner have known that? And is it enough for him and others now to say "Ooops! Guess we were wrong about 100 percent mortality?" Is there no one to hold accountable for the lie and its harmful effect on PWAs?

3

Terminal Velocity

Brian Gougeon started counting the purple spots on his legs in the spring of 1987. He consulted a doctor in Chicago about it, just as he did a few weeks later when thrush reappeared on his tongue and tonsils. If the doctor was piecing together a diagnosis, either he wasn't telling him or Gougeon chose not to tell his friends.

It had been months since we last spoke. He had stopped returning my phone calls, saying long-distance bills were outside his budget. Instead he answered via ornately decorated postcards, devoid of personal news. Then, just after his birthday in July, Susan Wild, a mutual friend from college, called to say he'd been admitted to the Illinois Masonic hospital with pneumonia and toxoplasmosis. "He asked me to come help him get to the hospital," she said. "He wanted to take a shower first, but didn't have the strength—he's so thin, David, I had to help him. He was embarrassed and apologizing the whole time. When we got to the ER, they ran tests and diagnosed pneumonia. They put him in the AIDS ward."

I had been waiting for, and dreading, and hoping against, this moment since AIDS first surfaced, when we were invincible twenty-two-year-olds, chain-smoking and reading the *Times* with Ray-Bans balanced smugly on our noses. I wanted to race to see him, but Wild said Gougeon had requested privacy. The toxoplasmosis left him somewhat confused. But he did want my advice. She read from a list of his lab results, a portrait in acronyms and ratios. He was very sick. I answered what I could and promised to research the rest. Most pressing was whether he should take AZT, which the physician had ordered. Given his low CD4 count and the high doses of pentamidine, I said I thought it was a good idea.

"He's going to need money," I added. He could be hospitalized for months, and unless he had savings he risked losing his apartment. I offered to pass a hat among his friends in New York and she accepted reluctantly, not focused on anything so long term. I spent the next week planning a gathering of his New York friends. The work gave me a feeling of usefulness. That Saturday, three dozen people convened at my apartment with small sums of cash in envelopes, a little over $800 in total. Someone brought a bulky camcorder and we wished Brian a speedy recovery through the newest technology.

When the videocassette arrived in Chicago along with the emergency funds, Susan Wild called to say he wouldn't be watching it. "I guess he's blind," she said. "It happened so quickly. He was talking to his mother yesterday and said, 'Norma'—he calls her Norma—'Norma, would you turn on the light? We shouldn't have to sit here in the dark.' But of course, it was the middle of the day. Sunlight was streaming in. When they figured out what had happened, and that the blindness was irreversible, he was really scared. He said to Norma, 'I'm a blind artist. What good is a blind artist?' And she said to him, 'Sculpture, honey. You could be a great sculptor.' By the time I talked to him, he had already begun to adjust a little, and I just cried."

His jar of AZT, delayed by shortages and high demand, arrived almost two weeks later. By then he was in no condition to take it, having slipped into a coma from which he never returned. He was twenty-eight when he died.

That call from Wild was the most devastating of my life. I'd spent six years gathering esoteric information, investigating every medical lead, ingratiating myself to scientists, doctors, activists, and patients. None of it made a bit of difference. Nurses gave Wild the chance to bequeath his unused AZT to a recipient of her choosing, but she suggested they just give it to the next person in need.

The Roman Catholic service was private. Norma Gougeon laid her second-youngest son to rest at the Holy Cross Cemetery in Alpena, Michigan, with six of his brothers as pallbearers. She kept the cause of death a secret from her priest and the local paper, attuned to the possible consequences. A memorial gathering for his friends in Chicago would take place in a few weeks.

I was back at ACT UP a Monday or two later. Like a wedding chapel or a movie theater, it was a place where you could cry without causing alarm. A man sitting to my left silently rested a hand on my rocking shoulder for a few moments. I was grateful for the stranger's gesture.

"Quiet, please!" said the moderator, calling from the front of the room. He wore a sleeveless T-shirt showing well-toned arms and stood with hands on hips. The room was restless, defying his admonishments. "Quiet! Now, we have Iris Long."

I looked up to see an awkward middle-aged woman standing shyly before the gathering, a wad of papers in her trembling hands and her mouth hanging open. Iris Long was a most unexpected arrival in the movement. With her suburban hair bob, she cut a figure that might have been perfectly ordinary on the subway, but not in this room, packed with fashion-conscious men and women. She favored a garishly bright-colored wardrobe belted through her soft middle with an overfull fanny pack. She wore sensible shoes and sun visors, and her eyeglasses, owlish panels rimmed in gold, were tinted a muddy brown. Everything about her pointed to the fact that she was a working-class, middle-aged heterosexual woman—a platypus among the swans. She had been attending since the first meeting, often rising to speak, in her thick outer-borough accent, when the agenda reached "Lifesaving." Her lack of erudition was distracting; she was all *ums* and stutters, with an enervating habit of introducing sentences but neglecting to provide their middles and ends. What words were intelligible tended to be arranged into pure scientific gibberish, or so it seemed.

It took weeks to discern her purpose. Iris Long, we learned, was a scientist. She had taken the long route to her degrees, earning a BS and MS in night school and returning years later for a PhD in pharmaceutical chemistry. That launched her into an unspectacular career. Her chosen specialty was nucleoside analogues—the esoteric study of altered sugar molecules trained to lure diseased cells away from healthy ones— but she had so far failed at finding work in the field. For many years, she toiled in a basement lab at Long Island Jewish Hospital studying phosphonates—linked to cholesterol, not cancers, which were her passion. She hated the work, hated her boss, and feared for her health in a laboratory where the exhaust fan was faulty. Reaching the end of her patience, she called in the Occupational Safety and Health Administration, which resulted in her termination. Though she had walked her résumé to every hospital and lab in the city, she never got another job offer. It was a soul-crushing end to her dreams.

Money was not an issue—her husband, Mike, had a good job at ITT. What she craved was to involve herself in something useful, some way to make a meaningful contribution. She was naturally curious about AIDS. But it didn't attract her serious attention until the science journals began reporting on AZT. She knew something about AZT. It was a nucleoside analogue, square in her wheelhouse. She called GMHC, because she remembered the name from the papers, and attended the very next volunteer training session at their expensive new headquarters in Chelsea. Though it was just under ten miles from her home in Jackson Heights in Queens, she had entered a world she had never imagined. A strict Lutheran background had kept her naïve about the sexual revolution. Before walking through the door she never had knowingly laid eyes on a homosexual. She told her husband that night how surprisingly normal they appeared, adding, "They're very interesting, actually."

At GMHC she was put to work in the file room, assigned to organize clippings into folders, something a high school dropout could have accomplished. When she appealed for something more challenging, she was transferred to the hotline, which, given her verbal limitations and unfamiliarity with the community, was even further from her expertise. But it put her in a place to hear about the excitement following Larry Kramer's incendiary speech. Knowing nothing about his fraught history, she sat among the three hundred who crammed into that first ACT UP meeting at Bailey House. The idea that the medical problem was also a political problem was new to her, but it made immediate sense. Having been shut out of the rarified world of research, she knew that a cold politics governed Hippocrates' world. These were outsiders with whom she identified.

The chore she assigned herself was to learn about drug trials in the city, evaluate the experimental compounds involved, and report back to the members. Unfortunately, her appearances in the front of the room tended to trigger a stampede for the door. A defiant din of chatter rose up against her anytime she spoke. This Monday was no different. She pressed onward valiantly, reporting about developments in clinical trials around the city. Vito Russo, the veteran activist, grew incensed. Jumping to be at her side, he turned angrily toward the energetic room.

"Shut up and listen!" he shouted. "Listen! I don't think any of you paid Iris Long the respect you should. There is no one doing any work in ACT UP that has a greater chance of doing real good for people with AIDS."

As the room settled down and people returned to their seats, he continued: "Nobody, if they succeeded, could help any more than Iris would if we could successfully monitor those clinical trials. Because in fact, we'd be monitoring how drugs go from the test tube to people's mouths, and whether those drugs were safe and effective."

While he was speaking, a wiry and intense man with an unruly black ponytail burst into the meeting and slid into a seat. Jim Eigo, a writer of experimental plays and literary fiction, was expecting to attend a forum to discuss gay rights and the Supreme Court. It took him some time to realize he was in the wrong room; the fascinating dynamics kept him there.

Until hearing Russo's speech, the idea that ordinary individuals could make headway against the deaths never occurred to Eigo. The role AIDS had given him was as a GMHC volunteer, helping the dying with financial planning. A few months earlier, he had tested negative himself, and expected to stay that way.

Eigo settled in for the show. The meeting cranked on for three remarkable hours, punctuated by thunderous applause, gallows humor, and, in one instance, a brutal shouting match on a topic of obscure significance. When Marty Robinson, another veteran of gay rights battles, proposed a particular demonstration, which he called a "zap," using the argot of long-ago radicalism, Vito Russo sharply challenged his strategy and goals from the sidelines. The vitriol these two middle-aged men slung at one another was jagged and outsized; their jousting palpably put the younger people on edge. Realizing this made both Robinson and Russo smile. "Don't worry," Russo explained to the room, "we've been doing this since we shared a jail cell in the early seventies."

When the meeting finally adjourned, Eigo presented himself to Iris Long. If she was the *deus ex machina* of the epidemic, as Russo seemed to say, then she needed a better speechwriter, and that job was more suited to his skills than his GMHC volunteer work.

"I want to find out more," he told her. "I want to help."

She glanced at him from a set of pages she was absent-mindedly shuffling. "I'm starting a study group," she responded. "Come Monday before the meeting."

THE PRESIDENTIAL COMMISSION on the HIV Epidemic scheduled its first public hearing for September 9, 1987, at the National Press Club in Washington. For ACT UP, this was a call to action. The group had spent the summer staging protests in New York over the panel's composition. Several Sundays in a row in July and August, ACT UP members distributed leaflets to Catholics as they entered St. Patrick's Cathedral, demanding that Cardinal O'Connor resign from the commission. Simultaneously, scores of activists staged what they called a "sustained protest" inside the cathedral. Each Sunday at precisely 10:10 a.m. during High Mass, when the cardinal began his homily, they rose and stood in silent objection. Calling the gesture menacing and frightening to worshippers, lawyers for the church won an injunction against standing, then called in police to make arrests the following week when the demonstrators moved to the sidewalk and knelt in prayer.

O'Connor was just one of their targets. They mounted an informational picket line outside the Midtown offices of *The Saturday Evening Post,* whose editor and publisher was Cory SerVass. She had a medical degree, but Reagan's main explanation for naming her to the commission was that she was a close friend of his wife's. Her experience in the epidemic was recent and contentious: when she wasn't needed at the magazine, she traveled the country in what she called her "AIDS Mobile," offering HIV testing and delivering the results by mail, bypassing the post-testing counseling that the American Medical Association and the Centers for Disease Control considered key in order to minimize suicides and other desperate acts. For two hours, protesters questioned her fitness to serve on the commission and followed a chant script that captured the media's attention with its ability to narrow complex issues through humor:

> *Cory SerVaas*
> *Makes us nervous*
> *With her mobile*
> *Testing service*

For the September hearings, the group chartered two buses to depart at 6:30 a.m. from the community center, and had no trouble getting a hundred people to sign up for a long day of travel and protest, including ACT UP members Michael Nesline, Avram Finkelstein, and Rebecca Cole, a twenty-nine-year-old frustrated actress who staffed the National AIDS Hotline. The Lavender Hill Mobsters Michael Petrelis, Bill Bahlman, and Marty Robinson enlisted, and even Larry Kramer planned to attend, a momentary break from his sabbatical. Bradley Ball, the group's unofficial secretary, sent word to D.C.-based AIDS organizations and to the gay paper there, the *Washington Blade,* seeking an outpouring of local support and promises of bodies at the demonstration. Nearly one hundred extra signs were made in anticipation.

None of this was known to commission members, who began arriving in Washington a day early, on September 8. It was the first time they were together since their chaotic appointment ceremony—a relaxed three-month interval during which another 2,281 Americans had died.

The chairman, Dr. Mayberry, organized a private reception for the commissioners, as much to outline the tasks ahead as to help build a spirit of cohesion before opening the doors to outsiders. What happened over supper took him by surprise. A number of appointees bitterly complained about his disorganization and dereliction, pointing out that Mayberry had yet to hire allotted staff for their headquarters. And he had barely been in touch with them. They heard of the hearing's agenda through media accounts. Subsequent calls to the commission's office were not returned.

A folksy man whose soft-spoken voice still carried hints of the Virginia Dells, Mayberry was uncharacteristically defensive. While it was true that his budget called for a staff of six, the entire war chest for their campaign against a virus that by now had infected as many as 1.5 million Americans by the CDC's estimate was just $950,000. By sorry comparison, the budget Reagan gave to a presidential commission just a year earlier for their work investigating the *Challenger* space shuttle disaster—in which seven crew members died—topped $3 million, exclusive of salaries for a staff of forty-nine.

"We are really worried that we are behind the eight-ball," said Admiral James Watkins, formerly a member of the Joint Chiefs and a veteran of such appointments. Even on a starvation budget, Watkins expected briefing books and background materials, both of which were lacking. "Where is the template that has been laid out? What is our final objective on the twenty-fourth of June to give to the president? How well has it been constructed? What is the hearing sequence that is going to lead us to the final set of objectives? How have we tried to lay this out?"

Staggered, Mayberry admitted that he had taken the job only after being assured that it would require his attentions merely two days a month.

"Gene," the admiral replied tensely, "I think this is one of the most unprofessional sessions that I have ever attended in my twenty years in Washington."

The antagonism still hung in the air the next morning when the commissioners approached the Press Club to find a wall of demonstrators, some in Mickey Mouse ears, handing out literature denouncing "this administration's blatant disregard for human life" and impugning the intentions of the members. "History will recall: Reagan did nothing at all!" the activists screamed.

Inside, when the day's session got under way, it became clear that still more activists had commandeered the gallery seats, jeering and heckling after the more outlandish comments from the panelists, and dominating the list of speakers during the brief public comment section. "Quite frankly, we think many of you would as soon see us dead," Kramer told the commissioners to wild applause from his comrades. "But sometimes the challenge makes the man or woman. There are many instances in history where the most unlikely heroes have emerged and triumphed over their perceived images. We pray this will be one of those rare and precious and God-inspired occasions." He added, "Right now we don't expect you to accomplish much or put aside your personal prejudices."

When Petrelis took his turn, dressed to impress in a crisp sport jacket and tight ponytail, he issued a stinging rebuke of his own, disregarding the time limit Mayberry had imposed. Petrelis touched on everything from the committee's medical ignorance and homophobia to his own brief life expectancy.

Mayberry beseeched the AIDS organizations—which he called "interest groups," to a fresh uproar—to allow the presidential appointees a chance to prove themselves. "I can assure you that the commission is devoted to bring to bear the very best," he told them pleadingly, "to make recommendations to the president and to the secretary of health and human services. I can tell you that this charge and this mandate comes from a concerned president for this problem and the commission intends to do its very best to try to serve the president, the secretary of health and human services, and society insofar as we are humanly able to do."

Settling into their seats for the long bus ride home, the protesters congratulated themselves for having gotten across their anger and desperation. News of their activist presence would lead the evening broadcasts. But the tenor of the coverage went against them, led forcibly by the HHS secretary who replaced Margaret Heckler, a former governor of Indiana named Otis R. Bowen. "To criticize this effort is counterproductive and mean-spirited," he said, "and tends to tarnish what is a solid record of accomplishment in modern medical science and health policy." Mayberry also pleaded with America to look beyond the panelists' significant limitations. "We believe we have the capacity to help or we wouldn't be here," he said.

In the area of message management, ACT UP had to acknowledge its own failure. But what most clouded their appraisal of the day was that fewer than ten Washingtonians stood with ACT UP on the sidewalk; ninety surplus posters sat unused in a pile on the pavement. Bradley Ball used the ride home to compose an angry letter to Washington's gay community. "We need to deliver an equally pointed and powerful response that this policy of benign neglect is not acceptable," he pleaded. "Otis Bowen has no compassion for the sickness and the death and the hate and the fear and the rage and the frustration that have become deep and daily factors in our lives during the last seven years. We must protest this administration's non-effort. We must make them listen to us. And we must do this together."

A WEEK LATER, on a crisp and still September morning in Chicago, a beautiful light slanted through the leaded windows of the Nazareth United Church of Christ, just blocks from where Brian Gougeon had lived with Doug Gould, his nearly continuous partner since college. I arrived early, slipping into the pew beside Katrina Van Valkenburgh, my college girlfriend, midway between the entrance and the altar. Gould sat directly in front of us, alone at first, appearing to be stunned. He wore a speckled wool jacket and a whimsical bolo tie—a Gougeon creation. His black hair, glossed tight over his temples, framed puffy and unfocused eyes.

The public memorial service for Brian Gougeon was surprisingly religious, with a Protestant prayer of grief as its centerpiece.

CONGREGATION: I am weary with moaning and every night I flood my bed with tears, I drench my couch with weeping.
PASTOR: Fear not, for God has redeemed you! God has called you by name, and called you God's own.

After a reading of scripture, friends were invited to share anecdotes while a slideshow of Brian's abbreviated body of work, his world of dreamy, faraway places, flashed on a large screen. But we soon turned back to hymns and psalms and, finally, "Amazing Grace," a stabbing reminder of the young man in Grand Rapids who had banned the song at his own pending funeral. I stood in stubborn silence, more opposed than ever to the disavowal it symbolized.

That night Brian's close friends gathered in an apartment in Ukrainian Village. Away from the trappings of pastors and relatives, Doug had gotten very drunk. Never much for talking, he was now muzzled as much by grief as by liquor, bumping his way to the kitchen for refill after refill. I learned from others that Brian had broken up with him a few months previously—"probably the first sign of his brain infection," someone surmised. Heartsick, Doug had tried suicide. He checked himself into a hotel room with a plan involving pills, and when he survived the night he returned to his parents' home in rural Colorado, morose and aimless. Having raced to Chicago too late to bid Brian farewell in person added considerably to his burden.

After one especially unbalanced passage through the living room caused worried glances, I followed him into the kitchen to find him wrestling with a bottle of vodka. Grateful for my help, he didn't notice that I filled his glass with tonic water instead.

"I didn't talk to Norma, I couldn't," he said, meaning Brian's mother. His tongue was thick and slurry. "She would hate me, blame me."

Having met Norma Gougeon only briefly, I didn't feel competent to disagree with him. I handed him his glass. "She would want to know what he meant to you," I suggested.

"I guess I got it too. I told Brian I didn't care."

"You've taken the test?"

He shook his head. "But this," he said, patting the back of his head. I reached over and put my palm against his Cherokee mane of thick, black hair and encountered what appeared to be a very large and moist scab. It encased most of his scalp. When I withdrew my hand and saw that it was red with blood, my heart pounded. I lurched for the kitchen sink and repeatedly splashed myself with antibacterial soap, wringing my hands like Macbeth's widow and scrutinizing my flesh for cuts and abrasions, weaknesses the virus might exploit.

"Doug, what is that? You're *bleeding*."

He shrugged. The liquor had put a childish look on his face, sadness crossed with amazement. I noticed for the first time that the collar of his shirt was pink from his wound.

"Do you have a doctor?" I asked. He didn't answer. "You need a *good* doctor, someone who understands AIDS. They know how to prevent the infections now. People are *living* with this. They can prevent death." Tears filled his eyes, but he still said nothing.

"You have to come with me to New York," I spontaneously added. "They've got way more experience there. I'll get you to the right people. Don't worry about money, I have a good job. I have room in my apartment. You can't stay in Colorado."

The invitation surprised me as much as it did him. But with Brian's death, I felt a need to stop rummaging through the epidemic as a journalist, with the illusion of agency. I had been sitting on the sidelines for long enough.

"Let me take care of you," I heard myself say.

Doug rocked unsteadily on his heels, then he kissed me drunkenly, which I took as his acceptance, though it may well have been an accident. I mailed him a ticket, and a week later I met his flight at JFK and escorted him to the East Village, where we would figure out how to fight his illness together. Along the way, we had to learn what role we would play in one another's lives. I wasn't surprised when our arrangement turned into an awkward romance. I felt the purest kind of love for him and what he had represented: our hopeful youth, our place in the world, life itself. I clung to him and he allowed it—he needed it maybe as much as I did.

Doug was stunned by the scene in New York. Below Fourteenth Street, KS lesions were as common as bug welts in the Central American jungle. There was now a permanent line of wheelchairs outside the Village Nursing Home, where bony young men napped in the sun. The gay bars, which had been the teeming hub of gay society during his last visit, were now lifeless and ghostly places.

As soon as he had unpacked, I made an appointment for him to see Dr. Waitkevicz. Then I got Michael Callen on the phone, the first time I spoke to him outside of my role as a reporter. He listened patiently to my conundrum, then tutored me in the specifics of prophylaxis and the practical use of the PWA Health Group's underground pharmacy. There now were twenty-four known opportunistic infections responsible for 90 percent of all AIDS deaths, many of which could be prevented.

"It's every gay man for himself," he told me. "It's not going to be easy—they want to see us all dead, and I'm not exaggerating." When he said this, he gave a disturbing little chuckle. By late 1987, you didn't have to be Chuck Ortleb at the *Native* to reach that conclusion.

On a bright fall day, Doug and I made our way over to the PWA Health Group offices. The group had grown significantly since it started making AL721. It occupied a large loft in an old industrial building in Chelsea, tucked behind the verdant sidewalk displays of the Flower District merchants. A banged-up elevator, operated by a bent old man, took us to the fourth floor. The PWA Health Group, with its long countertop and dusty air, was reminiscent of an old apothecary. A small staff scurried purposefully beneath a hand-lettered sign listing the available offerings. The group's stated mission was to seek out and make available "what-the-hell drugs," that is, compounds with some suggestion of efficacy and no evidence of causing harm. By far the most popular of these was dextran sulfate, a nontoxic blood thinner believed to slow the progression of disease. Considered an over-the-counter elixir in Japan, it lacked FDA approval in the States, so the group's volunteers flew to Tokyo once a month to fill suitcases with the stuff. When the FDA threatened a crackdown on unlawful importation, the group's director,

Derek Hodel, held a withering press conference vowing a protracted battle.

"In the absence of adequate health care, we have learned to become our own clinicians, researchers, lobbyists, drug smugglers, pharmacists; we have our own libraries, newspapers, drug stores, and laboratories," he said. "Today, we fight business with business."

Half a dozen people were ahead of us in line. When we reached the counter, a female clerk with tightly shaved hair listened to Doug's questions about preventative drugs. Nothing in the underground armamentarium could do what the mainstream drugs could, she explained. As an example, she described how doctors were using DHPG to prevent the blindness caused by cytomegalovirus retinitis. It was not FDA approved, so patients had to navigate the drugmaker's complex Compassionate Use program to gain access. And it was so hard on the veins that a special port, called a Hickman catheter, had to be surgically implanted near the heart. To date, only 2,500 PWAs had taken it and the rest were left without options. An epidemic of blindness had become a major problem.

The same was true for PCP prevention. Low-dose Bactrim was cheap and effective, for those who could tolerate it. For those who couldn't, many doctors had begun experimenting with dapsone, which had performed so well in Dr. Metroka's small study. In addition, some proposed using a nebulizer to deliver pentamidine—the same drug taken intravenously to treat PCP—directly into the lungs. A pilot study involving fifteen patients in San Francisco had shown that aerosolized pentamidine was "equal or better than" Bactrim. The promising results appeared in *The Lancet*, touching off a craze for aerosolized pentamidine in San Francisco and New York. The key to success was getting the misted drug down to the smallest possible particle size for distribution deep into the lung. Some doctors built elaborate nebulizing booths in their offices; others recommended home units marketed for treating other lung disorders, especially an ultrasonic version from West Germany and one from a Colorado manufacturer. The community showed keen interest in this approach, in large part because it was not a systemic treatment. The mist sat inside the lungs doing its defensive work without entering the bloodstream, leading to fewer side effects beyond coughing and wheezing at the time of administration.

But to know conclusively how well inhaled pentamidine worked would require a much larger study. Eventually, Fauci's people at NIAID began speaking to Lymphomed, the small pharmaceutical outfit that now controlled the exclusive pentamidine license, about putting the drug into large-scale trials. The company was keen, quickly preparing a trial protocol—and, in anticipation of positive findings, raising the wholesale price of the drug from $25 to $99 per vial. That's as far as things went. NIAID never advanced the trial. Under withering questioning by Congressman Ted Weiss months later, Fauci—who still refused to issue PCP prevention guidelines—blamed a lack of resources, admitting he "just didn't have the staff to take someone and say, 'The only thing you're going to do for the next X number of months is aerosolized pentamidine.'"

In frustration, a group of San Francisco AIDS doctors took matters into their own hands, enrolling patients in an eighteen-month-long community-based trial in anticipation of seeking FDA approval independently. No new drug or treatment had ever been evaluated in this way.

Callen and Sonnabend were impressed with the philosophy of the West Coast doctors. Because frontline AIDS practitioners had access to a vast population of potential trial subjects, they could enroll a study in a fraction of the time it took academic centers, and at a fraction of the cost. With the help of Mayor Dianne Feinstein, they accomplished this in San Francisco by uniting the city's biggest institutions into an ad hoc research network they called the County Community Consortium. With the consortium, they would undertake what frontline doctors considered high-priority research initiatives, bypassing Fauci.

Sonnabend and Callen immediately took steps to replicate the effort in New York, though with no help from city hall. Rather than creating a consortium of hospitals, the two envisioned a network of individual physicians and their patients under the auspices of the PWA Health Group. They called their network the Community Research Initiative, and empowered it with an impressive scientific advisory committee, a research department, nurses, and a staff of skilled administrators. They even formed an institutional review board to look after the well-being of the patients, modeled after the best academic centers, only in this case all board members would be people with AIDS themselves, a solid fail-safe against placebo trials or policies requiring anyone to discontinue prophylaxis.

In little time, the CRI recruited doctors representing two thousand AIDS patients eager to join studies—at a time when Fauci's research network, called the national AIDS Clinical Trials Group, had been able to enroll just a few hundred. Aerosolized pentamidine would be their first undertaking. They solicited a $400,000 grant from Lymphomed, and had everything in line to begin enrollment by the first snowfall. News of these desperate efforts reached editors at *The New England Journal of Medicine,* which endorsed their call for an era of PCP prevention. This increased the pressure on Fauci to issue the guidelines that Callen had begged him for. But Fauci still refused, instead setting up a committee to consider recommendations. He justified his inaction by reminding anyone who asked that it was the responsibility of individual physicians to keep up with the journals. He was confident that AIDS patients themselves would find the information about prophylaxis through their own means. Were he an AIDS patient, nobody could keep him from protections, he said. "I would go for what is available on the street for me."

IT WAS NOT EASY to adjust to Doug Gould's presence in the apartment. With no job to distract him and ladened with grief, he tended to wallow in daytime television, bales of marijuana, and frequent alcohol binges. In contrast to the garrulous and giggly young man I had known in college, he pushed people away, including those with whom he had been very close. He did not like engaging with any of my friends, even asking me not to bring them by the apartment. "I don't want people crying later," he said. "I don't want that responsibility." If not for his visits to the doctor and the frequent trips to a stairwell in the projects on Avenue D to buy his marijuana, he might never have budged from in front of the television.

He did keep in contact with two or three Chicago friends by telephone—gossip from the theater community there was his only joy. I was grateful, though not at all convinced, to overhear him describe his life with me as happy. We quarreled over things simple and complex. But as the weeks added up a sweetness crept into our relationship. Our sexual life was sparing and circumspect, but that was the case for everyone we knew. In some ways, I was less likely to contract AIDS from a lover I assumed was positive; I never felt tempted to drop my guard.

But there was the unnerving matter of the constant flow of blood from his scalp, emanating, we learned, from a virulent staph infection. Dr. Waitkevicz put him on pills and ointments, but he continued to ooze even after many weeks.

Soon his HIV test came back positive, to no one's surprise. Waitkevicz gave him a letter describing the full array of treatment she might one day prescribe for him, most of it available only on the underground market, but lucky for him his CD4 count was high, nearly five hundred, and he had none of the major opportunistic infections that would have earned him a diagnosis of full-blown AIDS. So far, AIDS medicine would not be needed. As things went, this was good news.

I had taken a job at *The New York Observer*, a new city broadsheet, covering AIDS, health, and politics. The pay was good enough to cover Doug's living costs and mine, but my health insurance could not cover him. It was imperative that he find work before a traceable diagnosis linked him to AIDS and gave him a "preexisting condition" excluded from coverage. The only thing worse than an AIDS diagnosis was the prospect of relying on public assistance. To cope with the thousands of uninsured patients, the city had opened the Division of AIDS Services to mete out welfare entitlements like Medicaid and modest disability allowances through Social Security. But from its inception the small office was dysfunctional and capricious and the staff was deliberately indifferent, requiring endless waits and repeated letters of requalification. Dr. Waitkevicz made a point of not writing Doug's anonymous HIV test results into his file, so he was still a pristine candidate for coverage.

Doug did not have a plan for employment. He had no interest in returning to the stage, nor of finding work on the technical crews. He said he would not do anything he had done before. But that wasn't indicative of a desire to broaden his horizons, just the opposite. After reading through *What Color Is Your Parachute?*, the job hunter's manual, he set his new sites low, ultimately taking a job alphabetizing records for a union pension fund. The pay was poor but the health benefits were a relief, and it gave me hope that he would reinvest in life.

NO ONE EXPECTED anything meaningful from the Presidential AIDS Commission, but few could have predicted the flamboyant mess it became. A full-blown coup brewed inside the ranks, with numerous commissioners militating for Mayberry's ouster. "I like the guy and he's sincere," Dr. Frank Lilly, the gay commissioner, told a reporter, "but he has had that job for four months and we are still exactly nowhere." Cardinal O'Connor offered the reasonable suggestion that he and several others on the panel should be replaced by "competent" experts. Public opinion was beginning to bend against their obvious incompetence, exemplified by an editorial cartoon in *New York Newsday* showing the commission spending its tiny budget on condolence cards.

On October 6, Mayberry went to his handler on Reagan's staff and demanded the power to clean house. Told he had no say over the commission's composition, he resigned the following day.

Reagan then offered the chairmanship to Admiral James Watkins, the blunt-talking commissioner with the temperament of George S. Patton and the tact of J. Edgar Hoover. Watkins, a staunch Republican and a personal friend of O'Connor's, didn't have the slightest interest in the job. He told the president, "I'm a sailor and a submariner, and I know nothing about medicine." But he capitulated when Reagan inexplicably replied, "You're exactly who we're looking for."

Watkins inherited an office staff that still consisted of just two secretaries. Ringing phones went unanswered. Unopened mail was piled in stacks several feet high. Applying his military discipline to the challenge, he quickly appointed an executive director, hired support staff and experts, and set up a hearings schedule. In quick succession the commission visited hospitals and research laboratories in New York, San Francisco, and South Florida, and for eleven packed days that winter took testimony from an ambitious lineup of bona fide experts.

Every time and anywhere the commission met, Bill Bahlman sat in the gallery, a lone activist inside the chambers. Tall and fastidiously dressed, with a SILENCE=DEATH badge fixed to his jacket and a stack of AIDS literature under his arm, he introduced himself to the commissioners and their staff, representing himself as not just an activist but also as an expert, someone to answer their questions on any aspect of the epidemic, whether scientific, cultural, or structural. As testimony was being given, he would rifle through his tower of background literature, plucking out scientific studies or ACT UP primers to circulate among the panelists to support or discredit the people giving testimony.

During recesses, he made an effort to speak to each commission member individually, impressing upon them, in his soft and patient tones, exactly what the community expected of them, and why. Most panel members had never met anyone like him—he defied the stereotypes of gay protesters put forth on television.

He waged his campaign on his own time, on a volunteer basis, but not a selfless one. A nasty case of shingles earlier in the year had convinced his doctor that Bahlman likely was immune compromised himself. To his relief, the test came back negative. But his closest friends and the people he most admired were not so lucky. Vito Russo, whom he followed into GLAAD, had AIDS. So did Marty Robinson and Henry Yeager, who led him into the Lavender Hill Mob and then ACT UP. The way Bahlman saw it, AIDS was testing the lesbian and gay community as a people, just as Francisco Franco had tested the Spanish.

· · ·

PETER STALEY had been living a fitful and exigent double life for most of the year, serving up growing profits to his Wall Street managers while pumping his financial knowledge into ACT UP, where he was secretly attending committee meetings several nights a week. He helped organize ACT UP's first ambitious fund-raising affair, which took place at the Saint, an East Village disco, and provided the largest cash influx yet, $8,000. He spent that night behind the merchandise table hawking SILENCE=DEATH T-shirts and buttons. For the first time since learning his HIV-positive status, he felt attractive and desirable. As the evening progressed, he found himself flirting seriously with Michael Nesline, his committee chairman, a decade older and HIV negative. They began dating thereafter. With the help of Nesline and weekly sessions with his therapist, Staley continued to manage the awkward balancing act of living in the closet with a fatal disease.

His test results showed no deterioration, so he took on more and more responsibilities, at work and at ACT UP. To the relief of Nesline, Staley assumed the chairmanship of the fund-raising committee and instituted an ambitious expansion of the group's war chest, to match the group's widening scope. He wanted no initiative to be stymied for lack of money. He instituted a large-scale merchandizing plan, promoting the iconic T-shirts and buttons in gay papers and magazines around the country. He convinced local club owners to give ACT UP the gate from several nights a month, helped program charity dance performances, and sought out a coterie of major donors. But it was still not enough. He wanted the group to launch a direct mail campaign, an expensive and controversial gamble for any small organization with no paid staff, much less one known for intentionally and flagrantly breaking the law. ACT UP wasn't even incorporated as a legal nonprofit.

He first presented the idea to Larry Kramer, who was enthusiastic; he personally agreed to pay the mailing's printing costs, $3,500. With Kramer on his side, Staley undertook an intense internal lobbying effort, pitching the idea to each of ACT UP's committees, subcommittees, and affinity groups, encountering varying degrees of resistance. The ragtag group Iris Long formed was as baffled by the language of money as Staley was by their dense scientific presentations. Jim Eigo gave him a reductive sobriquet, "Callow Young Stockbroker," like a character in a Bertolt Brecht play. Nonetheless, he proved to be an effective diplomat—a skill that might have fueled the political career he once dreamed of—and won them over handily.

With the groundwork laid, Staley brought his proposal to the

Monday-night meeting for debate by the general membership. The firm he planned to hire was the only one of its kind in the country, specializing in building a vast database of gay and lesbian consumers. Sean Strub, a co-owner, would charge $26,000, much of it for postage and printing, which he agreed, in a concession to Staley, to collect from the proceeds stream. The rank and file found the cost shocking. The more radical members were unwilling to feed a profit-making endeavor with money raised for AIDS activism. But before the night was over, Staley eked out a victory. More than fifty thousand mailing pieces were readied.

Then Kramer reemerged the following Monday. Angry that the group was sending Bill Bahlman to monitor each of the Presidential AIDS Commission hearings (paying for "first-class accommodations," he was sure), he withdrew his seed money and quit ACT UP again. Staley managed to replace Kramer's donation, and a follow-up went on to gross $300,000, enabling an impressive schedule of street manifestations. It was unlikely that any direct action grassroots movement ever enjoyed such ready finances.

Staley's magic touch prevailed at work as well, where his continued successes at the short-shorts brought him to the attention of a competing firm called CRT Government Securities. After a weeks-long courtship, including offers of a VP title and a huge base salary, he made the jump. Unfortunately, he foundered in his new job, and only weeks into it came Black Monday, one of the worst market crashes in history. The pressure took a steep toll. His night sweats intensified. The skin on his face became blotchy and flaky. His CD4 count went from 515 to 364, squarely in the danger zone. In November 1987, Dr. William convinced him it was time for AZT, 1,200 milligrams daily. Unfortunately, Staley was among the 50 percent of patients who could not tolerate it even for short periods of time. His AZT anemia was so severe that he nodded out at the trading desk. He stopped taking the medication. His CD4s plunged even further, putting him face-to-face with his own mortality.

He became more careful with his time, unwilling to allow a single day to slip past unproductively. His social circle narrowed, to the dismay of old friends. Tracey Tanenbaum knew he was fighting for his life, and wanted to support him in any way she could. But they quarreled about AIDS politics and activism and eventually fell out of touch. When not on the trading floor, Staley now passed his time with Nesline and other new friends from the fund-raising committee, plotting new campaigns.

• • •

THE DEMANDS of activism never eased. In the fall, ACT UP planned to descend on Washington, D.C., for the second national march for lesbian and gay rights. It seemed like everybody in New York was making plans to attend. Early on the morning of October 10, a bright and cold Saturday, Doug and I rode one of the ACT UP buses to D.C. It was amazing to see so many gay people in one place, colonizing the coffee shops, parks, and sidewalks and making the capital into a vast and colorful gay city. Protesters of all persuasions mingled with student groups and religious contingents standing on street corners singing songs. Women in tuxedoes applauded clusters of men disguised to parody Jesse Helms, Dan Quayle, and William Dannemeyer, "the leading homophobes in Congress." Hundreds of veterans in their uniforms banded together in support of gays in the military, while down the block was another group cheekily promoting "Gays in the Millinery" in their pillboxes, toques, and large-brimmed Gainsboroughs trimmed with organdy and tulle. We wandered through the Dupont Circle area like excited tourists taking in a show.

When we reached Constitution Avenue, a large crowd was forming in the middle of the street, forcing traffic to a standstill. There on a slight knoll near the IRS building, a purely symbolic "mass wedding ceremony" was taking place. Although the possibility of marriage was the furthest thing from our imagination, we stopped to listen as the officiant spoke about a fantasized future.

"I'm going to ask you to take a breath, totally release the past and take one step forward into that future and your place in the world," she said. The crowd surged ahead. The scene had an unexpected power; Doug took my hand, and we stepped forward too. "And so it is. You are together as friends, as lovers, as life mates, as partners."

A collective whoop rose up from the impromptu wedding party. To our left, a dark-haired man in his early thirties kissed his partner, then let out a shout. "We're married!"

Doug was characteristically less exultant, but in his own way moved. "We're Moonies," he joked before giving me a kiss too.

As police arrived and began making arrests to clear the avenue, we retreated hastily, heading back toward Dupont Circle, where the reverie continued into the night.

The next morning, about thirty thousand of us made our way through pockets of fog to the Ellipse, that section of the National Mall just south of the White House fence. From blocks away we could hear the dull cadence of a lone female voice reciting the names of the men and women whose elegies were stitched into a huge cloth tribute called the AIDS Memorial Quilt, making its debut appearance. Begun just months earlier in San Francisco, it became the immediate fulcrum of the nation's collective grief. Already it contained 1,900 panels and weighed three and a half tons.

We stood on the edge of the massive field listening to muffled sobs around us as a platoon of pallbearers, dressed uniformly in white, unfolded great colorful panels and slowly lifted them into their place on the grid. There, beneath the doleful roll call of names, they silently tied the panels together with ribbons. *Douglas Lowery. Gary Barnhill. Neal Yager. PaulSteven Quesada.* The speaker paused after each name, and you could sometimes hear combustions of grief from their loved ones roll across the meadow. *Bill Cathcart. Paul Castro. Félix Velarde-Muños. Bobbi Campbell.* The effect was overwhelming, combining the community's losses for the first time into a massive map of sorrow, an exponential tragedy. The cadences consumed the morning hours. *Dennis Oglesby. Roy Esquibel. Dick Gamble. José Ramírez.* The readers often choked on tears, for it was also personal to them. *My lover and best friend, Scooby Bowman. My brother Jack Alvez.* There were panels from around the world, each one carefully unfolded and laid down into the tapestry of the plague. *Rick Claflin. John Hall. Brian Gougeon.*

We scarcely believed our ears. Brian had only been dead a few months. We didn't know someone had made a panel for him. Yet his name had raced toward us from the enormous speakers, echoing throughout the Ellipse. *Brian Gougeon.* His death was an American loss. The sobs were ours.

When the whole quilt was in place and people were allowed to walk through the temporary graveyard by way of fabric pathways, we searched for his quadrant, picking our way square after square as through a body-strewn battlefield. We passed familiar names—*Tom Waddell,* founder of the Gay Games; *Willi Smith,* the great young fashion designer; *Liberace,* whose panel was fashioned from rhinestones and lamé. We passed by names of people who had accomplished too little in their short lives, whose squares were hung with words of farewell, or yards of sequins, or teddy bears. Some were primitive expressions, with names laid out in spray paint and snapshots stapled into place, but many were marvels of hand-stitched artistry. The overall impact was devastating.

It took us nearly an hour, but we finally found Brian's memorial square, a gorgeous three-dimensional panel with pyramids and palm trees just like in his artwork, and the words, as though written in his own distinctive hand, "When it rains, it pours." We fell to our knees.

In time, we wandered toward where the massive march was to take place, still half dazed. Everyone was as wasted with grief as we were; we mustered in silence, swelling into the largest gathering of gay, lesbian, bisexual, and transgender people in history. Though the Parks Service initially reported that 200,000 were in attendance, they later admitted it surpassed the size of any other Washington march in the nation's history. Organizers pegged the number at 750,000. If there was any fear that AIDS would push the community deeper into the closet, this was proof that the opposite was happening. Almost every constituency group sent representatives. Colleges and universities fielded contingents. Groups of Broadway performers, socialists, lawyers, feminists, teachers, clergy, and parents carried banners, interspersed with mute marching bands and choral groups and wheelchairs—hundreds of wheelchairs. The banner at the head of the march declared, "For Love and for Life, We're Not Going Back."

We fell in behind ACT UP, a couple of hundred strong. For a mile or so, Doug carried a poster depicting Ronald Reagan as a devil-eyed demon in a toxic green haze. It was mid-afternoon under a cloud-choked sky when we arrived at the rally's center. Michael Callen sang from the stage. Speakers demanded money for AIDS research and recognition of our relationships, in life and in death. Ginny Apuzzo from the Human Rights Campaign Fund spoke angrily. "How many must die for this administration to wake up? Other groups of Americans have gathered here before us, to speak of the dream. To them I say, If the dream is to become a reality, it must be shared."

Doug and I took a bus home to New York that night, feeling no less scared about the future. Almost four thousand stayed behind for a demonstration at the Supreme Court the next day. "Civil disobedience is not new to gays and lesbians," organizer Pat Norman told reporters on the courthouse steps. "Every day in our lives we commit the act of civil disobedience by loving another. We demand an end to this idiocy." Officers pulled on Playtex gloves and began detaining people. By noon, 840 people were in handcuffs, the largest mass arrest since the Vietnam era. The detainees responded hostilely to the gloves and the implication that their personhood was contagious. They settled on a rejoinder laced with ridicule, crafted as a put-down only gay men raised on Hollywood classics might appreciate: "Your gloves don't match your shoes / you'll see it on the news." That was the only chant to make the news, alas, leading the national television broadcasts and creating quite a bit of confusion among Americans. What, they rightly wondered, did police officers' shoes have to do with anything? Few people felt more empathy for our plight following the weekend-long protest, or had any better understanding of what it was we wanted.

BY NOW, there were so many people in need of AZT who could not afford it that Congress approved a one-year, $30 million grant program for state governments to supply the drug to the destitute. To win votes, sponsors had to promise that this was a one-time-only measure, though something permanent needed to be done about AZT's towering price tag. With considerable behind-the-scenes help from ACT UP in New York, the job fell to Congressman Waxman. He began an investigation, with Bill Bahlman providing resources to his staff. Bahlman also enlisted members of the Presidential AIDS Commission, eventually even recruiting Cardinal O'Connor, who held an impromptu press conference denouncing the price as usurious. Editorials followed.

With negative attention accumulating, Burroughs Wellcome preemptively sliced 20 percent off the cost of AZT in mid-December. Editorial writers quickly noted that AZT was *still* the highest-priced drug in the country—$8,000 a year—and one that had been essentially developed at taxpayer expense, undermining the company's claims that it had to recoup $86 million in expenses. Independent analysts put Burroughs Wellcome's profit margin for the drug at anywhere from 40 percent to 80 percent. According to *Barron's*, the company would bank "$172 million—$206 million in revenues a year, in the U.S. alone," partly footed once again by the taxpayer, thanks to Congress's emergency appropriation.

ON DECEMBER 17, 1987, Bahlman was on the cheap train to Washington—"the Milk Run," it was called, pulling out of Penn Station at 3:45 a.m.—to monitor another Presidential AIDS Commission session. The ACT UP leadership defended the cost of his undertaking after Kramer protested, but they also had misgivings about Bahlman. His dual membership with ACT UP and the Lavender Hill Mob created suspicions about his loyalty and about message control. Some underestimated his cleverness, wondering if he was equipped for the work. His working-class New York diction and rather slow locution, and his lack of a college degree, undermined their faith in him. They kept him on a tight leash, requiring him to request approval for each trip rather than for the whole campaign, and only approving meager amounts. Recently, when the commission convened in Miami, their appropriation was so low he had to ask local AIDS activists there to book a motel room for him. For meetings in Washington, he slept on the train down and back.

This week's commission hearing was called to address the particular challenges and needs of the IV-drug-using community. Bahlman had armed himself with a stack of scientific, social, and political literature—as well as a few strident leaflets of his own creation—to circulate to the commissioners. Even if they refused to read them, at least they would be forced to recognize that the AIDS community actually had a position and that their ignorance of it was willful. Nothing in his experience as a top club DJ had prepared him for this role, but he proved an effective diplomat despite his comrades' misgivings. The commissioners liked him, and after a time some of them actively looked to him for the latest findings or theories. Bahlman didn't leave much to chance. "They're not particularly cerebrally advanced," he reported back.

After the hearing that night, he did not hurry to the train as usual. He had received an unexpected invitation to dine with Tony Fauci and Dr. James Hill, the gay researcher who was Fauci's special assistant. Bahlman had met both men a few months earlier at a scientific conference while distributing a leaflet decrying the egregious underperformance of federal research. Fauci's national AIDS Clinical Trials Group was designed to accommodate 10,000, but the ACTG, as it was called, had just 442 patients enrolled to date. And none of the trials were for the countless number of drugs people with AIDS were already taking on the underground.

"I like your flyer," Fauci said to him. "One correction. It's not 442, it's 475."

"Are you sure, Tony?" Bahlman asked, bypassing formalities. "Because I called your secretary on Friday and that's the figure I got."

"No, it's 475," Fauci persisted in his rich Brooklyn accent. "But I'm glad you have the lower number, because the more you're protesting about what we're doing, the more money I'm going to get to spend on research."

Bahlman could see that the community and NIAID shared a goal, especially when Fauci spent the rest of the conference hunting down Bahlman to introduce him to various members of his staff. One of them was Hill, soft-spoken and deferential. With a glance they acknowledged one another's gayness.

But Bahlman and ACT UP, sensitive to the potential for cooptation, kept the pressure on. Fauci soon invited Bahlman and Larry Kramer to learn more about the ACTG and to take a tour of his domain at NIAID: the labs, meeting halls, libraries, staff, and patient rooms. This was the caliber of activism Kramer found most comfortable. He no longer attended ACT UP meetings on a regular basis. For all his obsequiousness that day, Fauci failed to win over his visitors. Several times during the tour, Kramer and Bahlman pressed Fauci to reveal what more he needed for prosecuting the AIDS war. Fauci said only that his team could use more physical space for his operation. The next time ACT UP made the news, they carried posters that read, "Fauci: Space Isn't the Answer. You're Killing Us." The accompanying flyer, handed out to hundreds of people and scores of reporters, slammed Fauci for "suppressing, strangling and eliminating" drug trials other than for AZT, "thus ensuring that the AIDS epidemic is allowed to grow and grow in its devastation!!!" Kramer was quoted accusing the government of genocide. The ferocity of ACT UP continued into the fall and winter.

Hoping to reset relations with the activists, Fauci invited Bahlman for a supper at Hill's Capitol Hill home—an off-the-record, air-the-laundry summit of sorts. By coincidence, the dinner was taking place a week after the National Gay Rights Advocates, a public interest law firm, filed a class action suit against Fauci's office, accusing NIAID of "arbitrarily and capriciously" delaying the testing and approval of AIDS drugs. Bahlman did not seek permission from ACT UP to accept Fauci's invitation, knowing it would sow needless discord.

He arrived alone at Hill's address, where he traded his coat for a glass of wine and the frigid night air gave way to a warm social conversation among adversaries. It wasn't until much more wine flowed that Fauci laid down his napkin and steered toward his agenda. "To be honest with you," he began, "one of the things that has been counter-productive in the past . . ." He searched for the right words.

Bahlman fiddled with a tape recorder, and when the red light came on he placed it on the table between them. "How friendly my leaflets are?" he offered.

Fauci wasn't open to levity. "Yeah, right," he said, growing brittle despite the presence of the tape machine. "Things have been taken out of context and used in a way that has really been, obviously, ad hominem to me. But also, I think, ultimately destructive to what I believe we are both trying to do." He shifted in his chair. "Many, many times I become reluctant to give you the background, so you will understand, because things get taken out of context and get thrown up on a sign somewhere."

He was specifically aggrieved by the poster ridiculing his need for more space. "What that really was, was my trying to give you people a *feel*—the people who were there at the meeting at the NIH—a good *feel* for what is going on. And when I was pressed for the kinds of things that could help, I mentioned that! And the next thing I know there are people demonstrating with signs."

Fauci was a tightly wound aggressor. "Do you really believe the things you put in the flyers? Do you really believe that this is a concerted effort on my part or the NIH's part for *genocide*? Or interfering with the effort of trying to get drugs out? Or is that just your way of calling attention—to try to get people moving a little bit more quickly? Certainly it is not, I think, the productive way to go about it if we want to be in a partnership of helping each other. It really works negatively, that's what I find. You know, it bothers me, in the sense that I am, believe it or not, one of the best friends you have."

"Larry Kramer is a bit of a loudmouth," Bahlman said by way of introduction. "Larry Kramer tends to blow things out of proportion. Recently he had sent a letter to ACT UP denouncing *me*, tearing *me* apart—"

"Join the list," Dr. Hill said. He passed the wine.

"He had completely distorted all the facts. He had everything wrong about what I had been doing," Bahlman continued. "That's kind of the way the man operates."

This was a spectacular denunciation, and gave Fauci more of a divide-and-conquer opportunity than he had dreamed possible.

"Well, actually, that saddens me," Fauci said. "Because I can see in him—which I thought when I first met him—in his own way, the same kind of passion for helping as I have in my own area." He shook his head. "I was really surprised and disappointed when it turned into a personal attack that I thought was counterproductive, 'cause it only diminishes his own credibility."

"Larry is known as a person to shame people into taking action to protect themselves," said Bahlman. "That's what he does best. And then he should get out of the way and let other people do the work."

"The fact is," Fauci laid it on, "there is a total commitment by me personally, for sure, and certainly by the NIH, in eliminating this epidemic. And we do it as scientists."

Now Bahlman was handed an opportunity. "We want clinical

research done," he said carefully. "I'm very concerned about the underground market. I'm very concerned that there is very little data being
collected. . . . Why can't you at least do some form of limited testing
of substances such as Imuthiol, Ampligen, AL721, Carrisyn, foscarnet,
and others, to determine their efficacy in fighting AIDS? You may say
they're useless but the public is demanding that they be tested. How
can the NIH maintain any credibility when it doesn't respond to public
outcry and investigate all possible AIDS treatment?"

When Fauci scowled, Bahlman gently added, "We're talking about
drugs that have been given out quite a bit with no great reports of heavy
toxicity."

This kind of argument, coming from an unschooled activist, offended
Fauci's sensibility as a scientist.

"The idea of a clinical trial is not correctly perceived by people," he
snapped. "If in fact you are looking at whether a drug is going to be safe
and effective, versus just giving somebody the opportunity to say, 'I'm
on something; I may be dying but I'm on something,' those are issues
that get clouded. Because you always bring in the idea of compassion in
that. The most compassionate thing would be to most quickly as possible get the right answer!"

Hill had been biting his tongue. "Let me interject one thing," he
said. "One of the points that Bill has made was, why didn't we do the
studies of all these drugs, just look at them and see if they're good or
they aren't good?"

"A minimum of fifteen or twenty people at least in a study," Bahlman
added.

"We have a limited amount of people who can do the studies," Hill
said. "And we had to set priorities. And the priorities were to prefer
to pursue certain things with AZT in comparison, because that drug
seemed to work."

"I don't complain about the AZT studies," Bahlman jumped in.
"What I wanna see is *more drugs in clinical trials*."

Fauci's tone turned a bit patronizing. He had just buckled to pressure to enroll a real study of AL721, the egg lipid–based home remedy,
which he considered a waste of time, only to have activists slam him
for designing the trial around a placebo. He had to draw the line somewhere. "You can't treat every drug candidate the same," he seethed.
"You can't treat a drug that has shown in animal testing to be safe, that
has been shown in vitro to block the virus, has been shown in a preliminary pilot study to be reasonable—you can't treat that drug the same

way that you treat a drug of somebody who gets it off a boat somewhere in outer Transylvania!"

Bahlman changed the subject slightly, pivoting to prophylaxes. Like Callen and Sonnabend, he was deeply engaged in the campaign to prevent the major opportunistic infections. "What do you think's going to happen with DHPG?" he asked Fauci. The anti-blindness drug was lost in a negative feedback loop. Despite intense pressure from activists, the FDA refused to give it full release without a clinical trial, something Fauci's NIAID had refused to undertake, forcing people to rely on anecdotes from off-label users to evaluate the drug.

Fauci's voice tightened. He stabbed the table with a finger. "Now there, Bill, is a classic example of what happens when the proper trial is not done, and I think you know that. Let's just say it, so that everybody else can hear it."

"We're talking over twenty-five hundred people over a two-year period," Bahlman pushed back. That's how many people had gotten access to the drug under a program allowing compassionate use even without FDA approval. Their doctors kept records—it would be possible to conduct a retroactive study by way of those charts, he implied.

Fauci exploded. "And you look at the data and it's uninterpretable! That's the point, Bill. That really nails down what we're talking about tonight. *The goddamn data's uninterpretable.*" He took a breath. "When you actually take away the television sets, take away the newspapers, and look at the data, the data isn't worth a *shit*! Because you have to do a *study* to get the data. That's the problem."

Smiling, Bahlman gently reproached Fauci, saying, "You got a little carried away here." Fauci apologized, and Bahlman moved on to other subjects seamlessly, though he wasn't going to let DHPG drop, not while gay men were going blind needlessly.

When he returned to New York, he transcribed his audiotape, made copies, and had stacks of them available at the next Monday-night meeting, touching off a fresh round of outrage about his unauthorized dinner party, which he simply ignored. In time, the whole of ACT UP would see the value of Bahlman's Capitol Hill confab, which concluded with a gourmet meal prepared by Jim Hill himself. It offered a rare glimpse inside the (slightly inebriated) mind of ACT UP's chief nemesis. Using convoluted logic, Fauci blamed the lack of clinical trials on the community itself. He was defensive and intractable but also fragile emotionally, which meant he had vulnerabilities that had only to be discovered and exploited.

• • •

BY THE START of the new year, Iris Long's study group had grown
to ten members. They met weekly at the impressive loft apartment of
a book publisher with AIDS, Herb Spiers, whose moody good looks
were matched by an organized and probing mind (he had earned a
PhD in philosophy). No member had any training in science. David
Z. Kirschenbaum was an architect, and Margaret McCarthy was a college student. David Barr was a gay rights attorney at the Lambda Legal
Defense and Education Fund.

Long proposed calling their group the Data Committee, but
Kirschenbaum thought their name should draw attention to treatments. Ultimately they merged missions and formed the Treatment +
Data Committee, which would become known as T+D. Long answered
question after question from her own body of experience: How did
the FDA work? How did new drugs get developed, tested, approved,
and introduced? How did the Centers for Disease Control work with
the National Institutes of Health? Who was in charge? Who did they
answer to? How did they set their priorities? How could they be influenced? Those were simple but important lessons. Long had seen the
proliferation of literature in the back of ACT UP meetings promoting
alternative medicines or smuggled pharmaceuticals and, as a scientist,
it troubled her. The drug underground was never going to solve the
important problems regarding AIDS. The health care system could not
be bypassed. It had to be conquered.

The one question she couldn't answer was the most important one:
Where was the next generation of AIDS drugs and how could someone
get access to them? Bill Bahlman's research revealed that the patient
spots at most trial sites were empty, while researchers looked in the
wrong places for patients and patients were begging the wrong people
for access. There was no simple way to match patients and trials. Long
called the city hospitals she knew engaged in research. To her surprise,
every one of them refused to confirm whether or not they were running a trial, calling that information proprietary. David Barr crafted
requests under the Freedom of Information Act and sent them to hospital administrators, claiming they had a legal obligation to disclose
how they were spending government-provided research funds. He did
the same to NIAID and the FDA. When these requests were denied, he
followed up with threats of litigation.

This was the fundamental work of ACT UP—to crack open the
secretive and illogical world of pharmacological research and close the

gap between scientists and patients. For many, AZT was too toxic and of limited use, and in the absence of any other drug on the market, access to experimental compounds was essential. Even an untested medicine offered a better chance than doing nothing at all. These trials were the only health care available. And health care was a fundamental right.

"Drugs into bodies" remained ACT UP's central call to arms; now they were plotting a strategy for making that possible.

Through this effort, by January 1988 ACT UP discovered that more than forty AIDS drugs were approved for clinical trials. This seemed like great news, and it meant that what Fauci was telling the community was indeed true. But a strange fact soon surfaced: 98 percent of patients participating in trials in New York State were enrolled in a small number of studies involving AZT. Since AZT was acknowledged to be too toxic for half the patients, ongoing trials were meant to test the drug at different doses and at different points in a patient's disease progression—to fine-tune a blunt-force instrument. Nationally, the picture was only slightly better: 83 percent of patients enrolled in drug studies were participating in AZT research.

Meanwhile, approved trials on the other thirty-nine drugs accepted for study had almost no enrollment. In the whole country, at a time when 49,342 people had AIDS, only 25 PWAs were in trials evaluating medicines other than AZT—"an unrecognized scandal," Jim Eigo and Iris Long wrote in protest. Exactly why this was became apparent when a group of Long's followers managed to arrange a meeting with administrators at the NYU Medical Center in January. There, Dr. Fred Valentine explained how tightly drawn most of the non-AZT studies were, requiring that trial candidates meet stringent clinical profiles imagined by the pharmaceutical companies that often didn't match AIDS patients in the real world. One study might require a history of PCP but a very high CD4 count, an improbable combination. Then participating research centers employed a haphazard system used for enrollment. Any NYU physician could refer a patient from his or her practice if, by chance, they met the requirements. They might have to screen a hundred patients to find one with the desired profile. The whole enterprise simply waited for more candidates to come along. This made little sense when nearly two hundred people were now meeting every Monday with ACT UP, perhaps half of whom were infected, and more than one thousand very sick patients were taking part in GMHC support groups every night of the week. Why was there no outreach to them?

That, Valentine explained, was just the way it was done. He conceded that it was a less-than-ideal system—quite an understatement—and admitted that NYU had two FDA trials set up with not one patient enrolled. It fell to Eigo to explain this to the ACT UP membership. Despite having earned his degrees in playwriting, the thought of speaking at an ACT UP meeting traumatized him. His heart raced, and his mouth went dry. In preparation, he wrote his speech out in longhand, pushed it through a computer, and rehearsed readings from the printout that afternoon as a mise-en-scène ran in his head.

Eigo made it through his report. And then he explained that he had been devising a solution to the impasse, something he called "parallel track." If scientists found it necessary to limit enrollment to a homogeneous patient profile, why not add another arm to that trial—a *parallel track*—allowing any willing party to partake. The stricter study would still go forward, giving the pharmaceutical company the information it desired, while the parallel track had the potential to yield data on the way a wide range of patients used the drugs—real-world data, useful to regulators as they contemplated approval. He had written to the NIH and the FDA about his proposal, but had received no answer. He vowed to continue promoting it.

This was how the activists' agenda was advancing, in big proposals that mostly went ignored. Nevertheless, in a few weeks came a breakthrough for preventing the killer pneumonia that even Fauci couldn't ignore. In February, Dr. Margaret Fischl, the Miami AZT researcher, published findings from a study using Bactrim as prophylaxis, proving to the satisfaction of skeptics that the drug performed in AIDS patients as it did in everybody else. She put sixty patients into a study, randomly assigning half of them to Bactrim and the other half to a placebo. Twenty-eight of the thirty patients on placebo died, eight of them with their first episode of PCP. There were no PCP deaths among those who took Bactrim.

When Bahlman read the results, he was mortified that anyone would deny patients prophylaxis in order to watch them die. "There's another twenty-eight killed by Margaret Fischl," he said. "First nineteen and now twenty-eight. Will there ever be a trial for these crimes?"

The only good to come of this latest deadly experiment was that Fauci could no longer deny the evidence supporting guidelines for preventing PCP. Yet the FDA never approved Bactrim as a prophylaxis, Fauci still did nothing to alert doctors, and a preventable infection remained the number one killer in the epidemic.

4

Against Nature

Peter Staley's health didn't improve after his failure with AZT, and the markets continued to vex him following Black Monday. It seemed that his whole life was off track. His bonus that year would be minuscule. He recriminated himself for changing jobs, and for having the hubris to ignore the death sentence hanging over him. The environment at CRT Government Securities, run by self-described born-again Christians, was even more hostile to gays than it had been at J. P. Morgan, something he had thought wasn't possible. The mounting weight of his predicament finally caught up to him one weekend night in February. He had only just arrived at the Bar, the popular gay tavern in the East Village. The closeness of the room—where cigarette smoke hung heavy and marijuana was passed hand to hand—turned his stomach. Was it something he had eaten? The flu? He looped back through the fog and tides of men, desperate for the door and a breath of air.

The next thing he knew, he was flat on the floor with a stranger tugging at his elbow. He had passed out. Later in the month, his CD4 count hit an all-time low of 171, signaling that his disease was so far advanced that opportunistic infections would follow shortly. His time had come. He discussed his circumstances with his psychologist, who began the sobering work of helping him reconcile with a limited future. He decided that whatever time he had left he wished to spend with his comrades at ACT UP, not battling the vagaries of the bond market. Six months to the day after joining the firm, Staley filed for disability leave.

It did not go well. The man who had hired him felt betrayed by Staley's news, accusing him of duplicity and even fraud for not disclosing during his interviews that he was marked for death. What's more, he sent over paperwork from the company's long-term disability insurance carrier showing a one-year exclusion for preexisting conditions. This came as a total surprise. Staley had studied the paperwork they'd given him previously, which did not contain that clause. He threatened to sue CRT. CRT threatened to sue him. The struggle cost him even more CD4s, pushing his number down to a perilous 103 and forcing him to capitulate. The best he could get was an out-of-court offer of $125,000, payable in five yearly installments of $25,000—assuming he was alive to receive them; his death would immediately end the payments. Everyone including his doctor believed the money would see him to the grave.

In March, marking the first anniversary of ACT UP's inaugural protest on Wall Street, the group returned to the financial district, this time with Staley among them for the first time. Freed from the corporate world, he had no further need for the closet.

The picketers were not as cordial as they had been the year before, when Staley first encountered them. Now there were more than three hundred of them, organized into dozens of semi-autonomous "affinity groups" that planned unique and complementary zaps designed to keep police on their toes and tie up all of Lower Manhattan throughout the morning.

Staley fell in with one of the groups and surged onto Broadway, blocking southbound traffic on Lower Manhattan's chief artery. It took some time, but police eventually cuffed him and carted him away without incident. He was one of 111 people arrested that morning. But in the chaotic choreography of the day, there was something about Staley that caught the media's attention. He alone was granted a tight close-up on the local news, as an officer tightened handcuffs on his wrists. The image of his beaming face—as smooth and innocent as a college freshman's—led the evening newscast beneath the words "Peter Staley, AIDS Victim."

Every bond trader from coast to coast (and, thanks to the gossip channels in the bond market, as far away as Tokyo) now knew Staley's most intimate details. There were no secrets now. Just a louder ticking clock.

WALL-TO-WALL COVERAGE in the city's media outlets followed the second Wall Street demonstration. The publicity more than doubled the size of ACT UP. Now nearly five hundred people crowded into the tight main room of the center every Monday night. A stable tone was set by the moderators: an articulate and beautiful young woman with long golden hair named Maria Maggenti, and a tall, angular former dancer, David Robinson, who practiced a form of cross-dressing meant as gender commentary and defiance more than identity: swooping earrings and muttonchop sideburns, Dr. Martens boots and a shimmering miniskirt.

It was always the same. "Welcome to ACT UP," Robinson would call out to quiet the masses. Maggenti would pick up the script. "We are a diverse, nonpartisan group of individuals united in anger and committed to direct action to end the AIDS crisis."

Robinson: "We protest and demonstrate, we meet with government and public health officials; we research and distribute the latest medical information; we are not silent."

Maggenti: "If there are any on-duty members of—or anyone gathering information for—the New York City Police Department, the FBI, or any other law enforcement agency, you are required by law to announce yourselves and we ask that you do so by raising your hand now."

Robinson, smiling brightly after a beat: "Just because we don't see hands in the air doesn't mean they're not here!"

As the group entered its second year, the pace it set was numbing. Each week brought expanding reports from Staley, whose efforts succeeded in making ACT UP–branded clothing among the city's most popular fashionwear. An intense man with a large voice named Bob Rafsky headed up the Media Committee, as good a match as Staley was to fund-raising. By day, Rafsky was spokesman for the real estate developer Donald Trump. He knew assignment producers and editors at the highest levels. Besides his work on T+D alongside Iris Long, Jim Eigo headed a committee called Issues, whose task it was to make sure that each person in the room could understand all that was being discussed, whether the topic was the potential clinical value of gamma globulin or the mechanisms by which the city determined its overall hospital bed count.

Another committee, called Actions, proposed and coordinated the large-scale demonstrations tied to the issues. These supplemented the many smaller zaps and quasi-independent efforts carried out by affinity groups, such as wheat-pasting subways and buses with safe sex messages, or setting up needle-exchange tables inside heroin shooting galleries in the Bronx and Harlem, or buying a block of one hundred Mets tickets to unfurl a banner—"MEN USE CONDOMS OR BEAT IT"—large enough to be seen across Shea Stadium and on ESPN worldwide. The co-head of Actions was a lighthearted actor-turned-office-administrator named Ron Goldberg, who found in ACT UP meetings the stage that too often had eluded him in his theatrical career.

He was responsible for, among other things, breaking down the week's issues into slogans fit for the evening news. There would be no more debacles about gloves not matching shoes. This earned him the title, "Chant Queen," though predictably he quibbled: "I'd rather be called 'Chant-*euse*.'" Goldberg was also the unofficial esprit de corps officer, organizing talent shows and the like when the ACT UPers needed a lift.

In its totality, ACT UP was an intoxicating mix of people and passion, with some occasional frustration. Meetings could last until 11 p.m., sometimes erupting into dramatic mudslinging, but more often than not sinking into mind-numbing exegeses about specific drugs or specific hospital policies. And there were torrents of numbers: how many bus tickets for an Albany sit-in to protest insurance denials; how many paid admissions needed for the benefit at the World; how many volunteer lawyers to appear at how many arraignments in which jurisdictions, whether Manhattan, Albany, Washington, or points west. It was a remarkable scene week after week. No one ever forgot the stakes. The personal tragedies on display were heart-wrenching. People stood before the room to offer surplus medicines, or to remember those who were there last Monday and buried since. Bequests from wills were read and acknowledged. Individual members begged for help with doctors, hospitals, landlords, employers, courts. As Bob Rafsky often reminded his audience, "The power of this room is available to each and every one of you."

Soon, as the epidemic grew to impact more people of color than whites, the challenges grew more knotty and systemic. A new committee was formed to respond to evictions from shelters, forced sterilizations, sick young orphans who needed volunteers to cradle them, and the many unique needs of gay African Americans and Latinos brought on by this crisis. They called it the Majority Actions Committee because the minorities were now the majority of newly diagnosed.

It surprised no one when, by late spring, the massive agenda threatened to spread the whole undertaking too thin. Members were burning out. Leadership positions were going unfilled. With demonstrations planned almost every week, some were drawing as few as thirty people. A new committee to conduct "burn-out workshops" failed to stem the tide. To deal with the problem, a special town hall meeting was called in May. Larry Kramer was the first to speak and, out of deference, was allowed to go well beyond the established time limit. The sole and towering purview of ACT UP, he extolled, had been to get drugs into bodies. While guerrilla armies were being fielded to zap William F. Buckley (because he said something offensive) or infiltrate the upcoming Democratic National Convention (because they weren't saying enough), where were all the drugs? He had just published an article putting the blame for this on Fauci's head. Without new drugs, he pointed out, everything else was moot.

Next came Vito Russo, who echoed Kramer's criticisms. "ACT UP has to renew its commitment to putting drugs into people," he said. "ASAP." Many in the room—in particular the men who either knew or suspected that they were positive—endorsed this view with ardent applause. But others argued that a broader mandate was needed. The strongest voice expressing this view belonged to Maxine Wolfe, a professor of environmental psychology and veteran of numerous progressive and left-wing movements. Drugs, she argued, weren't enough—the entire system of delivering and controlling health care in America needed rethinking, and to get there the group had to address politics, economics, class, and privilege. "Being out on the streets is how things are changed," she said. Her forceful oratory found a receptive audience. Even before the plague's onslaught, most of ACT UP's women, now sizable as a minority, and many of its gay men, had personally experienced systemic prejudice from the health care world. As a member named Allyson Smith pointed out, women and people of color were routinely excluded from drug trials—proof that confronting sexism and racism was a necessary precursor to gaining access to any promising drug.

Staley remained neutral throughout the discussion. Like Bahlman, he saw both approaches as complementary, if overly ambitious. Ortez Alderson, a fiery veteran of Chicago's theater community with past ties to the Black Panthers, spoke for everyone when he said ACT UP's overweening goal had to be saving every last person with AIDS. That was their shared millstone.

The tension between the two tendencies wasn't eliminated by the town hall summit. Week after week, Doug Gould sat beside me in the back row of the ACT UP meetings, trying to find his own place in the room. The stridency made him uncomfortable. He excused himself more than once to calm his nerves outside with a joint. He took up knitting as a distraction. After months of spooling yarn and clacking needles, he couldn't take it anymore and began to fill his Monday evenings with *Dallas* reruns instead of ACT UP drama. I didn't blame him, but carried on my weekly vigilance in his name.

Something of the ACT UP ethos did rub off on him, though. After being in New York for six months or so, he put himself on a diet and exercise regimen. He gave SlimFast a try, following the instructions to eliminate alcohol from his daily routine. Though he still smoked marijuana whenever he could, he never took another drink. The weight flew off him. His skin tightened up. He had the strong and angled face of an adult, finally. His mood improved as well. In sobriety, at least from liquor, a contented man with a ready sense of humor emerged. As his twenty-ninth birthday approached, he was happier than he had been when we first met as teenagers.

I overheard him discussing his transition as though some force beyond his powers had allowed him to escape the grip of drunkenness.

"Rehab? AA? Cold turkey?" the friend asked.

His eyes shot open with astonishment. "SlimFast!"

ONE SPRING AFTERNOON, in the checkout line at the grocery, Callen scanned the tabloids. *Weekly World News* was a hilarious tonic, with its in-depth coverage of Elvis sightings and extraterrestrial military plots. But it was the newest *People* magazine that caught his eye. On the cover was Ryan White, the teenager who had been violently hounded out of his middle school in Kokomo, Indiana. After Rock Hudson, White was perhaps the best-known person with AIDS in the country. The media adored his boyish indomitability and buoyant good humor. He made our exotic disease seem humdrum. Here was a carrier who loved junk food, Max Headroom, war games, and skateboarding. He was an everyboy with AIDS, the patient who linked gay Americans, however tenuously, with the rest of humanity. Celebrities in particular found his story useful. Conspicuous visitors to his modest rural home included Tom Cruise, Brooke Shields, Yoko Ono, and Elizabeth Taylor. The Olympic diving champ Greg Louganis—at the time deeply secretive about his own HIV infection—had White as his guest for the Pan Am Games, and even gave him one of his gold medals. Elton John sent his private jet to bring the whole White clan to Disneyland, and continued calling and writing weekly. Kareem Abdul-Jabbar and Michael Jackson called him a friend.

Despite all the attention and fame, and despite the boy's reported "courage," "serenity," and "goodness," White had suffered a medical setback, *People* reported:

Ryan White nearly died last January, one month past his 16th birthday. He was rushed to the hospital with pneumonia, the result of his AIDS. He has been taking AZT since last August, and it has helped him put on weight and generally improved his health, but it cannot stop his lungs from sometimes filling with fluid or prevent other opportunistic infections brought on by the disease.

Callen couldn't believe what he was reading. He'd met White once, at a photo session for AmFAR with Elizabeth Taylor, and hoped he might contribute to the *PWA Newsline*. He bought the magazine and ran it over to Sonnabend's office.

Sonnabend bent over his shoulder to take in the article.

"I can assure everyone he has AIDS and it's still fatal," says Ryan's doctor, Martin B. Kleiman of Indiana University Medical Center. "But all the scientific data we had would not have pointed to him being with us today and doing so well. Ryan has just blossomed, and I don't know why. I'd like to think it's because I'm a good doctor, but I can't take full credit."

He couldn't take *any* credit, as far as Sonnabend was concerned. Callen grabbed a phone, and, after strongarming his friends at AmFAR, GMHC, and elsewhere, managed to get a phone number for White's grandmother. Reaching her at home, he introduced himself as a representative of the National Association of People With AIDS, one who also sometimes appeared in the pages of *People* himself. He asked if the boy was on some sort of PCP prophylaxis. Callen glanced knowingly at Sonnabend. *Prophylaxis,* he repeated. *To prevent the pneumonia?*

She had never heard of such a thing. Callen offered to have Dr. Sonnabend call the youngster's physician, and she eagerly shared his number. Later that day, Sonnabend reached Dr. Kleiman, who was unfamiliar with the simple prevention techniques. This made Callen frantic with worry. As he said later, "If world-famous Ryan White didn't know about the importance of PCP prophylaxis, there are undoubtedly thousands of Americans who are at this very moment being denied what ought to be the standard of proper medical care for people at risk for AIDS." This was the reason Callen had pushed Fauci to set treatment standards. "It is a national scandal that Ryan's access to potentially life-prolonging treatments had to be left to such happenstance," Callen said. "It is a symptom, I assert, of a federal response to AIDS that to this day remains sluggish, inhumane, and frankly third-rate."

• • •

WHEN GAY PRIDE Month rolled around again, in June 1988, the Soviet Union's shaky economy led to giddy predictions that the cold war superpower was coming apart. Ronald Reagan was enjoying a spectacular finish to his presidency, at least in matters of state, and the evening broadcasts were as preoccupied with his legacy as he was. He had caused a quantum shift in global politics, to be sure, but the excitement accorded Reagan—an approval rating better than any president in a generation!—distracted from the realities on American soil. Heroin and crack cocaine had taken over the major cities, fueling gang warfare and creating another AIDS "amplification system," this time for the epidemic's march into poor communities. Impoverished and drug-haunted African Americans now made up the majority of HIV's new targets. In the East Village, the sidewalks were strewn with spent hypodermic needles and empty crack vials. Addicts slept in doorways. A vast, festering shantytown sprang up in Tompkins Square Park, where makeshift structures housed more than two hundred, many of whom had lost their homes after an AIDS hospitalization. Reagan's "shining city on the hill" was only a dream.

Like many New Yorkers, Michael Callen's day-to-day circumstances grew more dire. Having lost their legal battle, he and Dworkin were forced from their $700-a-month loft into an apartment on the edge of the industrial Meat Packing District that was smaller, less safe, and almost three times the price. The dislocation was one challenge too many for Callen. He retreated to the studio to finish his album, which he called *Purple Heart,* an often sad compilation of mostly original work, including the song that would become the anthem for the times.

Love don't need a reason
Love's never a crime
And love is all we have for now
What we don't have
What we don't have
Is time.

When organizers pleaded with him to give an address at the Gay Pride Rally, he was disappointed to realize that a new generation of leaders hadn't risen to take his place. Sometimes it seemed that there were only fifty people doing the business of AIDS politics, he thought. Nevertheless, he relented. On Saturday, June 25, he climbed the stage in Central Park and was able to see the AIDS Memorial Quilt stretching toward the horizon, darkening with rain clouds. He spoke passionately.

> We live in wartime and it's a civil war not a foreign war. AIDS is our Holocaust—and I do not use that analogy lightly. . . . We will someday be able to count the actual number of lives senselessly lost because of Fauci's and the federal government's inaction. Anyone who has died of pneumocystis at least within the last year needn't have died. There's no other word for that besides genocide.

A thousand heads nodded in agreement.

"We are imperiled from all sides," he continued. "I joke that I've managed to live this long by studiously avoiding federally designed treatment protocols, few though they be. I'm only half joking."

His jaw tightened. Beyond his audience, he could see large pockets of New Yorkers enjoying their Saturday afternoon. Baseball teams swapped turns at bat. Dogs chased Frisbees. A drum circle formed— business as usual, untouched by the epidemic.

Callen's voice was dry.

"AIDS casts its shadow over gayness itself," he said. "Loving another man is seen by many as an act of madness. Gay men are viewed as the Flying Wallendas of the eighties, performing death-defying high-wire acts merely by loving, while the 'general population' below turns away in horror."

A FEW WEEKS LATER, Griffin Gold arrived at Dr. Sonnabend's office on West Twelfth Street without an appointment. It was a Friday evening. He was not breathing well and complained of extreme pain. A rattling cough had gone on all week. More perplexing was what was happening in his belly. In a matter of hours, it had distended alarmingly, straining the skin and punishing his internal organs. It was hard to the touch. Through the stethoscope Sonnabend could hear fluids, but something else too, something unidentifiable.

Fearing the worst, Sonnabend called around for a hospital with an available bed—Gold was in no condition to languish on a gurney in the ER. It was not uncommon now to wait for days before being moved into a hospital room, not ideal for anyone sick, much less someone in so much pain. He got lucky. There was space at St. Luke's, in the shadow of the grand Cathedral of St. John the Divine on the Upper West Side.

A female staff physician met Gold and rushed him in for an examination. A test found PCP, suggesting not only that Gold's immune system was shot, but also that he hadn't been taking the prophylaxis prescribed by Sonnabend. The cause of his belly's growth was a very large and aggressive malignancy. This presented a conundrum. The amount of chemotherapy needed to fight the tumor could kill someone as sick as Griffin Gold.

The physician tried to comfort Gold, but he knew the situation was grave. "I have to ask you how much you want us to do for you," she said to him. "Things are going to be unpleasant. Ultimately, whatever we do will not save your life—only extend it."

She thought he seemed somehow both frightened and resigned. He listened intently, weighing his limited options. He was a thirty-two-year-old man contemplating the extraordinary measures that might give him a shot at thirty-three.

"I want more time," he told her halfheartedly.

She left to make arrangements. Moments later, his two closest friends arrived. He had met Michael Lesser and his lover, Ray Balsys, when the three of them first landed in New York as wide-eyed young stagehands, working together at the Roundabout Theatre Company. With a fractured tie to his biological family, Gold considered Lesser and Balsys kin. He was less afraid with them at his side, and was able to sleep.

As he dozed, his friends overheard the hospital's senior staff, gathered just out of sight, debating Gold's grim prognosis. They wrestled with the bleak fact that their ICU had only one open bed. "He won't make it through the night," one of the doctors predicted. No one contradicted him. It was agreed to keep the bed available for someone more likely to thrive.

Hearing this, Lesser and Balsys bolted to the hallway to beg for Gold's life. In time, they swayed them. Orderlies moved Gold into the ICU. A massive regimen of chemotherapy was begun that night and Gold was still alive in the morning, though just barely.

News about Gold's condition circulated through ACT UP, and hit Staley especially hard. He fixated on the pneumonia diagnosis. Staley had been taking prophylaxis every day for months, ever since his CD4 count suggested he was at serious risk. He was lucky that the little white Bactrim pills caused him no side effects. Why Gold had gone off them was inexplicable. A few days later, on a hot July afternoon, Staley visited Gold at St. Luke's, an imposing array of hulking, yellow-brick buildings. Gold was on the mend, but it was not a happy reunion.

"Why weren't you taking the Bactrim?" Staley demanded.

Gold shrugged.

"Did you ever start on Bactrim?"

Silence.

"Are you just going to let this happen? Are you just going to die without a fight?"

Gold had no answer.

BILL BAHLMAN'S lone campaign to bird-dog the Presidential AIDS Commission sessions was paying off in little ways. In February, Admiral Watkins moved the hearings to New York City, the heart of the epidemic with one in four U.S. cases and where AIDS was now the leading cause of death for all men aged twenty-five to forty-four. ACT UP sent an army of three hundred activists to join Bahlman, surrounding the hall with bullhorns and leaflets while tying themselves together with miles of red tape to protest the bureaucratic morass that mired the epidemic.

This time, Watkins made room on the agenda for leaders from the gay and AIDS community. Sonnabend, Tom Hannan, and Michael Callen were invited to explain that it took community-based research to break the stranglehold that AZT had over the federal research establishment. "Lipid research is a good example of this," Callen told the committee. "Lipids may or may not be anti-retroviral. But they seem to repair cell damage—something which certainly is happening in AIDS. Why has Dr. Fauci and the NIH only so begrudgingly begun trials? It's as if they don't want to believe *anything* does damage other than *the virus*. Another example is PCP prophylaxis. Preventing the number one killer of people with AIDS ought to have been the number one treatment priority." He looked up from his paper, catching Watkins's eye. "I believe that PCP prophylaxis will, in a single stroke, save more lives than all the AZT in the world."

Callen found it difficult to read the faces of the panelists to know what impression, if any, he had made. The answer came in the subsequent weeks when Watkins made a surprise visit to FDA headquarters to see how the situation Callen described had developed. He spoke with remarkable candor about what he found there. Scientists "pulled me into a back room" to plead for new staff, space, equipment, and money, he said later. He added, "We are not ready for this disease. This country is simply not ready for an emergency medical epidemic of this type, and we have got to do better because we don't know what the next mutation [of the virus] is going to be."

With the epidemic now in its seventh year, Watkins made an urgent call to the FDA to speed up drug approvals, and he promised to take up the question of distributing clean needles to junkies.

Then the commission went to work on its report for the president. In the end, it contained 576 recommendations, stunning in quantity and reach alike, including the need to triple federal spending on research, teach prevention in the nation's secondary schools, and give emergency powers to a single government figure for addressing the calamitous state of affairs—an AIDS czar of sorts. Watkins courted even more controversy by calling on Reagan to issue an executive order preventing discrimination against individuals who carried the virus, a measure he called "the key to the entire report."

Some of Watkins's fellow appointees quietly complained that they had been strong-armed by the admiral into accepting his conclusions as theirs. But nobody was as shocked by the report as the activists themselves. "I am very much surprised," said Mathilde Krim. The activists had clearly touched Watkins with their steady campaign. Bahlman more than anyone else deserved credit.

Bolstering the report were two government actions that followed within a month of one another. First, Reagan's surgeon general, a born-again Christian named C. Everett Koop, defied Reagan's inner circle by mailing an educational brochure on AIDS to every single household in the country, the largest such health-related public mailing in history, in which he called upon the nation to respond compassionately to the afflicted. Then a panel of experts convened by the National Academy of Sciences produced a report covering much of the same ground, and reaching a series of conclusions similar to the commission's. The political winds were finally shifting. The spring of 1988 brought the first glimmer of compassion and reason from Washington.

It was overshadowed, however, by the Reagan administration's forceful recalcitrance. A swift and severe backlash took hold. Religious activists called for Koop's head, denounced the Academy of Sciences' conclusions as biased and wrong, and branded Watkins a heretic. It did not upset Watkins that he was cast as the bête noire of the right, but given the seriousness of his mission he didn't expect to be shunned by the White House as a result. When he arrived on schedule to brief Reagan and Vice President George H. W. Bush on the findings, he learned that the event would be private. No reporters were alerted, and after a few minutes White House personnel ushered him past the press room and out a side door like an unwanted guest. His report was given a similar boot. Not one of the recommendations was acted on.

If Watkins felt any outrage over this treatment, he did not let on, not even to his family. He had done what he was called upon to do, then he never weighed in on AIDS politics again.

IT HARDLY SEEMED POSSIBLE, but the level of hostility against the afflicted increased dramatically as the summer of 1988 unfolded. More than six hundred noxious legislative initiatives had been authored around the country, among them a bill in New Jersey that would require anyone selling his or her home to inform potential buyers if a PWA had ever lived there. Similar developments were taking place in the private sector. The convenience store chain Circle K canceled health insurance for any of its 26,000 employees with AIDS unless it was contracted through a blood transfusion or from an errant spouse. "There are certain lifestyle decisions that we are just not going to assure the rights of," a company officer said. Public health advocates reacted angrily, but there was no recourse. As the AIDS caseload surpassed the fifty thousand mark, the country's major religions also turned sharply against the community. The Southern Baptists spent their convention that summer condemning homosexuality as "a manifestation of a depraved nature" and "a perversion," overwhelmingly passing a resolution blaming gay men for inflicting AIDS not only on one another but on "innocent victims" as well. Similarly inimical views were held by the United Methodists, the Evangelical Lutheran Church in America, and the Catholic Church.

Given the increasing power that faith leaders wielded in Washington and in America generally, a Hobbesian cycle of brutality and fear took hold. Nationally, anti-gay hate crimes had tripled over the previous three years, while in New York City marauding gangs had violently attacked gay men in 309 separate incidents since the weather warmed, including more than a dozen murders. Almost none of the crimes resulted in arrests, and the news media gave them very little ink. Many Monday-night ACT UP meetings were dedicated to discussing the inability of the so-called "general population" to see gays with any sympathy; AIDS had only made us more repellent to them. If we couldn't get society to extend one of the basic services of civilization like police protection, then we surely would never see a change in health care policy.

In searching for an effective response, ACT UP members entertained numerous proposals for civil disobedience, mass lobbying, die-ins, kiss-ins, and "fax zaps," a new strategy to send a loop of transmissions to opponents to deplete their thermal paper rolls (its effect on the other end was little more than frustration). Michael Petrelis floated the idea of lesbians and gay men going out into America to challenge the status quo the way civil rights Freedom Riders had twenty-seven years earlier. He circulated a memo that said, "When we, Lesbians and Gay men, remain in the closet we perpetuate and strengthen the hatred, violence and discrimination against us. If we allow others to define who we are by our silence, then the misconceptions about us will prevail." He envisioned buses filled with homosexuals going to some of the most dangerously anti-gay corners of the country, stopping to display panels from the AIDS Memorial Quilt and communicating directly with local reporters.

Only a small coterie of activists agreed to ride with Petrelis, but ACT UP funded it, and they set off for the South in July, with plans to attend the national conventions of both political parties. First came the Democratic National Convention—which opened in Atlanta, the city where Michael Hardwick was arrested and prosecuted for sodomy, and which pursued him all the way to a Supreme Court victory against gay sex. Convention organizers were not warm to the arrival of ACT UP, with its thirty-eight members dressed in black boots and earrings and T-shirts with slogans designed to remind Atlantans that sodomy was nearly as common as holding hands:

SO	SO	SO
DO	DO	DO
MY	MY	MY
Parents	Neighbors	Kids

They were immediately shunted to a "free speech zone" a number of blocks from the convention hall at the Omni Hotel, in a large pen devoid of reporters. They chanted and generally cavorted for hours, acting on the day's theme, "Queer Visibility Day." On the second day, the ACT UPers vowed to play by their own rules. The goal was a picket-style kiss-in at the Omni's doors. Marching slowly in an oval formation, they planted quick pecks on the lips of the person standing opposite them. It took the police a little while to realize that protesters had escaped from the designated area. Then hundreds of them descended on the band of smoochers. Outfitted in riot gear, plastic shields, and weighted black truncheons, they advanced in tight formation, in unison ordering the protestors to "Move! Move! Move!" and easily driving them back to the free speech cage. But when the police phalanx retreated, the kissers scurried back to their places to resume their smooching. Infuriated officers smashed their way into the crowd and violently scattered demonstrators and an equal number of journalists, many of whom complained of broken cameras and confiscated tape recorders. Nobody had anticipated the heavy-handedness. ACT UP staged two more kiss-ins during the convention, including one on the steps of city hall where they demanded and received an apology from Mayor Andrew Young for the actions of the riot squad.

The Gay and Lesbian Freedom Ride departed Atlanta the day after Governor Michael Dukakis and Senator Lloyd Bentsen became that party's standard-bearers—a bad-news team, as far as gays were concerned, because the former opposed gays as foster parents and the latter supported the restrictive amendments that Senator Helms attached to all AIDS spending. The Riders needed only a single van, unfortunately, having atrophied to just four men and one woman—Heidi Dorow, a Hampshire College student. Even Petrelis found a reason not to continue on.

That didn't dampen spirits in the van. The Riders headed first for Montgomery, Alabama, chosen for its symbolism, where they organized a roundtable dialogue with local activists and a touching display of about fifty panels from the quilt. Like their role models from a generation earlier, these Freedom Riders were keenly aware of the huge gulf between their goals and the facts on the ground. The political leaders of the South played to their reputation. "We'll guarantee them their rights of free speech, but we won't guarantee they'll be loved," the mayor, Emory Folmar, warned in a front-page *Montgomery Advertiser* story. "I have zero sympathy for them and zero sympathy for the cause of the Gay and Lesbian Freedom Ride. People who get AIDS from homosexual activities or illegal drug activities certainly don't deserve, certainly won't get, my sympathy."

Progressing through Birmingham, Nashville, Louisville, and Knoxville, the Freedom Riders sought out local gays in bars with names like "The Guest Club" and "Mabel's Beauty Salon and Chainsaw Repair." At night they slept on sofas in the homes of volunteers, sharing stories of homophobia and views on aerosolized pentamidine, the gay vote, drag queens, and the National Gay and Lesbian Task Force (the name had recently been amended to include women). By morning, chances were good that a local ACT UP chapter had been announced.

Activists marched against the Helms Amendment in New York. In

Boston, a group zapped Dr. Frank Young of the FDA at an appearance at a health conference. Eleven people were arrested—including Jim Eigo and Ortez Alderson—for taking over New York health commissioner Stephen Joseph's office and demanding his resignation. The "Joseph Eleven" were charged with criminal trespass and released in plenty of time to head to New Orleans for the Republican National Convention in August, where they met up with the Riders. Peter Staley and the T+D members joined as well. All prepared for police department violence when they staged their kiss-in in New Orleans, but it was the Republican delegates, not the police, who turned hostile. Fists flew. The riot squad unexpectedly jumped in to protect the activists, who sustained only a few minor injuries. The anti-gay chants left more lasting scars: "No God-given right for a sodomite," and "AIDS cures itself."

While in New Orleans, Staley visited the nearby headquarters of Imreg, a tiny biotech firm that had developed a promising therapeutic but did not have in place a pre-release access program for the very sick. He and about twenty-five other ACT UPers staged a protest there but were back in time to scream and shout when George H. W. Bush and his surprise running mate, Senator Dan Quayle, took the stage at 3:30.

In the aftermath of convention season, the Freedom Ride continued with stops in Jackson, Mississippi, Memphis, and Little Rock. The last stop was Arcadia, Florida, the small city south of Tampa where a local family sought a court order to allow their three HIV-positive kids to enroll in elementary school, only to have their house burned to the ground by arsonists. Joined by a handful of Florida activists, the Riders marched fifteen strong to the courthouse on the second anniversary of the fire, for which no arrests had been made. About a hundred counter-protesters greeted them with shouts of "Go back where you belong," and myriad anti-gay epithets. Though it looked at one point like the melee would become physical, a strong police presence kept the peace, and the subsequent news coverage let locals see and hear from articulate gays, lesbians, and people with AIDS, often for the first time in local memory.

It was an exhausting few months. But in mid-August came the first sign that all these efforts on multiple fronts were having the intended impact. In response to a push from T+D, the FDA loosened its rules on a new, experimental anti-pneumonia drug, trimetrexate, which would be available to anybody who did not respond to Bactrim or the other drugs, even without definitive trial data. The attorney David Barr, a

T+D member who played a principal role in bringing about this change, took a victory lap at that Monday's meeting. "This opens an entirely new approach to providing experimental treatments to people with AIDS and other life-threatening illnesses," he said.

A NEW FACE had appeared in T+D. Mark Harrington was a chain-smoking punk rocker who tended to dress all in white save for a pair of oxblood Dr. Martens high-tops. His ginger hair was shaved close, giving prominence to mug-handle ears, one of which was adorned genie-like with a single silver hoop. Nothing in his background had prepared him for the detailed scientific and medical discourse that drove the group. His degree from Harvard—in an individualized major amalgamating art, literature, and history—propelled him into years of drifting through love affairs, club hopping, and dead-end jobs. He dabbled in filmmaking, writing, and art in his free time and earned his rent money at a film archive, sorting and indexing the collection. He was drafted into the activist trenches when a close friend, Scott Johnson, passed out in his arms one Tuesday night at a popular Lower East Side club. Afterward, Johnson spoke of the vulnerability he felt as a man with a bad prognosis, no job, no insurance, no idea how to navigate the health care system, and no hope. Harrington went looking for answers at ACT UP and T+D specifically.

Mostly, he listened quietly. Afterward, he would go home to research the words and compounds that tumbled from Iris Long's and Jim Eigo's lips. When he had attended meetings for about three months, he broke his self-imposed silence and shyly announced that he had produced a glossary of AIDS terminology. He presented a forty-eight-page reference manual, beginning with an entry for "accrual" and ending with "Zovirax," the brand name of a herpes drug. On the cover page he included a line from Prince's newest album: "I'm going down to Alphabet Street . . ."

The glossary thrilled Eigo. "Taking control of the vocabulary is a prerequisite to our taking over the system," he said. The committee passed out hundreds of copies at Monday-night meetings that summer. Harrington had found his calling.

THE CRUSHING HEAT wave that summer gave rise to a bizarre plague of mosquitoes, triggering warnings from the public health sector of a possible outbreak of dengue fever, a temporarily incapacitating disease. The social whirl in the Hamptons suffered. Because the East Village had risen from swampland, the problem was even worse there. The talk on the street was whether mosquitoes carried HIV. After all, they transmitted malaria and yellow fever. All the science debunked the possibility, but that did little to quell the irrational fears. Forty cases in a town in Florida were said to have been spread that way—a discredited hypothesis that nonetheless dominated the AIDS news.

David Barr and Mickey Wheatley, a fellow staff litigator at Lambda, knew better than to be afraid. On a hot summer night, they chose an outdoor table at the Dojo Restaurant on St. Mark's Place in the East Village. A twenty-three-year-old HIV-positive associate named Gregg Bordowitz joined them. Bordowitz, a video artist and graduate of the prestigious Whitney Museum Independent Study Program, had been around ACT UP from the beginning, drawn by a desire to chronicle their demonstrations. He soon recruited other Whitney fellows. They had formed an affinity group called Testing the Limits, a video collective committed to making documentary films and other creative responses to the crisis. He held a unique place within ACT UP. His thick sideburns, dimpled cheeks, and fiery eyes put him on par with Peter Staley as one of ACT UP's male sex symbols. The fact that he was also the only open bisexual male broadened his physical appeal to include many women in the group. As he rose in prominence over the past year, he began to show great leadership skills. It fell to him and a small stable of others to instruct new members in the philosophy of civil disobedience and nonviolence. He conducted seven-hour training sessions in a room on the center's third floor, for twenty people at a time, lessons he infused with his thoughts on reading Derrida, Foucault, and Genet.

There was something Bordowitz wanted to discuss with Barr and Wheatley that night over dinner. With little concerted effort and no ongoing campaign, theirs had become a national movement, he said, "just sort of by word of mouth." Nobody knew how many cities were organized, or how many people they could mobilize.

"And it's global," Barr noted. This was technically true. Letters of affiliation had arrived from Toronto and Montreal.

Bordowitz said he had been mulling over the idea that AIDS activism had the potential for achieving critical mass. He envisioned a massive AIDS protest event, drawing PWAs and activists from dozens of cities into a single spectacular act of civil disobedience. There was no shortage of deserving targets, from the White House to the United Nations.

Barr and Wheatley had also been thinking about magnifying their reach. Hearing Bordowitz speak, the FDA immediately came to mind. Reforming the agency was high on the list of the disregarded Watkins report. Discounting the history of AZT, on average it took seven to ten years for a new compound to go from test tubes to medicine cabinets—or longer, in the case of the anti-blindness drug DHPG, which still hadn't been put into human trials. Instead of correcting that oversight, the FDA was instead now clamping down on AL721, the buyers club favorite. The PWA Health Group moved two tons of it every month in New York alone. Now lawyers for the agency had sent cease-and-desist letters to two companies involved in bootlegging it.

Lawyers at Lambda were girding for litigation. "They're not following their own regulations and they're keeping us from getting lifesaving therapies. That should be where our action is," Barr said. "ACT UP needs to go to the FDA. We need to take control of the FDA."

"Look," Wheatley added, "many groups have gone to Washington and protested in front of the White House. Many groups have protested in front of Congress. For our movement, we need to go to the Food and Drug Administration."

This made perfect sense to Bordowitz. If he had any doubts that such an undertaking were possible or that he could help pull it off, Barr gave him the confidence he would need.

"Gregg, you're becoming a very visible leader within ACT UP. When you speak, people listen to you, and your opinion carries a lot of weight within the group."

Bordowitz knew this was true. He put his name on the agenda for the following Monday night. The room was overpacked and uncomfortably hot. A photographer had arrived from *The New York Times*, touching off a tense debate over the paper's coverage and whether or not people could have a presumption of anonymity at these meetings. The personal costs of being revealed as gay or as a PWA were often intolerable. It was determined that the photographer could stay on the condition that he shoot only one side of the room. Those unwilling to be photographed migrated to the other side. When the din of chair swapping subsided, Bordowitz began speaking with David Barr at his side for support.

He reviewed the FDA's many failures and recent regression and shared his vision for "a major action" at FDA's headquarters, an army of sick people and their advocates pounding on the door to demand pills from uncaring bureaucrats. The visuals would surely stun Americans. Nobody had ever picketed the drug regulator before, making it even more attractive as a target. "We need to seize control," he said.

The response was electric. In the discussion that followed, a target date was set for October 11, and a list of demands started to fall together. When it came to a vote, hands shot in the air in unified agreement. Members subsequently approved a budget to send Bordowitz around the country building support, along with Robert Garcia, a high-energy young activist who identified as half Navajo and half Mexican and worked as a secretary in an insurance company.

It fell once again to Peter Staley to find money for transportation to the FDA, lodging, and food for such a huge undertaking. Because the first direct mail campaign was so profitable, he planned a second in July, this time without fees to Sean Strub and his company—Strub had been so impressed with ACT UP he was now a regular member, volunteering his time and talents like everyone else. Benefit soirees were planned for Fire Island and throughout the Village. Staley plunged $3,000 into more logo hats and T-shirts. He solicited money from other AIDS organization—GMHC sent over $10,000—and, while tripling the ACT UP bail fund, helped David Barr solicit a battery of volunteer attorneys to defend against an expected onslaught of criminal prosecutions.

From the start of the FDA campaign, it was decided to pursue a kind of good cop/bad cop approach with the agency. Barr would lead the good cop team, reasonably presenting the grievances to officials and demanding full and unconditional compliance with the Watkins Commission recommendations, while Bordowitz's strategy would be to menace the agency with news about the upcoming march on a regular basis. The implication was that an invasion of unruly activists could be avoided if the FDA capitulated.

In August, Barr secured a meeting with the FDA's consumer affairs unit. With a Lambda colleague and his college intern, Margaret McCarthy, he critiqued the agency's handling and mishandling of the drug-approval process in general, and in particular for AL721 and other treatments of great interest. He admitted that esteem for AL721 had begun to wane in the AIDS community. Sonnabend's study at the Community Research Initiative was inconclusive, and Michael May, whose miraculous rally after taking the drug in Israel fueled the wild demand, had died nevertheless. Still, the FDA's crackdown generated swift and angry objections not only from gay and AIDS groups but from the holistic community and doctors, who were convinced, at least, that it did no harm.

At a second meeting, on September 2, Eigo, Staley, and Bordowitz joined the negotiations, giving teeth to Barr's concerns. For Staley, this inaugurated a new stage of his activism. He was methodical and steady as he pressed for change at the FDA, helping to impress its consumer affairs director enough that she proposed ongoing meetings between the agency and ACT UP. Protest preparations continued through the month. So that all demonstrators would be capable of justifying the action and explaining its aims, Treatment + Data organized a series of "FDA Teach-Ins." Mark Harrington compiled a special issue of his famous glossary and gathered together a committee to produce an official ACT UP FDA handbook.

Taking charge of the media buildup to the demonstration was a former *People* magazine stringer named Michelangelo Signorile, whom Bob Rafsky had groomed for the job. Signorile's deputy was Chip Duckett, a club promoter known for creating buzzy events downtown. They devised a marketing push that made publicists for Madonna seem timid and dull. Reporters and editors at nearly every paper in the nation were on high alert. A crescendo of stories hit the radio, including a major piece on National Public Radio addressing the immorality of placebo trials.

Bordowitz spent the run-up to October 11 offering civil disobedience training, as did several other facilitators. Their programs included practice sessions for responding to simulated attacks, provocations, and arrests. In New York alone, nearly 250 people were prepared in this way.

As the day of the protest approached and with little progress on ACT UP's demands, the organizers requested a meeting with the FDA commissioner himself. In a sign of the agency's nervousness, Frank Young agreed, setting the summit for October 5. Jim Eigo and Mark Harrington would present the science for ACT UP. The issues of women and people of color would be addressed by Margaret McCarthy, the college student, and Ortez Alderson, the Chicago actor and director whose youthful political work helped hone a sharp rhetorical style. Staley and Bordowitz could speak as patients, but their main goal was to scope out the building in order to help with logistics; Bordowitz bought a video camera for that purpose.

When the six of them arrived at the meeting, they found that Young had gathered a large group of his senior staff, including Dr. Ellen Cooper, the agency's elusive point person on all regulatory matters associated with AIDS drugs. Cooper was spirited, intelligent, and young—at thirty-seven, she was just a year older than Alderson. She made no secret of her anger at being dragged into this meeting.

Eigo laid out the group's philosophy, and reviewed the list of demands in his deliberate and unadorned way. Young, as warm as Cooper was chilly, seemed understanding but on point after point claimed powerlessness. He saw no acceptable alternative to placebos, and was stubbornly noncommittal on any specific drugs, citing trade secrets and the rights of drugmakers, which were paramount, even in this time of dire emergency. When Alderson and McCarthy criticized the near-total exclusion of women, people of color, drug users, and children from the federal trials, Young was genuinely sympathetic. But drug companies were paying for these trials. Their beliefs—that people of color were prone to drop out of studies, and that women, because they might conceive a child while the experiments continued, posed unacceptable legal risks—were vulgar, but he could not force their hand one way or another.

Having said that, Young wanted his visitors to know that the regulators and the activists were "on the same team" about wanting to get these drugs evaluated and, where appropriate, released. When coffee and cookies arrived to signal the end of the summit, Harrington had reached the limit of his patience.

"The last decade has been a shameful one in the history of America," he snapped. "And history will record the names of those who have blocked access to lifesaving treatments to thousands of people with HIV and AIDS. At the top of that list will be those regulating AIDS drugs at the FDA."

ON A CHILLY October weekend, fleets of charter buses rolled toward Rockville, Maryland, from a dozen states. When the far-flung ACT UP chapters all came together for the first time that Monday night, the vast All Souls Church—a half hour outside Rockville—was standing-room only. More than twelve hundred activists had heeded Bordowitz's call. They shouted out their cities, and the names of the dead they came to honor. Maria Maggenti, reprising her moderator's role, was moved to tears and inarticulation.

"You're totally beautiful," she called to them. "Everyone here loves everyone! We should love each other because it's great!" Her effusion hit a chord. Everybody hugged and kissed and chanted back, reveling in that intoxicating blend of truth and force that Gandhi called *satyagraha*. "Seize control! Seize control!" they shouted. "ACT UP! Fight back! Fight AIDS!"

By far the biggest chapter came from New York, a turnout that happily surprised Bordowitz. The Testing the Limits collective arrived in force. There was a newly formed affinity group drawing special attention to issues related to women and AIDS, called the Delta Queens in memory of their adventures at the New Orleans convention over the summer. Maxine Wolfe, Maria Maggenti, and Heidi Dorow were members, as were the artist Avram Finkelstein and Costa Pappas, a videographer from Virginia. Mark Harrington came with his affinity group, esoterically called Wave Three, which also included a number of T+D members: Jim Eigo, David Z. Kirschenbaum, and Margaret McCarthy. Proving that ACT UP was now the most exciting thing happening in New York, Michael Musto, the *Village Voice*'s audacious nightlife columnist, tagged along. It seemed that everybody from the Village was there—except for Larry Kramer, who was back to keeping his distance.

The FDA building was a blocky, eighteen-story glass tower tucked awkwardly into the hillside of a quaint suburban neighborhood. The activists streamed toward the building after daybreak as slack-jawed locals stared from their driveways, unsure what was transpiring. Media coordinators pushed through the crowd recruiting geographically diverse spokespeople. "Anybody with AIDS from Atlanta?" "Is there a mother of a PWA from Ohio?"

Banks of television news cameras at the FDA doorway started recording when the noisy mob was still on the horizon. After a time, the protestors drew close enough that their words became clear: "AZT is not enough / Give us all the other stuff." A neighborhood resident who had been trimming his shrubbery took personal offense at the invasion of his quiet neighborhood, emerging from his garage with a roaring chain saw, but the police—in their dishwashing gloves—were quick to extinguish any threat of violence.

The event put on display the full range of activism being deployed within ACT UP and its spin-offs around the country. One group dressed as laid-to-rest corpses and on signal fell dead in the middle of the road to block traffic, holding aloft personalized tombstones: "I Got the Placebo—RIP," and "AZT Wasn't Enough." The Delta Queens hoisted a Reagan effigy up a flagpole on the FDA grounds while another faction, calling itself PISD (for People with Immune System Disorders), set up a lemonade stand to hawk dextran sulfate, a supposedly beneficial drug available over the counter in most of the world but kept from Americans by the FDA. People with AIDS hoped it had antiviral properties. The Forget-Me-Nots, the United Fruit Company, the Queer and Present Danger—there were twenty-five affinity groups with twenty-five plans, each one scripted, costumed, and improvised. Some of it was too profane for TV audiences: for instance, a sign that said, "FDA—Fucking Disaster Area," and T-shirts emblazoned with another acronym:

America
Isn't
Doing
Shit

Despite the anger there was a joyous, county fair–like tenor to the day's affair, unlike anything historians of grassroots movements had seen before. Through the windows, FDA employees laughed and snapped pictures. Even the police, seemingly unsure of the appropriate response, held off making arrests, to the chagrin of the activists. As the morning wore on, waves of demonstrators surged symbolically toward the doors, which were defended by two-deep lines of officers, taunting them. Harrington's Wave Three group grew restless. Huddling with the Delta Queens, they decided jointly to try to physically invade the building, literally to "seize control." Despite the physical risks, they linked arms and formed a wedge, ramming into the stolid blue line while screaming "Seize control! Seize control!" Even that failed to earn them handcuffs.

Staley had made his own plans, involving smoke bombs he had picked up from a fireworks store. When he was at the building to meet Frank Young, Staley noticed a solid awning over the entrance doors that jutted out like the brim of a baseball cap. At the first opportunity, Charlie Franchino, another activist, gave him a boost, literally hurling him onto the overhead structure. Scrambling to his feet, Staley threw his arms in the air and let loose a howl. The crowd below went wild—this was the closest to seizing control they would get that day.

Turning around, he realized he was eye to eye with the workers inside the building who had been glued to the window, nervous and titillated. What a sight he was, with a bandana tied Mishima style around his forehead, and wearing a black leather bomber jacket. He grinned broadly and mugged for the workers' cameras as he got his smoke bombs smoking.

And then from below he heard the booming voice of Michelangelo Signorile from the media committee. "Peter!" he called. "Peter! You've got to get down! I've got you on *Crossfire* tonight!" Signorile had convinced CNN's prime-time debate show, which pitted the right-wing ideologue Patrick Buchanan against a bumbling envoy from the left named Tom Braden, to weigh in on the FDA's role in AIDS drugs.

Looking down on the riot helmets aligned below him, Staley gave Signorile a shrug. "It's a little too late to tell me that," he shouted.

"Excuse me," Staley called to one of the police officers. "Can I talk to somebody in charge?" With a brief negotiation, he was allowed to dismount the building and slip back into the crowd.

The police finally began making arrests in early afternoon, starting with demonstrators who covered the windows of several patrol cars with SILENCE=DEATH stickers. Energized by the change in policy, the affinity groups went into overdrive, with a goal of maximizing the number of detainees. By 4 p.m., the total count was 185, hastily booked and released, with citations that carried $25 fines.

The press coverage surpassed anything Bordowitz had imagined. Signorile and Duckett had pulled off a staggering campaign. The protest and mass arrests led every newscast and made the morning papers in more than two hundred media markets. For Bordowitz, seeing the community reflected back through the television was a powerful affirmation—images of potent gay people were brand new in the popular media.

And there, suddenly, was the face of Peter Staley, wearing a SILENCE=DEATH sweatshirt, in the opening sequence of *Crossfire*. Though he felt his lunch in his throat, Staley looked entirely at ease, an impressive performance given that it was his first time in the gladiators' den of national television. Braden made the first move. "Peter Staley, you have the AIDS virus and I am sorry," he said. "But don't you think that the Federal Drug Administration has a responsibility not to let people such as you have *quacks* that could cause even more harm than you already have?"

"The problem is," Staley said, his voice a notch higher than usual, "the FDA is using the same process to test a nasal spray as it is to test AIDS drugs, and it's a seven-to-ten-year process." He looked boyish in his floppy curls. Nerves exaggerated his slight speech impediment—his tongue slowed as he maneuvered through the many sibilants.

"You have the FDA giving you a drug," Braden said. "So far you've got AZT. Why—"

"Which I can't take, because it's far too toxic," Staley interrupted. "And over half the people that have HIV can't take."

"Okay, but the FDA says there is nothing else that is worth anything!"

"Mr. Staley," called Buchanan from across the table, seizing the lead. "This is going to astonish you, but I agree with you a hundred percent." Staley spun in his chair to look into the large, white face of the man who wrote speeches for presidents Nixon, Ford, and Reagan. About AIDS, he had frequently made his prejudices clear. "The poor homosexuals. They have declared war against nature, and nature is exacting an awful retribution," he once said.

Yet here he was on ACT UP's side. He had not developed a sudden concern for gay plague victims. What interested him was extending the Reagan doctrine of deregulation to the FDA as well. He held that the marketplace, and not the exacting precepts of science, should determine a drug's future. "I think if someone's got AIDS and someone wants to take a drug, it's their life and it gives them hope—you ought to be able to take it. What I want to ask you is whether you know of anything that you think might be some kind of miraculous cure that you think they're sitting on at the FDA."

Staley answered cogently, not slowing when Buchanan tried to interrupt. "There are over 140 drugs out there that the FDA has identified as possibilities and are in some stage of being looked at right now. Among that 140, there's gotta be one or a combination thereof that can—that can slow down this virus or halt it in its tracks."

"What would you like to take?"

"I'd like to take dextran sulfate—legally," he said. "I'm taking it on the underground right now."

"Well, why not, Mr. Braden?"

Braden, tall and wrinkled, showed himself to be slow-footed. "Because," he said. "Well." He looked at Staley. "Oh, I don't know anything about dextran sulfate, and neither do you."

"I'll tell you this," Staley reproved him. "It's an over-the-counter drug in Japan and has been for twenty years. *Over the counter!* I'm only asking that they be released after there's a minimal amount of efficacy, not a 100 percent test."

That was the point Buchanan wished to make, laid out beautifully by his guest. Business done, he now turned to his base. "Looking in the camera," he said, "what would you tell some kid, say you had a younger brother, twenty-one years old who also, uh, might have homosexual tendencies. What would you tell him if you wanted him to live a long life?"

Here, Staley bested him. "Use a condom," he said. "And also to use a lubricant, by the way, that—"

Buchanan was apoplectic. "This is Russian roulette! Aren't you—"

"It is Russian roulette," Staley calmly interjected, a slight smile forming on his face, "to not give people the information when human nature dictates that they're gonna go out there and they're gonna have sex."

Buchanan never regained his footing against Staley. A star was born—the first true AIDS star. And through the long weekend of protests in Maryland, a nation was reached. AIDS activism moved from the defensive to the offensive. As Kiki Mason reported in the *New York Native,* somewhat fantastically, "In the long war on AIDS this past weekend may be remembered as Gettysburg. We still have much heartache and bloodshed ahead of us. We can take it. The tide has turned. Victory will be ours."

ACT UP followed up in the coming weeks with a letter, mailed October 31, 1988, to each of the 2,230 FDA employees, in an effort to explain, as the subject line stated, "Why I Demonstrated at the FDA." "Our action was not directed at you or your co-workers. We recognize that the employees of the FDA are working under the same endless rules, regulations and red tape that are killing thousands of Americans. We are in a desperate fight for lives—ours and yours. We are up against an unresponsive and destructive bureaucracy. It is conservatively estimated that a million and a half Americans are presently HIV antibody positive. By the inauguration of our next president, in January, the number of Americans who have died from AIDS will surpass the total number of Americans who died in the Vietnam War," the letter said. "One of the positive things that has become clear during this crisis is how powerful and effective an individual can be. We have learned that individuals joining together can make the difference. That is where you fit in. We'd like your support and understanding. We'd like your ideas and information. We'd like your help."

EXCEPT FOR HIS occasional appearances, Kramer had been gone from New York and the movement for nearly a year. He had rented a place in the country and kept a strict writer's schedule. When he returned to New York City, he had a new play, a venomous parody he called *Just Say No,* lifting a phrase from Nancy Reagan's famous anti-drug refrain. The action was framed in a Georgetown townhouse, with characters based on Ronald Reagan Jr., Mayor Ed Koch, and the first lady herself, depicted as a sex-hungry shrew. Kramer intended it as a "play about a farce."

It opened at the WPA Theater, an off-Broadway house in Chelsea, two weeks after the FDA demonstration. Far from the masterpiece Kramer had promised in his ACT UP farewell, the play was abhorred by critics and detested by audiences. "Imagine the worst possible taste," Mel Gussow wrote in the *Times*, "then take it several steps further." *The Christian Science Monitor* called it "an exercise in churlishness and scurrility." It closed in a few weeks, a colossal flop, and sent Kramer spiraling into self-doubt. Unlike the vitriol stirred up by *Faggots,* these critics focused scorn not on content but on lack of artistry. Mortified and brooding, he kept an unusually low profile. The anxiety triggered a congenital hernia condition and in November he went for a trip under the knife, life imitating art.

Unexpectedly, the hernia surgeon discovered that Kramer, never a drinker, had a liver ravaged by cirrhosis. A chronic active hepatitis B infection, something he likely acquired sexually during the 1970s, was the cause. And there was something else. Kramer was also HIV positive. That news stunned him. He had abstained from unsafe sex from the first days of the epidemic. Certain minor health complaints, mostly dermatological, made him wonder about his prognosis, but he had taken a firm personal stand not to be tested, not wanting a positive result looming over his head. Doctors performed the test anyway because the hepatitis B treatment he urgently needed was an immunosuppressant, so they needed to know his status.

The dual diagnosis put him in a medical bind. If he treated the hepatitis aggressively, AIDS would take him away in two or three years, but doing nothing would mean an even quicker death by cirrhosis. He immediately started on a regimen of colchicine, propranolol, spironolactone, and Mephyton, all of which slowly pushed his CD4s downward, as predicted. His gums bled and his intestines erupted, but the drugs improved his liver function and allowed him to return to his normal daily life. His infectious disease doctor wanted him to begin taking AZT, but Dr. Sonnabend, whom he consulted, spoke just as adamantly against it. It was an agonizing decision. Kramer filled a prescription, but ultimately decided against using the drug. He'd seen how it had debilitated others, and he worried that the side effects would interfere with what remained of his writing life.

Instead, Kramer turned his extreme will against HIV, coupled with more mystical forces. As an atheist, he rejected prayer. But he started wearing a trove of Native American jewelry because long ago a fortune-teller had said to him, "Always wear something turquoise, it will protect you and bolster your health." He crammed heavy amulets on his fingers, wrists, and neck. They rattled and clacked against one another when he walked and clashed with his Oxford-cloth shirts and Brooks Brothers slacks. Although they had little effect on the skin blemishes, eruptions, itches, and scaling that were haunting him, the jewelry (plus numerous vitamins) did allow him to feel he was taking care of himself. He felt he was in control of an uncontrollable situation.

GRIFFIN GOLD remained in the ICU for over a month. Not only did he survive the chemo and the pneumonia, but he gained strength and a modicum of his spirit. Soon, he was well enough to return to his small apartment on Christopher Street and resume his duties as a PWA Coalition board member. From time to time, he even made appearances at ACT UP meetings and events.

Staley had not visited him since their tense encounter at St. Luke's, kept away by his own gutlessness about death. Knowing he needed to make amends, he bought tickets to Key West for the two of them. They arrived on December 6 and checked into a magnificent room at the Cypress House, a historic mansion just off Duval Street. It was not an easy journey for Gold, who took to bed directly and resisted all of Staley's attempts to take him sightseeing, except for a single trip to the beach. One afternoon halfway through their time together, Staley gave Gold a pep talk. It only made matters worse. Gold sat listless on the edge of the bed and wept.

"I'm scared about dying," he admitted. "I'm really frightened."

Staley sat down beside him and put an arm over his fragile shoulder. Gold collapsed against him. "I know," Staley said. "We don't know what's going to happen. But we have to keep on fighting—we both have to keep on fighting." Staley didn't offer false hope. They were both marked for premature death, of that he was certain. He wrapped his arms around Gold. "This is frightening," he agreed.

They returned home a few days later, on a morning when temperatures fell below zero and icy gusts of wind tore at Gold's skin on the taxicab line. He declined precipitously and soon was back in the hospital, with time running short. Again, Peter Staley couldn't find the courage to visit.

Gold's estranged mother joined her son's bedside support network. She got to know his doctors and his best friends, Michael Lesser and Ray Balsys. And in her own way she was able to express her love for him genuinely, and just in time. On one of the coldest days of the frigid winter, a fungus swept into Gold's lungs and claimed his life at age thirty-three. That same week, five other members of the PWA Coalition died.

The *Times* ran a tiny obituary in which Gold was said to have been survived by his mother. But she didn't allow her name to be used, nor did she correct the writer on his true name: he was memorialized as Griffin Gold, his nom de guerre, not as Paul Frederick Griffin III, the name his family gave him then took back once he became a prominent gay leader. The obit was a fitting honor for a warrior of his stature, a Malcolm X of the plague.

Lesser and Balsys organized a "Celebration of Life" at Judson Memorial Church for Gold's friends and colleagues. The socialite Judy Peabody, one of Gold's GMHC buddies, was there. So were Dr. Sonnabend, Larry Kramer, and Michael Callen and the top leadership of the PWA Coalition, GMHC, and AmFAR. This was a send-off befitting a hero and martyr, as grand and historic as any AIDS memorial that had come before it.

In one of his last acts, Gold had called Staley to request a piano recital in his honor. Staley hated the idea, but he could not refuse the dying wish of the man who had been so important to him. He chose a heartbreaking farewell, Brahms's Intermezzo in A Major, op. 118, no. 2. His playing was rich and moving, with all of the emotional texture of his best years as a child prodigy, but his face was a steely mask of grief. When it was over, he rose stiffly from the keyboard and knew he would never play the piano again.

STALEY HAD no head for science. The first scientific article he ever read was in the *Discover* magazine he picked up on that day he was diagnosed, which despite being geared toward the general public was as opaque to him as the first time he looked at the compositions of Claude Debussy or the treacherous Charles Ives. By reading the article very slowly, he found he could vaguely grasp the differences between this type of cell and that kind of virus. He'd gotten much more agile with the discipline in the intervening years. With reasonable accuracy, he could now describe the diabolical action of reverse transcriptase and the ways in which AZT struggled to inhibit it. But he knew he would never master the technical details, not the way Mark Harrington had, or the rest of Iris Long's protégés, who seemed to thrive in the intersections of immunology, biology, virology, and chemistry. He had begun attending their meetings early on in search of his own treatment options, and continued going because of the forceful encouragement of Herb Spiers and Charlie Franchino, two ACT UP friends who were members.

The weekly discussion remained frustratingly above his head. He could scarcely comprehend Iris Long, who had not improved as a public speaker. Only Jim Eigo seemed able to decode her. So he took it upon himself to offer simultaneous translations of her insights. But as Eigo tended toward the obtuse himself, it fell to Mark Harrington to filter the science once more. Eventually Staley came to a reasonable command of the issues.

In the fall of 1988 the committee took on two extremely young members. Spencer Cox was twenty, though he looked much younger, a southerner by way of Bennington College, a school he chose specifically because its lack of a core curriculum meant he would not have to take any science courses. He majored in drama and the bygone gay art form known as camp. Cox came out when he was just twelve, and had a strong immediate identification with the community. He was back home in Atlanta when ACT UP descended on the convention, and was immediately enamored of the group's combination of theatrics and purpose. So when money ran out for his final year in Vermont, he headed for New York to find the group. It blew him away to see Susan Sarandon and Tim Robbins sitting in the front row one week, and Janeane Garofalo on another, to no particular fanfare. Activism was hot, and he was thrilled to take part.

He gravitated toward the media committee initially, proving himself adept at crafting press releases and answering questions. In order to help journalists with their more scientific understanding, he forced himself into an apprenticeship to Mark Harrington. All the T+D people intimidated Cox. It wasn't just their serious intellects that struck him, but also the reversed social strata they represented—"all the nerds from high school and they're cool now," he told me.

Despite his fear of science, he proved a quick study on everything but immunology. At the Strand Book Store he picked up a secondhand copy of an immunology textbook that he studied every night, hoping to disentangle humoral from cell mediated, innate from adaptive. Staley was impressed at the young man's capacity. When he heard that Cox had committed to memory the entire script of George Cukor's 1939 film *The Women*, he had no doubt it was true.

At about the same time Cox arrived, Staley noticed that a very quiet teenage girl with a funny-sounding name had started showing up. Intrepid and darkly beautiful, Garance Franke-Ruta had dropped out of school and had made her way to New York with dreams of becoming a hat designer. A drag queen she knew invited her to an ACT UP demonstration when she was seventeen, and she was hooked. When she discovered she had a head for the technical stuff, she gravitated to Iris Long's group. "Science club," she called it, like it was an after-school activity. Based on their closeness in age, Franke-Ruta felt an immediate affinity with Cox as well as with Derek Link, another young man who arrived before completing school. They jokingly called themselves "the chicken caucus" because of their young ages. Of this group, Franke-Ruta had the most to learn about gay culture, but Cox took her by the hand. "Let me introduce you to Bette Davis," he said.

The work of T+D was taken over by AZT. Iris Long had compiled a damning report on Burroughs Wellcome's recalcitrant pricing strategy, laying out the familiar chronology of taxpayer-funded research, corporate profiteering, and patient impoverishment. But while compiling her research Long discovered something nobody had known. The company had opened a program on its own to supply poor patients with AZT if they couldn't get it any other way. Nobody knew this because Wellcome never publicized the program. There was no press release announcing it, and it was never revealed to government overseers at the FDA or elsewhere. One had to call the company's North Carolina headquarters—specifically the office of public affairs, as Long had done—to learn of its existence. Only shareholders, whom the phantom program was meant to impress, had any clue.

She called the company's role in the epidemic "obscene."

With so much taxpayer money flowing to Burroughs Wellcome, it meant that the steady increase in federal allocations to fight the epidemic represented more of a corporate handout than anything that might help the sick or vulnerable. Representative Ted Weiss, continuing his investigative advocacy in Washington, held hearings on the 1989 AIDS budget, which the White House now claimed was $2 billion. He learned that one-third of that total represented Medicaid benefits that would have been paid out regardless of the administration's actions, and another third was for future spending, not available in 1989. Weiss determined that the amount newly allocated for AIDS in the coming year was just $585 million—less than the government spent on military outlays *per day*. Much of that went to enriching Burroughs Wellcome.

"The American people deserve more than a quick-handed shell game from the White House on AIDS," Weiss said. "Ineffective commissions, [inadequate] budgets, and stalled education and research campaigns will be the sad legacy of Ronald Reagan on AIDS."

• • •

A BITTERSWEET 1988 Thanksgiving celebration took place in Callen's new apartment. He and Dworkin laid out a meal for seven of their friends, all men with AIDS and all with very little reason for cheer. George Herbert Walker Bush had just been elected president—"Reagan's third term," the papers were predicting—meaning that the funding drought would likely continue. The convention that preceded the election was a festival of open hostility toward gays, with Senator Orrin Hatch winding up the GOP base against what he called "the party of homosexuals." No lawmaker on the left was bothered enough to complain. In the fall Congress kept a steady focus on legislation regarding gay employment: the peculiarly named Fair Employment Practices Resolution, which passed with a 9 to 1 spread, established the right of federal lawmakers to refuse to hire "anyone whose life style they decide is unacceptable," as *The New York Times* reported.

At least the dinner guests were all able to perambulate and hold down food, a small miracle. Two of them filled plates to take to their lovers at home, too sick or depressed to make the trip. Another came without his lover, who, in what was becoming a tradition in the community, had instead flown home to bid family farewell. One guest said, with as much pathos as if he were discussing the cranberries, "The saddest thing is, I don't cry anymore when someone tells me they've been diagnosed."

Callen forced himself to count his blessings: his beloved cookie-cutter collection, the imminent release of Streisand's next album, the pleasure of watching Julia Child videos, and the secure sensation of his lover coming to bed—it all made him want to weep with joy. "I should miss them so, if I died," he said sincerely. What he wouldn't miss was AIDS politics, now safely in his past. In his spare time, he committed himself to leading a new project he called PWA Singles' Teas: in essence, speed-dating events that had already produced a number of couples, but more significantly helped people address the idea of being "damaged goods," no longer romantically desirable or available because of their diagnosis. Among the many powers he attributed to love was survival itself. Six and a half years into his relationship with Richard Dworkin, Callen felt he could confidently predict that he would survive AIDS. Even so, he was never quite sure Dworkin would stay by his side if his health were to recede, and on regular intervals sought assurances that Dworkin would not leave him. "Never," Dworkin would promise, banishing that doubt momentarily.

When the table was cleared, Dworkin helped apply medicated lotion to Callen's recurring rash. There on the back of his lover's arm, Dworkin found the unmistakable outlines of a KS lesion. It was deep in color, the shape and size of a lima bean. It felt slightly leathery, like a misshapen mole, not tumor-like at all. It was hard to imagine it as the fearsome cancer he knew it was. He let his finger pass over the spot, wondering how KS would change Callen's confidence, how KS would change their lives.

5

Denial

Peter Staley and Mark Harrington asked Burroughs Wellcome for a meeting to discuss the festering price dispute. It was the first direct contact made with the company in the two years since it created gales of protest. Lisa Behrens from the company's public affairs department invited them to Research Triangle Park in North Carolina for a meeting and a tour of the pharmaceutical giant's massive headquarters, a cluster of pyramidal buildings evoking a fantastical colony on Mars. They flew down on January 23, 1989, a perfect pair for this mission: Harrington, with his debate-team-like skills; Staley, with his facility with the language of business and money.

Behrens, a short and wound-up woman fresh from college, personally retrieved them from the airport with nervous effusions about everything from the wonderful weather to the recently expanded airport. Her chatter continued on the drive to the facility and the march through the outcropping of Brutalist-style buildings and their perplexing floor plans. (Fittingly, the concrete colossus was the filming location for *Brainstorm*, a sci-fi thriller featuring Natalie Wood and Christopher Walken.) After a time, they were delivered to a sparkling greenhouse beside a luminescent reflecting pond, where a table was set for lunch.

There they were introduced to three men in dark suits and defensive smiles: Tom Kennedy and W. Thack Brown, corporate VPs involved in communications, one of them no older than thirty, and Dr. David Barry, the company's head of virology. Though young himself, Barry was already an industry legend, known as Mr. AZT for having collaborated so profitably with Sam Broder at the NCI. With his translucent gold eyes and tightly animated face, he was an arresting figure, intimidating and inscrutable—as much businessman as scientist. His body language expressed his conviction that the meeting was for amelioration, not negotiation.

Harrington had prepared himself by donning his trademark white jeans and a matching denim jacket, pulled over a rumpled ACT UP T-shirt—"punk formalwear," he called it. "Our goal," he explained rather grandly, "is not to target specific individuals for abuse, but rather to effect some kind of change within the entire system involving doctors, clinicians, researchers, companies, the community. The factor missing in all these deliberations is the community. For the first time in the history of medicine, a community is aroused around an issue, and in many cases knows more about the issue" than the experts themselves.

Harrington lit a cigarette, sending Lisa Behrens scrambling for an ashtray. "This is the basis for the lack of trust: people are being driven into poverty to pay for your drug," he continued. "People who lack access are dying because they can't get your drug. It's very ironic that the company which produces the first approved, effective treatment for this disease is held in universal hatred and disdain."

Barry regarded Harrington with bemusement. Matching his provocation, Barry lit a cigarette of his own. "Number one," he said, "if a patient is dying because he can't afford AZT, something's wrong somewhere other than us, because we have a program where if a person needs the drug—"

"Nobody knows about it," Harrington interrupted.

"—and none of the usual mechanisms for drug funding are available, we give them the drug."

"The patients most in need do not know about the program," Harrington repeated. For that matter, neither did their doctors or hospital administrators, who were incentivized to overlook an AIDS diagnosis in charity patients, treating only their opportunistic infections and not the considerably more expensive underlying disease. Harrington rattled off the results of a study by New York's chief epidemiologist that found that AIDS deaths among uninsured IV-drug users were underreported by 130 percent—2,520 deaths, which were attributed to causes like endocarditis or encephalitis rather than AIDS, might have been staved off by AZT.

"You have a fig leaf program which provides AZT for three hundred people but which nobody has ever heard of."

"If you can give me documentation of an AIDS patient going into a New York City hospital where he's being potentially misdiagnosed, that is *criminal*," Barry said. "And I would be more than happy to help you go to the New York district attorney."

"It's well documented. It's been in *The New York Times*," Staley joined in. Though he wore an expensive suit, with his small body and whiskerless face Staley looked more like a youthful Wall Streeter than a fearsome opponent.

"There are lots of things in *The New York Times* that may or may not be true," Barry said.

"It's not *mis*-diagnosis, it's *not* diagnosing. . . . And it's documented. They're showing that thousands of deaths of IV-drug users never got diagnosed. And that wasn't an accident."

What happened in a distant city hospital seemed of little consequence to Barry. The smile never left his face.

"Although you don't realize it, because you're far from the scene of the actual battles, people are dying," Harrington continued. "All the time. People are dying because they do not have access to the drug which is priced beyond the range of most of them, and which in many states is not available. And you're totally washing your hands of responsibility for it."

This angered Barry. He snubbed out his cigarette and immediately lit another. "I think it's really casting aspersions on our morality, which I don't think are appropriate, to say we're washing our hands of it," he said. "We're doing lots of things. Now, maybe we're not effective enough in those areas. Maybe we need to do more and we will be doing more, but believe me, we feel the burden of that illness and death every day." He shifted aggressively in his chair. "I do think we need to talk to each other. Because I don't think our goals are that much different."

"Well, if we don't get any price reduction, we're not going to get closer," Staley fired back.

"Tell us what we can do."

"Lower the price."

"I've got to have an income," Barry said impatiently. "We have all kinds of very, very sophisticated accountants working out how much is available for research, how much each product within our whole panoply has to cost. If you decrease the amount of money that comes in from any product, be it Neosporin, AZT, acyclovir, Septra, you name it, it's going to be that much of a decrease for the amount we have on research."

"Are you claiming that there's not enough profit that you're making off AZT?" Staley asked. "See, I've done a little arithmetic on my own." He snapped open his briefcase and pulled out a portfolio, which he dropped on the table between them. "We're hearing a profit margin in December '87 of about 60 percent."

"I don't know what you mean by profit. Is that gross revenues minus what the sales brought?"

Tom Kennedy, the top corporate affairs official, jumped in to confirm. "Classic GP," he agreed. "That's right."

Staley continued. "And this is what we're hearing from a lot of analysts: that it's increased over time to 80 percent."

Criticizing the margins on one drug misunderstood the way the industry worked, Barry said. "Ask those analysts what the profit margin has been on the four hundred other compounds that I've had more than fifty people working on over the last three years."

"You're talking about R&D again," Staley acknowledged. He got it. "That's the cost of R&D. But—"

"We'd only have less of a probability of discovering innovative new therapies for everything—Alzheimer's, multiple sclerosis, cancer, you name it. But also for HIV infection," Barry added unnecessarily.

Staley shot a look at Harrington, then lowered his voice to a firm, steady timbre. "There is this vague concept of excess profit here, and it's very hard to define, but you went point by point by point to try to refute that the world doesn't need that money as much as you," he said. "I think you can stand a price reduction without any problem. That's what I'm trying to say."

"Well, *I* hear you," said Tom Kennedy, hoping to diffuse the tensions while committing to nothing.

"Sure, it's going to hurt the price of your stock," Staley continued. "If I were a trader, I'd sell as soon as you reduced the price."

This concession struck Barry as unexpectedly forthright. He wasn't about to let it go without putting it center stage. "If our price goes down, then our ability to borrow or expand our operations and everything else will go down too," he said. "You've been on Wall Street long enough to know that that single thing affects a lot of other issues."

Staley shook his head. "I don't think it's going to affect your credit rating. It's not going to affect your ability to borrow." He said this with such deep authority that even Barry was sure it was true. He was momentarily speechless.

The conversation turned to trial designs and economic conditions in Africa, without resolving the issue at hand. When the meeting broke up, Barry left the New Yorkers at the elevator bank and Lisa Behrens and her two vice presidents walked them out the door, past the dull, heavy buildings and toward the vast expanse of parking lot.

"Just think," said W. Thack Brown, putting his gleaming teeth to the task of positive spin, "in a few years, we'll all look back on this and—"

Harrington spun around abruptly. "Not all of us will be around to look back," he seethed.

Staley wasn't paying close attention. He was silently memorizing the building's layout, its siting and visibility from the road, and the number of guarded checkpoints. He was already planning to return.

IT HAD NOW BEEN two years since ACT UP formed and seven months since the town hall meeting had sought to reset its agenda, and still they had failed in their main objective to get drugs flowing into bodies. Besides AZT, there were no other antivirals on the market or even in trials. In contrast, the underground marketplace was burgeoning. Buyers clubs around the country were pedaling unapproved drugs by the truckload, but none of them seemed to do any good. Certainly nobody was being cured. The one thing extending life dramatically wasn't AZT but the campaign to prevent opportunistic infections. And in that arena, ACT UP had gained some ground. The FDA still blocked full approval for the anti-blindness drug DHPG, and had not yet begun a clinical trial, but as a compromise the agency announced a special plan to allow for its limited distribution free of charge to people with CMV retinitis. The numbers of patients on the "compassionate use" program quickly jumped from three thousand to more than five thousand, with hundreds more signing up for DHPG every month, but the epidemic of blindness grew at an even faster pace.

Syntex Corporation of Palo Alto, California, DHPG's manufacturer, then gathered data from those patients' doctors, which is exactly what Bill Bahlman proposed at his dinner with Tony Fauci. On average, doctors administering DHPG observed an 80 percent improvement in preventing blindness. This was no substitute for a clinical trial, but it added to the overwhelming evidence in favor of the drug. Syntex took the data to the FDA with a plea for full approval, but the advisory committee refused to consider the anecdotal data. The committee's opinion was not subject to appeal. If the company hoped to release DHPG, it was going to have to conduct the controlled clinical trial it was lacking. It took most of the year for Syntex to submit a trial design to the FDA. When the details leaked out the community went wild. The study required half the patients with early CMV retinitis to be randomly assigned to placebos for a period of twelve weeks or until their sight measurably deteriorated. Treatment + Data sent Fauci a stinging rebuke. Patients voted with their feet. Instead of risking blindness, anyone in need turned to the compassionate use program instead. This put the research firmament in a bind. Unwilling to consider a trial without placebo controls, the FDA announced plans to cancel the expanded-access program, a move meant to coerce patients into the study.

The move nearly caused riots. Iris Long alerted a *New York Times* writer to the reversal while other activists wrote letters of outrage and complaint about the Public Health Service's inhumane policy. The standoff showed no signs of resolution. When Eigo learned of a meeting in Bethesda of a group convened by President Bush to study the AIDS drugs pipeline, he and about thirty ACT UPers boarded a bus on the morning of February 1 to offer unsolicited testimony. They formed a picket line at the doorway of the hotel where the meeting was taking place, handing out informational literature to panelists as they arrived.

Bill Bahlman was there under changed circumstances. He was now HIV positive. The news came without any sign of illness; he felt terrific. And since his negative test in 1987 he had kept himself as safe as a dog on a leash. In these times, sexual confinement was not especially challenging. Physical intimacy in the age of AIDS induced in him waves of anxiety and self-recrimination—protection by Pavlovian conditioning. But it had done him little good. He nearly fainted from the news. The doctor surmised that his previous test result was a false negative, and that Bahlman had been infected in the mid-'80s. He had two years to look forward to.

He retired as a prominent club DJ and reinvented himself as a freelance AIDS correspondent for a public-access cable show called *Out in the '80s*. This was not a wise financial move, given the meager pay it offered. His incessant activism had already put him a year behind in his rent and plunged his apartment into darkness after the power was cut off for lack of payment. The road now would entail even more sacrifice. But it put him squarely on the front lines, where he had a better chance at survival.

Standing in the morning breezes outside the Bush-sponsored meeting, wearing a tie and a tweed jacket, Bahlman gripped the microphone enthusiastically, like a lanky kid lip-synching to Diana Ross.

"We're with Jim Eigo of ACT UP, and there's a major protest going on here in Bethesda over the drug DHPG. Tell us what's happening," he said, blinking into the camera's eye.

Eigo, in his trademark brightly colored T-shirt and wiry black hair tightened into a bun, introduced the complex issues to Bahlman's audience. "This is the second meeting of the Bush Commission for reviewing procedures for approving AIDS and cancer drugs," he said. "And we thought, since the non-approval of DHPG is such a perfect example of how regulation has gone wrong, we'd bring it home to the commission itself by showing up here in force. And that's exactly what we've done."

Bahlman said, "Also, inside at the hearing itself I understand there's going to be an action in just a little while when Ellen Cooper speaks."

"I guess so," Eigo agreed.

Bahlman turned to Heidi Dorow. "What do you think it means to these government officials—these federal officials involved in research—when they see a demonstration like this right at their doorstep?"

Dorow, crisply attired in a leather bomber jacket, brushed blond bangs from her eyes with her thumb. "Obviously, they think of people like us as 'the fringe.' But I think they're also shocked by our knowledge, our expertise with the language, the information. And I think it scares them. Frankly, I think that's important, us scaring them, putting the pressure on them to act."

Inside, thirty members of the group were wedged into the small meeting hall, silently waving colorful placards reading "See The Light. DHPG Works," or else hoisting their watches aloft to underscore their urgency. They outnumbered the scientists in attendance, straining the capacity of the room and causing a heavy tension. It was their anarchic appearance, more than their message, that put the scientists on edge. Heavy stormtrooper boots and leather jackets were worn menacingly, though often accessorized with ostentatious earrings and asymmetrical haircuts. One young man added a SILENCE=DEATH sweatshirt and a long skirt, with a spray of beads in his curly mane. Spencer Cox, leaning against a wall nearest to the podium, brandished a flier declaring that the government had "blood on its hands." A shimmer of fear crossed the faces of the panelists.

The activists remained respectful for hours, awaiting Dr. Cooper's turn on the agenda, and they didn't interrupt her until she had finished her presentation on approval procedures at her division. As she headed from the rostrum back to her seat, activists lobbed questions from the edges of the room.

"What about DHPG?"

"Why are people being allowed to go blind?"

"Have you read our statements?"

Pulling a few pages from her files, she crossed back to the podium. Her face was tight as usual, but in an electric-blue suit with a contrasting velvet collar she appeared younger and more vulnerable than the activists had expected. "Anticipating this question, I've made a few notes. What I'll do is first recite what's happened with DHPG."

"It would not be compassionate to not give the drug," one of the ACT UPers yelled.

"Let me go on," she scolded. "We really felt—at the FDA—stuck between a rock and a hard place." A low salvo of boos distracted her momentarily. "If we . . . approved the drug on the basis of the widespread belief in the community, even though many of us shared that belief, without objective data, we feel that we would indeed be on treacherous grounds in defending that decision, and in fact would be wide open to the charge of arbitrary decision making. Although, we certainly wouldn't be accused of being inflexible."

A man with a high voice called out, "You did it with AZT, I don't see why you can't do it with DHPG!"

Cooper momentarily let her anger show. She raised a finger to the heckler, flared her nostrils, and snapped, "I have to say that the difference in the data between AZT and DHPG is the difference between night and day."

Timmy Vance, the man wearing the long skirt, corrected her. "Between sight and blindness," he shouted. A sprawling war of words broke out that only subsided when the chairman of the commission called in the guards. As the protestors were escorted out, they shouted, "Ellen Cooper has ice in her veins. Fire that woman!"

Thereafter they referred to her as "the Ice Queen."

Disheartened by the unproductive confrontation, Heidi Dorow and Spencer Cox led half the group straight from the meeting to the NIH campus, a short ride by metro, to request an emergency meeting with Fauci. They had no appointment, but Fauci received a small delegation fronted by Bill Monaghan, a redhead with a soft, calming voice. The meeting was brief. When the team reemerged, Monaghan gathered the ACT UP representatives on the lawn to give a report.

"We basically said, We need a White Knight in this situation. We need somebody to defend us. We need somebody to say, A mistake was made. People don't have to suffer because of that mistake. And he said to us he would talk directly to Frank Young today, and try to meet with him next week and ask him, Is there a way that DHPG could possibly be released?"

Fauci did as promised. The following Monday, Dr. Young told the senior staff at the FDA that he was reevaluating not only the cancellation of compassionate access to DHPG but the need for a drug trial at all. Then Young dictated a letter to Mark Harrington's attention at ACT UP.

"Many people believe there is sufficient evidence in existence to approve ganciclovir (DHPG) for marketing. Because that belief is so widespread, and because the first results from the controlled clinical trial will soon be available, I have decided to reconvene our Anti-Infective Drugs Advisory Committee on May 2 to examine the latest data on the drug's safety and efficacy. We will supplement the Committee with additional experts in AIDS virology and ophthalmology," he said. He even invited ACT UP to place a speaker on the meeting's agenda, which was unheard of in the history of drug regulation.

The walls had begun to tumble.

EVERYONE WAS SURPRISED to see Larry Kramer meander into an ACT UP meeting one chilly night that winter. He reserved a spot to speak late in the agenda. He had been devastated by the dire findings on most of the underground drugs. The drug that drew Rock Hudson and hundreds of others to Paris, HPA-23, made no difference whatsoever. Suramin, a fifty-year-old Swedish drug for treating parasitic infections that was believed to have immune-boosting properties, was inexplicably fatal in some PWAs. Even dextran sulfate, the drug Staley had advocated during his *Crossfire* appearance on CNN, was a bust. After the massive FDA demonstration, chastised researchers finally took that drug into the lab only to discover that it made a hasty trip through the urinary tract without ever being properly absorbed. It was the placebo effect that made Staley feel better on dextran sulfate.

Through all of this, Kramer had stayed out of the limelight. He was at work on another play, an autobiographical prequel to *The Normal Heart*. News of its focus on Kramer family foibles irked his brother and sister-in-law, and presaged a sharp estrangement. For many months the Kramer brothers didn't speak; for many more, they only yelled. After the eventual rapprochement, things were not the same, and Kramer chose to turn more of his attention to AIDS. Part of his motivation was personal and urgent. His own CD4s were declining, producing the first real evidence of his own infection.

AIDS was all that he could think about. Recently he had made love for the first time in five years, but ended the relationship after five dates, neurotically worried about spreading disease even despite precautions. He felt as toxic as Love Canal.

The Monday-night meetings had become standing-room-only events since Kramer last attended. A small anteroom on the eastern wall of the derelict meeting hall was also full, and still more people spilled out the back door to the garden. Microphones now were needed for the moderators to keep order and the committee reports to be heard. The gatherings were hyperactive assemblies touching on a wide range of subjects, from prospects for gay marriage to life insurance laws to the advisability of leasing versus purchasing a large copying machine. Squabbles were frequent and sudden, whipping up like tornados and skating off just as fast. There was a sense of purpose and urgency, but sometimes the showmanship could seem more important than the cause. Democracy, Kramer thought, is as wily as a virus itself: just when you thought it was advancing in an orderly fashion, it mutated—it built up resistance to the energy and ideas it once thrived on and began to feed on something else, often quite unrelated.

He held his tongue until a speaker used her time to discuss the Haitian refugees being held in Guantánamo Bay or a proposal to honor the anti-apartheid boycott movement. Kramer exploded. He demanded to know why nobody was talking about drugs. Now he claimed to have five hundred dead friends. In the early days, he kept a little green notebook of names—people in his circle, or in the circles of people in his circle (the hairdresser of his sister-in-law was one example). Thereafter he clipped obituaries with familiar names and tossed them into a box. Five hundred dead friends would not be dead if ACT UP had won effective drugs.

He waved a sheet of paper over his head. Does anyone know what's going on in San Francisco? he asked, adding, You're talking about making Xerox copies; they're talking about Compound Q.

A few heads nodded vigorously. Reports out of the University of California, San Francisco, suggested great excitement about the compound, which had a long history in traditional Chinese medicine as a late-term abortifacient.

Kramer said Compound Q had people dancing in the streets in San Francisco. They called it the long-awaited AIDS cure.

A hush fell on the room. Nobody had ever before used the word *cure*.

Kramer said he had been on the telephone with Martin Delaney at San Francisco's Project Inform. A very small Phase I trial was ongoing there, but the rumor mill was on fire. What's more, the protein extract—technically called trichosanthin, from *Trichosanthes kirilowii*, a common landscaping plant also known as Chinese cucumber—managed miracles in studies in vitro: it seemed to have a laser-like ability to kill infected cells but not healthy ones. Time-consuming efficacy trials were being contemplated, but where was the urgency? *Compound Q selectively kills HIV in a single dose! But it's not going to be available for two more years—or eight, or ten? Is there a better word than genocide for this? Why aren't you all going nuts?*

Nobody from T+D was on hand to hear him that night, as they had all been summoned to Washington. Had they been present, they might have brought a dose of skepticism to Kramer's breathless announcement. As it was, scores of people in the room instantly became mad for Compound Q, and, as Kramer urged them to do, they put an intense amount of pressure on their doctors for access to the drug.

In the weeks that followed, Compound Q was nearly the only thing on people's minds. Accounts in the community newspapers described it as forty times more effective than AZT. "It's possible," said a typical article, "that several doses will be sufficient to knock out HIV." The San Francisco Buyers' Club managed to get its hands on some Q. In New York, GMHC obtained a small amount. Dr. Barry Gingell, the young medical information director there, called his friend Dr. Barbara Starrett with a proposal: he would try it out on himself if she agreed to monitor the experiment. There was a long tradition among physician-researchers to experiment first on themselves. In 1900, doctors in Cuba proved that yellow fever was contagious by intentionally exposing themselves to the virus. A few years later, Dr. Werner Forssmann proved the safety of cardiac catheterization by running a wire through a vein in his forearm into his own beating heart. But Gingell's interest was not academic: he was waging a personal battle with HIV, having spent the last two months in a hospital bed, overrun by myriad infections. He didn't have much time.

Starrett was no stranger to the underground—she and her lover had flown to Japan for dextran sulfate for her patients, personally smuggling huge quantities back to the country wrapped up and disguised as gifts. In addition, she had prescribed ribavirin, an underground anti-flu drug smuggled from Mexico, and experimented with off-label compounds like antabuse and NAC, an antioxidant some hoped would amplify AZT's benefits. Even if the power of such drugs was all in the mind, she was committed to letting her patients try new things—even herbal poultices, even laying-on of hands. She knew little about Compound Q, but the side effects were said to include seizures and delirium. One of her patients had tried it, she learned. His mother somehow got a dose and surreptitiously injected it directly into his saline IV bag as he lay dying in the hospital. His rally was so unexpectedly dramatic that he was soon discharged.

Starrett agreed to Gingell's request. One evening in April, she and her sister Sheree, who worked as her office manager, set up an IV drip over Gingell's hospital bed. They kept the procedure out of Gingell's records and did not let the hospital staff know what they were doing. He was lucid, though very weak, and once he expressed his informed consent she opened the drip and let some Q into his bloodstream. When the sun rose, so did the patient, lucid and hopeful. But his newfound strength lasted only two days before he drifted into a quiet coma, weakened by disease and struggling for breath. He died at age thirty-four. A lung autopsy revealed that the cause was a common mold called aspergillus, more likely to cause allergy than death.

AS EXPECTED, Burroughs Wellcome did not lower the price of AZT in the wake of the tense lunch meeting with Staley and Harrington. After leaving messages for a few months, Staley managed to get the woman from the communications office on the phone again. "Dr. Barry was very clear that he felt the price was justified," she reminded him. She also said the company might consider sending out some sort of press advisory so that the existence of its assistance program for indigent patients would be less of a secret. "I think that's about all you're gonna get from us," she said.

Staley was disappointed, but not surprised. He called together a close group of activists, including a number of ACT UP members outside of T+D, and proposed a fitting riposte.

At sunrise on the morning of April 24, eight of them piled into a rented van and pointed it toward North Carolina. Armed with annual reports from the company and Staley's memory of the place, they mapped out the environs, looking for the location that offered the most media-ready setting for their plans. To them it seemed that the west side of the main building met those needs: it faced the highway, in plain view of thousands of drivers each day, and it was close enough to public property that the press could witness their protest even if they were escorted from the grounds. The workday was done by the time they reached the imposing gate at the company's sprawling complex. They conducted a swift reconnaissance (someone brought opera glasses), then trundled off to the less-than-luxurious Heart of Durham Hotel ($37 a night) for some restive sleep packed four to a room.

They rose with the sun. Two of them—Jay Blotcher and Steve Rosenbush, both even-tempered and tireless—began unpacking supplies to turn their room into a media nerve center. While they worked to hook up a fax machine for sending press alerts to their national media contacts, the six others helped each other smooth on the costumes they had brought with them—what they called "executive drag," coats and ties for the five men, and a handsome dress for the sole woman among them, Deb Gavito. They removed their many earrings, checked one another for visible leather or rubber wristbands or funky rings, and put their protest accoutrement on the dressing tables—lapel pins, medalions, and anything that might suggest "gay" or "downtown" or "AIDS." Beside Staley and Gavito, who would remain out of sight in a second vehicle—an alternate driver if needed—were Dan Baker, a young member of the fund-raising committee; Lee Arsenault, a forty-one-year-old import/export executive with advancing AIDS who looked the part of an itinerant salesman; James McGrath, thirty-two, a small-business owner originally from Providence, Rhode Island; and Blane Mosley, in his mid-twenties, a blade-thin interior designer and the group's only African American.

Today they were pharmaceutical sales reps.

Staley opened a briefcase and packed it with a brick-sized cellular telephone, the newest technology, and a supply of food and Evian water. The other men weighed down their valises with needed equipment as well, swallowed a high-protein breakfast, then piled into the van.

It was just before 10 o'clock when they entered Burroughs Wellcome's space-age campus. Dan Baker pulled up to the imposing door of the largest pyramidal building and headed inside to ask for directions, as they had rehearsed. He was convincingly befuddled. Once the guard handed him a map to trace his route around the wooded grounds, he asked to use the men's room and was allowed to do so.

Back in the driver's seat, Baker gave his surveillance report. There were three guards attending the front desk, he said, not one, as Staley had reported from his previous meeting. The men's room was located beyond the sentries, deep into the lobby. He drew a map showing that to get to the bathroom one had to pass an elevator bank.

Their plans were finalized.

When enough time had passed, they returned to the main building where this time all five men got out of the car, toting their heavy briefcases, and Baker reacquainted himself with the guards. "They sent us back over here," he said, scratching his head. "We're looking for"—he gave a false name. "Maybe he's in this building?"

The guards were solicitous, confirming spellings and trying diligently to untangle the visitors' conundrum. And as they did this, Staley interrupted, gesturing toward the unseen facilities and mentioning their long car ride. "Could we . . . ?"

As Dan Baker receded, the other men swept past the security desk and took a sharp right, following a woman into a waiting elevator. A guard shouted after them, but Staley pushed the top floor button and the door cranked closed. The female passenger, heeding the guard's cry, dutifully reached the doors-open button, but was deterred with a strong swat. The doors closed as the sounds of anxious footfalls drew closer. The close call set the men's hearts racing.

On the top floor, they walked toward the side of the building with the desired exposures, and entered an office chosen at random. It was small, approximately ten by ten. In it, a female executive was speaking on her telephone. "Ma'am," said Lee Arsenault, politely but firmly. "There's a situation on this floor. Please calmly proceed to the lobby."

"Joyce, I gotta go," the woman confided to her caller, before collecting her things and abandoning the office.

Staley closed the door behind her and unpacked his bulky modular device and placed a quick phone call to the hotel, confirming their location and triggering a cascade of events. Within minutes a press release was on the AP wire announcing that Burroughs Wellcome had been infiltrated and was being occupied by ACT UP. Reporters were racing to the location.

The other men opened their briefcases, which carried an assortment of equipment: two industrial glass cutters, three boxes of screws, a pocket-sized TV with backup batteries. In ACT UP's affinity group tradition, they gave their gadget-savvy group a name: the Power Tools.

James McGrath produced a drill and steel plates for sealing the door. He got to work cranking long bolts into the metal door jam, crossing the door in multiple places. It would take a bulldozer to get through when he was done. But he encountered an unexpected problem. Despite its small size, the office had a second door, one that inexplicably opened outward onto the hallway. Crossing the entrance with metal bars would be pointless, as guards could just open the door and duck into the room. McGrath rummaged through his briefcase. He was in luck. They had packed L-shaped iron brackets, which he used to fix the door to the doorframe. Meanwhile, Blane Mosley put himself to the task of sealing the transom windows above each door, glazed in Plexiglas. But they were out of hardware. Proving his resourcefulness, Mosley emptied a small metal bookshelf in the office, dismantled it, and bolted the back panels against the windows, closing off the last possible route for entry. In minutes, they had completed their self-entombment. There was no turning back. A lawyer had told them the worst-case scenario was a ten-year prison sentence.

The plan was to cut an opening in the window large enough to drop a banner—a visual for the reporters, eminently visible from the highway—then hunker down for the long run. In their briefcases was enough food and water—and the pharmacopeias that kept them alive—to hold them for a week.

But there was a new problem. They hadn't anticipated the remarkable thickness of the tinted window—no ordinary glass but something with structural properties. The cutters spun and spun and only scored the surface. The drill didn't work either. "Stand back," Staley shouted, swinging a heavy office chair with a growl. It thudded against the windowpane and fell to the floor. He tried again and again, managing only to warp the chair.

Luckily, the lack of a banner didn't seem to slow the media's interest. The mobile phone rang nonstop. In the parking lot, Dan Baker worked the arriving reporters and Debbie Gavito feigned ignorance.

All of this filled no more than eight minutes before the sheriff's deputies knocked on the door and demanded to know who the intruders were.

"We are nonviolent and unarmed," Staley shouted. "And we're not coming out until Burroughs Wellcome agrees to lower the price of AZT."

"You have ten minutes to open the door," the lead officer stated, "before we come in after you."

They were confident their barricades would hold. But just in case, they handcuffed themselves to a twelve-foot length of chain, and locked the chain to the radiator, all while fielding calls from reporters.

When the deadline passed, nobody from Burroughs Wellcome came to negotiate terms. Instead, the sheriff's deputies burst through the sheetrock like it was made of paper, a contingency that had not occurred to the activists—office walls in New York City were made of much more formidable stuff. The activists were extracted from the room just fifty-five minutes after arriving. Still attached to the long chain, they were paraded by police past about thirty terror-struck company employees and out the front door into range of a dozen television cameras. It was quite a spectacle. The deputies allowed them a moment to explain themselves.

"Burroughs Wellcome is profiting off of our lives. That's why we did today what we did," Staley proclaimed before entering the back of a cruiser. "And if they don't start listening to my community, to our community, the AIDS community, then we'll be back."

ACT UP bailed the men out of jail in a few hours, with $20,000 in traveler's checks they had stockpiled in the motel room. News of the action appeared on CNN and NPR; in the *San Francisco Chronicle* and *New York Newsday*; and on local radio and television around the country. The company didn't respond publicly, and when ACT UP offered to pay for the damage, officers quietly let it be known that Burroughs Wellcome wished to have the charges dropped. For the Power Tools, the drive back to New York was full of merriment and self-congratulation, the peculiar traditions of combatants in a subversive war. But as the weeks passed and the price of AZT didn't budge, their moods were tempered once again.

DR. FRANK YOUNG kept his word, calling an emergency session of Dr. Ellen Cooper's Anti-Infective Drugs Advisory Committee to review the status of DHPG. On May 1, with the cherry trees in full blossom, the same twelve experts returned to a windowless room in D.C. to consider the same old data. The only difference this time was that they also heard from the patient population. ACT UP selected Garry Kleinman to speak out against the bureaucratic blindness that had overcome common sense to block this drug. He called for including PWAs and advocates at all levels of decision-making, which now was ACT UP's mantra.

It was afternoon when the matter came to a vote. By a show of hands, the panel made AIDS-related blindness a thing of the past. Activists in the gallery erupted in applause. For the first time in history, patients had forced the FDA to reverse its position on a drug—and one that had undergone no formal trial, another first. But their delays and stubborn obfuscation over the previous years had resulted in needless loss of sight, making this a bitter victory.

A more troubling truth had become apparent. As Mark Harrington pointed out, there seemed to be nobody at the FDA—or anywhere else in the Public Health Service, for that matter—dealing with "the entire map of AIDS, the constellation of opportunistic infections, the gaps in research, the underrepresented populations, the fact that the diseases and the drugs required to fight them might be different in those populations. There was no guiding agenda, there was no leadership, there was no overall strategy for how to deal with AIDS" in the United States or the world. "It sort of felt like reaching the Wizard of Oz," Harrington said. "You've gotten to the center of the whole system and there's just this schmuck behind a curtain."

In the darkness of the ride home that night, the T+D members gave themselves a daunting assignment: *they* would compile the AIDS Treatment Research Agenda for the federal government.

They got to work immediately. A group of five began meeting twice a week in Harrington's sunny old tenement apartment. They researched what had gone wrong in drug development to date, and determined what in their opinion needed to take place going forward. They listed the "Five Drugs We Need Now" and the "Seven Treatments We Want Tested Faster." Every drug trial would be advertised to the afflicted community, they would be open to all races and genders, prophylaxis would be permitted, placebos avoided, and "efficacy criteria and end-points humane." They proposed innovative new guidelines for designing and conducting clinical trials, building on the experience of Callen and Sonnabend, whose aerosolized pentamidine study already had two hundred patients. Along with the Community Consortium in San Francisco, their Community Research Initiative was proving more nimble and responsive than Fauci's AIDS Clinical Trials Group, with no federal funding. Their experience would be promoted as a model for Fauci to follow.

Treatment activists from both coasts entered the summer of 1989 with a strong conviction favoring research carried out by community doctors. They saw the approach as a way not only to prod Fauci onward, but to rein in the proliferation of unregulated buyers clubs, some of which were less principled than others. The operation in Dallas was a chaotic enterprise being operated as a profit-generating engine for its founder, Ron Woodroof. Professional drug smugglers had joined the cause. A physician in Europe was charging $10,000 for a worthless injection of thymus-gland extracts and a clinic in Southern California charged $34 for a small vial of cow's colostrum—the first milk secreted by mammary glands—with promises of its immune-boosting properties.

And a former Vietnam helicopter pilot named James Corti found a source for Compound Q in China and made ampules of it available to the sick. Across San Francisco, patients were infusing themselves in their kitchens, their IV bags hanging from nails on the wall, while informal salons called "guerilla cliniQs" formed in Dallas, Atlanta, and elsewhere. To Marty Delaney, the Project Inform founder who was the leading treatment advocate on the West Coast, such haphazard self-medication posed unacceptable risks. There was no strong scientific reason to believe Compound Q was doing any good, for instance, though there was much encouraging anecdotal evidence. Many people reported looking better and feeling well, with better mental clarity. And almost all believed that their knobby lymph nodes had shrunk (no previous drug had helped with lymphadenopathy). Some noticed a rise in CD4 cells as well.

To put an end to the uncertainty and fraud, Delaney proposed that the consortium—the San Francisco network of hospitals undertaking community-based drug research—conduct formal clinical trials of Compound Q. But the consortium leadership, viewing the nostrum's early data as unconvincing, turned him down. So did Fauci himself. Nobody but an exploding legion of patients saw any promise in Compound Q.

Undaunted, Delaney began planning a clandestine, underground trial of the kind that had never before taken place. His own Project Inform would run the California arm. He recruited a husband-and-wife physician team—Dr. Vera Byers and Dr. Alan Levin—to serve as principal investigators. They were the perfect pair for this. Both were careful physicians. Theirs was one of the largest AIDS practices in the state. And they had determined that they had to take risks. They were joined by another local expert, Dr. Larry Waites. Delaney then put together a panel to help devise a program to protect the patients from unethical practices. They recruited a local attorney with AIDS to help design a vigorous system for informed consent. A script was readied for the doctors to use in explaining risks, and a consent form for the patients to sign—with a third party witnessing. To avoid any misinterpretation of the patients' desires, the entire consent process would be videotaped.

Delaney then turned to physicians in Fort Lauderdale and Los Angeles to recruit patients there, and to the Community Research Initiative to run the East Coast branch of the trial in New York. To his surprise, Callen and Sonnabend were not interested. They wanted more safety information than a few anecdotes from Bay Area kitchens and salons. At a fractious board meeting, their view prevailed and CRI rejected the invitation to participate.

But Tom Hannan, the CRI cofounder, broke ranks and immediately signed up to help. So, in fact, did most of the CRI staff, departing en masse from the high scientific standards they had hoped to set with CRI. "I have AIDS and I am painfully aware of the need to move swiftly," Callen said. "But it seems to me that people have charged ahead irresponsibly."

In fact, people in New York were already "Q-ing." After Larry Kramer's enthusiastic announcement, a half-dozen men mailed checks to Corti, the pilot, who shipped out Q ampules in padded containers. Once a month they gathered at one of their apartments, where Risa Denenberg, another ACT UP member, who happened to be a nurse, administered the doses. It was not something she did lightly. The range of side effects was daunting. She dealt with heart palpitations, high fevers, and fainting spells. But she was a nurse at plague time, doing what she felt needed to be done.

To run the New York arm of the trial, Hannan recruited Dr. Barbara Starrett. She knew she was taking a big risk to accept the responsibility. What the Office of Professional Medical Conduct might make of this, she had no idea, and she could well lose her license. Worse, she could lose her patients' lives. But like Denenberg she was AIDS hardened.

Starrett assembled a team of volunteers to run the complex logistics, including two nurses, each with a PhD, and a number of patient advocates from the People With AIDS Coalition. She reserved the same basement room at Judson Memorial Church in Greenwich Village where Michael Callen had distributed AL721. Church leaders carefully reviewed the study design before agreeing. They installed a number of backyard lounge chairs so that patients would be comfortable during the anticipated long infusion time, converting the large space into what looked like a calm, underground resort.

All this was being done in utmost secrecy. When news leaked to T+D, they forcefully echoed Callen's objections. They believed that the maxim they'd learned from Iris Long still held: the black market was not the answer to the drug bottleneck. What's more, they were critical of the specifics of the trial, from the administration of what seemed to them a particularly high dose to the meager patient protections in place. Nothing was known about how people with low CD4s would handle Compound Q, or what effect it might have on people with neurological manifestations, a common problem. To T+D, it seemed that Q was being treated as if it were as harmless as AL721, when it was anything but. They gathered their findings in a factsheet they had titled "Q Fever," which Harrington presented at an ACT UP meeting. While Kramer had called Compound Q a possible cure, to Harrington it was a dangerous toxin. "We're not talking about health food here—they are playing with fire."

The blowback was furious. One speaker after another accused Harrington of arrogance, obstructionism, and paternalism. An outraged

Larry Kramer crossed the crowded room and joined him at the front. "You're just like Ellen Cooper!" he screamed.

But for a while, it didn't seem to matter. Alarmed when the renegade human trial was discovered, the FDA shut down all access to the Chinese compound on July 14. For a moment, anyway, it seemed the issue was dead. But Corti, the Vietnam vet, soon developed alternative sources, and within days enrollment was back on track, to the measured relief of a desperate community.

Sixty-six patients volunteered, a quarter of them in New York. The first round of infusions was scheduled for one evening late in July. In another example of how the response of San Francisco gays differed from New York gays, the Bay Area's secret trial took place in a gorgeous art deco skyscraper at 450 Sutter Street, in the heart of the city's cable car district, amid a festive atmosphere. One subject arrived on roller skates and was dressed as Little Bo Peep. The doctors invited local reporters from ABC, CBS, and NBC to bank footage to use after the trial's completion.

In New York, the mood was as sober as a surgical suite. Except for the buzzing fluorescent lamps, the church basement was unusually tense. Patients milled about nervously. Starrett, dressed as usual in formless slacks and a block-printed blouse, turned on a video camera and handed it to her sister, who pointed it toward a pair of chairs. Starrett lowered her ample frame into one of them. She tapped on the empty seat and was joined by her first patient, a robust-looking man in his mid-thirties with a bristly moustache and eager energy. He smiled. They knew each other well.

"Hi Jim," she said. "Okay, I know you've tried some innovative treatments for being HIV positive."

He rattled off everything from AZT to an experimental immunomodulator called Imuthiol. "I read about Compound Q in *The New York Times* and I thought that it was a good, you know, *chance*."

"You're aware that this drug does look very, very promising in the test tube?"

He nodded self-consciously.

"But it's only in the test tube. So we do not know, one, whether this drug will do the same thing in a human being that it does in a test tube for HIV-infected cells. And, two, we don't know how this drug will respond to people who are HIV positive."

"I read that," he said, showing the informed consent form he'd been given.

"People have had fevers, joint pain, fatigue, sore throat, swollen glands—they've gone away."

Tom Hannan, sitting on the other side of Jim, interrupted. "Not the patients! The side effects!"

No one laughed.

Some patients had been known to have a seizure-like response to the drug, she explained, perhaps a result of the drug sending a wake of dead viral particles through the brain. But she had been informed that the reaction was transitory, seldom requiring hospitalization, but in some cases a dose of steroids was necessary to treat the inflammatory response.

"I understand that," he said.

"We do know there have been three deaths related to people who have had Compound Q—and this is not on the consent form—that I want you to know about. One patient committed suicide. One patient developed neurological symptoms, went into a coma, and developed pneumonia and died. The third patient, similar, had Compound Q, went into a coma, and went on a respirator . . . then choked on some fluids in his lungs."

"Yes," Jim said. "I am aware."

"Okay. And would you still like—"

"I would still like to continue with the trial, begin with the trial," he blurted out impatiently.

She watched him sign the written release. In an awkward ritual having to do with legal liability, Tom Hannan then turned to Jim. "You'd like to have the medication administered to you as a treatment?" he asked.

Jim stiffened with purpose. "Yes."

"I have to give you the actual medication, which now belongs to you—because I have just given it to you." He leaned forward and placed a clear plastic bag holding about a liter of fluids into Jim's hands. "And you have to officially request that it be administered to you." Jim, growing confused, hesitated until Hannan gave an encouraging smile and gestured toward the doctor.

Spinning in his seat, Jim offered the infusion bag to Dr. Starrett. "I request that this be administered to me," he said awkwardly.

"Okay," she said, then gave the bag to her nurse, who marked Jim's name on it.

Starrett repeated this clandestine Kabuki time and again—to a well-built African American man with a sharp nose and a tight polo shirt, to a hyperactive Slavic-looking fellow with spiked hair and a gold neck chain, to a ravaged white man whose crooked glasses hung above a weak moustache. They listened, consented, requested, handed over, and took their positions in the reclining chairs. When it was time, the nurses worked their way through the room, puncturing veins. They opened the spigots. And they waited.

The room was eerily quiet for the first thirty minutes, then slowly a sense of camaraderie tentatively took over. One patient shared a song. Others told long stories or else practiced the dark humor that was becoming a hallmark of the epidemic. An aproned deliveryman brought boxes of pizza. Through sheer force of will, as far as they knew they had entered one of the most promising phases yet in the seven years of plague. A scientific revolution was taking place. Dr. Starrett circled the room with the video camera, capturing the patients as they waved and mugged and rejoiced. There were so few moments of joy in these days, but this was one of them.

"Hi, Larry," she said to one. His right arm had been immobilized, strapped to a plank of wood with ribbons of gauze. He gestured to the emptying bag and gave a thumbs-up. He smiled so broadly his glasses rode up his nose.

"You'll have stories to tell," Starrett said, poignantly adding, "in the future."

"I'm sure we all will," answered her very first patient, Jim.

6

Madness

Doug's income lifted our living standards while simultaneously conditions in our building, which had never been very good, declined precipitously. Crack dealers now occupied the hallway and vestibule, and two empty units had been converted to shooting galleries, taken over by a parade of sooty heroin addicts. The other PWAs in the building had either died or moved to more healthful surroundings. We began looking for another apartment. It was Doug's idea to investigate home ownership. The prospects of life without a landlord energized him. He circled ads in the *Times* and the *Voice,* and made appointments for us to spend our Saturdays at open houses. It was good to see him excited about life. Ignoring the improbability of us ever landing a mortgage, I tagged along happily.

One evening in the early summer as we returned home from dinner, we encountered a small crowd that had formed outside the building next door to ours, and watched as paramedics pulled a gurney down the stoop and toward a waiting ambulance. Strapped to the stretcher was a body in a bag—the remains of Frank Barbier. We knew Barbier casually. A handsome, middle-aged African American who favored leather biker clothing and skullcaps, he spent his summers tending a rooftop garden. We spotted him there from our own roof one Fourth of July, and introduced ourselves from the distance during a pause in the fireworks display. A cloud seemed to hang over him. In fact, it was just a few months after the death of his lover of twenty years, Donald Corder. Sensing his grief, we made a point of saying hello thereafter, but had lost track of him recently. We watched numbly as attendants muscled his remains into the back of their vehicle. A woman explained that Barbier had been dead for a week.

Over the following days, his relatives marched up and down that stoop, always grimacing. One young man who said he was Barbier's nephew asked if I knew men in the neighborhood who could haul rubbish. "Nobody in the family wants any of his stuff," he said. "My mom can't even go in there."

"It must be tough losing her brother," I commiserated.

"They hadn't spoken since the sixties," he said. "She didn't approve. Nobody in the family did."

"Did you know he was sick?"

He waved a hand. "My mom's a cop. She's handling this the way she would handle one of her cases."

He invited me up to Barbier's apartment. I was surprised to find what a wreck it was. He and Corder occupied two small adjoining rail-road flats, one of which was used for a vast collection of books and opera records piled to the ceiling. The other reflected their appetites in healthier times. Snapshots and Polaroids of naked men covered one wall, probably souvenirs of various conquests. An S&M-like sling hung from the ceiling in the bedroom, which incongruously also held a motorized hospital bed, the sling to which Barbier had until recently been confined. The nephew shuddered. "You don't want it, do you?"

The question embarrassed me. "I've already got a bed," I said finally.

"I mean, do you want this?" he said, swinging his arm at the whole messy estate. "It's a co-op apartment. We asked a real estate agent to list it, but she wouldn't even come into this neighborhood." Even by East Village standards, the apartment was a horror. The wooden window frames had rotted clear through in places, and long nails held in place the mismatched sashes, which had apparently been harvested from dumpsters and abandoned buildings. So much plaster had fallen from the walls, you could see the dusty bricks of the building's hundred-year-old skin. And there was a sickening smell, the reminder of the heat wave that accompanied Barbier's first five days as a corpse.

The asking price started at $90,000 but quickly dropped to $19,000. Doug was determined to make it work. He borrowed $3,000 from his family. I approached our landlord for a buyout, and he offered $10,000 for us to vacate the apartment and withdraw from the various lawsuits that entangled us. We managed to borrow the rest and became the proud owners of a dilapidated bit of Manhattan, and everything in it.

Going through their boxes, we learned that Frank Barbier had been an acclaimed designer of fabric and cocktail napkins, among other things. Don Corder, white and mustachioed, had been a schoolteacher. Snapshots of their lives together went back to the early sixties, when they had lived on Christopher Street with a beautiful white standard poodle, and were members of the last pre-liberation gay society. Their cocktail party photographs were rich tableaux of caricatured poses and self-conscious accessories. On the wall of our new home was a haunting pen-and-ink likeness of Corder as a very young man, signed by the gay American portraitist Don Bachardy. They had met in Washington Square. Bachardy, whose life partner was Christopher Isherwood, had hoped to coax Corder out of his clothing, but he remained resolutely in shirt and tie, at least for the portrait, which we inherited.

When Corder took ill, their sexual lives became more circumspect. Barbier arranged for all of Corder's health needs, which mounted quickly and soon sent him to St. Clare's, a bare-bones West Side hospital entirely given over to AIDS care. Barbier mounted a one-man campaign to improve patient care there, pressing the administration to take out garbage more often, and, when nurses refused the many cries for ice from fever-troubled patients, he got the local McDonald's to donate an ice machine and then got General Electric to send a refrigerator.

Barbier never found peace after Corder died. When he got sick, there was nobody to fight *his* fights. Except to visit his rooftop garden, he seldom left the apartment thereafter. Meals came from God's Love We Deliver, attuned to the needs of homebound PWAs. When the final fevers arrived, he laid himself down on the floor of the apartment, surrounded by a vast selection of books on art, Judaism, civil rights history, and African culture. After they removed his body, a dark outline remained permanently on the spot where he had lain.

WHEN THE RESULTS of the CRI trial on preventing PCP were finally tabulated, as the community expected, they showed the benefits of aerosolized pentamidine for preventing illness, the third such study in backing prophylaxis. Sonnabend submitted the results to Ellen Cooper's AIDS drugs committee at the FDA, feeling a lot like Dorothy thrusting a burned broom toward the wizard. Cooper was still unimpressed, reluctant to approve the drug because the trial was done without a placebo arm, but agreed to schedule a hearing.

Callen lobbied to offer comments following Sonnabend's scientific presentation. His searing speech was entitled "AIDS and Passive Genocide."

In May of 1987, other AIDS activists and I met with Dr. Anthony Fauci—the closest person we have to an AIDS czar. We asked him—no, we begged him—to issue interim guidelines, urging physicians to prophylax those patients deemed at high risk for

PCP. Although it would not have cost the government much to have done so, he steadfastly refused to issue such guidelines. His reason: no data. So the Catch-22 was complete and many more people died of PCP who didn't have to.

I asked a CDC statistician how many AIDS-related PCP deaths had occurred between the date of our [first] meeting with Dr. Fauci and February 20—the last date for which cumulative deaths from PCP are available. The answer: 16,929.

I repeat: nearly 17,000 Americans died of a disease they probably shouldn't have gotten in the first place. In other words, thousands of Americans died who didn't have to die.

In May 1989, the advisory panel sent a unanimous vote to Ellen Cooper, who signed off on the approval. It was the first time that a drug had been released based on data generated by community researchers. The monopoly of NIAID and academic science was broken. Finally, there was an approved means to prevent the leading killer of PWAs. With FDA approval, insurance companies now covered the costs. (In a case of inexcusable torpor, the FDA did not see fit to approve Bactrim for this use until 1994.) It took another forty-five days for the Public Health Service to publish the long-awaited PCP prevention guidelines, after which the preventative was routine. Soon, a quarter of a million North Americans and Europeans infected with the virus were taking regular doses of aerosolized pentamidine. The era of preventable AIDS deaths was nearly over.

Callen was rightly exultant. "The AIDS community," he declared, "has done an end run around federal incompetence and indifference."

Lymphomed, the little company with the exclusive American patent on pentamidine, was naturally thrilled to finally have access to the wider market, thanks to the sacrifices of the PWA community. They celebrated by increasing the price again. "Everybody is out to make a buck," Dr. Starrett said when she heard about it. "Why should the price of a drug double when so much more of it is being ordered? You would think that with the increased demand prices would go *down*."

So much was upside down in the AIDS crisis.

THOUGH ACT UP had managed to exercise some influence over America's views of the plague, the organization itself often fared poorly in the public's perception. Their actions were derided as "deplorable" and "dishonorable" by critics, and editorial writers at *The New York*

Times felt they actually made matters worse by their rage-fueled antics, providing "another reason"—besides, presumably, homophobia— "to reject both the offensive protesters and their ideas." If the activists hoped for a kinder reception in the gay papers, they were equally thwarted. Coverage in *The Advocate,* driven by an older and more conservative generation, was typically at arm's length and often critical. And the foundering *New York Native* ignored the group's activities almost entirely.

Chuck Ortleb's paper had sunk even deeper into paranoid convolution in recent years, infused with his own now-solid conviction that HIV and AIDS were a twisted hoax concocted to sell AZT and enrich Big Pharma, while the real culprit stalking the community was, depending on the week, either African swine fever virus, untreated syphilis, a brand-new herpes virus, a mysterious "virus-like" particle recently discovered by a young Army researcher, or some combination of them all. Even Callen and Sonnabend, still strong proponents of the idea that it took more than just HIV to cause AIDS, were appalled by Ortleb's views, going so far as to call a press conference distancing themselves. That the paper remained in business was owed to the wild proliferation of phone sex ads, which promoted the perfect new industry in the plague years: callers were charged by the minute to encounter one another over the telephone lines, sanitarily. Those ads helped bring a record $2.4 million to the paper the previous year, though circulation was down to 5,000 or fewer.

Native reporters still managed to provide important coverage of civil liberties battles arising from the epidemic, and Phil Zwickler, hired to fill my old job, was an aggressive thorn in the side of politicians. But on matters of pharmaceutical science—and therefore on anything having to do with ACT UP's drugs-into-bodies campaign—it was infuriatingly silent. Peter Staley wrote a letter of protest, moved by the blackout on news about his derring-do with the "Power Tools" affinity group at the Burroughs Wellcome headquarters. Receiving no reply, he attended a panel discussion organized by PEN, the writers' group, at which Ortleb was a scheduled speaker. During the question-and-answer period, he confronted Ortleb on his editorial biases.

In the tense exchange, Ortleb admitted that it had been a mistake to ignore the attack on Wellcome and promised to remediate the lapse. But when Ortleb's piece appeared in the May 29 issue, he condemned the protest action as a waste of time and money. "The costly Burroughs Wellcome demonstration ($8,000 paid to plasterers to repair the damage to the Burroughs Wellcome building!) asked the company to reduce the price of a costly, profitable, and toxic AZT by twenty-five percent, a move the company was planning anyway," Ortleb wrote, without evidence.

The following Monday night, Peter Staley took the microphone at ACT UP. He was not a regular speaker at the main meetings, considering them unnecessarily gladiatorial, but now was an exception. He waved a copy of the paper. "They're irresponsible," he said. He rattled off egregious examples, which included cartoons depicting leading AIDS researchers in Nazi uniforms, doggerel poetry about Gallo and Fauci ("rhyme," Ortleb explained, "is contemptuous"), and a raft of befuddling editorials steering readers away from the NIH, the CDC, AIDS doctors, and all AIDS drugs. He made a motion to declare a formal boycott of the *Native*, saying, "We have to say 'Enough is enough.'" Everyone agreed.

In response, Ortleb cut back his public appearance schedule and let his surrogates defend the paper. ("A boycott by gay people of a gay publication," wrote one editor, is "an expression of self-hate. Not only that, it's tacky and dumb.") Paid circulation vanished, advertisers fled, and the legitimacy and esteem the paper once enjoyed had long disappeared. Chuck Ortleb, one of the first and most pivotal activists in the plague, was now a tarnished footnote. It was the sad denouement of a brilliant man. What AIDS did to others virally it did to him intellectually. Though he continued in business for many more years, the *Native* only attracted the tiniest readership. I never saw Ortleb again after that; few of us did.

SHORTLY BEFORE SUNRISE on a moist morning early in June 1989, ACT UP members filled three buses and headed toward Montreal, where they would be uninvited and unwelcome guests at the Fifth International AIDS Conference. After many months of planning, they were ready to provoke the "full frontal assault on the research/regulatory establishment" that Jim Eigo had promised. The group had worked over the spring to develop a ten-point "Declaration of the Universal Rights and Needs of People Living with HIV Disease." Dubbed *Le Manifeste de Montreal* and co-endorsed by Montreal's ACT UP affiliate, Réaction SIDA (SIDA is the French acronym for AIDS), and by the Toronto-based group AIDS Action NOW, it enumerated a call for unqualified access to any drugs, approved or not, and for full freedom from prejudice, threats of quarantine, and the maddening refusal of researchers to stop using placebos in research.

When they reached the showy Palais de Congrès, the convention center was preparing for the largest gathering of AIDS experts in history, some 12,000 of them from around the globe, armed with 5,302 new studies to discuss, including those on a raft of drugs being ignored or mishandled by the National Institute of Allergy and Infectious Diseases. Despite a budget that now reached $74 million a year—thanks in large part to the actions of AIDS activists—Dr. Tony Fauci's operation had not completed a single drug study. And now there were more young Americans dead from AIDS than from the Vietnam War.

Several hundred activists ringed the front doors, dispensing protest literature. They chanted, "The whole world is watching," hoping it was the truth. Guards stood in an orderly cordon before the multicolored glass building, observing the activities with good humor. It took little time for one American demonstrator to test their mettle. Holding a sign above his head, he sauntered past the dumbfounded guards and spun through the revolving door into the center's spacious lobby. Nobody pursued him. Shortly the activists were all inside, riding the escalators to the cavernous meeting hall on the second floor where the opening ceremony was to take place in a few hours. It was an entirely unplanned action, without script or leader. Tim McCaskell, a prominent Toronto activist, found a microphone. To rapturous applause, he declared the conference open "on behalf of people living with AIDS in Canada and around the world." Soon the delegates began arriving, and it became awkwardly clear that the protesters lacked an exit strategy. They chanted and sang deep into the afternoon, delaying the convocation address by Prime Minister Brian Mulroney by two full hours, until they simply ran out of steam. Many of the conferees were mortified by the more unruly manifestations of the protesters' rage. An article in *Mother Jones* called the event destructive and the demonstrators petulant, a tragic distraction from the important work of the experts.

But that would not be the lasting impression. Once serious matters began to be discussed, what unfolded was an unforgettable first meeting between AIDS activists and the rank-and-file scientists charged with keeping them alive. The highlight came at an electrifying summit called by the Treatment + Data Committee to release their National AIDS Treatment Research Agenda. They laid out four thousand copies of the booklet for scientists to take. Speaking from a makeshift dais, Larry Kramer invoked the memory of those who had died needlessly from PCP. "That's the kind of business-as-usual mentality that ACT UP is fighting against. That is why we are so angry, why we are here in such numbers, and why we make so much noise. That is why I beg of all of you to listen to what is being presented to you here today. We have educated ourselves, we know more than the system knows. And somehow we have to make the system listen to us so that your sons and daughters, brothers and sisters, and all of us may live."

The agenda envisioned a full reconsideration of the way drugs were tested, evaluated, regulated, and released. It demanded an end once and for all to trials that required people to stop protecting against PCP and other preventable opportunistic infections—the so-called "death trials"—and exhorted Jim Eigo's concept of "parallel track," through which any patient could be assured access to any experimental therapy while tightly controlled clinical trials proceeded.

But it was their list of promising new treatments that reflected the sense of urgency the T+D members felt. At the dais, Staley, dressed in a T-shirt and a baseball cap emblazoned with ACT UP's logo, held a copy of the booklet in his hand. "The reasons I can't get any of these drugs is 'cause for nine years now the leadership in [my] country has failed to come up with a plan of action. They failed to come up with a plan of research, a national research agenda. People With AIDS and their advocates have finally done this for them. This is it." He hoisted the booklet high over his head, a gesture reminiscent of the Black Power movement. "This is the plan we're presenting. We need our government to read this plan. We need them to work with us. If they want to change it a little, we'll talk to them. But I want them to adopt it. I want them to get started on it. I want them to save our lives."

A few reporters sat through the presentation, listening politely and asking a few questions. In general they considered the activists an off-color sideshow to the week's events. Most of the scientists thought the same way. But at least one of them was curious enough to want to learn more. Dr. Susan Ellenberg, the top American biostatistician working on AIDS drugs, was terrified of encountering an ACT UP member (she wasn't convinced of their nonviolence), but she snuck up to the table in the front of the room and pulled a copy of the booklet off a pile, retreating as cautiously as she had approached.

"I was sitting through meetings and thumbing through it, and it was very interesting," she admitted later. Some of the group's ideas made her say to herself, "No, no; they don't understand," but her response to many suggestions in the agenda had her thinking, "You mean this *isn't* the way we're doing trials? You mean people *aren't* allowed to do this or that? You know, what's going on here?" When she returned to her office, she made copies and passed them around to a small working group of statisticians meeting quarterly to review study designs. They got as excited as she did about the ideas for humanizing drug trials. Quickly, the news of their enthusiasm reached ACT UP in New York, and a T+D member named Bob Huff called her directly. "We understand that you are discussing our Treatment Research Agenda, and if you're having these discussions we should be there," he said.

Her first thought was to panic, she later confessed. "These are people who at this international AIDS meeting were standing up and interrupting presentations, and using profane language and calling people the worst kinds of names," she said. "These people [want] to come to our meeting? How are we going to be able to deal with this?" But her fellow statisticians, energized by the challenging discussions they had been having about these novel proposals, encouraged her to extend an invitation. After getting Tony Fauci's permission, she opened up the working group meetings to AIDS activists. The researchers were hungry to engage in the direct dialogue. About twenty statisticians attended the next meeting, a record, and a hundred people attended the one that came next.

Tony Fauci emerged from the Montreal convention as a wounded leader of the country's AIDS efforts. Hoping to reset the dynamics with activists, he accepted a request to meet a formal delegation from ACT UP in Bethesda on June 20, expressly to defend his sluggish AIDS Clinical Trials Group. Some of his NIH colleagues thought he was too kind to the New Yorkers, that he was indulging them to "play science," wasting everyone's time. But he was starting to see it differently. He needed them to have faith in his institute or his drug trials were doomed. He was convinced that their differences with the AIDS Clinical Trials Group—and single-minded preference for community-based research initiatives—could be assuaged through Socratic means, something he had learned from the Jesuits who schooled him. Besides, his irritation with the activists was giving way to a growing fascination.

Peter Staley, Bill Bahlman, and Jim Eigo led the group that day; four others joined in, all thrilled to engage the ACTG directly. Two years had passed since Iris Long's and Bahlman's analysis proved the inability of the vast system to enroll patients, despite its two thousand researchers and enormous budget. The ACT UP representatives were prepared to demand that people with HIV or their designates be at every ACTG meeting, conference, laboratory, or break room where their lives were being discussed. As Long explained it, Fauci's findings were unreliable without their input—everyone knew that patients were gaming the system by falsifying medical records to gain enrollment, then testing their drugs in private labs and quitting if they turn out to be placebo.

The individuals involved in operating the trials met three times yearly in an enormous summit, drawing together literally thousands of scientists, statisticians, and technicians involved in the enterprise. The next meeting—the sixth since the new system took shape—was coming up in three weeks.

"The July ACTG meeting has got to be open," Long declared.

Choosing his words carefully, Fauci gave credit to Long's arguments and acknowledged that input from ACT UP might indeed be beneficial, despite its reputation for disrupting scientists. He thought, "If I close my eyes and stop being influenced by the theatrics that surround them, the things that would intimidate very conservative, stuffy scientists, and just listen to what they're saying, it makes absolutely perfect sense." But ACT UP traveled in a pack—a sometimes cross-dressing, often disrespectful, alien pack; there was no ignoring that.

He told Iris Long it would not be possible to include them in July. However, he would present their request at the July meeting and, if he found agreement among the ACTG leadership, ACT UP would be invited to monitor the subsequent summit, scheduled for near Thanksgiving. "You'll have to wait till November."

Staley spoke for the delegation, sounding nearly apologetic. "Like it or not, we're going in July," he said. "You'll just have to live with it—or arrest us." Even Long nodded her head, though she prayed it wouldn't come to that.

The meeting ended at loggerheads. Fauci called Staley at his New York apartment the next morning. He had already spoken to his deputies, chief among them Dr. Dan Hoth, the ACTG director. Hoth was a stubborn man, methodical and conservative. But he had agreed to accommodate their request for direct representation on the panels, if the activists would let the July meeting go as planned and wait until November to be included. The way Fauci saw it, it was a fair compromise.

After caucusing with his T+D colleagues, Staley got back to Fauci and begrudgingly accepted his terms.

Iris Long was relieved. When she returned from D.C., she told her husband about the tense standoff and the threat to face arrest. Michael Long had only a superficial grasp of what his wife had been up to for the last two years. He once saw an official-looking publication in a pile of her things called *AIDS Treatment Registry*, and was impressed to see the bold type listing "Iris Long, Ph.D." as its editor. But the late-night meetings and Milk Runs to Washington, the lawyer letters from hospitals and packages from the FDA, were all part of her world and not his. He was just glad his wife had found something to keep her challenged.

But getting arrested?

"Don't you dare," he said with unnerving vehemence. "The police are not gentle. You're going to get poked with a stick and pushed down and possibly hurt. Stay away from that, you don't need that." He tried to imagine the repercussions at Sunday services or family Thanksgivings. "Nobody wants to be associated with a convict, Iris."

She promised, and they never discussed it again.

FOR MOST of the year, Jim Eigo continued speaking and writing about his parallel track proposal, refining his thinking about expanding drug access outside of clinical trials, and cementing his conviction that it would serve both patients and scientists equally. It was promoted at demonstrations large and small. He wrote to Fauci and Ellen Cooper about it, and Harrington got the leading AIDS and gay organizations to sign a consensus statement endorsing the proposal, but the idea was not getting traction. Then in June, Eigo picked up *The Wall Street Journal* to find Fauci extolling the idea of parallel track trials, using Eigo's own words. He was quoted in an article about a medical meeting in San Francisco saying, "It makes sense from both a public health and a humanitarian standpoint to make a drug available to individuals" who don't qualify for clinical trials. Fauci made similar comments to Bill Bahlman for his cable access news program. This was a signal breakthrough.

Wasting no time, they requested an appointment with Fauci and his staff to discuss logistics. On July 7, 1989, Iris Long and Mark Harrington, Jim Eigo, and David Z. Kirschenbaum met with Fauci at Columbia University on Manhattan's Upper West Side, in the Mental Health Services Center. Fauci brought Dan Hoth, the obstinate ACTG head. An ample man with a thickly bearded chin, Hoth wore a dark suit and an expression as cloudy as a cataract, unhappy to be forced into a meeting by a ragtag group of homosexuals from Greenwich Village.

Though wary, Fauci was in a voluble mood. "What we say here today is off the record," he began. "I need your emphatic acceptance of that." He didn't want a repeat of the time Kramer called him a murderer because of an offhand comment. Harrington, who had planned to tape the meeting, took longhand notes instead, and though he and his team agreed to the conditions, they did so in ACT UP style: they intended

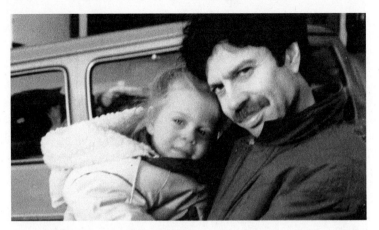

Bob Rafsky, who famously confronted presidential candidate Bill Clinton on his nonexistent AIDS plank, became a prophetic leader in ACT UP. Pictured with him is his young daughter, Sara.

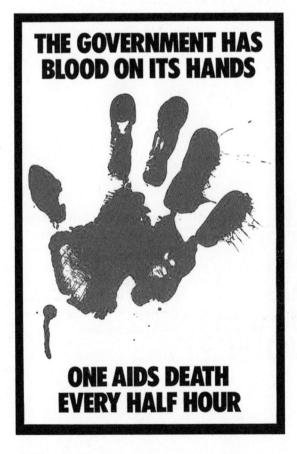

THE GOVERNMENT HAS BLOOD ON ITS HANDS

ONE AIDS DEATH EVERY HALF HOUR

The artist collective Gran Fury, an ACT UP offspring, used the visual tools of advertising and commerce to "fight for attention [to AIDS] as hard as Coca-Cola fights for attention," in the words of member Loring McAlpin.

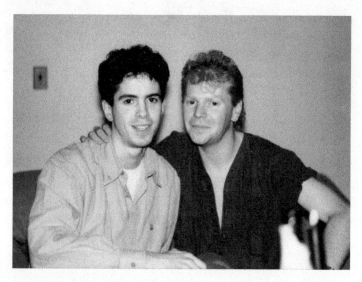

Peter Staley (left, March 1987), a former bond trader who rose to help lead ACT UP, credited his political conversion to Griffin Gold (right), a founding member of the People With AIDS Coalition.

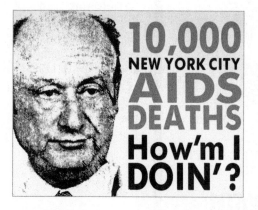

10,000 NEW YORK CITY AIDS DEATHS How'm I DOIN'?

New York City Mayor Edward I. Koch, whose response to the epidemic paled compared to those of heads of other cities, though New York remained the epicenter, was the target of much of ACT UP's political ire.

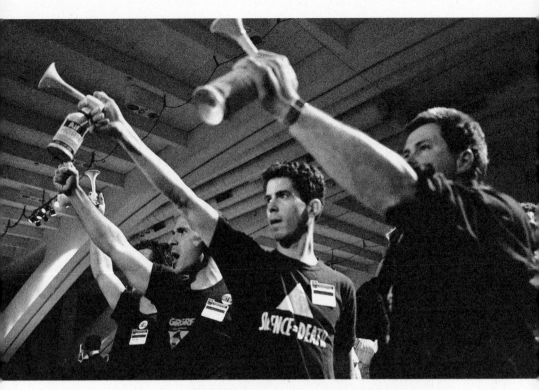

When the International AIDS Conference convened in San Francisco in 1990, activists boycotted in protest of United States restrictions that denied entry to homosexuals and people with AIDS, but ACT UP/NY elected to attend, with Staley (center) and others disrupting Health Secretary Dr. Louis Sullivan's closing remarks.

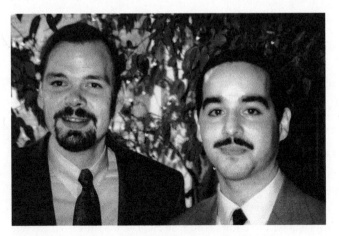

Me (left) and Doug Gould, who succumbed to his infection on November 18, 1992, at age thirty-three

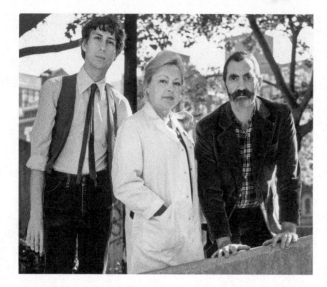

Michael Callen (left), Mathilde Krim, and Dr. Joseph Sonnabend, in 1983, the year they organized the American Medical Foundation to help fill the gaps in federal research. In 1985, AMF merged with a Los Angeles initiative founded by the actress Elizabeth Taylor to become the American Foundation for AIDS Research, AmFAR.

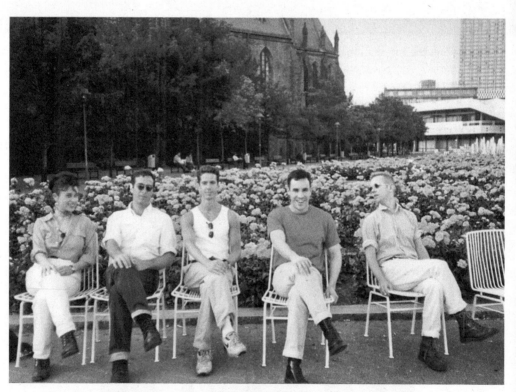

Leaders of Treatment Action Group, an ACT UP spinoff—from left, Garance Franke-Ruta, David Barr, Peter Staley, Gregg Gonsalves, and Mark Harrington, in 1993

Frank Barbier, a neighbor of mine, who died of AIDS in his apartment in 1988 at a time when HIV was moving deep into communities of color, both gay and straight. Doug Gould and I preserved his legacy.

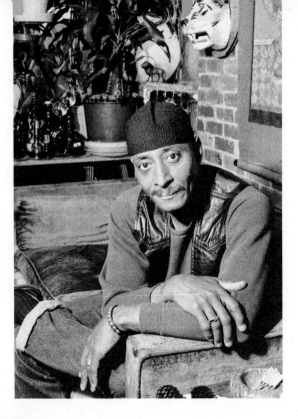

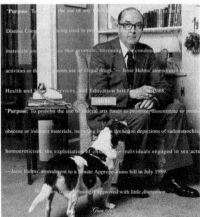

Senator Jesse Helms (R-North Carolina) opposed federal AIDS funding, which he said would "promote, encourage, or condone homosexual activities." His "Helms Amendment" passed year after year, blocking prevention measures, and limiting research.

Failing to sideline Helms politically, activists hoped to draw attention to the human cost of his bigotry with a daring action. On September 5, 1991, they wrapped his suburban Virginia home in an enormous condom, paid for by the entertainment executive David Geffen.

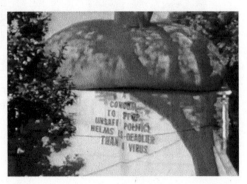

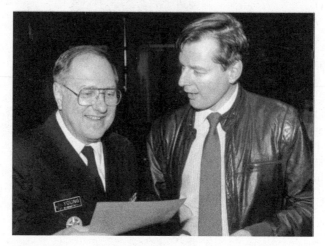

Waging a one-man information campaign, Bill Bahlman
(right) doggedly pursued the FDA Commissioner
Frank E. Young and members of the president's AIDS
Commission, papering their meetings with leaflets of his
own design.

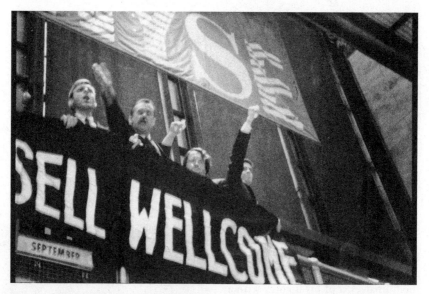

Having left Wall Street, Peter Staley (right) returned in 1989 to lead a
campaign against Burroughs Wellcome, makers of the first AIDS drug,
AZT, for pricing it higher than any drug in history.

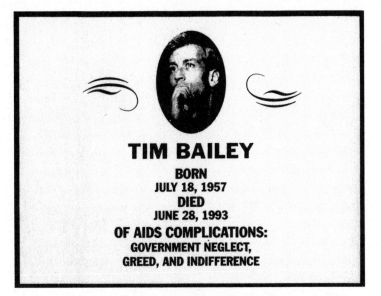

TIM BAILEY

BORN
JULY 18, 1957
DIED
JUNE 28, 1993
OF AIDS COMPLICATIONS:
GOVERNMENT NEGLECT,
GREED, AND INDIFFERENCE

By 1993, with ACT UP's ranks thinned by conflict and death, weekly meetings included announcements of the casualties. The fashion designer Tim Bailey, called "as close to ACT UP royalty as anybody can get," died that June.

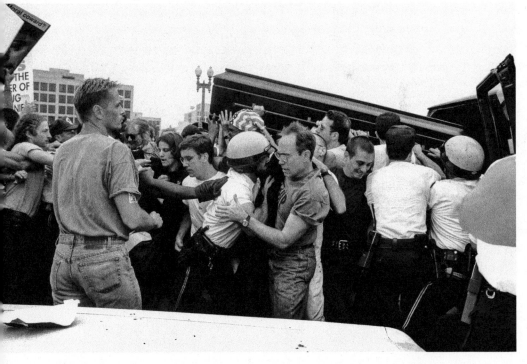

Bailey asked fellow activists to hold an angry service for him at the White House lawn, but local authorities created a chaotic scene when they sought to block the July 1, 1993, spectacle.

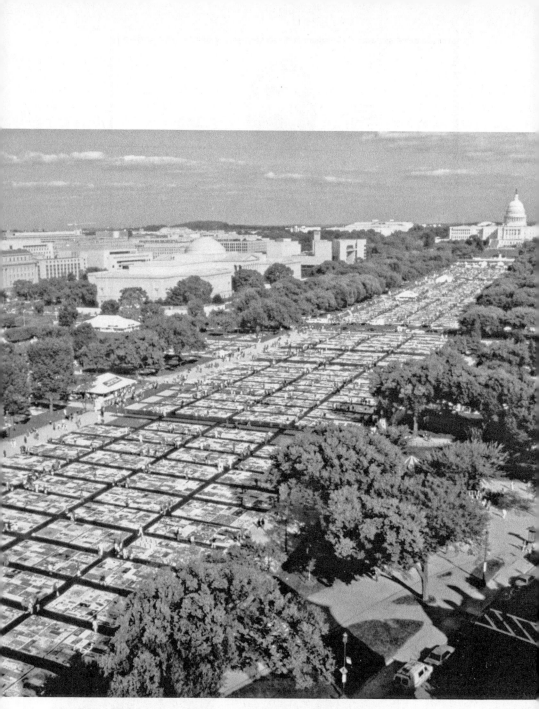

The AIDS Memorial Quilt as it appeared in Washington, D.C., October 1987, when the American death toll surpassed 21,000

to write up a detailed report for delivery to the members the following Monday regardless.

Fauci began with the bad news. Much as he liked the idea, he didn't see a way to bring parallel track online. It would be up to the FDA, not anyone at NIAID or the ACTG, to change the way drugs were studied. And after his remarks in San Francisco, Dr. Ellen Cooper "screamed at me saying it'll never work," he said.

This confused the ACT UP delegation. Just weeks earlier, Cooper had told them she supported the parallel track. In fact, they had tape-recorded her unequivocal remarks in favor of simultaneously releasing experimental drugs to any patient who wanted them. According to Fauci, she still felt that way. What she couldn't abide was Eigo's proposal for collecting "real-world data" from those patients. The way science had always generated data was to compare homogenous groups of trial subjects, all closely monitored to eliminate outside variables that might skew results. In her view, "real-world data" were "dirty data" and therefore of little use.

"It must be a distribution system," Fauci said. "It can't be primarily set up to gather information." He added that he was prepared to put a modified parallel track into place for all ACTG trials. He would appoint a panel of representatives—from the FDA, the NIH, Big Pharma, and "the AIDS constituency" of patients and activists—for deciding which drugs should be available on the parallel track.

This was an enormous victory for activism, though Eigo didn't love the idea of pumping experimental drugs into the community without a formal study or monitoring system in place. He had fully adopted Iris Long's commitment to the scientific process. But for the sake of the very sick, he embraced Fauci's compromise. A tenet of their philosophy, that "drug trials are health care," as Eigo once said, was finally being addressed. It would require a series of hearings and months of negotiations before parallel track became a reality. But there was no underestimating the significance of this moment. The activists and the establishment were now working together.

Eigo welled up with pride in his community, and the fighting organization they had managed to pull together. "None of what we did could have been done by individuals," he said later. "ACT UP did what it did because it had those of us who were thinking seriously about these things and coming up with good solutions, but we were backed by hundreds of people who would put their body on the line." But there was still much more to do. The most logical candidate to push out on parallel track would be a drug developed by Bristol-Myers, a big company with little previous AIDS experience. Called ddI, the drug topped T+D's wish list of the "Five Drugs We Need Now." The company had completed Phase I studies, putting it further along than any other contender. Its mechanism against the virus was similar to AZT's, but it appeared considerably less toxic. The ACTG, with its obsessive attachment to studying AZT over and over, had so far not fully enrolled a Phase II efficacy trial for ddI.

The activists decided on an aggressive strategy toward Bristol-Myers. They hand-delivered a letter to Richard Gelb, the company's chairman, introducing their vision for parallel track and demanding a meeting. When they discovered that Gelb was a Yale graduate, like Larry Kramer, they asked their founder to call Gelb and press for a meeting date. It worked, and Gelb—a Republican stalwart with deep ties to the Bush administration—was an immediate convert. It was unclear whether this was because he saw parallel track as weakening the FDA's regulatory authority, a GOP priority, or because he hoped the parallel track might speed ddI's approval. To ACT UP, his motives didn't matter. On July 13, Bristol-Myers announced it would immediately "make ddI available to all AIDS patients for whom treatment under an emergency or compassionate drug program would be appropriate."

Overnight, the number of anti-HIV drugs doubled, and the thousands of patients for whom AZT didn't work—or had stopped working—had hope again. As Mark Harrington would later note, "The summer of treatment utopianism was in full splendor."

ON A HOT Friday night later that month, Barbara Starrett was settling into her loft apartment after a long day when one of the nurses from the Compound Q study called about Scott Sheaffer, an attractive but very sick actor who had already survived two bouts of PCP. He had received his first Q infusion one evening earlier in the week. Everything seemed to go well. But now, three days later, he'd suffered a seizure. His roommate, John Sefakis, had arrived home from work to an extraordinary scene. There was evidence of fire—the halogen lamp had crashed against the sofa, singing the upholstery. A glass coffee table was shattered. Sheaffer was slumped on the sofa, babbling incoherently into the broken lamp as if it were a microphone and attempting to form random numbers into a sentence. He couldn't move his legs.

Sefakis, an ACT UP member, recognized the psychosis as the feared side effect of Q. He grabbed the phone and dialed the nurse, who called Starrett.

She reached Sheaffer's Midtown apartment in a matter of minutes, finding the young man still thrashing about on the floor. She managed to restrain him long enough to set up a saline drip. For a moment, this seemed to help, but his shouts and senseless ravings quickly resumed.

"You're having a reaction to Compound Q," she called out to him. "You're gonna need to go into the hospital just to monitor everything." She turned to Sefakis. "Call 911," she said.

The ambulance took Sheaffer to St. Clare's, three blocks away, rather than St. Vincent's, where Starrett was affiliated. She called to warn the emergency room staff to expect an AIDS patient who was having a seizure reaction to an experimental drug—she didn't say which one, because there was no known protocol for handling a Compound Q seizure. "He just needs support," she said. "It's gonna be less than twenty-four hours and he will be okay."

Her prognosis was more or less accurate. After a rough night, he fell into a deep slumber, and when he awoke he remembered very little. He was discharged after about thirty-six hours and, though weakened, made it home under his own steam. By the following Tuesday, he was back at his doctor's office as scheduled for his second infusion of Compound Q. Starrett was ecstatic to see him. But she was not about to tempt the fates: if Q did this to him once, she had reason to believe it would again. Sheaffer pleaded with her, believing Q was his last chance. He grew very angry; Starrett held her ground. Though denying his wishes violated a principle she had adopted at the start of AIDS, that a patient should have the right to take whatever risk he felt was necessary, she concluded that it would violate her Hippocratic responsibilities to give him another infusion.

She made an announcement to the other patients that day—and every day of the study thereafter—explaining what had happened to Sheaffer. Not one of them withdrew from the study.

IN AUGUST, Fauci's research network finally published some of the data being produced by the numerous AZT trials. The most interesting finding suggested that AZT was effective in people at all stages of the disease, even well before CD4 cells had begun to vanish. For people with relatively intact immune systems, the drug seemed to halve the risk of developing symptoms, at least over a short period of time. This meant that a lot more people should be taking AZT—up to 600,000 from the current 40,000. That would mean $4.8 billion *per year* in sales for Burroughs Wellcome. The company's profits, already doubled thanks to AZT, would surge. Its stock price leaped 32 percent when the results of the study were announced, triggering dozens of biting editorials, including in *The Journal of the American Medical Association,* which echoed ACT UP's criticism of the drug's unbudging price. Immediately, ACT UP began planning a new demonstration.

Staley saw another opportunity to confront the chain-smoking Dr. David Barry, and his team. He requested another meeting, a gutsy move given the takeover stunt, and the company, cornered by the drumming press, agreed. Understandably, they changed the venue to a hotel out near the airport. Three others from ACT UP joined Staley, who brought leaders from the more mainstream organizations as well, including David Barr, an ACT UP member who was officially representing the Lambda Legal Defense and Education Fund; Jeff Levi of GMHC; and Jean McGuire of the AIDS Action Council in Washington.

Barry was even less amiable than before. He scolded ACT UP for alerting the local media; a bank of television trucks clogged the hotel parking lot, hoping for a dramatic reprise of their last encounter. Staley was equally unwavering. Before the meeting ended, he gave Barry an ultimatum. "The pressure's just gonna get worse and worse, and we're not going to give up. We're doing a massive demonstration against Burroughs Wellcome on Wall Street. You've got a few weeks. Lower the price before then."

Barry glowered. Lisa Behrens from public affairs took a note. "I appreciate the heads-up," she said.

ON A NIGHT early in September, Mark Harrington took the narrow elevator up to his seventh-floor apartment on East Eleventh Street. He was tired. His activism had taken him away from his creative pursuits and cost him his job. For some time, his finances had been painfully tight, but in ACT UP circles this was not an unusual story. AIDS activism was impoverishing many people. A friend at AmFAR threw him a lifeline, giving him a two-month gig organizing a conference on community-based research. After eighteen months as an AIDS activist, he had been adopted by the most powerful research advocates fighting the epidemic.

He was not home long when the telephone rang. It was John Sefakis, who got right to the point. Scott Sheaffer had died. He told Harrington the whole story. In the weeks following his Compound Q seizure, his weight dropped to 130 pounds. His doctor prescribed AZT, which did little good. Sheaffer died in his sleep just after his thirtieth birthday. The death came forty days after his infusion, but it seemed pretty obvious to Sefakis that Q was cutting lives short, and he wanted Harrington, T+D, and the rest of ACT UP to know.

Over the next month, Harrington undertook an investigation of the surrounding events. From what he could piece together, it seemed that the illicit drug coupled with a poor monitoring plan had caused Sheaffer's death. Sheaffer had a preexisting neurological condition that should have excluded him from the trial, and he probably had fewer than a hundred CD4 cells at the time of his Q dose, making him arguably too frail for such a toxic regimen.

One Monday morning, Harrington called Gina Kolata at *The New York Times*, alerting her both to the underground trial and to the Sheaffer case. That night, he made a strident presentation to his ACT UP colleagues. "People who give their bodies for research deserve the very best care, whether the sponsor of the trial is the government, a pharmaceutical [company], or people from within the community," he said in a written report. "If we are going to support unofficial studies, we will share the blame for avoidable harm that occurs to people in such studies unless we can prevent it at the outset."

Next, Peter Staley took to the floor to defend the trial, exposing an intense rift with ACT UP. An angry debate followed. Some in the room were in the secret study or else taking Q on the underground; for them the results of the study could be a lifeline. Larry Kramer was dismissive of the scandal. "People always die in trials," he said. "Grow up."

Michael Callen took a similar position, despite the fact that he had so strongly opposed the underground trial in the first place. He knew Scott Sheaffer from one of his speed-dating events. From what Callen knew, Sheaffer, who was in the terminal stages of AIDS, had joined the trial of his own free will, and clearly was not discouraged by his adverse reaction or he would not have pleaded to be "Q'ed" again the following week. The bottom line for Callen was respect for the absolute autonomy of every PWA.

After the meeting, Harrington bought an early edition of the next day's *Times*, which he knew would carry an article by Kolata about the whole affair. The headline was "Critics Fault Secret Effort to Test AIDS Drug." More than two-thirds of the way into the story, Kolata quoted Sheaffer's personal doctor saying the proximate cause of death was "'cardiorespiratory arrest' secondary to an AIDS virus infection," not Compound Q. Much more prominent were quotes from physicians with no connection to the case who blamed the trial and fired an accusing finger at Dr. Starrett herself, painting her as careless, subversive, and frankly half mad. In this narrative, Sheaffer had been as healthy as a long-distance runner before falling to Starrett's toxic elixir. The reporter got this impression from Harrington himself, who, though he never met the man, pronounced him "healthy and stable" when he entered the trial. "His decline was so rapid. It was like nothing I have ever heard of in AIDS."

Harrington regretted saying this, but that didn't help Dr. Starrett. Probes began that would tie her in knots for the next years; she barely managed to save her license. Kramer furiously condemned Harrington, as did many inside ACT UP. The group's coordinating committee quickly issued special guidelines to limit public disclosures around Compound Q, expressly meant to rein in Harrington.

In this atmosphere, the Q experiment limped along. Curtis Ponzi, a patient from San Francisco, was sure the drug had saved his life. "The difference of how I felt before and after was like twenty years of weight lifted from me—absolutely euphoric," he said. But when the trial results were quickly tallied that fall, the data didn't confirm the anecdotes. Though CD4 cell counts were up slightly after two months of dosing, the evidence of its power as an antiviral was weak, a "mixed but intriguing picture" in the rosiest estimation. Marty Delaney called a community meeting in San Francisco on September 19 to release the findings. Some five hundred men filled the hall, their desperation palpable. When Delaney was finished speaking, the room emptied in near silence.

And then a surprising thing happened: demand for Q skyrocketed anyway. With the trial completed, the PWAs once again were attending Q transfusion salons set up like Tupperware parties in people's homes. Large groups formed in Boston, San Diego, Miami, and points in between, as well as in Holland and Australia. For the cost of a round-trip ticket, a nurse in LA offered to travel anywhere "from Maine to Baja" to infuse any groups of four or more. Q Fever was unstoppable.

WITHIN ACT UP, a small but influential number of activists were looking outside of Western medicine for answers to AIDS. Holistic advocates had been around from the very early days of the epidemic, promoting macrobiotic diets, acupuncture, and other alternative approaches. An organization called Health Education AIDS Liaison—HEAL—formed in 1982 to popularize Reiki, Chinese herbs, garlic, urine, and bee pollen therapies for boosting immunity. When ACT UP first formed, some HEAL regulars joined to create the Alternative and Holistic Treatment

Committee, a kind of naturopathic antidote to T+D. A natural antipathy smoldered between the two committees. Harrington was sometimes overtly hostile toward their proposals, but for the most part T+D and the Alternative Committee coexisted in complementary opposition, occupying separate realms within ACT UP.

The Alternative Committee didn't militate against pharmaceuticals generally. Many of its HIV-positive members were taking prophylaxes. And they didn't have blind faith in health food store offerings. Like their parallels in T+D, they put their faith in empiricism, demanding that their treatment options be rigorously tested. By this standard, acupuncture proved a disappointment, as a study of patients at a New York clinic saw little more than an "improved sense of well-being." Aloe vera juice scored significantly better in a Dallas trial, showing that dramatic results were produced in 71 percent of patients, including an end to fevers and night sweats and relief from diarrhea.

Holistic medicine didn't much appeal to Staley, despite his disastrous experience with AZT. It was true that his rapid CD4 decline seemed to stabilize once he left the workforce and all the pressure that went with it. But no amount of "improved sense of well-being" was turning those numbers in the opposite direction. He tried everything on offer at the buyers club. Nothing made a significant difference.

Frustrated, he returned to his doctor with his old jar of AZT, making a proposal to slash the dose from twelve pills a day to just three. "If it's suboptimal, so what," he said. "It's better than nothing."

Out of ideas, Dr. William was game.

Staley had no trouble tolerating the quarter dose. As a result, his CD4 numbers more than doubled, and held steady for months. Staley had stumbled on one of the first errors in the AIDS treatment era: the AZT dose being prescribed was wrong. He and his doctor became vocal advocates for slashing the FDA recommendations. Their campaign caught on. Soon there were fewer transfusion-dependent patients and, though AZT still had many detractors, it was no longer easily dismissed as poison. For some, it was a lifesaver.

He did not mistake his good fortune for a cure. But his CD4s were in the normal range. "I figure that buys me another year or two," he told a friend. "And I know there's other stuff—I'm always looking in the pipeline."

PLANS FOR THE Wall Street demonstration against the price of AZT were advancing, and were not undermined by the pending release of ddI, a direct competitor. On the contrary, it was more important to the activists to keep pressure on Burroughs Wellcome so that Bristol-Myers would not feel encouraged to price its own drug out of reach. Activists formed into affinity groups and made independent plans for actions within the demonstration. Peter Staley and the Power Tools wanted to make a spectacular impact on Burroughs Wellcome. The idea to infiltrate the New York Stock Exchange was Staley's, and once details were worked out it included a plan for a small group in "executive drag" to enter the Exchange on the corner of Wall Street and Broadway and chain themselves inside.

In the weeks leading up to the event, Staley scouted the building with two other men, both of them HIV negative—Charlie Franchino, a chiropractor, and Robert Hilferty, a writer and filmmaker. They posed as tourists with a video camera. Back home they studied Hilferty's footage. Each of the traders they encountered wore a pocket badge, which the guard at the door scrutinized only glancingly. Hilferty zoomed in on several badges. They were plastic-coated white tags, about three-by-five inches, and contained the name of the firm along with a series of large, bold numbers. Franchino knew a place that would copy them exactly. They decided to masquerade as traders from Bear Stearns, because that firm seemed to have the greatest representation on the floor.

The replicas looked spot on, but to be sure, Staley and Hilferty gave them a dry run one day after lunchtime, when a thousand traders streamed back to work. Wearing dark blue suits and gripping chunky pads of paper for effect, they walked right past a guard without a moment's hesitation. The trading floor was a cavernous place, with an eight-story-high ceiling and massive wooden kiosks placed periodically along the marble floor, crowded with telephones and electronic ticker screens and clerks in red jackets. Staley and Hilferty walked to the center of the room. At one end of the floor they saw a dense cluster of throne-like enclosures rising in a gentle slope—the original, famously expensive exchange seats. On the other end was a small, disused balcony, reached by an extremely narrow wooden stairway.

"There," Staley said, glancing at the balcony. His co-conspirator nodded inconspicuously.

From over their shoulders came the startling voice of a stranger. "Well, hello!" A broad-faced man approached. "You fellows must be new here!" He slapped his hand into theirs.

A welcoming committee was the last thing they had anticipated.

"Bear Sterns," Staley said, offering his hand. "Nice to meet you."

The man tapped Staley's badge. "Three thousand? That's strange.

I've never seen a number over two thousand. That's the most traders they've ever had on the floor."

Staley forced a laugh. Their badges contained arbitrary numbers, all apparently outside the expected range. He looked down at his own lapel. "Well," he shrugged, "that's the one they gave me."

"Strange," said the older man. "Anyway, welcome."

The reconnaissance team beat a path straight out the door and back to the printers for new badges.

On the morning of the Wall Street demonstration, the guards were jittery. Leaflets and news accounts predicted the noontime arrival of a thousand ACT UP protesters. Staley and his affinity group members slipped inside the Exchange with the morning crowds. The opening bell was set to sound at 9:30 am. At 9:20, five of them climbed to the balcony, locked a chain to the balustrade, and handcuffed themselves to the chain: Staley, McGrath, and Arsenault from the Power Tools, and filmmakers Scott Robbe and Gregg Bordowitz. No one had yet noticed them up there. When Staley saw the electronic clock read 9:29:45, he signaled to the others to unfurl their banner. It said, "Sell Wellcome," using the Wall Street shorthand. Then they pulled portable marine fog-horns from their pockets and pointed them in the air. For Staley this action had deep personal meaning—payback after having endured the homophobia of the trading desk for so many years. He gave the signal.

The noise was deafening. At the same time, they pulled big stacks of fake money from their pockets—in homage to Abbie Hoffman, who had protested the Vietnam War inside this building years earlier—and threw them into the air. The slogan printed on the bills bypassed diplomacy: "We die while you make money. Fuck your profiteering."

Once the traders realized what was happening and why, they exploded in outrage. They surged angrily toward the balcony's staircase. Pens and other projectiles sailed through the air accompanied by cries of "mace the faggots" and worse. In the confusion, nobody realized the opening bell had sounded, and trading was delayed by many minutes, the first time in the 197-year history of the Exchange.

Down below, the two remaining protesters—Hilferty and Richard Elovich, a former IV-drug user—snapped a few photographs and hastily retreated toward the door, sprinting the last several yards after someone bellowed, "Who the fuck are you!" and twisted-faced traders lit out after them. When they were blocks away, the photographers passed their film to designated runners who headed straight for the AP offices to have the images developed and copied for the wire. Police took their time extracting the five from their chains. They dragged them out of the Exchange and into the thunderous applause of fellow activists. As Staley stepped onto the running board of the police department van, he allowed his eyes to turn toward the windows of the old J. P. Morgan trading floor. He pictured his former colleagues pressed against the glass, and smiled.

When lunchtime came, nearly 1,500 other ACT UP protesters descended on Wall Street, likewise armed with air horns and placards and banners decrying the cost of AZT. Their angry voices echoed through the narrow canyons into repetitive, blurred cries: "How many more must die? How many more must die?"

That same day, ACT UP chapters staged satellite demonstrations in London, where Burroughs Wellcome's parent company was based, and in San Francisco, where the company's major U.S. warehouse was located. Papers throughout the world carried news of their feat, following *The Wall Street Journal,* which played the story above the fold. Only the *Times,* continuing its aggressive stance against covering gay news, let the historic event go unmentioned in the morning papers.

The following Monday, admitting to being pinioned by protesters, Burroughs Wellcome slashed the price of AZT for a second time, finally reaching the price range demanded by ACT UP. It took another seven months for the criminal trespass case to come to a head. A judge, ruling that the defendants had acted "in the interests of justice," dismissed all charges.

TONY FAUCI'S taxi pulled up to the door of the Lesbian and Gay Community Center in New York one rainy October evening in 1989. There had been a sharp change in the balance of power between him and the activists that year. Now he was being called to the telephone sometimes several times a day, not just by the T+D members but by other branches of New York's ACT UP, and even by far-flung chapters. The Provincetown affiliate took twenty-five minutes of his time the previous week interpreting the raw data for Peptide T, a drug he didn't consider worthy of anyone's attention. Others had demanded he study St. John's wort, an herb sold in health food stores, and oral alpha interferon, a natural human protein that for some reason Louis Farrakhan's Nation of Islam was selling as an AIDS cure on the streets of Harlem.

Now he was about to meet T+D on their home turf, at their behest. They had timed the summit to take place just weeks before the first ACTG quarterly meeting they were to attend. The invitation made it clear that they wanted to be fully up to speed as they joined the AIDS clinical trials system, but they also felt that a far-reaching conversation would help Fauci better understand them as a community. Fauci accepted, suggesting a day when he and his senior staff would be in New York anyway. His assistant, Dr. Peggy Hamburg, joined him.

They could not have anticipated the disheveled surroundings at the community center. The building was covered with graffiti, with crooked windows and a flaking brownstone facade. Inside, the worn linoleum flooring was reminiscent of the schools of Fauci's youth, spent a short subway ride away in the Bensonhurst section of Brooklyn. He walked past the busy information desk through a set of double doors to the main meeting hall, with its fluorescent lights and whirling ceiling fans. The floor was covered in cigarette butts. A spray-painted mural stretched across one wall, including the window, blocking outside light; it featured what appeared to be naked wood sprites.

About fifty activists had pulled folding chairs into a tight circle, resembling a kind of tribal council. Most were wearing tight jeans and shirts that showed their arms. Jim Eigo wore a bright orange T-shirt that was snug at his thick biceps and thin waist. His shiny black hair was pulled into a ponytail. Richard Elovich, the former IV-drug user who had served, variously, as personal secretary to Allen Ginsberg, John Ashbery, and Jasper Johns, was chosen to moderate. He showed the stiffly attired Fauci and Hamburg to seats, bringing the room to silence.

"Here's how we planned this," he said. "What we want to do is run this like a Treatment and Data meeting. A number of times we've had people come to a Treatment and Data meeting and speak on certain issues. We try to get in-depth, we try to nail issues down. This isn't a free-for-all; let's call it a 'working confrontation.' So, why don't we start." He turned to the guests. "This," he said somewhat dramatically, "is Dr. Anthony Fauci."

Fauci looked up from a notepad on which he had been writing to smile at Jim Eigo, Mark Harrington, Iris Long, and a number of other ACT UPers he had come to know well over the past year. David Barr and Jay Lipner, who had tangled with his legal department, and Rebecca Pringle Smith, a medical student working at AmFAR, slid into their chairs. Spencer Cox eyed Fauci warily. Seeing a friendly face, Fauci waved to Bill Bahlman, who was operating a video camera. "Bill! How you doin'?" he called. Being back in his hometown brought out the Brooklyn in Fauci's voice. Bahlman responded with a brief glance.

The tight agenda was drawn up by Garance Franke-Ruta, who,

though still a teenager, carried a full workload of activism. They would address pathogenesis, drug trials, and opportunistic infections in segments of equal length, she said. Then Elovich called on Bob Rafsky, who rested his elbows on his knees in a gesture of weariness. Coming face-to-face with Fauci for the first time made Rafsky's mind go to the past, not the future.

"I may be wrong, Dr. Fauci," he began, "but it's my understanding that thousands of people died from PCP because there was no priority within the government or within the medical system as a whole to push the known preventative treatments for a long time. And it was only because of pressure from the community, and work within the community, like CRI, that a full spectrum of prevention for PCP became available, and the rate of deaths began to slow. Now those thousands of people are dead, are gone. There's nothing we can say or do in this room that's gonna bring them back."

Though he continued speaking in measured tones, his disdain grew more apparent.

"It would seem to me that someone who was within the government while that took place, as you were, would be *seared* by the knowledge that that happened on their watch, as we're seared in a different way by that knowledge—and would be moving heaven and earth to see what's the next leading cause of death, the other opportunistic infection, and dealing with that. But it's not happening. The data isn't even gathered. Whatever push there is still seems to be coming from the community.

"My question is, Why? Is it because the people who are dying are gay and people of color? Is it because science is blind in some way and can only perceive certain paths? Why?"

Fauci, who had been nodding along, had prepared for this question. "The thing about PCP and aerosolized pentamidine was really a bad scene," he admitted. "It was really awful."

Someone from across the room shouted, "It goes back years before that. I think he's talking about how Bactrim had been used in the '70s. The fact that they knew that there was something that could prevent PCP pneumonia—and no one ever thought to prophylax people with AIDS."

"There was an incredible amount of delay on that," Fauci agreed, as if critiquing someone else's work. "When I went back and looked at that, it was just really ridiculous—it was a matter of people haggling with each other about who was gonna do what. What I did at that point was to tell the people in the program that I wanted someone specifically to look over the shoulders of any of those studies that get hung up for any reason at all. Hopefully it will never happen again."

Jim Eigo, upset at this self-spun hero's narrative, gripped his elbows as he stalked the back of the room like a caged animal.

"I guess we're looking for more than 'suggestions will be quickly considered,'" Rafsky continued. "What we're saying is that people, including yourself at some level, must have on their conscience these deaths. Why isn't there a more aggressive movement to ask, *Why isn't there prophylaxis for this or for that? How can I fix that?*"

"That's being done," Fauci said, his voice rising. "There's a very heavy priority on opportunistic infections right now in the institute. I'm telling you, there is."

This was not a room without a memory. Rafsky scratched his head in disgust. Mark Harrington, in a worn flannel shirt, jumped in. "Two years ago, Larry and Michael Callen and a bunch of other people sat with you and asked *you* to put aerosol pentamidine into studies. And it was still thirteen more months!"

"That's a tough one," Fauci said, explaining that he received no good proposal in those thirteen months. For the first time all evening, the room erupted in a rustle of hostility, demanding to know why he didn't actively solicit a research proposal. "The reality of the situation," he said defensively, "is: There was a great reluctance among the community of everything from the scientists to the Congress [to] . . . telling investigators what to do, [that] we should allow them to do what they feel is the most important. Now, that sounds awful when you're putting it in the context of what we're talking about here. But the whole world isn't in this room."

This was exactly why ACT UP felt it needed to take part in the ACTG meetings—to infuse the sentiments of this room in every level of the research effort. Another member, Ken Fornataro, maneuvered to get Fauci to reiterate his invitation, here in this public forum, recorded on Bahlman's video, to attend the November meeting. "If I remember correctly," he said to Fauci, "you did agree that you would encourage and strongly support the inclusion of either a person with HIV or AIDS and/or an AIDS activist on the AIDS clinical drug development committee, that's correct?"

"Correct," he said.

"As well as allowing interested parties to attend the AIDS Clinical Trials Group meetings so we could have that educational exchange between us. Is that also correct?"

"Correct," Fauci said, quickly adding, "They're not happy about it." His message once again had a subtext of his own self-declared heroics.

"Well, I think *we're* all not happy about really *any* of this," Fornataro snapped back as Fauci tightened his grin. "But what I want to know is—"

"I'm just telling you, the answer is Yes! *Yes! They're not happy. It will happen.*"

Relieved, Mark Harrington called Dr. Hamburg the next day to make all the necessary arrangements. She appeared unprepared to talk to him about the ACTG meeting, though, asking if she could call him back after speaking with Dan Hoth. She got back to Harrington with unacceptable news: Hoth now said he needed to discuss ACT UP's attendance with the ACTG's executive committee, which meant the November date was out. Hamburg was embarrassed. When she suggested the invitation be pushed to spring, Harrington lost his temper.

"We've exhausted our patience," he said.

Shortly, his phone rang again. It was Fauci himself, full of excuses for the behavior of Hoth and his investigators. "I didn't recognize the strong reactive feelings. Hoth has got to deal with these guys every single day," he said. The investigators were mortified at the prospect of contending with activists, whom they thought of as politically radical and scientifically facile. "All they think is guys with banners and earrings in their ears."

He continued, "Dan went back on his commitment." With apologies and all due respect, they would not be allowed into the meeting after all.

Harrington ended the call quickly in order to discuss the development with other members of T+D. The next day, he wrote Fauci a letter to express the group's resolve. "It is vital that commitments made between ACT UP and NIAID be honored," he wrote. "Only by scrupulously honoring our commitments to each other can ACT UP and NIAID's AIDS Program have a fair and constructive relationship." He reminded Fauci that his promises had been recorded and witnessed "before fifty members of ACT UP and the New York AIDS community," and rescinding them would "vitiate the trust" that they had been building between ACT UP and NIAID. Welcomed or not, they would hold him to his word and attend the meeting as planned.

Their delegation would include Harrington, Fornataro, Iris Long, and Rebecca Pringle Smith. Additionally, Jim Eigo would attend as a member of a new Institute of Medicine panel reviewing the NIH's AIDS program, and ACT UP member Jon Engbretson would serve as an envoy from AmFAR.

"AIDS research, as I am sure you would agree, is a matter of the most urgent public concern. Science cannot function well in an atmosphere of secrecy. It is (or is supposed to be) based on an open exchange of information and opinion. Closed meetings which exclude the very people with the most to gain from the AIDS research enterprise do not embody the scientific ideal. We have far more to gain from working together than from being divided by bureaucratic considerations."

Harrington fixed a SILENCE=DEATH sticker to the letter and pushed it through a fax machine on November 3.

Three days later, the small delegation of disinvited guests arrived at a hotel ballroom in Rockville wearing their usual storm-the-barricades uniforms. Some eight hundred researchers filled the ballroom, the brain trust of the nation's emergency response to the plague. These were the scientists concocting drugs to study; researchers designing the testing protocols and recruiting the patients; and statisticians and analysts assessing the compounds that might one day save lives. They were not much older than the activists themselves. That realization did little to assuage their anger with the AIDS establishment. It was as if they had peered into the window at Cape Canaveral to discover frat brothers in Hawaiian shirts and beer-guzzler hats.

Dr. Hoth took the rostrum to open the meeting. He looked out at the young activists sourly. "The issue of *constituency representation* at the ACTG has been precipitated by ACT UP New York," he said. "Against our will, they have sent four representatives who are here today. We did not invite them. We wish they were not here. Nonetheless, we did not wish to provoke a physical confrontation by attempting to secure their exit."

He added, "They will not be permitted to talk in any of the meetings."

Harrington and his team expected that Hoth would be furious about being outmaneuvered. Following his opening remarks, they approached him to firmly reject the restrictions. Hoth upped the ante. Now he held that two-thirds of the scheduled meetings were private, closed-door sessions from which they were to be strictly excluded. This included every meeting on opportunistic infections, ACT UP's keenest interest, and on ddI, despite the fact that Jim Eigo was deep in negotiations with the manufacturer Bristol-Myers regarding its parallel track program.

Despite the sting of the frigid reception, the activists went about what business they were allowed, on the margins of the meeting. What they witnessed was a fascinating education for them, a window onto the idiosyncratic culture of the enterprise that might save their lives. They took copious notes, indexing the alien and colorful language like ethnographers. Here was Dr. Thomas Merigan, the Stanford virologist chairing the Primary Infection Committee, who described upcoming trial results as "the iceberg effect—the effect on gross disease," whatever that meant. Much of what they observed was entirely lost on their untrained ears.

But they learned more to further their main objective—drugs into bodies—than in any previous setting. They learned of eighteen planned studies, another eight that had been canceled, and four that had been completed, though not yet published. They heard interesting reports on drugs that had been included in their much-discussed AIDS Treatment Research Agenda, including one to treat cryptococcal meningitis and another for CMV retinitis, as effective as DHPG and far easier to administer—but, it turned out, significantly more toxic.

And by stealthy means, they managed to get an insider's view of the study of ddI, despite Hoth's obstructions. Dr. Larry Corey, a Seattle virologist who chaired the Executive Committee, reported that only thirty-nine patients were by now enrolled in the Phase II study, which put half on ddI and the rest on AZT. By comparison, 1,001 had already signed up for the parallel track, where they were sure to get the new drug. Researchers called this proof that parallel track was "drawing patients away from our trials," according to Dr. Merigan.

This threatened to trigger a reversal for ACT UP, though in truth the principal reason that the ddI study was undersubscribed had to do with last-minute changes in the protocol, drug packaging, and delivery schedules. It simply was further behind schedule than the parallel track.

But the more disturbing revelation was yet to come. Dr. Corey announced, with a voice as calm as if he were revealing a change in the lunch menu, that all new human trials had been temporarily halted. The reason for this was devastatingly simple: the ACTG had canceled a contract for data monitoring with the Research Triangle Institute in North Carolina and was beginning a new one with Harvard's Cambridge campus. During the transition period, which was expected to last nine months, there was no provision for drug trial enrollment or oversight. During that time, an estimated 22,875 more would die of AIDS in America and many times more than that in Africa, where the explosion of cases had led a foreign aid doctor to predict "an apocalypse." The cost in human lives of this ham-fisted management decision was staggering.

The mood was dark on the train ride back to the city. Mark Harrington was deeply traumatized by the blithe disregard for gay and black people's lives. He received a call from Scott Johnson, whose illness had propelled Harrington into AIDS activism. Initially deprived of aerosolized pentamidine, he had come down with a hideous case of PCP. Having survived that, he now had the wasting syndrome, presumably associated with a massive AIDS-related intestinal infection caused by *Mycobacterium avium-intracellulare,* or MAI. The mycobacteria are present in everyday drinking water, of little concern to most people. In PWAs, the organisms disseminated wildly, destroying intestinal linings and eating away at the lungs, spleen, and lymph glands. The condition was increasingly common, and AIDS experts from Texas predicted that MAI would eventually imperil most, if not all, PWAs who did not die from another HIV-related event. Yet in the chaotic and random federal research effort, there was not a single MAI study ongoing or planned.

After a grueling four months of diarrhea Johnson didn't think he had more than a week to go. He called from San Francisco to say farewell. "It's too late for me now," he said.

Harrington jumped on a plane as soon as he could. When he saw Johnson on Christmas Day, he was shocked by his shrunken appearance, his straw-like hair, and his eyes opened wide by malnutrition. Johnson had enough energy to sit up on his sofa for a visit that day. On January 3, he no longer did. "I wish it were over," Johnson said during their second visit, sipping liquid morphine and squirming painfully in bed. In a few days, his wish came true.

At the following Monday's ACT UP meeting Harrington revealed a boiling rage. "We had some useful information," he said, referring to the ACTG conference. "But the whole network is not going to be enrolling any new patients for months *because they're changing their data center.* They're not going to be able to start any new trials. They're not doing any opportunistic infections studies. They're at a standstill, *because they're changing their data center!*"

From the back of the room, someone called out, "We have to have a demonstration."

For the next many months, the activists talked about almost nothing else. There was a hunger for vengeance. *Who will be held accountable for these unnecessary deaths,* Harrington wondered, *this slaughter by unaccountable bureaucracy?* Their opportunity would come in the spring.

THE YEAR DREW to a close in a maelstrom of ACT UP actions, running the organization deep into debt. Peter Staley met the new challenge ably. He helped Sean Strub stage ACT UP's first art auction on December 2, with donations from Andy Warhol, David Hockney, Keith Haring, and Julian Schnabel, among others, netting $315,000, enough to keep the war effort in bus tickets and leaflets for another six months. The group's battlefronts had multiplied significantly: for the first time including a vast Speaker's Bureau for sending activists into schools and community organizations, fighting the policy for conducting strip searches of detained activists, and sending a team to the Marriage Bureau to demand a marriage license for Matt Ebert, twenty-four, and Alan Klein, twenty-five, a provocation made necessary by city hospitals that still refused to allow men to visit their dying lovers. They staged zaps against *Forbes* magazine, the Corcoran Gallery of Art, the Immigration and Naturalization Service, a Connecticut pharmaceutical company called Astra, the socialite Pat Buckley, and the *Times*, an ongoing target of frustration. They hounded the paper's publisher, flooded the home mailbox of its AIDS news reporter, and affixed $900 worth of stickers to the paper's sidewalk vending machines that declared, "Warning: This Tells Lies About AIDS." They were mounting needle exchange operations in shooting galleries, developing policies on housing issues, taking issue with the government's definition of AIDS for excluding manifestations common to women, and fighting the epidemic in communities of color.

Their many messages found a large audience as the epidemic continued to expand. Mail poured in from the farthest reaches of the globe, including from a twenty-six-year-old Parisian who had seen a news clip of ACT UPers chanting, "The whole world is watching." "This is *true*! You have to be sure about this. Your action is not only American, it concerns the whole world! And, American gays are the most numerous and the best organized. You must go on ACTing Up."

It was entirely too broad an agenda for Larry Kramer, who had cautiously returned to activism after the wounds from theater critics had somewhat healed. His time away from the organization didn't make him less curmudgeonly. He condemned the lack of focus. He interrupted speaker after speaker, blaming them personally, through some convolution, for the government's continued inaction. He hurled a bomb over the fence of a late November meeting in the form of a febrile memo he titled "We Must Make Tomorrow Happen Today," which he duplicated and stacked on the literature table in the back of the room.

"I believe we are suddenly in more trouble than we have been for some time," he wrote. "The horrid possibility exists that the main reason the ACTGs are changing data base centers is because the one they have been using (at Research Triangle in Raleigh-Durham) has been unable to adequately process or interpret all the data collected up to this time. This means that there is a good chance that everything NIAID and the ACTGs have told us about all the treatments they are shoving into our bodies may be based on USELESS OR FLAWED DATA. This means THERE IS A GOOD CHANCE THAT AFTER NINE YEARS OF AN EPIDEMIC THEY KNOW ABSOLUTELY ZILCH ABOUT ANYTHING."

He claimed that all of this had been allowed to happen by a weak movement. Too few people were doing too much work, the group as a whole was too timid, its goals too plentiful, its verve too limited. "What we are entitled to—what is just out there, over there—is being denied to us and we demand that it be ours. It's there, still out of reach, but coming closer. We can't stop now. We've started the revolution. We can't quit until we finish it."

His hectoring resonated with some, but not all, of the exhausted members. "Larry is being unfair," Marty Robinson said. "Sometimes I really think he doesn't understand anything about gay and lesbian liberation. He's too elitist and concerned with stars. Of course we're going to make mistakes. But we're learning and we're wonderful and I love you all." Garance Franke-Ruta and Peter Staley felt similarly.

"I'm concerned that there is very little room for a 'centrist' political position in ACT UP anymore," Staley said. "And quite frankly, a lot of very good people who had centrist political views or even conservative ones, were very good workers and they were dedicated to ending the AIDS crisis, and they're gone. I don't think that's good."

In fact, the group's most radical action to date was already in the works. On a Sunday morning when the mercury fell well below freezing, I took a subway uptown to St. Patrick's Cathedral, where a huge protest was already under way. At issue was Cardinal O'Connor's redoubled efforts against the use of condoms in any context, which he said had no place "in a pluralistic society or any other society." He invented a scientific basis for this belief, arguing that the molecular structure of latex allowed as many pregnancies and infections as it blocked.

The scene was chaotic. The sidewalk in front of the cathedral was crowded with 4,500 demonstrators, including some from the new organization Women's Health and Action Mobilization, a cosponsor. The scene included ACT UP's typical mix of rage and ridicule. A group of clowns charged the church with buffoonery, goofily spinning into Fifth

Avenue traffic and forcing their arrest one slapstick gesture at a time. In homage to the Macy's Thanksgiving Parade, another affinity group held aloft a forty-foot-long, helium-filled condom, which bore the inscription "Cardinal O'Condom." Dozens of other demonstrators carried more provocative images besides the ubiquitous SILENCE=DEATH banner. One poster, using the inscription CURB YOUR DOGMA, included a line drawing of the cardinal doing a dog's business. Another paired a photo of the cardinal in his miter alongside the coincidentally similar shape of an unrolled condom: the harsh caption read, "Know Your Scumbags."

Ray Navarro, a young artist and videographer with shoulder-length black hair, pushed through the crowd in the persona of a telecaster from a different era. He wore a white toga and a crown of thorns, setting off a delicate face. "This is Jesus Christ, I am in front of St. Patrick's Cathedral on Sunday," he intoned. His microphone, which revealed his affiliation with the "Fire and Brimstone Network," nearly disappeared behind the frost from his breath. "We're here reporting on a major AIDS activist and abortion-rights activist demonstration, which will be taking place here all morning. Inside, Cardinal O'Connor is busy spreading his lies and rumors about the position of lesbians and gays. We're here to say: We want to go to heaven too."

I left the throngs on the sidewalk and with a number of other reporters entered the large nave. The pews were almost all full. Because ACT UP had announced the demonstration in advance, the faithful had shown up in militant defense of their leader, joined by heads of other religious institutions as well as by Mayor Koch. After the rich pipes of the organ fell silent and O'Connor began his homily, individual demonstrators who had been scattered in the pews popped up simultaneously and fell to the floors in the aisles—a silent die-in involving scores of protesters. They did not intend to halt the service, but to disrupt the idea that O'Connor's policies had no victims. The effect was eerie and drew the wide-eyed attention of congregants, some of whom prayed openly and wept. A phalanx of priests strode up to the prone and the supine, dropping flyers with the day's prayers on them.

Undaunted by the commotion, O'Connor continued his prayerful sermon until Michael Petrelis broke the agreement among affinity groups to conduct the demonstration in silence. He rose from a shadow-hidden pew and shouted, "Why are you killing us? You're killing us! Stop it! Stop it! Stop it!" His voice tore through the nave. Another protester, Neil Broome, joined the chorus. "Stop it! Stop it! Stop it!

Stop it!" Voices from across the cathedral adopted the chant. Someone began to blow a whistle, and the chaos multiplied. A squad of police officers with yammering walkie-talkies on their belts marched in from side doors wearing their dishwashing gloves. Anticipating this, many protesters on the floor handcuffed themselves to the pews or pillars.

Forty-three people were carted out on stretchers to waiting police vans. As the officers climbed over Spencer Cox with lock cutters, he shouted, "Prayers won't save the one to one-point-two-five million people infected with the human immunodeficiency virus!" But when the service resumed in earnest, it was apparent that others had been quietly waiting their turn, like sleeper cells, dressed innocuously in their Sunday best. Another affinity group rose and turned their backs to the altar in protest. Later still, two people, both former Catholics, allowed the cardinal to place a communion wafer in their palms—one of the holiest sacraments in the church—only to throw them to the ground, an act of unimaginable cruelty and desecration in the eyes of the faithful.

The press coverage was scathing, complete with pictures of O'Connor alone in his cathedral conducting a kind of exorcism and cleansing ritual to remove the unholy stench of the ACT UP protesters. Every lesbian and gay organization in the nation denounced the action. Many of ACT UP's own members shared the opinion, most of all the stalwarts of T+D. Three days later, ACT UP's leaders were forced to call a press conference and explain themselves further, arguing that O'Connor had crossed from religion to politics, making him a fair target for protest. But it did little to calm the uproar. "Somewhere in that Cathedral, sitting in those pews, was a young Latina from the Bronx who found her only solace in life in the comfort of the church. I worry that she would not now listen to us, or would be much less likely to now," lamented Jim Eigo, an ex-Catholic.

Among the treatment group, only Larry Kramer welcomed the calamitous press. "It's the best thing we ever did," he said. "They're all afraid of the sissies now."

•

PART 4

Revolt of the Guinea Pigs

New Beginnings

As 1989 drew to a close, Callen was traversing the country conducting further research on long-term survivors for a book that HarperCollins had commissioned, a far cry from his days begging for space in the *Native*. Writing, he had come to think, was a form of activism best suited to Callen. He intended to address some of the fatal errors of the movement in his book, which he was calling "Surviving AIDS." Rereading his old articles and speeches triggered in him a broad reappraisal of his own life and political work, an introspection further motivated by Sonnabend, who over the summer bitterly accused him of seeking fame through the plague.

"It is too brutal and I am too raw," he explained to a group of students at Yale. "Joe Sonnabend once told me that KS lesions are very similar, physiologically, to bruises. He suggested that I think of my KS as bruises that don't heal. This image stuck with me and I knew I had to get out when I started naming lesions for the particular battle I was fighting when each new lesion appeared." He lifted his shirtsleeve. "This, for example, I refer to as my Compound Q lesion. I simply cannot sustain another body blow and so I leave the fractious fray to others."

He and Griffin Gold used to joke that the only way to extricate yourself from AIDS work was to die. Callen hoped to go out on his own terms. He stepped down from the PWA Coalition and resigned as editor of *Newsline*. He left the PWA Health Group, too, which under his leadership had sold an astonishing $2 million in underground treatments. "That's $2 million worth of desperation and frustration," he said.

He even planned to quit the Community Research Initiative, which he considered his crowning achievement. In its brief life, CRI had enrolled more women and people of color in clinical trials than all the testing sites the ACTG controlled in the city combined. It was true that the group was beset by financial problems, as was common in projects involving Sonnabend, but Callen felt confident he had put an effective succession mechanism in place. As a last act, he expanded the board and recruited Mark Harrington, aligning CRI and T+D.

It was a move Callen came to regret bitterly. Working on his own initiative, Harrington took on a top-to-bottom institutional appraisal of CRI. He presented his findings at what was to be Callen's final board meeting. They were devastating, snide, relentless, and unforgiving. He charged the medical director, a psychiatrist named Bernard Bihari, with managerial bumbling and scientific incompetence, noting that few of the nine studies completed to date had resulted in publishable findings. Despite objections from the others on the board, Harrington pressed on against Bihari. He found what he considered to be instances where Bihari had misled the board, and the board had misled the PWA population, characterizations the board strenuously denied. He concluded that CRI had squandered the confidence of everybody from the FDA to the gay community itself, as evidenced by its inability to raise funds and by the rising criticism of it from the city's AIDS doctors.

As Harrington spoke, Callen slammed his fist on the table in a frightening explosion. "This is my last meeting and I will not have this! Not after three years of blood and guts."

Harrington took a breath and continued his eviscerating appraisal. When he was done, Callen let years of frustration and exhaustion erupt.

"I think you are a Nazi, fascist pig who does not know how to do anything but destroy organizations, and I resent every word out of your mouth and every action that you ever took, and I never want to speak to you again."

Callen's raw and personal censure brought Harrington unexpectedly to tears. But it did not end his campaign.

Soon, Larry Kramer piled on against CRI, demanding that the board of directors resign en masse and appoint a receivership of sorts—he named the only candidates he would accept—or face his public wrath. The ultimatum helped Kramer's sinking reputation to decline further. *The Nation* called him "mad as the Ayatollah" and to *New York* magazine he was now no more than "a volatile man at turns wrathful and weepy." The board ignored him.

Within months, though, Harrington's campaign had succeeded in shutting down CRI and opening a reborn agency called the Community Research Initiative on AIDS, or CRIA, unburdened by the old group's debts. Callen's legacy had been erased, for which he would never forgive Harrington. Nor did he intend to discuss it again in public. Now he was just "one more lowly Person With AIDS," and that's the way he hoped he could remain. He needed to conserve his energy. At the very least, he hoped to be around long enough to witness Nuremberg-like trials in which politicians (and a few activists) would be made to account for their decisions regarding AIDS. Until then, a new a cappella group he formed called the Flirtations would get his attention.

But retirement wasn't going to be that easy. His telephone never stopped ringing. Friends of friends needed pep talks, doctors needed advice on patient outreach, and everybody knew where to find him. He started talking more about wanting to leave New York, the city where he had been infected. He begged Dworkin to go with him to California, but the geography conflict exposed fissures in their long relationship. Physical intimacies between them had been fraught since the beginning. Callen never disentangled sex from the imagery of death, nor even from the messages of shame indoctrinated in him throughout childhood. For more than two years he had avoided sex entirely, employing a series of reasonable health explanations. No one was more surprised by Callen's chastity than Callen himself. "If you had said to me ten years ago when I was having sex so much that a day would come when I would not want to have sex and when life would be perfectly fine without sex, I wouldn't have believed you," he told a friend.

Dworkin was generally understanding. He adored Callen and believed wholeheartedly in their partnership. But being in relatively good health, Dworkin felt his sexual drive as urgently as ever. At Callen's urging, he indulged in anonymous sex from time to time, an arrangement that soon led to an open affair with a vivacious and quick-talking schoolteacher named Carl Valentino. Throughout, Dworkin reassured Callen of his love and devotion. Callen feigned equanimity, but he told friends that Dworkin's divided affections left him feeling like a failure "as a partner and as a person."

OUR TELEVISIONS that winter filled with images of the Berlin Wall coming apart. Young people danced atop the cold war's tumbling emblem, the sound of swinging hammers and popping champagne corks drowning out the weepy speeches from politicians. It wasn't long before chunks of the wall made their way around the world as souvenirs, carried joyously through Checkpoint Charlie, suddenly with no guard in sight. It was tempting to see in that thrilling moment a sign that history did indeed bend toward justice and that for homosexuals and AIDS patients it was just a matter of time.

But the barriers around the halls of science proved many times more durable. A lopsided war of letters followed the showdown with Dan Hoth at the fall ACTG meeting. Mark Harrington bluntly accused the ACTG gatekeeper of slander and sabotage for implying that the activists tended toward violence. Garance Franke-Ruta slammed the agency for continuing to exclude blacks, women, and active drug users from trials. ("It is never an argument," she wrote, "to design trials that do not take into account who the eventual patient population for the drug will be.") Jim Eigo followed with a sharp year-end assessment of Hoth's empire, which he cc'd to "all the AIDS organizations I can think of and a few members of congress & of the press." He pointed out that the ACTG had evolved into the most lavishly endowed clinical trials system in world history, thanks in no small part to the work of ACT UP. Its budget had expanded to $90 million for 1990, and the cumulative federal commitment to AIDS research hit $1 billion. Yet in three and a half years, the ACTG made no progress whatsoever with regard to treatments, and AZT, the often toxic nostrum that predated Hoth's empire, remained the only approved drug on the market. By painful comparison, in January Washington announced a launch date for the Hubble Space Telescope, the culmination of a massive effort involving thousands of the country's sharpest minds. Nothing remotely like that existed for AIDS. "With a past & present this bleak, & the prospect not much brighter," Eigo wrote, "it should be obvious: At the ACTG there need to be changes made."

None of the letters elicited an expected reply from Fauci or Hoth. Not even a flurry of Freedom of Information requests for internal records provoked substantive responses (forcing Franke-Ruta to recruit the ACLU to ready a suit). While the NIH stonewalled, Harrington embarked on a thoroughgoing analysis of the AIDS Clinical Trials Group. He was dismayed by what he uncovered. Years after AZT was introduced, and even after evidence showed positive benefits from the drug lasted only about six months, 80 percent of all ACTG trial participants were still corralled into AZT-centric studies (for instance, testing AZT against AIDS dementia). Despite the promise Fauci made to T+D, only 17 percent were currently enrolled in studies for one or two of the opportunistic infections. The rest of the OIs, as they were collectively shorthanded—including MAI, the likely cause of Scott Johnson's death—were still of no interest to anybody but the dying.

Harrington learned that determining where the money would be spent was the responsibility of five researchers, appointed by Hoth: Dr.

Margaret Fischl from Miami, Dr. Larry Corey from Seattle, Harvard's Dr. Martin Hirsch, Stanford's Dr. Thomas Merigan, and Dr. Douglas Richman from San Diego. They assigned a huge portion of the budget to themselves for trials conceived in their own labs, which seemed of questionable ethics at best. Each had made his reputation studying acyclovir, the anti-herpes drug. That meant that all had existing allegiances to the blockbuster drug's maker, Burroughs Wellcome.

Were Burroughs Wellcome and the ACTG's powerful leaders engaging in what Harrington, in uncharacteristic light-handedness, called "a genteel form of intellectual and moral corruption?"

He put the question to the NIH directly, asking for any information on financial arrangements between Hoth's five advisers and Burroughs Wellcome. Martin Hirsch, who chaired Hoth's committee, gave a partial, and telling, reply. "Nearly all ACTG principal investigators have some industrial consultative arrangements," he wrote. "Such consultations facilitate, rather than impede, proper conduct of ACTG trials by serving as a channel for communication and concerns for both industry and government." Any specifics about Burroughs Wellcome and AIDS research would be permanently elusive, though. "[T]he privacy or other interests of investigators, key employees, consultants (etc.) would be jeopardized" by any further disclosure.

As Harrington pressed on, a feeling of embattlement pervaded at the NIH. Fauci and Dr. Jack Killen took evasive action in December. In what they hailed as a major concession to the AIDS community, they announced the formation of a formal Patient Constituency Working Group within the ACTG system. This would be a mechanism for activists, patients, and community physicians to engage with the research process. Fauci and Killen reserved for themselves the power to name those who would join the Patient Group. When invitations went out for a preliminary meeting, to be held in San Francisco on January 14, 1990, nobody representing T+D or even the larger ACT UP was on the list.

Those selected did not lack credibility. They included Debra Fraser-Howze, a tireless and effective organizer representing New York's Black Leadership Commission on AIDS; Dr. Pierre Luddington, from the national coalition of gay physicians that Dr. Barbara Starrett helped found; Chuck Mayer from the National Association of PWAs; Marie St.-Cyr Delpe representing the Women's AIDS Resource Network; and Mario Solis-Marich, a policy analyst at AIDS Project Los Angeles, a GMHC-styled social service agency and the leading AIDS nonprofit on the West Coast. David Barr was also invited, but as a representative

402 HOW TO SURVIVE A PLAGUE

of the Lambda Legal Defense and Education Fund, his employer, not T+D.

ACT UP was not about to be shut out. They dispatched Harrington to San Francisco to crash the preliminary meeting, and he encouraged Jesse Dobson, a member of the ACT UP San Francisco chapter with nerves of steel, to join him. Harrington appealed to the appointed members to vote the two ACT UPers in, which they eagerly did. Through enterprise and skullduggery, Harrington was on the inside now, whether Fauci, Killen, and Hoth liked it or not.

After returning to New York, Harrington finished his ACTG critique in time to board the plane for the March 4 ACTG meeting, the first time the new Patient Group would attend. But when they arrived at the Hyatt Regency in Bethesda that Sunday afternoon, they discovered that Fauci, Hoth, and Killen had once again barred them from the bulk of the sessions, including any time policies and priorities would be discussed and new trials set. Officious personnel from the conference management company stood guard outside the meeting rooms to block unauthorized access.

To respond to this affront, the Patient Group convened a meeting in David Barr's hotel room at 5 p.m. As Harrington rushed to join them, he bumped into David Gold, another member of ACT UP, who had crashed the meeting on his own initiative, as did a number of his compatriots. Gold, who worked as head of an investment group, jabbed a thumb toward a placard announcing where the results of the highly anticipated ddI studies would be discussed shortly. "Are you going, Mark?"

"It's closed," Harrington said bitterly.

Shrugging, Gold pushed past the sentry and took a seat inside. After a brief and angry standoff, the moderator summarily adjourned the event rather than proceed in his presence.

Meanwhile, upstairs in David Barr's room, the Patient Group members, which now included Marty Delaney from Project Inform in San Francisco and Richard James of the National Hemophilia Association, expressed outrage over the researchers' stubborn recalcitrance. They developed a list of demands for Jack Killen, who had organized the event, and were of one mind about the road ahead.

The closed-meetings policy never lifted. Garance Franke-Ruta and David Z. Kirschenbaum attempted to sneak into a few sessions, only to be escorted back out. One T+D member, Bill Snow, a schoolteacher, managed to evade security by wearing an official badge someone had abandoned. He attended several sessions through this ruse. It was hard for him to understand why the conference organizers worked so hard to defend their bunkers. Much of what he heard was technical jargon incomprehensible to laymen.

The main plenary session, which Harrington was free to attend, revealed a number of new trials in the pipeline, each of which Harrington diligently listed in his notebook. At the meeting of the Primary Infection Committee, to which he was also welcomed, he learned that researchers for the first time were testing two drugs in combination—AZT plus an experimental compound called ddC. It was not just theoretically possible that combination therapy offered a synergistic advantage. Scientists could now see that AZT's impact was short-lived because the virus mutated wildly. Attacking the virus with two drugs, even as smiliar as ddC was to AZT, appeared to slow down mutation. But in what combinations remained unclear.

Then Harrington saw David Gold approach the microphone. Looks of panic crossed the faces of the assembled researchers when they realized that an uninvited outsider was going to speak.

"There aren't enough trials of AZT and ddC together, or alternating, in the New York area," Gold said. What centers there were in the city were already fully enrolled. Would it be possible, he wondered, to open others?

His question created the kind of pandemonium that might have followed the spotting of a sewer rat. The meeting was immediately brought to an end, forty-five minutes ahead of schedule. In the hallway outside, a very agitated Jack Killen grabbed Harrington.

"What happened in there," he said testily, "was inappropriate."

"Worse things have happened in the AIDS epidemic than someone who wasn't invited to a meeting asking a question."

"That's not the point," Killen snapped.

The sides were as far apart as ever. Disgusted, Harrington handed Killen two copies of his report, which he called "Critique of the ACTG," one for him and the other for Hoth.

A feeling of defeat prevailed as the New York delegation packed bags and reams of scientific literature into several cars for the drive home. To get her duffle into a friend's trunk, Franke-Ruta was forced to remove a pile of old ACT UP posters and leave them behind. As she waited at the wheel for her other copilots, she watched Susan Ellenberg, the government's lead AIDS statistician, break away from colleagues to pull a couple of SILENCE=DEATH posters surreptitiously from the trash.

She scurried off with them under her arm. A stream of researchers snuck away with the rest of them. This was the first positive development in the otherwise unhappy three-day affair. It meant the activists had the researchers' attention.

THE ACTG CRITIQUE, which Harrington formally dedicated to the memory of Scott Johnson, was annihilating. It identified case after case of institutional failure, and tallied the lives lost as a result. It called the ACTG's leadership delusional, narcissistic, and ethically barren, and decried the entirety of federal AIDS research as "corporate-driven," thoughtless, secrecy obsessed, arrogant, and "narrow." The bizarre AZT obsessions of the five top researchers earned special invective. "It would not be unfair to characterize the ACTG, in its first three years, as an enterprise in which Burroughs Wellcome behaved as the majority shareholder."

He offered a blueprint for reforming the mess. But the report's broadsides against Hoth and his deputies were all that anyone reacted to, with outsized condemnation. Jack Killen telephoned Harrington to deliver his own angry verdict. "It's the . . . the *innuendo*," he said. "And the theme that researchers are motivated by things that are somehow less noble." He was livid with Harrington for insinuating that scientists placed their career advancement over patient longevity. "Character assassination," he called it, in another telephone call later in the month.

He demanded that Harrington resign from the Patient Group. He saw this as the only way "to repair the damage that this has done," adding for emphasis that Fauci agreed with him on the necessity of Harrington's departure. "I'm quite willing to negotiate with you about an alternative person," Killen said, but "I'm asking that Mark Harrington not be part of this—for what I think are good reasons."

Harrington responded by convincing *The Village Voice* to publish an adaptation of his critique. It carried the withering headline "Anatomy of a Disaster." Upon publication, Killen removed him by fiat. One ACTG official even suggested that the activists themselves were responsible for the lack of scientific advancement, explaining in *The New York Times* that their tactics scared scientists away from the AIDS field.

"They should be afraid of our power," Harrington said in a bitter reply. "The rapidity with which the F.D.A. has changed is a testament to our power. That's what we intend to do now for the research process itself: speed it up. It's time for the community to help call the shots."

Amid the escalating fracas, a well-regarded researcher at the ACTG called Harrington to say he supported almost every one of his observations, adding that the silent majority of his peers felt similarly. He asked to remain anonymous. "I get nothing out of the system. We just don't think it's workable," he said in a friendly rant that lasted three hours.

The reason, he said, was the total domination of the five individuals Harrington had identified.

"We call them 'The Gang of Five,'" the caller said. "A lot of us don't share [their] view." He could not speak publicly, he said, explaining that he needed the relationship with the ACTG both for funding his lab and "to meet our quotas" at the academic institutions that required publication for advancement.

He took issue only with Harrington's caricature of ACTG scientists as being indifferent to the fact that thousands died every month from opportunistic infections. He and others were keen to study OI treatments and preventions. But their proposals routinely went unfunded in favor of anything involving AZT. "PCP, CMV, MAI—the third common pathway [to death], and we don't have an agent for it? That's obscene," he said. "If they abandoned #116, #117, and #118," he said—numbers designating the three largest studies on the table, all involving AZT—"the entire ACTG would have enough resources to do all the other OIs, cancers, and the rest."

This was why T+D needed to be involved in setting research priorities.

In the period of deafening recrimination and whispered support surrounding the release of the critique and the *Voice* article, most people missed a key passage they both contained. With ACTG policies obsessively analyzing AZT and its antiretroviral cousins ddI and, now, ddC, Harrington suggested, all the scientists were trying to find a drug that inhibited reverse transcriptase, that unique process through which retroviruses infected cells. "Why not more aggressively test antivirals that attack HIV at different stages of its life cycle?" he wrote. "Why not mount innovative studies combining antivirals?"

Harrington's proposal was not the first to hypothesize the value of using multiple drugs to target the virus at different stages, but his was perhaps the most prominent platform the theory had occupied. Dr. Steve Miles, a UCLA specialist in reconstructing the immune system, got Harrington on the phone to share his excitement about alternate viral targets, including protease inhibitors and integrase inhibitors, two brand-new theoretical approaches. Harrington had seen an NCI presentation on the protease gene in January and had written about it favorably. Neither approach was being studied by academic researchers, but Fauci or the ACTG could change that through what Miles called a "very, very directed approach, which the Federal government has been unwilling to do." For example, they had the power to tell administrators at SmithKline and Merck, "Here's a $5 million request for studying protease inhibitors," and to tell another pair of companies, "Here's $5 million for integrase," Miles said. Instead, with Fauci allowing the companies to advocate for pet projects, major areas of research were overlooked, and drugs compounds with potential were falling through the cracks.

Miles was a high-ranking ACTG researcher. It was obvious he was disgruntled and frustrated. He didn't think an effective protease inhibitor would be available for years, given the current state of research affairs. "Two years minimum," he said. "Integrase inhibitors, even further away."

It was tempting in the years to come to imagine what might have happened if Harrington's excitement for complex combination therapy had found champions then, or if Miles's fascination with protease inhibitors had attracted the funding he coveted. These ideas, though, found no traction. It was time to change that. The New York activists began planning a large-scale demonstration on the campus of the NIH, where Fauci, Hoth, Killen, and the national research leadership worked every day. If AIDS scientists wanted posters for their collections, ACT UP was going to bring a mountain of them.

THIS WAS the season when AIDS testing finally caught on. Within a few months, some of ACT UP's most influential members came to a reckoning with their own health. Derek Link, who was twenty-two, was not shy about telling people about his death sentence. He took the test because a former lover had fallen sick, a common trigger. Mark Harrington accompanied his ex, Jay Funk, to see Sonnabend. Funk was infected. Harrington avoided the HIV test in favor of a CD4 count. He had 565 CD4s, close enough to the healthy range, but his ratios were inverted—a reliable sign of infection. In addition, he had a dangerously low number of platelets, an HIV-related condition called idiopathic thrombocytopenic purpura. It was, he knew, only a matter of time. Funk was in more immediate danger. He had a CD4 count of just twenty-four, unexpectedly low given that he had no signs of illness. Sonnabend put him on Bactrim the very next day. Harrington absorbed the double blow with solemn purpose: he would focus on

Funk's health, not his own. His activism would become a very effective form of avoidance.

David Barr was just as stoical when, at the urging of Marty Delaney, he finally sent his blood to the lab. He had the telltale antibodies and 385 CD4s, putting him immediately on the AZT track, though toxicity forced him to stop after just a few months. He went public immediately as the only HIV-positive member of the Lambda staff—and, when he left to become GMHC's assistant policy director, one of the few remaining infected staff members there as well, after multiple waves of die-offs. Shortly, Barr took Spencer Cox to the doctor for his own moment of truth, joined by another friend, Gregg Gonsalves, who was uninfected. The counselor delivering the bad news was grave almost to the point of parody. Cox let out an involuntary laugh, which brought to his memory a quip of Oscar Wilde's at the expense of Dickens: "One must have a heart of stone to read the death of little Nell without laughing." Cox was now twenty-one years old and facing his shortened life expectancy the only way he knew how, with bon mots from the gay canon. His worried friends took him straight to lunch and a movie to take his mind off things. Cox chose *Defending Your Life*, a dark comedy about death—a decision they all quickly regretted.

All around the city, the ranks of the newly diagnosed grew so profoundly that GMHC could no longer keep up with client services. Already strapped, they now projected a 300 percent increase in clients and costs in 1990.

There was now one AIDS death in America every twelve minutes. So many prominent leaders in the arts were perishing that the dailies in New York, San Francisco, Miami, and Los Angeles ran AIDS obituaries almost every day. The dancer Ian Horvath, the sculptor Scott Burton, and the actor Ian Charleston, who won international acclaim for the film *Chariots of Fire*, all succumbed in January, followed by the artist Keith Haring, a regular at ACT UP meetings, in February. Countless others were dying in obscurity, or recalled only in the gay papers. The tiny *Bay Area Reporter* in San Francisco, the most conscientious periodical about honoring the dead, ran 112 obituaries in just the first two months of 1990, and those were only the deaths directly attributable to AIDS. At Cedars-Sinai Hospital in Los Angeles, Philip Saylor sat quietly on the edge of his dying friend Steven Jenkins's hospital bed for some time before using a pistol to end their shared suffering. Both were thirty-five. A spokesman for AIDS Project Los Angeles said such events were now weekly affairs.

A new urgency took hold at the Monday-night meetings as the massive demonstration was planned for the NIH campus. The group's demands had become a mantra: an end to scientific secrecy and the open inclusion of IV-drug users, women, and children in all studies. Inspired by something an ACTG source told them about the capacity of the system, they would also demand that thirty or more new compounds be tested annually in small, rapid efficacy trials—*drugs into bodies.*

On March 17, a Saturday, Peter Staley joined Charlie Franchino for a reconnaissance mission in Bethesda. By coincidence, Harrington planned to be in D.C. at the same time, for a series of meetings during the day and that night for one of Jim Hill's now-famous gourmet summits. Staley felt it was important to divulge their plans to Hill and Fauci, to lay out the group's demands and give them a chance to capitulate beforehand—to use the threatened demonstration as a negotiating tool, not an end in itself. Harrington concurred. At his suggestion, Hill agreed to set a plate for Staley and Franchino as well. They would all convene at the townhouse after sunset.

Franchino was behind the wheel for the four-hour drive to the towering iron gates of the NIH campus. Posing as tourists with Polaroid cameras around their necks, he and Staley made it onto the grounds unquestioned, cruising slowly around the rolling campus using a printed map as their guide. When they reached iconic Building 1, they parked and walked around it to take a closer look. With its broad steps leading to the entrance and a large plaza that could accommodate thousands, it was the ideal mustering point. And the building was the only structure on campus with the words "National Institutes of Health" carved into its cornice—a photo-friendly backdrop for their press coverage.

They were surveying the nearby security gates and documenting the various routes for arrival and egress with the Polaroid when a car bearing NIH's security insignia approached, followed by three unmarked vehicles. An officer asked them a few questions in a manner that suggested he knew who they were and what they were planning. This should not have come as a surprise, they had to admit; the protest had been discussed openly at ACT UP meetings, and fliers had already been distributed around the streets of New York and to ACT UP's fifty chapters around the country. The interrogation was over quickly. The intruders were never directly asked about protest plans, and they made no admissions, but as they left the officers said, "See ya later," and smiled knowingly.

They made it to Dr. Hill's at the designated hour. Fauci was already there, accompanied by his wife, Christine Grady. Her participation was unexpected, but not unwelcome. Grady, an HIV nurse, was a former staff member of Reagan's cartoonish Presidential AIDS Commission, where she was among the most level-headed voices. The evening began genially enough in the living room with pretzels and beer. Hill's dinner was his usual high caliber and the wine was free-flowing.

Staley turned the conversation serious. "ACT UP is planning a major national action—the biggest since we marched on the FDA," he told Fauci. "May 21, at the NIH campus. We're down here now to scope out the site, and we thought we should meet with you to let you know why we're demonstrating."

A smirk crossed Fauci's face. He locked his fingers behind his head and swung back in his chair. "Don't you think there are more effective ways to make your point?" he asked.

Peter shook his head. "We've tried everything else. We asked to attend ACTG meetings last July, and your staff tried to prevent us from going in November, so we had to force our way in. ACT UP members were escorted physically out of the meeting in March. Now, after Mark distributed his report, your staff are trying to throw him off the Patient Constituency Working Group. NIH and the ACTG don't seem to be open to activist attendance or participation. Maybe this will wake them up."

Harrington put down his wineglass. "These are our demands," he said. He reached for a list that he had composed and ACT UP had approved, and he slid it across the table.

Their vision was very specific, with a somewhat utopian flourish: "We assert that in any society worthy of the name *humane*, health care would be a right, not a privilege; that all people living within the borders of the U.S.A. are entitled to their government's protection against disease and death; that treatments for deadly diseases should be developed for public health and not for private profit; and that the AIDS communities must play a guiding role in the planning and execution of a coordinated, national effort to end the HIV epidemic and save the lives of all those infected. This is why we are bringing our demands, with our bodies, to the NIH on May 21, 1990."

The document laid out sixteen specific ultimatums, including an end to secret meetings, a restructuring of the ACTG around the mode Harrington had developed, a ban on consulting arrangements between federally funded scientists and pharmaceutical companies, and an immediate change in focus away from AZT in favor of new drugs, especially those aimed at the twenty-four opportunistic infections and cancers. The demands sheet reiterated ACT UP's recognition that experimental trials were the only chance people had to survive the plague. For this reason, they called on the NIH to immediately begin enrolling women, people of color, and children proportionate to their numbers in the epidemic.

"Medical apartheid," they called it. "Open trials to ALL HIV-infected people."

Fauci struggled to maintain a polite demeanor; only his wife showed any discomfort. Fauci hoped to convince Harrington to defend what hard-won access he still enjoyed. His message was: Lie low for now and win back trust over time.

"A lot of people are mad at you, Mark," he said.

"We have issues with a lot of them, too," Harrington answered stonily.

The mutual tension never left the room, despite Hill's arrival with more refreshments. Of the many meals they would have together, this one would be their least productive.

By Monday, everybody in NIH's leadership knew about the planned demonstration, including Jack Killen, who called Harrington. He was unusually contrite. "Unilaterally dismissing you from this committee," Killen said, carefully choosing his words, "was probably a tactical error on our part."

Harrington was savoring Killen's effort at peacemaking. It wasn't exactly a mea culpa, but it was more evidence that ACT UP's home-grown experts benefited from having an army of foot soldiers at their command.

THE PLANNING for the demonstration required ACT UP to operate at full throttle. Monday-night meetings were consumed by logistical work. Every Wednesday, T+D met in Charlie Franchino's apartment on Downing Street, reviewing scientific developments to refine their demands and perfect their "inside" strategy. By now the committee that Garance Franke-Ruta once dubbed "Science Club" had two dozen members, all versed in the arcane shorthand of science despite their unrelated vocations; they had enlisted a photographer, a chiropractor, a former Peace Corps volunteer, a performance artist, and a recent grad with a history degree. Most were white men, and most of them were HIV infected, though six uninfected women took central roles, including Rebecca Pringle Smith, a program officer at AmFAR, and Suzanne Phillips, an AIDS physician.

Just one member was African American: Keith Cylar, a preppy-looking social worker who had arrived a few months earlier. As had by now become a plague-era tradition, he shared his personal AIDS history from the floor of an ACT UP meeting in direct, unpitying fashion. Two years earlier, his lover, a New York City police officer, fell ill with a wicked cold. When it stretched on into its third day, Cylar took him to the emergency room at St. Vincent's. He never saw him again. His lover had never told his family he was gay; when relatives arrived at the hospital, they blocked Cylar from visiting and, after their son's death eight days later, locked Cylar out of the apartment they shared, leaving him homeless and—he soon learned—infected himself. This trauma pushed him into a serious cocaine addiction. He never hoped to become a citizen-scientist on Harrington's level. His interests in ACT UP took him to the Housing Committee and to Majority Action. But he began attending T+D as well because no one there was speaking for drug users and people of color. In this way, he served as the committee's social conscience and cultural ballast.

Over six weeks, which saw the death of five thousand more Americans, including the beloved Indiana teenager Ryan White, T+D members were dispatched to lead teach-ins about Fauci's world at the NIH with far-flung ACT UP affiliates. They convinced the country's leading AIDS organizations to endorse ACT UP's research demands. Meantime, other committees were plotting the "outside strategy." Monday after Monday, affinity groups reported their expanding itineraries to the floor, which now swelled so full that people in the back of the room complained about handouts reaching them long after the relevant matters were discussed. A subcommittee was formed to find a room that could accommodate a thousand bodies every week. Money was pouring in, $55,000 each month. The ACT UP videography collective was editing "how to do a demonstration" videos to ship out to the affiliates.

Meantime, work on other fronts was undiminished. One busy Monday-night meeting was interrupted by an announcement that a young couple had just been assaulted inside St. Vincent's, where they had gone for emergency care. The assailant was a hospital guard, offended by the tenderness one man had shown the other. In an explosion of outrage, the meeting hall spontaneously emptied as hundreds marched toward a confrontation with hospital administrators. Taking over the admitting lounge, they staged a kiss-in to demand sensitivity training for hospital employees. It was long past time for the flagship Catholic hospital to address its homophobia. There were more openly gay men in St. Vincent's beds at any one time than in most towns across the country. If the neighborhood hospital couldn't offer them effective treatments, the least they could do was keep them safe from violence.

The urgency driving the movement had never been more consuming. But at the same time, internal tensions ran high. Shouting matches erupted inside committee meetings and even in nearby restaurants where members gathered for post-meeting meals. Inflaming the situation, one member, Bill Dobbs, began publishing a weekly newsletter called *Tell It To ACT UP*, or *TITA* for short, as a platform for anonymous "suggestions box"–type comments. Some messages were humorous, inspirational, or flirty. But behind the cloak of anonymity, nastiness entered the energy mix for the first time. Much of it was directed at Peter Staley, from people who resented his now-frequent television appearances and what they considered his inflated ego and bristling hauteur.

"Who elected Peter Staley ACT UP poster boy?" one TITA commenter wondered. Another wrote about being snubbed after complimenting Staley's turn on *The Phil Donahue Show*. "His eyes never met mine, he smiled ever-so-faintly and coyly into the air and brushed by me like yesterday's trash." Staley was blamed for some of the same things that had bedeviled Michael Callen years earlier: hogging the limelight, coveting "fame" through AIDS, and, in this case, for constituting, along with Larry Kramer, Ann Northrop, Mark Harrington, and a few others, a kind of undeclared leadership in the supposedly leaderless organization. As David Robinson, the regular meeting facilitator, put it in a four-page open letter to members, "in ACT UP as a whole the situation is no longer 'We are the experts' but rather 'We have our own experts.' That change *must* be reversed."

Disastrous fault lines were forming.

WITH THE MAY 21 demonstration approaching, Dr. Fauci told a radio station that the threat of protest had surprised and injured him, describing himself as the best friend advocates could hope for. He authorized publication of a new NIH AIDS newsletter, devoting the May edition to refuting ACT UP's allegations, distorting its demands, and misstating the agency's accomplishments. Harrington and Eigo countered with a point-by-point rebuttal and mailed it to every name they found in an official NIH employee roster. "Federal officials with the power to redirect our nation's AIDS-research effort must listen to and work with us," it stated. "We will not rest until they do so."

Their organizing efforts proved more effective than Fauci's. When they finally converged on the Bethesda parking lot, ACT UP chapters from twenty states were represented, reflecting the epidemic's spread across America. For the first time, New York City was no longer the epicenter. Infection rates per capita now were higher in San Francisco and in San Juan, Puerto Rico, while two cities in New Jersey (Newark and Jersey City) and three in Florida (Fort Lauderdale, Miami, and West Palm Beach) were closing in fast on New York's caseload.

Some 1,200 activists stood together on the NIH campus that morning, and their numbers grew throughout the day. One man arrived directly from his hospital bed at the NIH AIDS ward, having seen the protest out his window. In his gown and slippers, and tethered to an IV poll, he joined in the chanting: "Ten Years. A Billion Dollars. One Drug. Big Deal."

Like earlier ACT UP demonstrations, this one was characterized by carnival-like theatrics and symbolism. An affinity group from Oberlin, Ohio, performed a piece of political theater, calling out lines in the manner of moustache-twirling melodrama. An effigy of Fauci was burned. A SILENCE=DEATH banner was run up the flagpole. A group of twenty-one made it inside the building to occupy Dan Hoth's empty office, scribbling demands on his chalkboard. Reporters took much of the action for churlishness, and even a number of gay leaders considered ACT UP's drama ridiculous and embarrassing, but given the worsening crisis no one came to the NIH's defense.

When the throngs moved on toward Fauci's office at Building 31, Staley, who was his own affinity group, once again catapulted himself to the awning above the entrance. This time, though, he was aggressively subdued. As distressed witnesses shouted, "The whole world is watching, the whole world is watching," an officer mounted the awning and approached him with his truncheon drawn. Staley held his hands in the air, which did nothing to defuse the situation. The officer grabbed him around his chest and slammed him onto his belly, planting a knee in Staley's back until backup officers arrived. They then lowered him by his armpits into the gloved hands of arresting officers on the sidewalk below. Television cameras captured the scene, like Rembrandt's *The Descent from the Cross.* Garance Franke-Ruta fought back tears. Had the world gone mad, she wondered, arresting the sick and not the heartless?

Officers wrenched Staley's arms behind his back and cranked zip cuffs on his wrists, signaling the beginning of a round of brutal arrests. In all, eighty-two were carted off in police wagons, and scores more were nursing injuries from pepper spray, batons, or trampling horses. The violent images on the evening news would be hard for Americans to ignore.

As he was being hustled away, Staley heard a familiar voice calling his name.

"Peter!" Dr. Fauci signaled for the officer to slow down. "Peter, are you okay?"

"Just doing my job," he replied.

An hour or so later, the NIH mounted a hasty press conference. A smiling Fauci said, "It was interesting theater. But it was not helpful."

To which Keith Cylar replied: "I think Fauci understands, and at times appreciates, what we do. Fauci himself understands that he does not have the power himself to do what needs to be done. That's why the system has to be opened up."

Fauci told reporters of bruised feelings and said a heightened skittishness on the part of scientists was the demonstration's main outcome. There was some evidence of this. Dr. Paul Volberding complained of "intimidation" and John Ziegler, the chairman of UCSF's AIDS task force, felt as embattled as a Kuwaiti soldier. "This is the Middle East," he said. On the Hill, where lawmakers were now wondering why AIDS merited more money than cancer, ACT UP's reputation was for insolence and brutishness—"a gangster group," in the words of John Leo, the influential columnist with *U.S. News & World Report*.

But in the coming days, true reform began. Fauci announced a commitment to include more women and people of color in drug trials, and said that priority in the coming year would finally be given to drugs focusing on opportunist infections. It was about time. Worldwide, 386,588 cases had already been reported in 151 countries, and more than half of them were already dead, killed by opportunistic infections.

Then, suddenly, Bethesda in 1990 was like Berlin in 1989. Activists found that all the barriers at the NIH and the FDA vanished in a blink. ACT UP members were appointed to dozens of committees, not only to review the results of studies but to approve the studies' designs and to help set priorities for which drugs to investigate and in what populations. People with AIDS and their advocates were integrated into every element of government's response to the epidemic, expected to give meaningful contributions.

"These are intelligent, gifted, articulate people coming up with good, creative ideas," Fauci told a reporter.

The activists took time to savor the victory. "Never again could any of this be done without taking people with AIDS and their advocates into consideration," said Jim Eigo. "This would be public business from now on."

JUST FOUR WEEKS stood between the NIH protest and the sixth International AIDS Conference, scheduled to open on June 20, 1990, in San Francisco. Since the previous summit in Montreal, ACT UP had been organizing a presence there. At least one of its committees—on youth prevention efforts—had been invited to present its experience in the massive poster hall, where important findings were displayed on large boards. But with their sudden traction with the NIH, Peter Staley saw an opportunity to keep momentum on their side. He argued that the New York group needed to build strong relationships beyond the small cadre of federal researchers they had been engaging in the ACTG. This conference would be a gathering of what Mark Harrington called "the very *heart* of the AIDS establishment"—the anonymous men and women toiling away inside pharmaceutical companies and biotechs, the bench researchers from Europe and Asia, the epidemiologists, the biostatisticians who reviewed trial protocols, the psychosocial experts, prevention innovators, and program administrators—and it was important to engage with them.

The other ACT UP chapters agreed in principle, but had voted to boycott the conference in protest of a new law, written by North Carolina's Republican senator Jesse Helms, that barred travel to the United States by anyone carrying the virus. There was no medical or scientific justification for the measure, which *The Lancet* called "remarkable mainly for its purposelessness and its ugliness." No reputable authority still feared casual transmission of HIV. Helms's amendment meant that AIDS patients from around the world, the specific beneficiaries of AIDS research, would be excluded from attending the conference. Compounding matters, the Immigration and Naturalization Service announced that it would strictly enforce the seventy-three-year-old ban on homosexuals at the border.

Their call to boycott quickly gained traction. Many rank-and-file scientists announced their intentions to spurn the proceedings if the exclusionary clause remained in effect. They were quickly joined by the International League of Red Cross Societies, whose secretary general worried that participation in the conference might be construed as condoning discrimination. Soon, more than eighty-five entities fell in step, including the governments of Switzerland, France, and the state of Hawaii. The American ACT UP network decided to appear in San Francisco in large numbers, but its members would remain outside of the conference, making their voices heard from the street.

This put the New York branch in a bind. Having turned their focus toward basic science more than public policy, everyone in T+D agreed on the importance of being inside the meeting hall. "More information about AIDS research and treatment will be available at the S.F. Conference than anywhere else this year," they wrote in an open letter circulated to members. "If we do not go, we will lose the opportunity to attend scientific panels, see posters about lab research and clinical trials, talk to researchers and clinicians at the conference, and obtain the *Abstracts*. Last year's Montreal *Abstracts* contained many obscure papers which greatly facilitated the work of T+D and other activists."

What's more, for the first time ever, their participation was being actively solicited. Robert Wachter, a young AIDS doctor at UCSF who was the program coordinator for the San Francisco event, and his deputy Dana Van Gorder, the highest-ranking gay man working for the conference, traveled to New York to personally invite the activists. They asked ACT UP to nominate candidates for a speaking spot at the opening plenary. This was an enormous development, and it came just one year after Montreal organizers called police to remove the PWAs. The "inside/outside strategy" was producing solid results. It made little sense to Staley not to take advantage of the opportunity.

The rift in ACT UP was wide open now. On one side were members who saw the epidemic's social and political challenges as indivisible from matters of science and medicine. On the other side were those for whom the need for effective treatments was so urgent that it took priority over everything else. Most of this latter group were T+D members, and significantly, most were HIV positive. "Joining the Boycott is a bad idea," they wrote. "Joining the Boycott would be the hallmark of an activism which puts the 'defiant gesture' before our well-known ability to infiltrate the scientific establishment and obtain life-saving information for people with AIDS and HIV."

Ultimately, two separate and opposing proposals made it to the floor one rancorous Monday night in May. Surprisingly, a resolution prevailed that met with the satisfaction of both sides. By a show of hands, ACT UP New York determined that half its committees would "support the spirit of the boycott" on the sidewalk while the rest—including those working on housing, needle exchange, Latino issues, and alternative and holistic treatments—would follow T+D through the door.

Staley returned to his fund-raising bunker. Hundreds of New York members planned to attend the week-long event, including dozens who needed full subsidies. The media operation required two video cameras and three Mac computers, as well as a number of fax machines, televisions, VCRs, and rented mobile phones. It would be a large undertaking, costing $100,000 or more.

Harrington got to work on an updated AIDS Treatment Research Agenda. This year's "Drugs We Need Now" would lead with a treatment for MAI, the intestinal marauder that claimed Harrington's friend. Protease inhibitors were on the wish list, too, as were experimental therapies that intrigued the activists, with names like hydroxychloroquine and aromatic polycyclic diones. The overall tone of Harrington's agenda was no more optimistic than the previous edition had been. He chose to open with a quote from Larry Kramer: "We have lost the war on AIDS. Millions who need not die so young will die so young."

It made Kramer proud watching the T+D stalwarts grow into respected experts. Thanks to T+D, ACT UP had become the juggernaut he had dreamed of, and though he was an inactive member over the winter—his prequel to *The Normal Heart* absorbed his time—he made sure to attend the meeting where ACT UP developed its nominating list for plenary speakers. The movement had by now produced many able orators, Kramer knew. But as the epidemic's first Cicero and the man whose words had conjured ACT UP into existence, he believed this opportunity rightly fell to him. He was certain it would take a public voice of his caliber to cement ACT UP's victories and forge new goals.

But to his dismay, the members chose Vito Russo. It was a betrayal on the magnitude of the time GMHC didn't pick him to meet with the mayor. He admired Russo, but not for this job. He took the news acidly.

He called Dr. Wachter the next day. "I should be the choice," he argued. "Don't pick somebody safe."

Wachter had met Kramer twice in the past, and found him at once obsequious and manipulative. In private conversations with other ACT UP members, he had heard that Kramer was "a loose cannon" whose veneer of civility was paper thin. He also knew there was no more recognized figure in the community. He promised Kramer that he would take his appeal into account. The consensus, though, settled on Russo, an inspiring speaker. The news provoked one of the ugliest bouts of petulance from Kramer, which he expressed in a regrettable letter to conference organizers:

> Everyone had hoped that your conference, of all conferences, in your city, of all cities, would allow the chance for divergent opinions to be aired publicly. Evidently such is not to be the case; and once again we face a conference homogenized, made bland, and blanched of open discussion of the many divisive issues that prevent AIDS from being cured. . . . You have, in effect, thrown down the gauntlet, and I intend to see that it is taken up. If you wish to view this letter as a threat, please do so.

As consolation, Kramer was invited to present at a workshop, a role he rejected. When Wachter stopped responding in any way to his stream of appeals, Kramer seemed to go over the edge.

"The same Doctor Strangeloves who control the ACTG system are the same Doctor Strangeloves who are controlling the agenda of, and shutting out any dissident voices from, the Sixth International Conference on AIDS," he wrote in *OutWeek* magazine, a new *Native* competitor where he was now a columnist. "HOW MUCH MORE EVIDENCE DO YOU NEED? DO YOU HAVE TO BE LINED UP IN FRONT OF A FIRING SQUAD BEFORE YOU FIRE BACK? *WE HAVE BEEN LINED UP IN FRONT OF A FIRING SQUAD AND IT IS CALLED AIDS.* WE MUST RIOT! I AM CALLING FOR A FUCKING RIOT!"

The bizarre fulmination triggered headlines around the globe and brought a steady stream of reporters to Kramer's apartment on lower Fifth Avenue, whom he took to greeting in a T-shirt with Malcolm X's famous motto, "By any means necessary." "It hurts me to say I think the time for violence has now arrived," he told Marilyn Chase of *The Wall Street Journal*, adding, "I don't personally think I'm the guy with the guts to do it, but I'd like to see an AIDS terrorist army, like the Irgun which led to the state of Israel." On *The MacNeil/Lehrer News-Hour*, he said, "We are up against a wall. There is no avenue left to us *except* terrorism."

At the next ACT UP meeting, which descended into chaos upon his arrival, Kramer and his call to violence were universally condemned. In its founding documents, and at the beginning of every Monday-night meeting for more than three years, the group had explicitly committed itself to nonviolence. Its members considered themselves heirs to Gandhi. They aligned themselves with Henry David Thoreau and Dr. Martin Luther King Jr.; with the anti-apartheid, anti-nuclear, and pro-feminism movements; with the nuns who empowered Salvadoran peasants and the Argentine mothers who stood silently in Plaza de Mayo. All of Kramer's followers seemed now to abandon him.

Kramer typed up his defense in the form of a letter to the members and placed a stack of copies on the literature table the following Monday night.

> You can ignore what I'm saying. You can say I've finally flipped out. (That's been said about me often.) You can slit your wrists. Or you can fight harder than you have before.
>
> The Sixth International Conference on AIDS is being put on by the very system that's killing us. It's their annual Big Show. You think [conference cochair] Dr. Paul Volberding is a saint, and I think he's a very efficient supplier of bodies to your local undertakers. . . .
>
> You are free not to riot and you are free to criticize my call to riot, and I am free not to comprehend your criticism.
>
> And we are all free to die.

Then Kramer went silent, quitting his monthly *OutWeek* column and ceasing to attend planning meetings for the conference.

About five days before the opening ceremonies, Dana Van Gorder from the AIDS Conference reached Peter Staley by phone. Vito Russo had come down with the dreaded pneumonia, he reported, and had to remove himself from the speakers' roster. Van Gorder asked Staley to take his place.

He was flattered by the invitation but asked for time to think it over.

"You need to tell them I should speak at this," Kramer said when Staley reported the offer. "You need to tell them that it should be me."

Staley considered Kramer the closest thing the movement had to a leader, mercurial and volatile though he was. He knew that a Kramer speech could have enormous impact. He called Van Gorder, and yielded the invitation to Kramer as promised, but the organizers were even less amenable now. Kramer gave Staley his grudging approval, then decided privately that he would not attend the San Francisco conference in any capacity. Larry Kramer was skipping his own riot.

• • •

THE CITY by the Bay was prepared for the worst. By chance, the conference was coinciding with San Francisco's Gay Pride Parade, which drew hundreds of thousands of marchers every year. Mayor Art Agnos pictured every last one of them joining the protests at the Moscone Center, where they would outnumber researchers forty to one. Additionally, an anarchist group was gathering for its own national convention, as was a group of animal rights militants from the University of California, Davis, who had turned against the medical use of animals, even in AIDS research. The potential for a perfect storm of radical protest activity had the city on high alert.

The San Francisco Police Department prepared 1,750 officers to handle Kramer's militia. Wild rumors wafted through town: that desperate PWAs intended to spray the police with infected blood, that AIDS-crazed radicals planned to kidnap new HHS secretary Dr. Louis Sullivan or jab Dr. Margaret Fischl and the other "Gang of Five" members with infected needles. Some five thousand articles about AIDS appeared in the world's press in the months surrounding the conference, focused almost entirely on the dangerous tensions. Conference organizers hired a top security firm, the same one that had protected the pope on his recent American tour. Hulking bodyguards were assigned to Volberding, Fischl, and Wachter, to their own embarrassment and relief. Never before had a scientific conference taken place under such ominous clouds.

Peter Staley kept his own counsel as he prepared his remarks. He had read that some scientists were leaving AIDS for fields including cancer and other infectious diseases, where they might feel more appreciated, or at least less reviled. Dr. Fauci was talking about mass defections. Staley saw his unexpected platform as an opportunity to build lasting bridges to the vast AIDS establishment. In draft after draft, he reached for the language of grace and inspiration, but found it maddeningly elusive. Though he had become proficient in television interviews, little had prepared him for this particular task. He wanted to show ACT UP as an imperfect amalgam of desperate human beings who sought a dialogue with another flawed slice of humanity. He wanted to convince the people filling the enormous hall that their goals and convictions were indistinguishable from ACT UP's.

On a sunny afternoon in June, Staley walked into the Moscone Center with several copies of his speech in hand. As required, he delivered his remarks to conference organizers for review, and they approved what they read. But Van Gorder's grapevine informed him that Staley was planning to invite all ACT UP members in the hall onto the stage with him, something the security team wouldn't allow. He and Wachter approached Staley.

"Nobody but you can be on the stage," Van Gorder warned. "Don't test us. It would be a *very* bad idea."

Staley excused himself for a quick consultation with his colleagues and returned to the organizers. "Done," he announced.

Moments before the opening music was to begin, someone whispered into Wachter's ear that Staley had unexpectedly submitted a slide to be shown during his speech. Fearing it might contain Kramer's call to violence, Wachter sprinted to the back of the room, clawed the slide from the carousel, and held it up to the light. It was an official White House portrait of the president. Relieved, he dropped it back into the tray just as the UCSF orchestra struck up Dvořák's Symphony no. 8 in G Major and the twelve thousand people in the audience settled into their seats.

Wachter ushered Staley backstage. When his eyes adjusted to the darkness, he was amazed to see in the wings a line of one hundred police, riot shields in place, batons drawn. Mayor Agnos was back there too, manning an emergency command center. Staley heard them discussing what they knew about the protests outside. Things had escalated precipitously. Waves of arrests were being made. Injuries were reported. Staley was mortified. *This is because of Larry,* he thought. *This is the cost of wild rhetoric.*

Staley was brought to the lectern about forty-five minutes into the program. Powerful spotlights glinted off his earrings and the ACT UP button on his chest. The reception from the audience was polite. The large screen above his head filled with a close-up of his own face, shot from a shoulder-mounted camera on the edge of the stage. He smiled almost angelically for a long moment, then leaned into the microphone.

"In an effort to bridge the gap that now seems to exist between AIDS activists and you—members of the medical and scientific communities—I would like you to join us in an act of activism," he began. From behind the stage he could hear the police squads shuffling into formation. "Trust me, you'll enjoy this," he said quickly, drawing nervous laughter from the audience. "But first, I would like to be joined in front of this stage by my fellow AIDS activists. Would you all come up?" From the darkness, ACT UP members streamed toward the stage, over three hundred in all, silently raising signs and banners.

"At this moment," Staley said, "there are others just like us who are trying to get into this conference but are being barred by the billy clubs of San Francisco police. And there are still others like us who are trying to get through customs at the San Francisco airport but are being detained instead because they are gay. And these same custom agents are under orders to keep a lookout for AZT in people's luggage. If you're found with any, you're put on the next plane out of the country. There is a man that could have prevented these absurdities. This man has said that he would like to see a kinder, gentler nation."

The enormous image of George H. W. Bush landed on the screen. "If you believe that the present INS policy barring people living with HIV disease from entering this country is useless as a health policy and discriminatory as well, please stand now and remain standing."

This was a huge gamble: if no one stood up, his speech would fail. A few people sprang up in eager solidarity, then a few more, and then whole quadrants of the auditorium clambered out of chairs. When the audience realized what they had done, a deafening cheer rose up in the cavernous hall. Over their enthusiasm, Staley called out, "I'd like to ask you to join us in vocalizing our collective anger. Join us in a chant against the man who could bring down the INS barriers. Join us in a chant against the man who has decided to show his commitment to fighting AIDS by refusing to be here today. Instead, he is at this very moment in North Carolina, attending a fund-raiser for the homophobic author of the INS barriers, that pig in the Senate known as Jesse Helms. Join us in this chant: 'Three hundred thousand dead from AIDS, where is George?'"

A full minute of spirited chanting followed. The world's leading AIDS scientists were in full catharsis, shouting out their frustration, anger, and fear. "Where is George? Three hundred thousand dead from AIDS!" Knowing his time was short, Staley waved his hands over his head in an SOS sign, only to ignite a new round of cheers when he beamed and said, "You can all now consider yourselves members of ACT UP."

When it was quiet again, he addressed them as a person with AIDS, a twenty-nine-year-old man who was dying.

I have always been painfully aware that, in order for me to beat this virus and live, I will need a great deal of help from all of you as well as from my government. Cooperation between all of us is the fastest way to a cure. However, recently I've begun to lose hope in our ability to work together to end this crisis. If anything, the gap that exists between all of you and AIDS activists seems to be widening. From your side, we're being constantly told to butt out. In a meeting I went to last week with other members of ACT UP New York's Treatment and Data Committee and NIAID's top brass, Dan Hoth, the director of the ACTG, told us that our participation at ACTG meetings—as observers only—could possibly scare the pharmaceutical companies away and bring the whole system crashing down. [The NCI scientist] Robert Gallo has said publicly that many of his fellow AIDS researchers are talking of leaving the field due to the antics of AIDS activists.

On my side, the level of anger and frustration is reaching such a point that attitudes claiming that all of you are uncaring and in it for greed are now widespread. I'm being taught to hate the Gang of Five—Doctors Corey, Merigan, Fischl, Hirsch, and Richman—without ever having met any of them. My good friend Larry Kramer has been trying to talk me into being an AIDS terrorist. Is there any way we can avoid all of this? I'm not sure anymore.

I do know that we have judged you at times unfairly. I believe that many of you care deeply about ending this crisis and that greed is not your motivation for fighting this disease. I also know that you have frequently judged us unfairly too. Yes, ACT UP has made mistakes, such as choosing an inappropriate target for a demonstration or using an offensive tactic. Communion wafers come to mind. But let's be fair here—when we make mistakes, what's the fallout? Some people become offended and begin to hate ACT UP. Whereas, when government or the scientific community makes a mistake, such as the now-legendary delays in bringing aerosolized pentamidine to market, thousands of people can die.

While at times we may offend you, remember as well that, like you, ACT UP has succeeded in prolonging the lives of thousands of people with HIV disease. An accelerated drug approval process, marketing approval for DHPG, early access to ddI, parallel track, a lower price on AZT, our own needle distribution programs in New York and San Francisco—these are just some of our victories in the war against AIDS.

Can we all, before it's too late, begin to understand each other? Will we realize that we share similar motivations? Can we try, at least this week, to bridge the widening gap between us?

If ovations had the power of peace treaties, Staley had ushered in a new era. The following four days of the conference saw a new kind of working relationship flourish. Tensions never went away altogether, but there would never again be a canyon of suspicion and hostility between activists and scientists. They were all on the same team now, all praying for the same miracle.

The work ahead, however, looked as hard as ever. No scientific breakthroughs were revealed at the conference and Fauci said he didn't expect anything significant in the epidemic's second full decade. "For the 1990s, [the challenge] is simply to fill the gaps in our knowledge that remain from the 1980s, and indeed there are significant gaps," he told Laurie Garrett from *New York Newsday*. In fact, the epidemic seemed to be getting worse, with an expanding list of AIDS-related ailments. Experts reported alarming rises in cases of B-cell lymphoma, anal carcinoma, cervical carcinoma, and Hodgkin's tumors in AIDS patients. This led to unsettling speculation that AZT might be causing malignancies. Dr. Robert Yarchoan, the drug's earliest champion, studied the records of the first AZT patients and found that those lucky enough to live for three years had a 46 percent chance of developing lymphomas. There was enormous work still to be done.

WHEN STALEY BOUNDED into the Gay Community Center the Monday after the conference, on July 2, 1990, he was stunned to learn that his speech had ignited a maelstrom among the activists. A line of passing criticism of ACT UP—in which he called the protest inside the St. Patrick's "an offensive tactic"—was seen by his critics as betraying ACT UP in order to create some vague feeling of kinship with the scientists. The attack on him was brutal, and only ended when Charlie Franchino yanked him from the room. Frustrated and amazed, Staley could do nothing but cry.

"The worst night of my life," he said later.

Still, Staley's peace accord with the scientists proved durable. At the next meeting of the ACTG network, which took place in Bethesda from July 10 to July 13, Dr. Jack Killen greeted the activists with genuine warmth. On the first night, Harrington and Rebecca Pringle Smith spotted Dan Hoth across the lobby as they sat sipping martinis, and sent him a drink. He wandered over to thank them, then chit-chatted for ninety minutes, embracing their participation in the redesign of the ACTG and showing by the second drink that the prior animosity was disappearing.

"Science thrives on doubt," he told them, "and you are bringing doubt into the system."

The following afternoon, Harrington apologized to the Gang of Five's ranking member, Dr. Martin Hirsch, acknowledging that his rhetoric had gotten out of hand. It was much appreciated. "I've never come closer to leaving the field," Hirsch confided.

"That would be counterproductive," said Harrington.

Pockets of frustration remained. In one of the sessions, Dr. Thomas Merigan, a stern and remote Gang of Fiver, blasted Harrington as impertinent and dangerous. But for the most part a new mood was prevailing.

"Unlike most politicians, bureaucrats, and journalists, many scientists are actually capable of rational discourse and sometimes even change their minds," Harrington wrote in *OutWeek*. "None of this could have happened without the efforts of thousands of people with AIDS over the last ten years and those of the hundreds of activists who stormed the NIH on May 21."

Harrington's renewed sense of optimism had the unintended effect of inflaming the Women's Caucus of ACT UP. They had been monitoring the ACTG for its treatment of women with AIDS, a population growing at six times the rate of infected men. The unique way the disease manifested itself in women was receiving no attention. Recent studies for new oral thrush treatments, for instance, didn't address the common occurrence of vaginal thrush in infected women.

"*We* don't have access or input," Heidi Dorow, a Women's Caucus member, wrote in response to Harrington's article. "We are ten years into this epidemic, and we still have no clue as to how many women have HIV, how it will manifest itself in their bodies, or how to treat it."

It took the Women's Caucus months of formal appeals before Hoth and Fauci agreed to a meeting. Seven women went to Bethesda that summer in a delegation headed by Maxine Wolfe, who had become a guiding figure within ACT UP given Larry Kramer's absence and Vito Russo's deteriorating health. Wolfe was a fiery and powerful speaker with an ingrained distrust of authority. She lacked Staley's interest in compromise as a strategy for gaining ground.

The meeting did not go well. The women confronted Fauci and Hoth for their "criminal negligence and ignorance concerning women with HIV/AIDS," as Wolfe later wrote. They laid down a series of demands, beginning with a call for a national conference on women and AIDS "within six weeks," and ending with a demand to halt a specific ongoing ACTG trial—pregnant women with AIDS were being given short courses of drugs in order to assess the protective benefits for the fetus. In their view, the trial treated pregnant women as mere vectors of infection, administering drugs without regard for the impact on them—their own health wasn't even being charted. Hoth made no effort to mask his contempt for the new ACT UP faction.

Fauci replied in a tone that was both officious and condescending. He let them know he had consented to receive them in his conference room not because of the letters they had written him, which he found rude, but because of his friendship with T+D members. "I can guarantee you one hundred percent, if you threaten, you will get nothing," he told them. "Zero."

The women let him know that, lacking a "basis on which to trust" him, they had no intention of easing up.

DOUG CALLED ME at work the afternoon his doctor diagnosed KS. We were already pretty sure that the kidney-shaped splotch on his thigh was the harbinger we had dreaded. "Dr. Waitkevicz says it's the best opportunistic infection to have and I should be happy it's not PCP." Doug's voice was tightly controlled. With a KS diagnosis he now met the official definition of AIDS, and the clock was ticking. In 1981, the average time from diagnosis to death was eighteen months. Now, nine years later, in a terrible indictment of the lackluster war on AIDS, it was only twenty-two months.

"I guess it's on my cheek, too," he added.

"What?"

"I got it a couple weeks ago. I've been putting makeup on it."

My heart pounded. "You weren't going to tell me?"

He ignored the question. "Waitkevicz said there's a doctor doing interesting things with shooting chemo directly into lesions. She got me an appointment." The doctor in question was Craig Metroka, the same oncologist whom Dr. Krim snuck into her lab night after night in order to treat his patients covertly in the early months of the plague. He had since cowritten the standards for treating KS in AIDS patients. No one could claim to know KS better.

"Did she say anything about AZT?"

"She gave me a prescription," he said. He made a maraca sound with the jar.

We fell silent. This was the moment we had been building toward inexorably. Every scene in our years together had pointed us to this one. I cried quietly at my desk.

"I'll go with you to Metroka's," I said. Though Doug had never asked me to accompany him to his doctors before, he accepted; our relationship had already changed.

A few weeks later, in a nondescript examining room on Central Park South, Metroka shot a needle full of chemicals into Doug's cheek and thigh, and we went back to the apartment together to watch the purple skin turn dark and flaky. That Saturday night, Doug spilled his first AZT capsules into his hand. They were smaller than I'd expected, bright white pellets banded across the waist by a bold blue stroke: Hockney's blue, the mazarine shadows in a Hollywood swimming pool. Incongruously, each capsule also bore a tiny illustration of a prancing unicorn with one hoof lifted in a high salute, and the abbreviated name of the company, which read like a macabre and misspelled convocation: WELLCOME.

He counted out four pills, the dose still recommended by the drug-maker and favored by his doctor, 1,200 milligrams daily. In order to keep to the demanding regimen, he bought a cheap digital watch on Canal Street and set the alarm to go off every four hours.

Metroka's continued efforts against the two lesions gave them a rutted texture that could no longer be masked with makeup. At the bodega or the laundromat or as he strolled down the block, the knowing eyes of gay men locked onto his cheek, and magnified his mortification. The AZT was punishing as well. Every morning at 3 a.m. he awoke for a dose, which left him exhausted. He was unable to hold down food and was almost always nauseated, but he was intent on persevering.

When he returned to the doctor, his blood test proved the immediate benefits of AZT, with a substantial boost to his CD4s. But within a few weeks, he was perilously anemic, which added to his debilitating exhaustion. Dr. Waitkevicz dispatched him to the hospital with a note for two units of blood. For a while thereafter, he was his old self. But the anemia quickly returned, followed by another trip to the transfuser, which was less successful. A spiking fever boiled in his veins.

Then came the gurgling cough: the dreaded pneumonia. Waitkevicz found him a bed at Beekman Downtown, the small hospital on the Lower East Side where she had privileges. The whole ninth floor was given over to AIDS. Starting on pentamidine quickly cleared his lungs over the course of a week, but because he hadn't gone a full day without a fever, the hospital couldn't release him. This was the common conundrum on AIDS wards. There were patients entering their sixth and seventh month on the ninth floor, young men wearing the unfocused gaze that Solzhenitsyn described, pale and sagging.

After failing the thermometer test for the twelfth day, Doug reached a breaking point. We tried a trick I learned from another patient in the reading lounge. While waiting for the afternoon thermometer, Doug kept a cracked sliver of ice below his tongue, replenishing it from a cup hidden in the bureau. It worked. He was out the door so fast he left his Walkman behind, a small price for freedom. Other patients blew kisses and applauded his good fortune. "It was just like the end of *One Flew Over the Cuckoo's Nest,*" Doug told a friend later.

Waitkevicz wanted him back on an antiretroviral drug, but couldn't risk another bout with anemia. She got him on the parallel track for ddI. Switching proved a mistake. A burning electrical sensation developed in the soles of his feet when he put any weight on them. This was called peripheral neuropathy, caused by nerve damage—a known side effect of ddI. Waitkevicz switched him back to AZT, this time at half the recommended dose, which he tolerated with fewer complications. But the feeling of needles in his feet never diminished.

His CD4 results remained "not bad," Waitkevicz told him. But the AZT anemia persisted, forcing him to begin injecting a blood-boosting drug called Epogen. He did this at home three times a week, jabbing a thin needle into his belly without complaint, and stockpiling the spent syringes in a big red biohazard container that now shared space with our toothbrushes on the bathroom vanity.

To deal with the many challenges he now faced, he returned to ACT UP. The group now met in the Great Hall at Cooper Union in the East Village, a college auditorium with nine hundred upholstered chairs, ample standing room, and a singular place in American history. On its proscenium stage, presidential candidate Abraham Lincoln gave his famous first speech against slavery. Despite the grand surroundings, the group was as low in decorum as ever, in Doug's estimation, the battling constant and mostly internecine.

He turned instead to GMHC, which now had 130 full-time employees. With a seemingly endless supply of sick New Yorkers turning there for help, GMHC was forced to institute what its executive director euphemistically called a "growth-management plan." Only one hundred new clients a month would be allowed through intake, selected from the first hundred callers on the first Monday of every month. Doug got only busy signals through the fall and winter. At the end of his patience, he called one Thursday afternoon to complain bitterly about the process, only to be told that GMHC had also set a cap on the number of complaints it would take.

"It's not trying to shirk responsibility," the executive director Tim Sweeney told *OutWeek*. "It's trying to be honest" about unfortunate but very real limitations. The problem vexed AIDS service organizations across the country.

Now there was a new HIV diagnosis every minute in America, and four AIDS deaths per hour.

Doug turned to Michael Callen's book, *Surviving AIDS*, which hit stores that summer. Part self-help and part wishful thinking, the book included profiles of fifteen people who, like Callen, were long-term survivors. Callen picked over their life stories for strategies and inspiration, but no clear lesson emerged. "If I had to describe in one word the common characteristic of the PWAs I interviewed," he reiterated, "it would be grit." Grit was not Doug's strong suit.

Callen's own grit was showing its limitations. New KS lesions were popping up regularly. He complained of being "soul-weary." His arrangement with Dworkin remained unsteady and painful. Though Dworkin's affair with the schoolteacher had fizzled, with Callen's express but sullen encouragement he was dating another man, a nurse from St. Vincent's named Patrick Kelly.

Right after Labor Day, 1990, with Dworkin in Europe performing a gig, Callen packed his things into a rental car and drove west to Los Angeles without a word of farewell. Dworkin felt betrayed by Callen, who had urged him to take a sexual partner and now left him because of it. It broke the pact Callen had made Dworkin repeat over and over, that the relationship would never end. The two exchanged long and emotional letters, filled with love and anger. The separation became an estrangement, a hurtful close to the most important relationship in either man's life. After eight productive and emotionally fulfilling years together, the relationship that Callen credited for his very survival was over.

In Los Angeles, he began work on a final album he planned to call *Legacy*, for which he hoped to record fifty songs. He also began a touring schedule with the Flirtations that would have exhausted someone with four times his CD4 cells. He knew his time was short. In a single week that fall he noted the death of the prominent AIDS activists Ray Navarro, Tony Cosarto, Kevin Smith, Oliver Johnson—who was a co-creator of the SILENCE=DEATH campaign—and Vito Russo, whose death was the most devastating blow of the year.

That those men died during the very week Senator Jesse Helms won reelection was too painful for many. The hundreds of mourners who gathered for Russo's memorial service were handed an anonymously produced flier that charged Helms with the endless stream of deaths.

Its author closed with two questions: "If I am ever brave enough to murder Jesse Helms, will you hand me the gun to carry out the deed? Will you hide me from the law once it is done?"

THAT DECEMBER, Bill Bahlman felt compelled to take his activism to a new level: he focused on his own functioning immune system, signing up as a volunteer in the study of a new drug from Merck and Co. Though infected, he had an enviable abundance of CD4s at the time, 748 per cubic millimeter of blood, so his motivation for signing up was not the usual one. He wanted to learn the ins and outs of drug trials firsthand.

Merck had been in the AIDS drug development sweepstakes since 1987, right after AZT proved that AIDS could be profitable. Dr. P. Roy Vagelos, the company's chief executive, named a charismatic young chemist named Irving Sigal to head the efforts. Vagelos made clear that this initiative came with limits. Under his guiding hand, the company had grown into the largest pharmaceutical manufacturer on the planet, minting wealth for shareholders. He expected the keel to remain steady.

Sigal recruited an impressive team consisting of medicinal chemists, virologists, and molecular biologists. His idea was to avoid competing head to head with Burroughs Wellcome's AZT, but instead to identify a whole new approach for attacking the virus. Quickly, his team proved the existence of a unique protease gene in HIV and set about trying to understand its function, character, and physical structure. The findings surprised them. The gene played a key role in HIV's replication, functioning as a kind of cleaver to slice apart long protein strings that then reassembled to form new infectious viral particles. Building a three-dimensional model of the protease molecule, he and his colleagues could see exactly how the snipping was accomplished—as by a pair of scissors. If they could find a way to neutralize that action, to jam something between the molecule's blades, viral replication would become impossible. It was unlikely that they would find a compound to do this by randomly pulling chemicals from shelves and seeing which might work. They were going to have to sculpt a unique molecule and fuse it to the protease in order to prevent the slicing. No pharmaceutical scientist had ever taken on a more difficult challenge.

Unfortunately, the work was derailed almost as suddenly as it began. At Christmastime in 1988, after finishing his work early at a scientific conference in London, Sigal changed planes to take a seat on Pan Am Flight 103, which came down in Lockerbie, Scotland, the result of a terrorist attack. Sigal's death devastated the team, and set back their efforts for months; ironically, it also bought them some leeway with Vagelos. When the team came under the new direction of Dr. Emilio Emini, the focus shifted away from inhibiting protease to inhibiting reverse transcriptase, the same approach AZT had pioneered. The initiatives on protease inhibitors were put on hold.

Tall and ambling, Emini was ideally suited to take on the responsibility he was given. Even in a shop known for its towering egos, his was the subject of much conversation and admiration. Senior management had collected the opinions of subordinates, colleagues, and supervisors on the leadership qualities of each of the top candidates. Emini far outscored the pack. In the few years since earning his PhD, he had done battle with polio, hepatitis B, and the exotic Venezuelan encephalitis virus, making him, as he liked to say, "a card-carrying virologist." Taking on the wily AIDS virus was one of the most thrilling assignments he might ever draw. "A head rush," he called it.

He turned the team's attention away from protease inhibitors in favor of the AZT-like compounds that had been proven profit-generators. Working with renewed focus, they reverted to the time-honored approach to drug discovery, throwing chemical after chemical into test tubes. In short order, they ran a staggering 23,000 theoretical agents through the laboratory to see which impeded reverse transcriptase. To his surprise, the few effective ones were not like AZT or ddI, the so-called nucleoside analogues, but rather a brand-new drug class— "non-nucleoside reverse transcriptase inhibitors," they called them, because they used a different method to thwart HIV's invasion of human DNA. After this thrilling breakthrough, Emini brought all his resources to bear on the non-nukes. One hundred experts joined the campaign. They quickly synthesized two versions, code named L-697,639 and L-697,661.

In December 1990, two years after the Lockerbie explosion, Bill Bahlman joined twenty-three HIV-positive volunteers at the NIH's hospital for a three-day exposure to Merck's L drugs. Bahlman was randomly assigned to the one ending in 639. Each patient received the same number of pills on the first day, and each was observed carefully over the next forty-eight hours, including near-hourly monitoring of blood and urine. He had no way of knowing if he was on the actual drug or a placebo, which was still being used. None of the patients on the ward experienced ill effects. Apparently, the L drug was as well tolerated as the sugar pills.

When Bahlman returned a few weeks later for a second dose, Dr. Fauci paid him a visit. Bahlman enjoyed the proximity to Fauci's world. It also gave him something that ACT UP had not yet developed strongly: close contact with the pharmaceutical industry. As a trial subject, he wrote to Merck requesting a meeting to discuss their research plans; he wanted to press for diversity among the patients in the trial, as his time on the ward at NIH revealed few women or people of color.

An appointment was arranged with Dr. Gordon Douglas, the Merck senior vice president for medical and scientific affairs, as well as his counterparts in policy and corporate communications. Because they were wary of Peter Staley–like antics at their headquarters, the meeting, set for a Friday that winter, would take place at the National League for Nursing offices in Lower Manhattan.

Bahlman arrived with Michael Becker, a lawyer who was also a T+D member and a trial subject. Tape recorders were produced by both sides. Bahlman put Dr. Douglas and his colleague, Linda Distlerath, the senior director of public policy, at ease with his quiet voice and gentle manner. Then he got down to business.

"We want a seat at the table," Bahlman told them. "We want to talk about the development of your drugs."

The request would normally have been anathema. The pharmaceutical industry was among the most secretive in the world, cloaking its research and development work from competitors—and regulators, when they could. Few outsiders were ever given access to a company's unpublished data. Dr. Douglas, though, was not immediately opposed to the idea. As the meeting progressed without raised voices or threats, the Merck team actually warmed to it. They revealed some details about the size of their gamble in AIDS, which now included one team working on vaccines and another that had returned to study protease inhibitors after two years. This was encouraging to the two activists.

Unfortunately, the Merck officials then revealed that the experimental drug both men had been taking was a disappointment. Compound L-697,639 was indeed well tolerated, as they had surmised, and it showed good absorption into the bloodstream, but the company's other experimental non-nuke proved far superior in all categories and that drug, not 639, would be going into Phase II efficacy trials.

The good news, at least for Bahlman and Becker, was that both men qualified to be part of the new study as well. That study would be conducted outside of the ACTG system, however, as Merck felt the advantages of running it through their own academic networks allowed them to move more nimbly. Details were still being worked out about the length of the trial, whether six weeks, as Merck was proposing, or eighteen weeks, as the FDA suggested, but either way they intended to begin by early April, an ambitious time frame. When the meeting came to a close, all sides pronounced it a success.

Within a few days Merck formally committed to future consultations with ACT UP. "Our discussions with you," a representative wrote,

> as well as our responses to your questions, speak for our company's willingness to openly communicate with your organization. For we understand that, while the development of new investigational medicines of Merck's discovery will remain Merck's ultimate responsibility, both ACT UP and Merck are working to defeat the same disease. So long as ACT UP can meet and talk with us in a cooperative, non-threatening way, as both of you have, we will welcome the organization's input.

No pharmaceutical company had ever before agreed to collaboration with the patient population.

Still, one obstacle after another delayed the Phase II study, drawing angry reprisals from ACT UP. No patients were enrolled until late the next year. Despite this, Bahlman was grateful for Merck's overall commitment to the activists. When he pointed out irregularities in the informed consent form he was asked to sign that September, various Merck officials invited Bahlman and Becker to formally review all future protocols while they were still in development.

Here, finally, was the seat at the table that ACT UP coveted.

LIFE INSIDE the plague's bubble left little time or inclination for mourning. Tears, once on copious display in the Village, had become rare as laughter. Jim Eigo was one of the few people who felt compelled to offer formal eulogies when colleagues fell. Every Monday as necessity dictated, he would deliver a brisk appreciation to the assembled activists, focused on the dead man's contributions to the movement. It made a kind of sense that ACT UP made little room for processing the experience of death. Opening a vein to the staggering loss could be paralyzing. In the group's activist ethos, one only looked angrily ahead. And that view was as bleak as it had ever been, as Eigo noted in a World AIDS Day speech. "It's a common observation that, at the end of his tragedies, Shakespeare, after the final body has fallen, makes a gesture toward the restoration of order," he said. He did not believe order would ever return. Nobody did.

David Barr's CD4s fell back to baseline, 235, at the end of his first year as a patient. The drugs had worn out for him and although he had no symptoms, he was haunted by a feeling of increasing vulnerability. On the battlefield, one cannot step over so many bodies without imaging one's own lifeless cheek on the ground. For the first time in his years of full-time AIDS work, he felt a need to plan for the end.

Beginning late in the fall, Barr invited a few of his closest confidantes to his East Village apartment for supper. Peter Staley, Derek Link, Spencer Cox, Mark Harrington, and Gregg Bordowitz were the first people Barr spoke to every morning and the last he called at night. All dealt with HIV politically and personally as well—they were fighting at the highest levels for their own lives. Bordowitz, the only one not directly affiliated with T+D, worked with Barr at GMHC—he ran the agency's media lab, producing public service announcements and other educational content.

Over takeout pizza that night, Barr proposed a formal support system, a structured forum through which they would discuss their private feelings about AIDS in a way that broke the unspoken rules of AIDS activism. He wanted his closest friends to take care of him when the end came, and vowed to do the same for them.

The others tended to be far less sentimental than Barr. Staley hadn't attended a support group since the one where he met Griffin Gold. Self-pity was not Harrington's style. Though he was still reeling from the news about his own health, the only concession he had made so far was to improve his diet—fewer meals at Odessa, Kiev, Leshkos, and Veselka, all the East Village purveyors of gravy-soaked Ukrainian food. He had nothing else to share about his status. He still had not identified himself publicly as a marked man.

For his part, Spencer Cox mocked the very idea of a support group, channeling a monologue from the Mt. Everest of camp movies, *Valley of the Dolls:* "I licked pills, booze, and the funny farm! I don't need anybody or anything!"

Still, with varying degrees of disinclination each of Barr's friends accepted his invitation. They mostly discussed and debated the escalating tensions within ACT UP, much of it focused on them. Writing in *TITA*, fellow activists anonymously accused them of entering secretive

deals with the ACTG and with Fauci specifically, of "hiding information" from readers of their weekly *T&D Digest,* and of suppressing
divergent opinions, especially those concerned with non-Western
treatment approaches. Calling themselves the Renegade Caucus, a new
group issued a list of demands to T+D in an effort to rein in their perceived arrogance, to which Harrington replied arrogantly, "They aren't
worth responding to."

Embracing their perceived superiority, Spencer Cox named their
support group the HIVIPs.

This wasn't the only battlefront for Barr's group. The gulf between
activists on the East Coast and on the West Coast had stretched wider
since the Compound Q debacle, and came to a head over an unlikely
flash point: the "Ice Queen" herself, Dr. Ellen Cooper. Marty Delaney
at Project Inform was pushing her for the immediate approval of ddC,
the Hoffmann–La Roche therapy that worked like AZT and ddI. Little
about its efficacy was known. Cooper would not consider it. Harrington
shared her concerns about the drug's data and called for more study.
Delaney pummeled and cajoled Cooper in letters and telephone calls.
After one especially tense call, she reached a breaking point. Her bitter
letter of resignation cited pressure from unnamed activists. "My situation in my current job is untenable," she told Marilyn Chase from *The
Wall Street Journal.*

Delaney was thrilled. For the activists in New York it was a disaster. Nobody knew AIDS science better that Cooper. Nobody was
more influential in that world. In three years she went from defending "death trials" to defending most of ACT UP's innovations in trial
design, including parallel track for wide distribution of experimental
compounds. Coming to her defense, ACT UP organized a nationwide
telephone campaign, urging members to call the FDA commissioner to
demand her reinstatement and suggest she be given even more authority. Larry Kramer, who once had called her "a murderer," sent her a
large bouquet of flowers and a note begging her to reconsider. "She's
been like Joan of Arc," he said later. "She's impossible to replace."

She did not return. Thereafter, Delaney and his colleagues would
share FDA committee assignments with Harrington and his group, but
mutual suspicion and doubt defined their encounters.

IN DECEMBER, the National Women and HIV Infection Conference
took place in Washington, D.C., the first tangible victory of ACT UP's
national Women's Committee and the Women's Caucus of ACT UP

New York. In the major cities, AIDS was now the leading cause of death for women ages fifteen to forty-four. Some 1,500 researchers attended, as did dozens of ACT UP members, including all of the female leadership from around the country. Tensions remained high. In protest one morning, two women barged noisily out of one contentious session only to collide with Mark Harrington and Rebecca Pringle Smith in the lobby of the Sheraton, though neither of them were attending the conference.

Risa Denenberg, a licensed nurse and Women's Caucus member, demanded to know what they were doing there.

Harrington explained that they were in town to attend a Christmas party being hosted by Dr. David Byar, a statistician inside the ACTG who had become one of T+D's key defenders. Byar was also a gay man who was dying of AIDS. Over their shared years in the trenches, Harrington and Smith had grown close with Byar. Now he was in and out of the hospital, and down to seventeen CD4s. With his remaining energy, he called his activist friends together to celebrate what they had managed to accomplish together, a valedictory feast. Fauci and his deputy Jim Hill were invited as well.

Danenberg could not believe her ears. That's the power of co-optation, she thought. That's what destabilizes a movement. From a nearby phone booth, she reported this to Tracy Morgan in New York, who was likewise outraged. "I find this revolting," Morgan wrote in the following week's *TITA*. "We must *stop* these private meetings and commit ourselves to acting publicly, where we reach more people with our message. . . . I resent the lack of thought behind the planning of this secret tête-à-tête."

Morgan, a formidable foe, kept the issue alive for weeks, galvanizing a small but influential army to her side. Nothing anybody tried could still their anger, not even shrieks from Kramer himself, who was in the unfamiliar position of condemning the internal discord (like "Mrs. O'Leary's cud-chewing cow condemning the Chicago fire," as one *TITA* writer wryly noted).

Heartbroken by the civil strife he had inadvertently caused, Byar sent an explanatory missive directly to "the members of ACT UP." He spoke of the power of his friendships with activists. "You must realize that talking to one another is not collaborating with the enemy—but simply opening up a very useful and often productive dialogue. I would be most happy to talk to and entertain in my home any time the author of the attack on Mark and any others who are sincerely interested in searching for ways to focus constructively on how to help us with our common goals to accelerate and improve the search for effective treatments."

In a rejoinder threaded with sarcasm and senseless allegations, Tracy Morgan called Byar "the enemy," Harrington a liar, and Fauci a pompous obstacle to reason. She found a vein of sympathy among the larger ACT UP membership who increasingly found themselves dismissed as mere rabble-rousers, deserving of none of T+D's credit or respect. Staley caught the arrows of opprobrium, as did David Barr, Derek Link, and the other male members of the "inside" wing. For the time being, Garance Franke-Ruta, Rebecca Pringle Smith, and Iris Long escaped their attention.

THE RANCOR was perhaps understandable as 1990 drew to a close. ACT UP was numbed by loss and exhausted from a frantic schedule of activism that produced only minor and inadequate victories. On every front, the country remained stubbornly indifferent to the epidemic and its targets. While Congress approved a record $800 million for treatment and prevention in the country's hardest-hit areas, not a dime was ever released. Hospitals in every major city were full to overflowing. Research was as chaotic as ever. Drugs that the NIH had called promising in 1985 remained untested five years later. The coordinating bodies were in disarray. Though the NIH had created a new Division of AIDS, designed as a coordinating body, it managed only to add a new layer of difficult personalities as "branch chiefs" for the various reporting areas. One, in the Pharmaceutical and Regulatory Affairs branch, was so disagreeable as to prompt mass resignations in December. Half the Division of AIDS positions remained empty.

Two days after Christmas, Franke-Ruta secured a meeting with Fauci and Hoth to discuss their personnel problems. It was a strange power inversion—a teenage high school dropout in thrift shop clothing and jewelry she fashioned from hardware store purchases trying to solve a problem for the two most senior men in antiretroviral research. In advance, she had requested a list of the jobs they were unable to fill. It was eleven pages of tiny type. Had they thought, she wondered, about securing a qualified headhunting service to help find candidates? Would they consider an agency to design more attention-getting postings and ads? What about the terrible reputation for workplace subterfuge and backbiting that the Division of AIDS had already earned; what was being done to counter the impression that it was a thankless place to work? She left despondent about the government's abilities generally.

This despair helped to fuel a project that she had been developing with Derek Link, who had become her roommate on East Seventh Street. Activists had for years been demanding research into opportunistic infections, with little success. Sitting in a coffee shop over a three-ring notebook, the two youngest T+D members could easily list a number of promising drugs for each of the OIs that were being ignored by the establishment. With a little more research, they identified the companies that would be most likely to push their candidate drugs forward if ACT UP could help clear the way.

This became the basis of an initiative they called "Countdown 18 Months." The two would give pharmaceutical companies eighteen months to evaluate drugs for treating and preventing the infections, or face a firestorm of protest. Franke-Ruta had reports from Burroughs Wellcome showing that their pretax profits had risen 26 percent in the previous six-month period, thanks entirely to AZT. AIDS drugs were big business. And she could help other companies claim a piece of the pie.

Derek Link was her ideal collaborator, an intense and clever activist with a time bomb ticking within him. He confided in Franke-Ruta that a KS lesion had appeared on his genitals. When the members of the HIVIP support group heard the bad news at one of their monthly meetings, they held him and wept—he was the first among them with a major OI, a reminder of their shared future. Link was just twenty-two.

Countdown 18 Months drew a core group of about a dozen activists. ACT UP gave them a travel budget, thanks to a second successful art auction with pieces donated by Richard Serra, Herb Ritts, Jenny Holzer, and Barbara Kruger. The Countdown volunteers were divided into groups, each specializing in just one of the OIs. Link and San Francisco's Jesse Dobson took toxoplasmosis. Partnering with a new member named Scott Slutsky, Franke-Ruta took on the dreaded MAI. There now was a drug being used against MAI, quite imperfectly: Sonnabend had found that an old leprosy therapy seemed to prevent onset of the disease, but it lacked a trial to test the hypothesis, and the necessary approvals to merit insurance coverage.

Franke-Ruta and Link unveiled the initiative at the National Press Club in Washington. "Committee after committee has reviewed the AIDS crisis in this country and come up with the exact same conclusion, that there is no plan, there is no one in charge, there is no coordination," she told journalists. "Well, here is a plan. It is doable. It is realistic. And it can save thousands of lives now and in the coming decades." Although punctuated by some of ACT UP's typical bravura

("What if progress isn't made?" "Then we'll do what we always do"), her presentation won wide endorsement, including from the nation's top opportunistic infections scientists and even Dr. Jack Killen, ACT UP's old foe at NIAID.

Only Fauci opposed the campaign as unnecessary and unworkable, saying he didn't believe in deadlines. "Science isn't done that way," he said.

After the holidays, Franke-Ruta went to Boston to discuss an MAI trial with representatives of Adria Laboratories, makers of a drug called rifabutin that had drawn the interest of PWAs. She brought Staley and members of Boston's ACT UP. Adria had said it would not make drugs available on a parallel track, citing cost. Franke-Ruta had a proposal. She believed she could convince the NIH to manage the distribution through parallel track, just as they had for pediatric studies of AZT, if Adria would agree to supply the therapy free of charge. They still turned her down. But they were impressed enough with her description of the marketplace to put the drug on a fast track. Luckily, rifabutin proved to be a powerfully effective tool for delaying and preventing MAI infections. In combination with other drugs, it brought relief to patients with disseminated infections. The scourge of this deadly opportunistic infection had finally been addressed.

2

Days of Desperation

W hen the calendar turned to 1991, 100,000 Americans were dead from AIDS, twice as many as had perished in Vietnam. And then war broke out. President George H. W. Bush mounted a massive international campaign against Iraq for invading Kuwait, and in January authorized aerial bombardments that went on for six weeks and leveled parts of Baghdad, leaving 10,000 dead. The war pushed the epidemic off the national agenda. Frustrated ACT UP members printed a bumper sticker—"The AIDS Crisis Is Not Over"—and pasted it around town. On January 23, the group declared a "Day of Desperation," staging a staggering array of angry, barely focused protests around the city. Teams of three and four from an affinity group called Action Tours fabricated name tags and ID cards and illicitly made their way into the soundstages of the major television news shows. As Dan Rather began his newscast, the blurry face of John Weir, a talented young novelist, appeared in the unlighted foreground, screaming, "Fight AIDS, not Arabs!" Similar scenes played out at PBS and NBC.

In the East Village, someone in an apartment near Avenue C protested the war by turning an arena-strength loudspeaker out a window and playing a soundtrack of crisscrossing helicopters and gunships erupting in machine-gun fire. Night after night, the thunder of war reached deep into apartments like mine, where Doug was mostly immobile due to the pain in his feet. Now a new viral condition, molluscum contagiosum, vexed him. Sprays of small, barnacle-like papules covered his belly and thighs. The infection was not uncommon in toddlers and pre-adolescents and typically resolved without treatment. Doug's spots wept continually, and several became inflamed by bacteria. He settled into a routine of disinfecting his body several times a day in an effort to resolve the infections. Several grew painful and were so deep they required surgery, leaving disfiguring divots and welts here and there.

The KS meanwhile was mapping a grid on his skin. He was no longer seeing Dr. Metroka for shots of chemo, which only seemed to make black necrotic-looking blemishes out of the magenta splotches—it did nothing to stem the appearance of new ones. He had decided, based on his reading of Michael Callen's book, that staying away from oncologists was the most promising survival strategy. Callen, who now had lesions on his legs, treated them only cosmetically. Doug bought a small aloe vera plant and painted his lesions with the sticky, cool residue as the guttural thrum of chopper blades rattled outside.

We took a vacation with friends that winter: two weeks on the beach in Puerto Rico. Other than trips to see his family in Colorado or mine in Michigan, we had not traveled from the city in over three years. Being on the beach without the infernal soundtracks of war was a relief, but joy was in short supply. The one time Doug removed his shirt, a nineteen-year-old on a nearby towel made note of all the marks on his flesh.

"Are those mosquito bites?" he asked, with genuine concern.

Doug glanced down at his marred chest and moved a finger from one spot to another, lesion to lump, virus to cancer, not sure how to answer. He opened his mouth to reply but no words came out.

We had been back in New York for a few weeks when I returned from work one night to find him in the stairwell halfway up to our apartment. He was covered in sweat. "I can't make it," he said, looking square in my eyes. "My feet are killing me. My lungs hurt."

I took his canvas backpack and looped a hand around his waist to hoist him from one step to the next. "I'll find us another place to live. A place with an elevator," I said.

"No," he snapped, steadying himself on the handrail. Grimacing, he took the next step himself, and the next. "Not yet."

LATE IN MARCH, ACT UP's national network of women's caucuses arranged a conference call to deal with the lack of respect they felt from the treatment activists around the country. In New York, Monday-night meetings had descended into nasty brawls. After four years, a type of "concentration camp syndrome" overtook them. All trust was gone. Similar fissions existed in the other chapters. Plague-weary representatives of twenty-eight cities joined the call. Most, but not all, of the voices were female. High on the agenda was a proposal from Tracy Morgan designed to keep T+D members from undermining their authority in the future: a mandatory six-month moratorium on any meetings with government officials on matters relating to women. In that time, she hoped that a consensus would develop within ACT UP allowing them to speak in one voice. The proposal passed 27 to 1.

Maxine Wolfe brought it before the Monday-night meeting in New York for ratification. She had to have known it would be a serious provocation, although for years to come she claimed to think of it as just another business matter deserving a vote. The reaction was ugly among the people who had fought so hard to infiltrate the ACTG system, to create and then populate the community advisory boards, to seek appointments to posts at the FDA, the NIH, and within pharmaceutical companies. They went ballistic.

At the height of the argument, someone defended the six-month moratorium by thoughtlessly saying, "It's not like it's the rest of your life."

Derek Link rose up in moral indignation. "Six months is not a lifetime? But guess what. For those of us with low T-cells, *it certainly is*," he said. *"Either help us fight for our lives or get the fuck out of our way."*

Debate over the moratorium raged on for weeks. It took a month before it came to a vote. In that time, a blanket of madness seemed to flutter down on the group. Larry Kramer opened a box in his mail to find it filled with human excrement. A half-dozen ACT UP lesbians complained of receiving threatening or mysterious calls late at night. Tracy Morgan changed her telephone number because of the harrassment, but it somehow continued without pause. Reports were made to the police.

It all stopped as soon as the moratorium went down in defeat. This was not a pure victory for the T+D people. The process left deep and lasting wounds. Thereafter, each side only spoke to the other in spasms of moral outrage. This, of course, soon depressed turnout at the Monday meetings—down 60 percent from the peak of more than one thousand. The movement was crippled.

THE INTERNECINE BATTLES were doing Staley's CD4 cells no favors. Or maybe AZT had just lost its effectiveness. But after more than a year on low doses of the pills, his blood test brought bad news. After consulting with his T+D colleagues, he decided to give ddI a try. He picked up a prescription from the PWA Health Group, which had supplies of the drug donated by friends of patients on the official trial who had died.

He thought of leaving them what was left of his AZT, but thought better of it. He remembered what Dr. David Barry had said during ACT UP's first trip to Burroughs Wellcome's headquarters. He predicted that one drug alone could never work against the disease for long. "A final real management, or a step to real management of this disease, is going to depend on multiple drug therapies, period," he had said. "That's been true with other infectious or transformational diseases for years. That was true for tuberculosis, it's true for leprosy, it's true for leukemias and lymphomas. . . . Wherever you have prolonged infection and patient immunosuppression, your best management is going to be with multi-drug therapy."

Staley concocted his own daily drug cocktail of 300 milligrams of AZT and 187 milligrams of ddI, an arbitrary choice. No trials of this combination had yet been reported, so nobody knew if the compounds would interact poorly. Taken by itself in the recommended quantity, ddI could cause pancreatitis, severe diarrhea, or liver disease on top of the peripheral neuropathy that crippled Doug. In combination, it could be even worse.

Luckily he experienced no side effects. The next time he sent blood for a workup he was amazed at the results. His CD4 count was way up, reaching a normal 606 per cubic millimeter. He rejoiced, sharing the good news in an unusually personal disclosure at the next ACT UP meeting, on an extremely hot Monday night.

"As far as I'm concerned, ddI has brought me an extra year of life, if not more," he told the few hundred members in attendance. "Now, I would never presume that my success with nucleoside analogs can be repeated by anyone who tries them. I've said it a thousand times and I'll say it here again: These are mediocre drugs that only offer a short-term benefit to some people. . . . I have simply made a choice between mediocre treatments and no treatment at all." He added, "I would never have gotten my hands on ddI if it weren't for ACT UP's having pushed for the drug's expanded access. Once again, I feel I owe my life to this group."

When I got home after that meeting, I found Doug shut in the bedroom with our roaring air conditioner. I mentioned the potential of combination therapy. He agreed to talk with his doctor. "I'm leery, though," he told me, pushing a pile of articles across the coffee table. "Michael Callen won't touch the stuff. He's all about 'blood cleansing' now."

AROUND THE CORNER from our apartment, in the sparsely furnished flat Garance Franke-Ruta and Derek Link shared, there was no reprieve from the fierce summer heat. Franke-Ruta was only marginally more comfortable at her office in the cramped PWA Health Group offices, where as the publications associate she was writing drug fact sheets for a salary that forced her to subsist on thirty-five-cent cheese sandwiches. Only the bracing corridors of St. Vincent's gave any relief, and, sadly, she was there nearly every day. She assumed principal care partner duties for Jerry Jontz, a friend and Countdown 18 Months colleague who was sitting out his last New York summer on the seventh floor. He was in a rapid decline. During one of her visits, he no longer recognized her; on another, he'd lost his speech. Swelling of the brain, the doctors told her. As a last resort, she, Derek Link, and Gregg Gonsalves snuck into his room to spray an experimental compound from the PWA Health Group shelves up his nose, something called Peptide T. It didn't help. They frankly didn't expect it would.

She thought, at nineteen, that she was hardened to the cycles of mortality, but when Jontz died that month it hit her hard. Another blow came in June, when Tom Hannan, her boss at the PWA Health Group, also gave up the fight. He asked Dr. Sonnabend for a large prescription of the anti-anxiety drug Klonopin, enough to end his life. This wasn't the first such request from one of Sonnabend's patients. AIDS doctors across the country were grappling with similar appeals. Sonnabend empathized with Hannan, whom he had come to admire since their days manufacturing AL721 together. But helping end a life was antithetical to his training and beliefs. Since that first summer day in 1981 he had dedicated every ounce of his energy to keeping people alive. He was perhaps the most vigilant AIDS clinician in the country, in constant warfare against the opportunistic infections. In New York it was said that his patients lived longer than anyone else's. He couldn't possibly switch gears. As sick as the young man was, Sonnabend apologized and gently denied the request.

Hannan hadn't anticipated this. He cursed Sonnabend, and later left him a phone message threatening to kill him if he wouldn't relinquish the drugs. For the next few days, Sonnabend traveled uneasily between his home and office—for a spell he took refuge in Mathilde Krim's Uptown mansion. Then he got a call with news that Hannan had ingested a large bottle of morphine and swallowed everything else he found in his medicine cabinet.

Sonnabend found Hannan unconscious in his bed, surrounded by evidence of his suicide mission. A small man to begin with, Hannan looked like a porcelain doll propped up on the pillow. His skin was translucent and his strawberry hair had gone thin. A faint heartbeat fluttered and his breathing was erratic and slight. Suddenly his eyes popped open and he looked around the room, giving Sonnabend a start.

"Oh hi, Joe," he said. "Did you use your key to let yourself in?"

The question made no sense. "Yes," he lied. "You go back to sleep."

He sat with his patient for most of the day. By nightfall there was no heartbeat. Sonnabend filled out the necessary paperwork to pronounce Hannan dead.

WITH HIS CD4S rebounding, Peter Staley spent much of the summer on Fire Island seeking calm. But he was fixated on Jesse Helms, the powerful North Carolina senator. Because Helms was personally unwilling, as he often said, "to spend one penny of the American taxpayer's money to encourage, condone, or promote sodomy," he blocked or neutralized nearly every bill providing AIDS funding on research, treatment, or prevention. More than anyone else, Helms was responsible for the fact that the CDC still had no national HIV containment plan. Every country in Europe and many in the developing world had comprehensive approaches for preventing the spread. The world's leading public health experts condemned the measure as misguided and disastrous. He was not moved.

"We've got to call a spade a spade," Helms said from the Senate floor, "and a perverted human being a perverted human being."

To many of Helms's colleagues in the Senate, his work on the epidemic cemented his position as the conscience of Washington. They passed his so-called "offensiveness rule" amendments with little debate, usually 48 to 2. The AIDS movement needed to undermine Helms's power, not only in the Senate but with the American people, who viewed his bigotry as unnoteworthy.

Taking on Helms directly seemed impossible, so Staley turned to ridicule as a weapon. The disarming power of mockery had a long political history, from the student movements of the 1960s to Shakespeare and beyond. Thomas Jefferson called it "the only weapon which can be used against unintelligible propositions." Staley's idea was to symbolize the deadly consequence of Helms's animus by equating his spewed hostilities to infection and disease: he wanted to drape the senator's suburban Virginia home in an enormous condom.

With his friend Twilly Cannon, Staley took a road trip to Arlington to check out the feasibility of the plan. Cannon, who had learned the art of protest stagecraft first as an anti-nuclear activist and later at Greenpeace, snapped photos of the senator's house, a modest saltbox, and showed Staley how to use the pictures to glean the dimensions for the prophylactic design. Staley faxed the specifications to a number of companies specializing in large-scale display pieces like those inflatable animals in front of car dealerships. The cheapest was $3,500, unaffordable by ACT UP, whose funds had depleted because of all the infighting.

Disappointed, Staley was weighing other options on Fire Island one afternoon when a middle-aged stranger interrupted his thoughts.

"I hear you need some money," the man said. Staley recognized the mogul David Geffen, who owned a large house on the waterfront. News of Staley's plot had begun to spread. Before he could say anything, Geffen passed Staley a thick roll of bills. "Don't ever tell anyone I gave you this," he said with a quick smile.

The prop arrived in August. In a dry run in a field upstate, it inflated perfectly with a pair of compressors and a small gas-powered generator. So on September 5, the team Staley had assembled led a convoy of news trucks out of a motel parking lot—all anybody knew was that an enormous condom would be unfurled somewhere—toward the sidewalk in front of the Helms home on South Glebe Road. Reporters roared with laughter as the team went to work. In seven minutes, the house was fully encased. The police, when they arrived, waited in stunned amazement—some doubling over in laughter—for the reservoir tip to fully inflate.

On the side of the condom, Franke-Ruta had stenciled the day's slogan:

A
CONDOM
TO STOP
UNSAFE POLITICS.
HELMS IS DEADLIER
THAN A VIRUS.

Immediately, the process was reversed. The condom was folded and bagged and except for bent blades of grass, the Helms residence was unmarred. When he learned of the shenanigans, Helms snapped his head in disgust, saying, "They don't like me and I don't like them." No arrests were made. There was much less coverage of the event than expected because news directors considered the image of a condom unsuited to family viewing. But within months, a federal court struck down the "offensiveness rule," and Helms was unable to pass a modified replacement.

· · ·

THE FRAYING COALITION limped into the fall, making showy but unproductive efforts at reconciliation. They held town hall meetings and strategy sessions, and organized goodwill brunches. Overtures were even made by T+D members, who joined in the next big ACT UP action, a massive protest at Kennebunkport, Maine, during President Bush's family vacation, but the public squabbling continued. Differences festered over two ACTG trials that pitted T+D and the Women's Caucus against each other. Harrington's patience, sparse in the best of times, had reached its limit. Between the spats, he was spending more and more time caring for his ex-lover Jay Funk, who had developed wasting syndrome. The fighting in ACT UP was taking too much of his time.

At the T+D meeting in the first week of November 1991, he snapped. Almost seventy-five people were present, including Simon Watney, who had become a leading AIDS activist in London—England's Michael Callen. It was a Wednesday night; T+D had been meeting every Wednesday for years. As he arrived at the rundown community center, Harrington stumbled on the fact that ACT UP's leadership had convened a simultaneous meeting elsewhere in the building to discuss "the troubles." How could freezing T+D out of the session begin to resolve anything?

Overwrought and smelling of cigarettes, Harrington addressed T+D with full fury.

"I don't want any part of the factions. I want to get away from it. I'm not willing to do work where half of my time is spent immobilized by ACT UP infighting and by infighting between ACT UP in New York and other groups around the country. And I feel," he said, scratching his head, "I mean, I'm going to put up a hypothesis and a suggestion. I am not saying this is what I feel. I just want it to be out there. I want people in this group to very seriously think about separating from ACT UP New York as we know it."

Garance Franke-Ruta's heart raced. Larry Kramer sank in his chair, pinching his lower lip between forefinger and thumb. The room that had been the noisy fulcrum of AIDS activism fell eerily silent for the first time in five years.

"I would like everyone to go home and really think very seriously about it," Harrington continued. "I think that we're bogged down. I think that we're at an impasse. I know that I, myself, have been *immobilized* for great stretches of time for the last eighteen months because of infighting and the attacks that have been done against me and against the people I have tried to work with. There's a group of people in ACT UP who are stuck with a set of tactics devised in the seventies that are essentially separatist in nature, and totally irrelevant to our work in the scientific and research infrastructure. We have to go *into* the infrastructure—*into* what I was talking about . . . as *the gray area*—and work there. And we have to accept the ambiguity that comes with that and to realize that we have just as much potential to do harm as any greedy researcher. We can kill people with AIDS too, just like we say they can.

"We have people who want to use this old-style M.O. of always being on the outside, always being right, and the enemy is always wrong. Well, you know what? We have more in common with Thomas Merigan"— the Gang of Five strongman—"'cause Thomas Merigan really does spend—however greedy he may be, and however much we may not like his research agenda—he spends his life working on AIDS. And that's what we do." With breathtaking speed, Harrington ran down the T+D agenda, which included "the six major areas of pathogenesis: HIV, immune reconstitution and immunology, OIs, neurology, wasting and nutrition, and opportunistic cancers," as well as challenging government agencies, pharmaceutical representatives, and public health authorities. "We have been spending too much time putting out our brush fires," he said, almost shouting. "We have to focus on the work and develop the structures that are appropriate to the work and no longer be wedded to the structures from which we have come, whether that be ACT UP or whether that be T+D as we now know it."

There was a smattering of nervous applause, then all eyes turned predictably toward Kramer, their often maligned but always revered patriarch. His face mapped a deep anguish.

"You're at your best when you get all riled up," he said finally. A few people laughed sadly. "I think we have to change, too. I started to talk about this last week. I don't have anything as specific as all that except that I have spent now a month in Washington and I know that we just have not penetrated that city. We have not. For all our work, we have not affected half as much as we think we have affected."

His voice was shaky and thin. "The only thing that's going to end this fucking plague is a cure, and that is the only thing I'm interested in fighting for. Let somebody else go out there and shake the masses. Let somebody else go out there and give the condoms."

It was resolved. Their new group would be called TAG, for Treatment Action Group. They left ACT UP behind. The great experiment in democracy and inside/outside activism had come to an end. After five years, ACT UP New York broke apart. Though it continued meeting regularly and staging some spectacular protest actions, it lost its strong traction on the scientific community and its connections to its founding battle cry: Drugs into bodies. The generals had deserted the army.

For several weeks, the knottiest question before the new group was how they saw TAG being structured, whether as an open membership organization like ACT UP or a professional think tank, a place where TAG's brain trust could be supported and kept free from financial pressure and political second-guessing. They elected the latter, eventually incorporating TAG as a nonprofit and handpicking who would be part of it. Harrington would handle policy, Staley took charge of management, and Spencer Cox would coordinate media. Many of the others were put on a board of directors to set strategy. Eigo declined to join them. In his mind, his validity as an HIV-negative AIDS activist stemmed exclusively from ACT UP's broad mandate and even broader base. It was hard for him to articulate, but without the group's rank and file, he felt illegitimate as a treatment activist. He began to recede from AIDS activism and soon resurfaced as the editor of a gay porn magazine, deviously hiding his messages of HIV awareness along with his Elizabethan prose inside the covers of *Playguy*.

A more difficult juncture arose with Kramer. The general membership deemed his histrionics too much of a distraction and voted to exclude him. Straws were drawn to pick who would bring the news. The unhappy task fell to Charlie Franchino.

3

Life

Bill Bahlman was not invited to join TAG, so he stayed in the dwindling ACT UP and kept his attention focused on the Merck trial he'd signed up for. The multiple delays frustrated him and Michael Becker. They didn't get their first "mysterious capsules"—code-named L-697,661—until nearly a year after enrolling. The study was small as Phase II efficacy trials go, enrolling 120 patients in total. At the insistence of Bahlman and Becker, Merck made sure to recruit at least a small number of women and active IV-drug users. None were on placebo and all were allowed access to prophylaxis and regular medical care, a major victory for the activists.

The patients were flown to Washington, D.C., every week for physicals at the NIH's hospital in Bethesda. By introducing himself to everyone he met there, Bahlman managed to compile a roster of contact numbers so that the patients could compare notes among themselves. Most reported feeling well. Over a mean treatment period of nine months, nobody in the study contracted PCP or CMV retinitis, though four did die, three of them suicides. This boded well for L-697,661.

In one of his many interactions with the drugmakers during this time, Bahlman suggested that if Merck felt it had benefited significantly from the input from the two ACT UP advisers, the company should consider instituting a formal community advisory board (or CAB) comprised of AIDS treatment activists from around the country. Merck's spokesman John Doorley liked the idea, as did Emilio Emini, who headed the research project. Given their good working relationship to date, formalizing the dialogue seemed beneficial to all sides. Doorley made Bahlman the inaugural member. Marty Delaney from Project Inform in San Francisco was another logical pick, as was John James, who published the influential community newsletter *AIDS Treatment News*. Soon the group grew to about a dozen, with representatives from several cities.

For Emini, the opportunity to work closely with patients was a powerful incentive. He rarely saw his work in terms of an individual's health. "It may sound strange to say, but I'm doing the science 'cause it's fun to do, you know? I'm not a medical doctor. I work with molecules." Getting to know the recipients of his efforts affected him profoundly. Still, in an industry known for sharp competition and a history of corporate espionage, the business risks were considerable. Emini had the CAB members sign confidentiality agreements. But he trusted that they were there to help, and he treated them as colleagues. The CAB members did the same, sharing insights garnered from their meetings with the FDA about upcoming regulatory issues, or with the ACTG about parallel drug development efforts. Their interactions were lively, sometimes heated, and always productive. Similarly, ACT UP, TAG, Project Inform, and the other treatment activists established CABs at almost all of the major and minor pharmaceutical companies in the business.

Despite their joint efforts, no good news was on the horizon. About seven months into the Merck study, John Doorley called Bahlman with a heavy voice.

"It's not good, Bill. We're finding resistance," he reported. "We need to have an emergency meeting."

A limousine collected Bahlman in the Village and delivered him and Becker to Merck's headquarters, nearly an hour away in Rahway, New Jersey. The company's compound was separated from a sleepy neighborhood of small one-story homes by an imposing wrought-iron fence. Inside the gate, a dozen office buildings, factories, and warehouses were nestled between rolling hills and endless slabs for parking. The limo took them straight to the CEO's helicopter for a brisk flight to a building north of Philadelphia, where a grim team of researchers awaited them.

Emilio Emini addressed the assembled community representatives, ticking through a succession of slides projected onto a large screen. Merck's first anti-HIV drug to go into Phase II studies had triggered rapid and virulent viral mutations. "It happens in everybody," he said. "We've got to stop the study immediately, because of the concerns for the harm it might be doing to people. We're very worried about safety moving forward."

This was excruciating news. Becker and Bahlman had had the same drug exposures, and probably the same mutations. Whether any future antiretroviral would work for them now was an open question. (For the moment, Bahlman wasn't worried about his own health. His CD4 count was 958, as high as it had ever been.) This spelled the end for Merck's line of non-nucleoside reverse transcriptase drugs.

Merck's commitment to financing AIDS research now hung in the balance. Emini's personal view was starkly pessimistic. The team was out of ideas. He wondered if long-term suppression of the virus would ever be possible.

"I don't think we can do this," Emini admitted to his community advisers. "It might not be possible."

The room fell silent. Bahlman scanned the faces of the Merck researchers anxiously. They wore expressions of surrender. The implications for the community were awful. If Merck pulled out of the field, the other Big Pharma giants were sure to follow.

"Look," Bahlman said. "We're in this for the long haul. We have no choice. But I am a firm believer that the efforts that you have already put in will pay off. We *are* going to find a cure for HIV. To me, it's like: You got to go home, get a good night's sleep, dust yourself off, and rededicate yourself to the lab tomorrow. We need you for the long haul too."

Emini felt ashamed. As he left the meeting, he thought to himself, *Emilio, you've got no right to say to yourself, I don't know if I can do this. We'll pick ourselves up. We'll go back at it.*

IN THE GRAY days of February, Michael Callen was on his first Midwest tour with the Flirtations. They had a gig at the grand Walker Theater in Indianapolis, where they were billed as "the world's most famous openly-gay politically aware a cappella doo-wop singing group." Indianapolis was a manageable drive from Hamilton and the modest house Callen grew up in, yet his parents, who had not seen him perform since grade school, would not be attending. They explained that they were "not comfortable" watching him sing as an openly gay man. It's not that they were hostile toward him personally, but they were devoted to their faith community and worried about what ramifications his flamboyance might bring to them, in Hamilton as much as in the hereafter. When Callen was a child, they sent him to a congregation where the faithful tugged at him and babbled in tongues to rid him of the devil that made him girly. Later, every Sunday for a decade, they had a prayer group calling on divine powers to get their son married to a woman, ignoring his angry objections. Barb and Cliff Callen didn't see these actions as contradicting their love for their son.

Growing up in the 1940s, the only sexual instruction Cliff ever received was an admonition from his parents: *Don't embarrass us.* He passed the same counsel on to his three children. What Michael Callen was planning to do at the Walker Theater was embarrassing. So was the fact that, when their son drove to Hamilton for a visit and turned up the driveway for the first time in years, he was tailed by a documentary film crew exploring homophobia in America.

Cliff, a former merchant marine now in his late sixties, was stunned by his son's appearance. Michael's skin was deep orange, the consequence of one of his medications, and he was as thin as a cadaver. His cheekbones created sharp creases on his skin.

After the filmmakers got what they wanted and left, Michael made it known this would be his farewell visit. He intended to speak his mind.

"Let me be really clear," he said to his father. "What hurts is that you would not consider my ten-year relationship with Richard to be exactly equivalent to Linda and Bobby and Barry and Patty," naming his younger sister and older brother and their mates. Though Callen had not spoken to Richard Dworkin in some time, the sting from his parents had outlived the relationship. "That has been a constant source of pain."

Cliff Callen shrugged and said, "I believe it, I believe it. But just as some of the things that you have done are a constant source of pain to *me*."

Michael knew that being seen as "a big old sissy" had deeply humiliated his father ever since he'd entered puberty.

"Anything recently?" he asked. "I mean, anything that I might be unaware of?"

"Well, I don't know how you'd modify them because, you know, just as I am what I am, you are what you are. And I have to accept that, whether I like that or not. And you have to learn to accept what I am, whether *you* like it or not."

Cliff added, "I know that you're disappointed and hurt that I could never accept Richard in the sense that I said. You didn't have to tell me that. I know that."

"I should say, to your enormous credit . . . you have never been rude to Richard when you spoke to him on the phone. I couldn't have maintained a relationship with you if you were rude to the person that I love."

"I am not rude to anybody," said Cliff.

"Yes, but I was always acutely aware—as was he—that you were not talking to him in the same way that you would talk to Patty or Bob."

"Because in my mind, it *isn't* the same. And I'm sorry it's that way."

Michael's wristwatch announced it was time to take his meds. "Okay," he said. "I want to go on down the list, because I have a whole list of things I want to talk to you about." The phone rang, and no one moved to answer it. "Mom said that she did not hear or know of the existence of gayness as a concept until she was twenty-five. So I'm interested in your—"

"I knew the concept as a sophomore in high school. As a *concept,* now."

"I'm interested in—"

"Even in every small town, there is a gay person that everybody knows about. In the small town that I lived in there were like two or three."

"Flamboyant?" asked Michael.

"Yeah. I mean one of them was an announcer for fairs and stuff like that. Everybody knew him. He was a newspaperman. But he also liked little boys. He was always trying to—"

"Just for the historical record, what do you mean by 'little boys'? Sixteen? Eight?"

"Oh no, not that little. Puberty. Puberty," said his father.

"You assume he had affairs with adults as well?"

"Well, yeah. I assumed that, but I knew that he tried to pick up fifteen-, sixteen-, seventeen-, and eighteen-year-olds because he very often, well, I knew kids that he had tried to pick up."

"Do you remember those people as being severely traumatized by it, or was it—"

"I don't remember that, Mike," Cliff snapped. "Now, you asked about a concept. And knowing the concept is not the same as saying I knew all the activities of homosexuals. I didn't. And by the time I went to sea, being around people who *did* know all the activities that homosexuals normally engaged in, they talked about it. By that time, then, you knew about gay bars and you knew about bathhouses and you knew about some of the more bizarre practices, based not on what you had observed but just simply on hearing them talk. They talked about places—I believe it was in San Francisco, and I'm sure there were other places too—where women dressed as men and men dressed as women. Floor shows, that kind of thing."

"Are there any people from your childhood or from sea or whatever that eventually came out to you, that you remember?" His father went silent. "You don't have to name them, but somebody that you went to school with that you presumably didn't have a clue?"

"Yeah, I did have a clue. I did. Because he had some of the characteristics at that time that you normally associate with somebody being gay."

"Which were? . . . I'm very interested in the details of how heterosexuals talk about us. Because it's my experience that in almost every instance, everyone knew all along anyway. But gay people go through a period when they maintain the fantasy that they've hid it so well no one knows."

"I knew you were gay from the sixth grade on."

This didn't surprise Michael. He remembered the time in the car when his father slapped his face for singing a Lesley Gore song, using a fluttery soprano and all of the original pronouns.

"There was no doubt in my mind that you were going to be gay. I talked to Mom about it to this extent. When I would mention, early on, 'Do you think Mike might be a sissy?,' she would say, 'Don't say anything about it or you might make it worse.' That was her tactic."

Callen didn't blame his parents for their hostilities. It would have been surprising if they had acted differently in the 1960s. It would be different for a gay kid in Hamilton today—but still not easy. "We gay activists have done a lot of work," he said. "The progress is achingly slow for us, but that's the nature of—"

"I don't doubt that you have made progress," Cliff Callen interrupted. "But I don't know how much more progress you're going to make."

"Time will tell," Michael said crisply. "And I won't be here for it."

That was the invitation to begin talking about AIDS. But nobody under the Callen roof was willing to go there.

BOB RAFSKY, the stentorian-voiced genius behind ACT UP's media machine, snuck into the campaign event for Bill Clinton by buying a ticket. In his suit and tie, he was indistinguishable from the other donors except for the telltale signs of AIDS. The KS lesions made his nose bulbous and somewhat misshapen, and something had turned his breath sour. He was thinner than he had been since his days at Harvard, but not yet the knobby skeleton he would become.

Rafsky was a member of TAG, but he continued on in ACT UP as well, one of the few straddlers. His strength being public relations and not science, he served both groups as a kind of Old Testament prophet, becoming their eloquent voice of reason and purpose, not just in fiery speeches from the floor but in ornate and soulful personal essays published in *OutWeek* and *The Village Voice*. Even *The New York Times* had offered him space, on the op-ed page. AIDS had launched the writing career he'd dreamed of claiming since college. "Imminent death," he jokingly told me, "has turned out to be my best career move."

With the Democratic presidential primary in full swing, he joined ACT UP's "AIDS Campaign '92," organized to push Governor Jerry Brown or Senator Paul Tsongas to address the AIDS crisis, without success. This was his first time lobbying the Clinton camp. He slipped past his colleagues picketing outside the Laura Belle, an art deco supper club in Times Square, and moved to the front of the room.

When Bill Clinton arrived, Rafsky felt the governor's rock-star powers. More than a thousand young party loyalists crowded the hem of the stage. A jolt of excitement rose up when Clinton began to speak. Rafsky wasted no time. He pushed toward the stage with such a look of crazed purpose on his face that Secret Service agents moved between him and the candidate. His voice rang out as never before. Nobody in the club missed a word.

"We're *dying* in this state. When are you going to talk about AIDS?"

Clinton turned to him midsentence and stared. The audience leaped to the candidate's defense with a polite smattering of applause. "First of all," Clinton finally said, "it will become part of my obsession as president."

"Bill, we're dying of neglect!"

"That's why I'm running for president—to do something about it." He walked toward Rafsky as he said this.

Rafsky was disgusted. If the epidemic were Clinton's motivation, it was odd that the candidate had yet to utter the word AIDS in public.

"What you're dying of," Rafsky bellowed, "is ambition."

This angered the Arkansas governor. His eyes narrowed, and he pointed a bent finger in Rafsky's direction. "Will you just calm down?"

The crowd aligned with Clinton, who began stalking the stage like a prizefighter, then spun toward Rafsky, stabbing his finger in his direction. "*I feel your pain*," he shouted. "I feel your pain! But if you want to attack me personally, you're no better than Jerry Brown and all the rest of these people who say whatever sounds good in the moment. If you want something to be done, you ask me a question, you listen. If you don't agree with me, go support somebody else for president. But quit talking to me like that. This is not a matter of personal attack. It's a matter of human loss."

It was a breathtaking performance, one that political candidates would seek to emulate for years to come. In those few sentences Clinton cast himself as a better friend to people with AIDS than people with AIDS themselves. He would become the "I feel your pain" politician. That night, the clean-cut Rafsky looked like a hothead on every news broadcast in the nation, but it didn't matter. He had forced Clinton to make a plea for compassion and action in the epidemic, the foundation for an AIDS agenda. In follow-up interviews, Clinton promised a "Manhattan Project for AIDS" under the direction of a cabinet-level "AIDS czar," if elected. Finally, a major candidate for office was talking about the epidemic as though it were an epidemic.

Rafsky was pleased, but not at all convinced, as he told ACT UP the following Monday. "It looks like what we have to do is to keep forcing these clowns to say the right thing so that if one of them happens to become president we can hold them accountable for doing the right thing. But it's always important to say that we all know that the names of the people who might save our lives are not Bill Clinton, Jerry Brown, et cetera. The names of the people who might save our lives are Iris Long, Mark Harrington, Peter Staley, et cetera. And they're the ones who will be remembered as the heroes of this epidemic, as well as those who have gone before."

THE TALK of a "Manhattan Project for AIDS" awakened Larry Kramer's faith that the country had come to its senses at last. The original Manhattan Project brought together over 130,000 people at a cost of billions; with leadership from the White House, it managed to cut through complex bureaucracies and produce a deadly atom bomb in less than four years. If such a monumental campaign were to focus on HIV and the immune system, Kramer had no doubt, a cure would come along just as quickly.

With Clinton leading the polls, Kramer took a break from writing to help divine what this strategy might look like. One weekend that summer, he swallowed his pride and hosted a group of TAG activists in an East Hampton house he was renting from a friend, a startlingly grand, castle-sized structure with multiple turrets and chimneys. "Spoiled children," he called his guests. But he knew a united front would be necessary for this plan to work. Besides, he had mellowed somewhat since moving to the country. His health improved as well. When he first arrived, he had three hundred CD4 cells; the ocean air and the country sun helped push them up substantially.

Mark Harrington agreed to Kramer's weekend invitation. He brought along fellow TAG members Gregg Gonsalves, David Gold, and Mike Barr, a research associate at St. Vincent's. Kramer laid out his plan, in which the renegade surgeon general C. Everett Koop would be put in charge of the massive Manhattan Project. People like the FDA head David Kessler and James Watkins, the admiral who rescued Reagan's AIDS commissioner, would join as ranking officers, sequestered alongside bench scientists and Nobel Prize winners in a remote desert lab with a towering budget and an Oval Office mandate. Kramer had discussed these possibilities with Dr. Bernadine Healy, the current NIH head, who hoped to retain her position regardless of the election's outcome. She agreed to solicit further thoughts. Separately, the reconstituted Science Committee of ACT UP was also looking at an ambitious proposal. However, in deference to the victims of atomic warfare in Hiroshima and Nagasaki, they rejected the Manhattan Project as a name and called their initiative the Barbara McClintock Project to Cure AIDS, named after the first female scientist ever to win an unshared Nobel Prize in medicine, an iconoclast in her field (the chromosomes of corn). Mark Milano, a film editor by training, and two other ACT UP loyalists, the psychology professor Maxine Wolfe and a botanist named John Riley, fleshed out the broad strokes of a plan that would cost a billion dollars a year for five years.

The TAG people wanted nothing to do with either plan. Tensions that weekend ran high. Harrington had studied Richard Rhodes's book *The Making of the Atomic Bomb* and concluded that what worked in physics couldn't work in biology. It made sense to lock the world's top minds in a bunker for them to puzzle through the challenge of atom splitting, he said. They knew what they needed to do, and had only to learn how to do it. In AIDS research, there were nothing but questions in multiple fields, from pharmaceutical chemistry, cellular biology, immunology, and even neurology. It required blood samples but also many thousands of patients at various stages of deterioration. Even if they were willing to leave behind their jobs, lovers, friends, and families, it would be logistically impossible to hole up so many people with AIDS in one location.

What's more, Harrington and his TAG colleagues were now convinced that in the chaotic and undirected search for effective medicine, too little attention had been paid to the basic science of the epidemic.

There was only a vague understanding of HIV—how it did its damage, why it killed different people at different speeds. Only slightly more was known about the mechanisms of human immunity itself. What was needed was the active engagement of the entire community of scientists, not just the few "celebrity leaders" on Kramer's wish list. Harrington called Kramer's idea "foolish, grandiose, and absurd."

The TAG team presented Kramer with a counterproposal: instead of building a whole new research system, parallel and distinct from NIH, they advocated for improving the way the existing one worked. Harrington and Gonsalves were already sketching out a reform plan. Since early in the spring, they had been requesting vast amounts of information from every branch of the NIH—on budgets, staffing, corporate reporting charts, and much else. The work of analyzing the records soon proved too daunting for the two to carry out on nights and weekends, so TAG's board put them on the payroll, the first time they had received money for their activist labors. They fired off even more detailed demands for public data. Fauci instructed his division heads to comply with their requests as thoroughly as possible. Cartons of dot-matrix, z-fold printouts were soon leaning in perilous towers along the walls of Harrington's apartment.

They discovered that eighteen separate institutes and centers at the NIH were engaged in AIDS research, all more or less independently, some overlapping or else competing outright with one another. The total yearly cost to taxpayers was $800 million. Roughly half of that was invested in the world that Tony Fauci controlled directly—the infectious disease institute and its ACTG system, for clinical trials under Dan Hoth's control. The rest was scattered among the branches devoted to cancer, childhood health, eyes, neurological disorders, and the circulatory system. The entity created to make sense of all this, the so-called Office of AIDS Research, which Fauci also ran, in fact competed for its own budget in ways that at times cannibalized from the other institutes. The two men were identifying ways to streamline the NIH by eliminating duplications and waste, adopting an official national agenda, and creating a top-down leadership structure—in effect, imposing order on the chaotic system.

Harrington and Gonsalves invited Kramer and ACT UP to endorse TAG's reform efforts and abandon their own, which only revived the old friction and hostilities. While their conversations continued into the fall, the sides hardened around competing agendas.

· · ·

IN THE MEANTIME, Harrington was planning a scientific experiment on his own body that would change the way scientists looked at HIV disease.

Since his first blood test hinted at infection two years earlier, he had closely monitored his CD4s, watching as they rose and fell within a fairly stable range, settling most recently at 660. He was one of the lucky ones, apparently able to keep a working immune system. Most doctors considered this a period of latency. But like Callen, Harrington suspected that something else was at work in his body, perhaps a special biological mechanism capable of holding back HIV's powers. If his CD4s were engaged in some sort of genetic trick, or if some other cells unique to him behaved in extraordinary ways, his body might harbor the secrets of a cure. So that April he went to Roosevelt Hospital in Hell's Kitchen, signed an informed consent form, and under local anesthesia had a rock-hard, walnut-sized lymph node removed from under his left arm. It was not an especially painful procedure, and he healed quickly as he awaited the analysis.

The findings were significant. In July, he took the data to the International AIDS Conference in Amsterdam, where he was placed on the official agenda alongside PhDs and Nobel Prize winners. It was the first time an AIDS patient had addressed questions of basic science in this forum, and more than five thousand scientists and clinicians packed the room for his talk. He wore his trademark white jeans, a single loop earring, and a green thrift-store blazer. His hair was buzz-cut on the side and floppy on top, the hot style of the summer. Looming on a big screen above his head was a twenty-foot-wide image of his infected node.

My tissue samples were sent to various laboratories for analysis. I went through several weeks of preoccupation with what they would find. Of course, I wanted to know the answers to the pathogenesis questions. Of course, I really wanted to know *what was going on inside my body*. But there were no answers, only a profusion of questions which crept up on me in a somewhat devastating way.

My doctor filled me in every few weeks. "They've found a signal." Oh. A signal of what? Later: "It's crammed with virus."

He looked out upon his audience, for whom news of his infection was a shock. Nobody in ACT UP or anywhere else knew he was sick. Friends sitting in the hall broke into tears.

He showed slide after slide, all depicting a very active hive of HIV replication. There was no such thing as HIV latency. His relatively stable CD4 count did not mean that HIV was at rest somewhere. On the contrary, HIV had commandeered his body, pressing it into service as a high-volume factory manufacturing thousands and thousands of new HIV viruses.

The slides also extinguished one of the reasons to doubt that HIV was the sole and essential cause of AIDS. Sonnabend and other researchers had noted that in blood samples of the sick there was a curiously low concentration of HIV—not enough, they assumed, to cause disease on its own. Now it was clear why that was. The bloodstream, it turned out, was not the main battlefield. The virus wreaked havoc inside the lymphatic system, a parallel network of vessels.

Turning back to his audience, who were fascinated into rapt silence, Harrington used the rest of his talk to beseech researchers to follow his lead back to the basic science of HIV infection. "There are a host of questions which could be answered by further investigation of my tissue and that of other volunteers," he said. "Activists and people with HIV can help to make this happen. In return, basic researchers must figure out how to work with—and not just on—people with HIV. That way, it will not take thirty years to finish this campaign, and the numbing litany of our losses can end at last."

Two hours later, TAG called a meeting with the press to deliver Harrington and Gonsalves's eagerly anticipated NIH report. The media event—the first of consequence since TAG spun off as a separate entity—was well attended and clamorous. Both Harrington and Gonsalves were in coats and ties, a sign of their new professionalism. They sipped water at a cloth-bunted table as Spencer Cox circulated copies of the critique to the journalists. The incongruous setting distinguished the three activists from what remained of ACT UP. Looking more ragtag than ever, ACT UP's delegation to Amsterdam marauded through the conference hall's exhibition area, overturning booths manned by pharmaceutical company representatives, affixing stickers to their computer screens, and generally expressing profound frustration.

TAG's report showed a blueprint for bureaucratic ineptitude. The removal of Hoth was their first demand, but they went after Tony Fauci as well. What Fauci had proved exceptionally adept at over the dozen plague years was seizing all the ceremonial trappings of authority. In addition to his duties at NIAID and the Office of AIDS Research, he ran his own research laboratory and served as the top NIH official for directing AIDS research. This made him his own supervisor, division manager, area vice president, and CEO; in essence, the fight against AIDS was a one-man show. As much as TAG members had come to like Fauci personally, they held him responsible for the devastating lack of progress against the disease. The reason there still were few treatments for the opportunistic infections was because of his continued insistence on "investigator-driven research" and refusal to set goals and priorities—his refusal to *lead*. They wanted somebody else—frankly, almost anybody else—to take the helm at the Office of AIDS Research.

Spencer Cox quieted the room and took the first question, from a female reporter who had arrived in a wheelchair.

"I noticed that you're both sitting up there in suits and ties," she said. "Do you feel that your approach is better than circling NIH buildings and so forth?"

Harrington leaned into the microphone with a slight smile. "I think that we like to keep our options open, but it's silly to risk arrest and the hassles that are attendant upon it if you can get serious attention and negotiations going with other measures."

Whether those other measures would be sufficient to unseat Fauci was anyone's guess.

MICHAEL CALLEN had been coughing for weeks. It seemed he suffered a bacterial pneumonia almost every year, an affliction probably unrelated to his disease, but this time something was different. While in Amsterdam, he coughed up a quantity of blood. X rays soon confirmed that the KS had moved to his lungs. Lesions were multiplying quickly. Within weeks, the pulmonary involvement was extensive. The latest medical reports suggested a person in his condition could expect to live for barely four months.

The news didn't depress him as much as he'd expected. Back in California he found himself appreciating life more thoroughly—that first aromatic spoonful of minestrone from Café Benvenuto, or the discovery of a kitschy new salt-and-pepper set. One of the first people he took into his confidence was Richard Dworkin. Though they hadn't spoken in many months, he had always pictured Dworkin at his deathbed. When an answering machine clicked on, he felt lucky that Dworkin was away, and left the news in a breezy report, no more gravely than if he were saying he had a new job.

Callen didn't dread the prospect of death. Maybe the decade he spent living in death's shadow had helped him find a way to accommodate it.

What upset him was the timing. He was nowhere near completing his ambitious *Legacy* album; in fact, in his two years in California he had managed to write just one song. Instead, he'd spent the time touring with the Flirtations. He felt sure he was finally on the verge of real acceptance as an artist. He'd been invited to sing in two feature films, one of them starring Tom Hanks as a person with AIDS.

So he did something he had counseled so many people against: he started chemotherapy, a staggering round every two weeks. He still believed it might hasten his death, but in the meantime it was the only way to keep his lungs clear enough to allow for singing. Briefly, he even contemplated AZT, the drug he once famously compared to Drano, but to his great relief his cancer responded well to oncology treatments alone, and slowed its progress.

To Callen's surprise, Dworkin didn't return his phone call. He called and left a second message, this one biting. Both came while Dworkin was touring Europe with another band. When Dworkin returned to New York and Callen's messages, he was devastated. His lover, Patrick Kelly, was also battling KS now. He called Callen right away, only to be accused of abandonment. There would be no rapprochement.

Friends sent Callen encouraging notes, urging him to "keep fighting." Some were limned with a subtle hostility, as if accusing Callen of betraying his followers by succumbing to cancer. "Re-read your own book!" said one note. In recent years, much of his time in therapy was devoted to shaking his "sick sense of obligation to others." While in California he had struggled to reestablish some measure of privacy in his health battles.

Now that he was truly dying, he thought, *Why bother?* He reopened his medical charts to public scrutiny, this time in an article he wrote for *QW,* a new gay weekly.

> It's begun to dawn on me that some people misinterpret my message of hope to mean that everyone with full-blown AIDS won't necessarily die of it. *I have never said any such thing!* Instead, what I've racked up 180,000 air miles trying to explain is that *no one diagnosed with AIDS needs to die on cue!* . . . But I'm definitely dying; I know it in my bones. I can't say when, but soon. *And it's truly OK.*

Doug read me these last lines out loud one evening when I returned home from work. He walked painfully to the window, gazing down to the littered streetscape below. "Michael Callen is dying," he said. "I'm screwed."

THE PRIMARY CAMPAIGN careened toward the convention with Bill Clinton holding an easy lead, with the gay and lesbian vote in his pocket. Exuding confidence, his team began drawing up a list of potential speakers for the convention, set to take place in New York City. They planned to include a gay speaker with AIDS.

Thus began what Bob Rafsky bitterly dubbed "the latest contest for people dying from AIDS." Résumés began flying as some activists promoted their candidacies for the convention lineup. Larry Kramer, of course, coveted the platform, as did several other ACT UP members. Ironically, it was Rafsky whom the Clinton people first contacted. Once he realized what the call was about, he hung up the phone.

In the end, the two PWAs who spoke were Bob Hattoy, a gay Clinton adviser, and Elizabeth Glaser, the HIV-positive wife of a television actor who launched the Pediatric AIDS Foundation in memory of her daughter, who had died from AIDS complications at the age of seven. Both gave sterling speeches. But none was as memorable as the AIDS speech given at the Republican convention in August. Worried that Clinton had gained an advantage, President Bush opened up a prime-time spot on the program for someone battling the virus. He chose Mary Fisher, the daughter of one of the GOP's top fund-raisers and heir to a large Michigan fortune. The AIDS community ridiculed her bona fides—a conservative, heterosexual woman from the middle of America—yet her remarks were anything but toneless. She brought her party, and the listening nation, to silence. It was one of the most powerful pieces of oratory in a generation.

"We may take refuge in our stereotypes," she said, "but we cannot hide there long. Because HIV asks only one thing of those it attacks: 'Are you human?' And this is the right question—are you human? People with HIV have not entered some alien state of being. They are human. They have not earned cruelty and do not deserve meanness. They don't benefit from being isolated or treated as outcasts. Each of them is exactly what God made: a person, not evil, deserving of our judgment; not victims, longing for our pity."

She then spoke of her two young sons, whom she feared would still be boys when HIV took her away. "To all within the sound of my voice, I appeal: Learn with me the lessons of history and of ignorance, so my children will not be able to be afraid to say the word 'AIDS' when I am gone. Then their children, and yours, may not need to whisper it at all."

IN THE FALL, Doug reluctantly filled out disability papers at work. He had come to love his job and his colleagues—African American women from the outer boroughs, not at all the theater crowd of his early career. He would have done anything to keep to his routine. What did him in were the stairs—at our apartment building and to and from the subway platform. His first few days at home were mind-numbingly monotonous. He spent more time in front of the television ("steeping," he joked, "in the healing power of the cathode ray") and on kitchen projects. He was an able cook, and for a time I was arriving home to the smells of rich sauces and savory vegetables. But his appetite, never reliable, declined further, and he soon ended his experiment in the culinary arts. Instead, he took up a massive sewing project that filled the apartment with bolts of dark fabric. He was making a log cabin quilt, which he hoped to finish before a long-planned visit by his parents from Colorado, their first to our home in the city.

On a bright morning in November, we descended the stairs slowly and headed to the polls. He stood weakly in the line outside the community center on East Third Street. The whole neighborhood was abuzz with excitement about an end to Republican rule. It was easy to daydream that Clinton's promises for AIDS research would produce quick results.

Doug was buoyant when he emerged from the booth. "Tax and spend, tax and spend," he said cheerfully. "I can't wait."

Unfortunately, he was right about that. Two days later, we awoke at 3 a.m. in a soggy bed flooded in his sweat. His temperature was careening wildly. Dr. Waitkevicz was baffled. Doug soaked the sheets the next night, and the next. On November 9, his breathing grew labored and he had trouble getting out of bed. "It feels like pneumonia again," he told me. His voice had the same strange reediness it had had during his first bout with PCP. He had been taking Bactrim religiously, but infections sometimes occurred in spite of that. I called Waitkevicz. She wanted him hospitalized immediately, and since Beekman Downtown was full she asked Dr. Metroka, Doug's old oncologist, the original pioneer in the KS battle, to admit him at Roosevelt Hospital. Doug hadn't seen him in nearly two years, but Metroka's office agreed to make the arrangements.

We packed him a small bag and hailed a cab. Clouds slid slowly across the sky as we made our way uptown in heavy traffic. Roosevelt's lobby was bright and airy. Metroka was not there to meet us, as we had expected, but Doug was admitted regardless, though not to the HIV floor, which had filled to capacity in the half hour it took us to get there. Rather, he was placed in a room at the end of a very long corridor on a post-surgery unit.

I came by the next morning with bagels and coffee. Doug was sound asleep, despite the irregular symphony of beeps echoing through the room. He was attached to a big bag of yellow fluids. A clamp on his index finger calculated his blood oxygen levels, which were low enough to trigger frequent electronic squeals, none of which earned the attention of staff.

I sat in a chair at the foot of his bed and snapped open the paper. The news was of little consequence, considering: Clinton was putting together his cabinet, New York had a new police chief, the Church of England was voting to ordain women. I couldn't concentrate on any of it. I began to cry. Doug, who had awakened, looked at me brusquely. "What's that about?" he whispered, sounding angry.

I shook my head. "I'm tired," I apologized. "What does the doctor say?"

"I don't know. I haven't seen anybody."

I slipped out to the nurses' station to find out more. "We're not treating him with anything, he doesn't have a diagnosis," said one of them, a West Indian woman with hair braided into a substantial architectural structure atop her head. She opened his file and drew a fingernail across a densely printed page, humming to herself. "The test results aren't in yet," she said finally.

"When is Dr. Metroka coming?"

She consulted a different form. "He was here already," she said, "very early. He'll be back again tomorrow."

I resolved to beat Metroka to Doug's bedside the following morning.

It was an hour before sunrise when I turned the corner into Doug's room. From the light of the hallway I could see that something grim had taken place there. A great arc of blood marked his privacy curtain and spattered the wall behind his bed. Crusty footprints tracked into the bathroom, where blood had puddled on the sink and the toilet seat. Doug was bent awkwardly on his bed, in a deep sleep, with dried blood on his hands and neck. I couldn't rouse him. I pumped the call button, then ran to the nurses' station when no one came.

"He was a bad boy last night," said the nurse with the hair, narrowing her eyes disapprovingly. "Pulled out his IV lines and took himself to the toilet. We found him passed out on the floor." She could not tell me whether he had called for assistance first, how long he was unconscious, how much blood he had lost, or why he remained caked in it.

"Please don't let Dr. Metroka leave without talking to me," I said.

"He's gone already," she said, before disappearing into a room behind the nurses' counter.

I looked at my watch. It was 5:30 a.m. "Call him back," I shouted, but she was out of range.

I decided not to go to work that day.

When Doug awoke, he was groggy and confused—and as shocked by the bloodbath as I had been. He had no memory of the night. I located a pair of rubber gloves and gave him a sponge bath. A janitor eventually came and cleaned the floor. But nobody from the medical staff arrived the rest of that morning. At lunchtime I left a message at Metroka's Central Park South office. In the late afternoon a young doctor entered the room, an intern or resident, whom I bombarded with questions and bitter complaints. He explained that test results weren't back, but agreed with me that it was likely PCP.

"Why don't you start him on pentamidine anyway," I asked, "while you're waiting for the results. He's just getting sicker and sicker."

He gave a look that said *That makes sense,* then pored over the dense graphs on the chart that hung outside Doug's door. "That's a question for Dr. Metroka," he said.

"But this is our third day here and Doug hasn't spoken to him yet."

"It looks like he makes his rounds at about"—he paused, consulting the chart again—"two in the morning? Hmm. Probably your friend was asleep."

Visiting a patient in the middle of the night made no sense to me. I was determined to stay in the room as long as it took to see the elusive doctor. I left only once, at midday, to lay in a supply of fruit from the cafeteria. Then, that afternoon, the pentamidine arrived. Doug and I were both relieved. He had never been sicker. He had taken to using the urine collector hanging from the bed frame since he had lost confidence that his legs would get him to the bathroom.

"You'd better call my parents. They're getting in the car," he said, consulting the calendar on his watch. "They should postpone the trip till I'm out of here."

I knew they had trouble dealing with his health. Whenever he tried to give a meaningful update, his mother, whose mystical belief system included the Ouija Board, stopped the conversation short, saying, "Don't talk about disease. Talking gives it power."

"They should still come," I insisted. I needed their help.

I spent that night in an uncomfortable chair in his room, dozing no more than a few seconds here and there. Metroka never came through the door. At sunrise I asked a new nurse if she had seen him. She looked through her paperwork. "He signed in at two," she said.

"But he never came into the room! Did he leave any instructions?"

She stared at the page intently. "Nope, sweetie."

CHAR AND JACK GOULD drove straight to the hospital from northeastern Colorado. Manhattan intimidated them. Though they had traveled the world with the Army—Jack retired as a staff sergeant and Char as a clerk—they epitomized the people of the Great Plains, wholesome, direct, and uncomplicated. They had adopted their son—Dougie, they called him—as an infant on a Cherokee reservation in Texas.

When they cracked open the door to his hospital room, they found me holding a urine bottle for him as he leaned on the bed unsteadily. His bony, polka-dotted body fully exposed, he looked frightfully older than thirty-three. No greetings were exchanged before Char spun on her heels and retreated to the waiting area, dragging her husband by the shirtsleeve. I followed them out.

Char had tears in her eyes. "David, would you tell me something? And be honest." She twizzled a pearl in her earlobe. "Does Dougie have AIDS?"

The question floored me. She had spent so much energy denying AIDS its power that she had removed the fact of it from her mind. I nodded sadly.

"I'll tell you what," Jack interrupted, forcing a note of cheer. "We'll just get on back to Colorado and you'll let us know a better time for a visit. Maybe in the spring."

Their vehement naïveté scared me. "*Now* is the time for a visit," I said a bit too aggressively. I gave them a set of our apartment keys and sent them to the East Village to await further instructions.

I resumed my vigil for Dr. Metroka. When a nurse insisted I could not stay past visiting hours because I was not immediate family, I challenged her to call the guards. None came. Neither did Metroka.

The next morning, I decided to go find the doctor. Doug's parents met me in the lobby of his Midtown office building, just after nine. The doctor's secretary buzzed us into his waiting room, but she encouraged us to make an appointment if we wished to see him, since he wasn't there. Over her nervous objections, we sat down and waited.

It was nearly noon when Metroka appeared. A short man with a broad, pink face and spotty scalp, he wore a bow tie and small, wire-rimmed glasses. He barely glanced at us as he swept past, with his secretary scurrying behind. After another twenty minutes without word from inside, we went hunting for him. Most of the place was disused and fallow. We finally found the doctor sitting at his desk in frozen silence. The secretary retreated. He looked up at us with a blank face.

"Come in," he said. "Sit."

I stood over his desk. "What the fuck is going on? You've got a very sick patient in the hospital. We've been waiting for days to see you." My anger was crossed with exhaustion and fear; tears flew from my eyes.

"We're doing everything we can," he said.

"You haven't even seen him!"

"Of course I've seen him," he said, fluttering his black eyes slowly. "It's just that I get there later than most doctors, after the"—he stammered a bit—"after the opera."

"Doug's never seen you, I've never seen you," I snapped. I surmised that he must leave his signature at the nurses' station for billing purposes then withdraw, leaving Doug to his death business, like the *Muselmänner* in the barracks. "You've never ordered one test! Do you even know what he has?" His expression didn't change. I clamped my hand on his elbow. "Let's go," I said, tugging him toward the door. "We're going to the hospital."

Metroka twisted free. "I can't now," he said in his flat affect. He was shaking slightly but not otherwise engaged in the moment. "I can get there at three."

He didn't. By then Doug's condition had worsened. I called GMHC and begged for advice. A counselor there recommended I ask to be assigned a social worker from the hospital's staff. Instead I called Dr. Waitkevicz. After learning of Doug's abandonment, she had been traveling to Roosevelt Hospital every night after rounds at her own hospital. The nursing staff let her read his chart, as a professional courtesy, and from her I learned that the test for PCP I had requested had come back negative. X rays showed pneumonia, but exactly what kind, and how to treat it, remained undetermined. On her recommendation, I asked the intern or resident to order a new round of tests. He started infusions with a powerful antibiotic concoction. Doug's lungs were so filled with fluid now that he wasn't getting enough oxygen to his blood.

A nurse brought a nasal cannula, then traded up to an oxygen mask. Doug was lightheaded and confused, and complained of ripping lung pain. Because of the narcotics administered for relief, he saw gelatinous purple orbs floating through the room. He poked at them anxiously with the clamp on his finger.

"One's on your cheek," he shouted into his mask.

I put my hand on his neck. "It's the pills, Doug. You're hallucinating."

The next morning, his oxygen meter was bleating dire warnings. We were forced to consider intubation. Doug and I had discussed this before, when hospitalization was still a worst-case scenario. At the time, he signed a living will allowing for two weeks on life-sustaining machinery, no more—and only if he had a chance of responding to treatment. Now he seemed confused. "Two weeks!" he objected. "Two weeks?"

"Remember, we talked about this? It will give time for the antibiotics to work."

He nodded. "Oh," he said. I showed him the form he needed to sign. His scrawl was unrecognizable and floated hazily above the signature line. An attendant took away the document and all the beeping equipment, plunging the room into silence for the first time in days. We had fifteen minutes before he would be wheeled away to the ICU. The afternoon sun cut through the window and warmed the room. As I held Doug's hand, he dozed fitfully. From time to time he gave my hand a weak grip, and I gripped his back.

When two attendants came for him, I stroked his hair.

"I love you, Doug."

His eyes were squeezed shut. He whispered into his mask, "I love you, too."

An hour later, his father and I were allowed a ten-minute visit with him in the ICU, a large, windowless room with nine beds arrayed in an oval around a central nursing station. What we saw there was horrific. After being listless and depleted for days, Doug was thrashing ferociously in his bed, driven to violent protest by the tube in his throat. We immediately saw that his ankles and wrists were tied to the bed rail with lengths of gauze. The restraints, the attending physician explained, were necessary because no matter how much sedative they pumped into him he kept yanking out the tube. Being hog-tied hadn't solved the problem; he fought back with his teeth alone, biting down on the plastic tube that carried air into his lungs once every few seconds. They had forced a foam block between his teeth.

What on earth had we done?

"This is a normal response," a woman in green scrubs said. "Some people don't like having that thing in them. But this one's a fighter."

When put that way, the ugly scene gave us a bit of hope: Doug Gould was a fighter. It was good to see evidence of this, even if what he was fighting was the thing keeping him alive. I held his agitated hand and watched his chest rise and fall mechanically, wishing I could do something for him.

"Does he know we're here?"

"With what we've given him, no chance."

I spoke to him anyway, apologizing for the intubation and reminding him of our Thanksgiving plans. He had arranged a large party, with guests flying in from around the country. I promised to take over the preparations. It would be his homecoming.

When our time was up, we moved into the floor's small, windowless waiting room, a place resembling the cabin of a submarine, until the next permitted visit; we were allowed ten minutes each hour. *60 Minutes* played on a small television suspended from the wall, and I hushed Jack Gould when a report on AIDS began. By bizarre coincidence, it was all about ACT UP and featured Peter Staley and Bob Rafsky along with Marina Alvarez, a full-time mom in her forties whom I had seen around ACT UP meetings. When asked by the correspondent, each said they expected to die of AIDS.

Rafsky talked about the book he was writing for his daughter, Sara, so she'd know what her father did to fight AIDS. A number of times over the previous months, he had asked me for help with his prose. I knew what his daughter meant to him from the paragraphs he read over the phone, though I had never met her. Knowing she would be left fatherless wracked him with sadness.

"Bob's a friend of ours," I told Jack Gould.

He found the coincidence astonishing. "You mean, you know someone *else* with this disease?"

When we saw Doug next, he was fully sedated and the cuffs had been removed. We all went home with a fund of hope. The next morning, his body had swollen to a shocking size and the ICU staff conceded that the antibiotics weren't working. During our visiting intervals, I rubbed his inflated hands without trying to speak to him. Soon, Jack Gould would not leave the waiting room, unable to see his son in such violent decay. Every hour brought worse news. By afternoon my bedside visits became a vigil. I saw Doug one last time, during the final visiting block of the night. My old college girlfriend, Katrina Van Valkenburgh, accompanied me; she had arrived early for Doug's Thanksgiving party. When our time was up, I leaned my body next to his and whispered farewell against his ears. I prayed he couldn't hear me.

"I'm sorry," I said. "I'm so sorry."

Back at the apartment, a small group of friends met to share stories about Doug with his mother and father, swallowing our pain with copious amounts of alcohol. We had just turned out the lights when the phone rang with news that Doug had died at 3:25 a.m.

Tests ordered by the ICU staff came back with a posthumous diagnosis: cytomegalovirus pneumonia, hard to treat but treatable. Metroka, having never pursued a diagnosis while he was alive, kept Doug from getting the medication that might have saved his life. That hideous fact was almost impossible to comprehend. In my shock, I lacked the frame of mind to pursue Metroka for abandoning us. It took me nearly a year to begin a complaint. By then he had left his practice, though temporarily.

Eventually, I was willing to mark Metroka down as one more victim of the plague, a gay man who had been a hero in the early days, who presided over years of unrelenting death despite his best efforts. I could not forgive him for abandoning Doug, but it made some kind of grotesque and infuriating sense to me that Metroka could not set foot in his hospital room. He had run out of steam. He had no more life in him than the *Muselmänner* in his charge.

One week after Doug died, I filled a paper bag with his unused medicine and headed for the People With AIDS Health Group. The young lesbian working behind the counter didn't pause to offer condolences. "Good," she said, turning to stock the shelves. "More Epogen."

DR. FAUCI was surprised and hurt by TAG's indictment of his record, and indignant at their campaign to have him removed as director of the Office of AIDS Research. He demanded a meeting in Bethesda. He was defensive. Respectfully, they let him speak his mind, keeping channels open. Neither side changed their view. TAG pushed a ten-point plan for reorganizing AIDS research, and Fauci replied with diplomatic obfuscation.

Late in the fall, the tensions seemed to subside somewhat when Fauci signaled a willingness to replace Dan Hoth and promised a nonspecific "five-year plan" to improve management. No concrete action came. At a subsequent gourmet summit he was unwilling to address the other items on the group's list of demands. So with Clinton's transition staff in place and a new era dawning in Washington, TAG pushed ahead unilaterally. They would attempt to incorporate their plan into the periodic legislation reauthorizing the NIH—imposing order on the research world through Congress. The key element of the plan was to shift all AIDS authority over to the Office of AIDS Research, putting a single entity in charge of overseeing and directing the entire national endeavor. The OAR would require a full-time dedicated director. Nothing in their plan barred Fauci from that position, but TAG correctly surmised that he would not leave his laboratory and his institute for the narrowly focused campaign.

For help on Capitol Hill, TAG turned to two deft political operatives. One was Tim Westmoreland, the AIDS adviser for Congressman Henry Waxman, Democrat from Los Angeles. On the Senate side they approached Michael Iskowitz, a policy staffer for Senator Ted Kennedy. Both agreed to introduce the TAG language into the NIH reauthorization bill. By the end of the year, AmFAR was onboard with them, as were the Pediatric AIDS Foundation and a majority of the other groups.

On January 8, 1993, Harrington flew to Washington to pay a courtesy call on Dr. Bernadine Healy, who was by now expecting to be held over as head of the NIH. Healy looked the part of a conservative politician in her pearls and crisp suit. Yet she was instantly at ease with Harrington. Besides her obvious political ambition, Harrington found her to be practical about medicine and science, and open to new ideas. She was cautious about TAG's reorganization plans, but not a hardened opponent. She professed an eagerness to hear more.

Next, a group of TAG people convened a January 10 meeting at the Dallas–Ft. Worth airport with thirty treatment activists who had flown in from around the country, hoping to build even broader support within the community. There was some opposition. At Fauci's instigation, Marty Delaney aggressively lobbied against the TAG measure, and Larry Kramer joined key parts of ACT UP to condemn it as a dangerous distraction from his call for an AIDS Manhattan Project.

It didn't matter. Senator Kennedy introduced the NIH reauthorization bill on the first full day of the new Congress, earning it the title "Senate Bill 1." Late that afternoon, a copy of the bill reached the NIH campus, and by nightfall Harrington's phone was ringing off the hook, as reporters called for a comment. The next morning, Dr. Healy called an emergency meeting in her office of all her institute directors. Recognizing that the two-day-old Clinton administration intended to shake up AIDS research, they knew that criticizing S.1 would be politically dangerous to them individually. Fauci offered to draft a memo for them all to sign. In it, he suggested putting the restricting provisions on hold for a year and commissioning a study of how it might impact AIDS research.

After reviewing Fauci's draft, Dr. Healy got Mark Harrington on the phone. "I'm working on S.1," she told him. "The [institute directors] wanted me to walk the plank on this. I told them it was partly their own fault for not having their act together."

Harrington had won her over. She did not join their protest.

Thereafter, the political work fell to Kennedy and Waxman, who introduced a tandem measure in the House, labeled H.R.4. Clinton's new health secretary, Donna Shalala, fell squarely in line. The battle-front moved to the rank-and-file AIDS scientists. Fauci slugged it out with TAG for their support—he faxed a fifteen-page memo around the country denouncing the reorganization plan, which was matched by TAG's faxed reply, addressed to 112 leading AIDS scientists.

On February 17, by a vote of Congress, Fauci was out as head of the Office of AIDS Research, and a campaign to streamline, reorganize, and prioritize the entire federal AIDS research machinery was under way. It was the first bill of Clinton's presidency. TAG wanted Dr. William Paul, a leading immunologist, to take over the newly elevated Office of AIDS Research. Clinton finally gave him the job, but not for another year, and Paul then ordered his staff to develop a comprehensive blueprint for AIDS research, the first ever. Leading his agenda was the "revitalization and expansion" of basic research.

THAT SAME FEBRUARY, Bob Rafsky entered the hospital for the last time. His KS had defied standard therapies and had moved into his lungs. ACT UP waged an international campaign to force a small pharmaceutical company to release an experimental chemotherapy for him, the only time the group was mobilized in this way for a single patient. When the drugs arrived, though, Rafsky would not give them a try. He was exhausted. He had lost his entire immune system and a hundred friends. It had been a while since anyone considered him a possible survivor. Even strangers saw him as the walking dead. One day as he limped past a street corner, a woman who had been talking to a friend interrupted herself to say, "I know you have AIDS." Her tone was neither hostile nor friendly. She was just stating the obvious.

He blamed himself. He didn't contract HIV until 1987, long after condoms were ubiquitous. In many ways, AIDS changed his life for the better. He loved the gay men and women in the community he found, the marches, the crystalline purpose. AIDS gave him a public life, and he was proud of his community standing. He sometimes thought it had all been worth the trouble. And then he would think of his daughter. In recent months, he had written and rewritten his long letter for her to read when she got older, his apology for leaving her fatherless. He knew his days were few, and his letter needed to come to an end. "[N]ow comes the reign of terror," he wrote in conclusion. "The pain will be overwhelming. Take refuge in celebrating the justice of my fate. Find room in your helpless love to hate me and my story."

Bob Rafsky died on the last Saturday of February 1993. With him were his ex-wife, her husband, and Sara, who was eight.

AFTER A LONG weekend in New York City, Michael Callen returned to Hollywood on March 31, sick as a dog. Doctors advised him against the trip, and even he thought it was a bad idea. He was down to 130 pounds, weak and frail. His right leg was swollen with edema and purple with KS, which had also spread through his lymph system. Painful ulceration of the esophagus made eating excruciating (burping even worse). Thrush had invaded his voice box. He gasped for breath, as the KS had shut down three-quarters of his lung capacity. But he was being given a lifetime achievement award at a big New York AIDS gala called "Night of a Thousand Gowns." His grace survived the whole night thanks in part to the new antidepressant imipramine. "A miracle drug," he called it. Prescribed by his doctor recently, it immediately ended what he now saw as the deep clinical depression that governed most of his life.

He was, ironically, in marvelous spirits.

He had a car take him directly from LAX to the hospital, where his symptoms were treated and doctors switched him to an experimental new chemotherapy, Doxil. It was less debilitating than what he'd been taking, but for the first time since his KS spread, he began to lose his hair. "It's gross," he wrote to friends, "but whenever I'm finished eating, my plate is always full of hair. And it's in the drain, and on my pillow, etc."

Being so sick led Callen to call Richard Dworkin to offer an olive branch, proposing that they resuscitate the parts of their old partnership that didn't involve sex, including their committed love for one another, their dependable friendship, and their shared musical projects. He had his legacy—and his *Legacy*—in mind.

"Look," he said to Dworkin. "I really want to do another album, but I don't know if I can. Will you help me?"

Worried that the end was near, Dworkin immediately flew to Los Angeles to arrange studio time. Meanwhile, in New York, Patrick Kelly—the man Callen had seen as his rival—launched a fund-raising campaign to cover the costs, even though he was sick himself. Finishing the project became the only thing that mattered to any of them. Callen's job was to keep his voice intact, which he accomplished by popping the Doxil religiously. On April 8 he shaved himself bald, solving the hair loss problem.

That week he opened a package from David Corkery, a friend in New York, to find a slew of articles on AZT. In Europe, a huge multicenter investigation called the Concorde Study, three years in the making and including almost two thousand patients, had finally asked the question that all of Dr. Margaret Fischl's truncated American studies had avoided: Did AZT extend life and, if so, by how much? The answer was unequivocal: It did not. It made no difference if you took it early in your infection or late or not at all, the final outcome was the same.

The bad news lifted Callen's spirits further. "Can you believe I lived long enough to see TOTAL vindication on this point?" he wrote back to Corkery. He drafted an article as a kind of victory lap, though he would never see it published. "Given that nine out of every ten drugs that reach any phase of human testing in the U.S. fail as either too toxic for human use or don't work, it never made sense to me to push for the kind of drug deregulation that so many AIDS activists seem to favor. And yet, I wonder where all the AZT-pushers are now," he wrote.

The Concorde Study had followed patients in England, France, and Ireland, half of whom were on AZT, the other half on placebo. Unlike the U.S. studies, which were terminated early based on preliminary results, Concorde was allowed to run its course. In the end, there were no statistically relevant differences between the groups on progression to AIDS and death. In fact, 93 percent of people taking the placebo survived the three-year span, compared to 92 percent who had taken AZT.

This destroyed the central myth about AZT, which was now generating a staggering $388 million a year for Burroughs Wellcome. It also destroyed faith in the AZT-like compounds that ACT UP had helped drugmakers sell, with similarly abbreviated data.

But the biggest casualty by far in the wake of Concorde was the tactic of AIDS treatment activists to race drugs to market, complicit with corporate marketing campaigns and in opposition to FDA oversight. As

Peter Staley explained to a television reporter, "It's been a huge expenditure, a waste of money for the U.S. taxpayer, and it was a naïveté on our part to think that the magic bullet was out there, it just had to be tested in humans and given to us as the cure."

Mark Harrington cast the blame on the ACTG, the AIDS clinical trials group he had invaded. He lambasted them for conducting trials that were too small, too short, naïvely overoptimistic, and which failed to generate clear answers about new anti-HIV drugs.

The scale of the mistakes they had made weighed on the members of David Barr's HIVIP support group. On a hot summer evening, they gathered for their fortnightly session, this time in Peter Staley's East Village living room. Derek Link was chain-smoking. "A couple of doctors at St. Vincent's said they were afraid of people committing suicide now, and I've been trying to figure out, like, what *is* that?" he said. "Because I just don't understand that argument. I don't know what despair is, and maybe I think sometimes I'm trapped in it." He tugged and twisted an earlobe. "You have to look at things really clearly, and it just doesn't look good right now."

Staley also lit a cigarette, a rare indulgence. "We've lost three acquaintances, three friends in the last two weeks," he said. "Larry Kramer said there's going to be a flood of deaths now, because the hope is gone . . . this massive pessimism is spreading now. And I don't doubt it."

There was general agreement around the room, which angered David Barr. He never believed that AZT was any kind of miracle drug. In fact, two years earlier he had reviewed a VA-run study as part of an FDA advisory committee that also showed AZT provided no survival benefit. That erased any lingering faith he had in the compound, although in an unusual piece of twisted logic, the VA researchers felt it said more about the veterans than about the drug—because a third of the study was black or Hispanic, they guessed that the drug worked differently in patients of different races.

Barr felt it was essential to keep a positive attitude despite the new headlines.

"Maybe it sounds corny, but I like being alive," he said. "It's really true! I don't feel like, Oh now I want to give up, now I want to stop living because AZT doesn't work."

"But we're a rare breed," Staley protested. "I mean, we had a hefty amount of skepticism and pessimism. Our hopes weren't flying high before."

"But do you think there are people walking around saying, 'AZT, yay. I'm okay'?"

"No, I think there were definitely people that were hearing, over the years, 'There's stuff in the pipeline,' hearing the drugs-of-the-month, and that was feeding their hope."

"I don't think people decide to live because a drug might come along."

Spencer Cox sat cross-legged on an armchair, resting an elbow on his knee. He understood the point that Barr was making, that the men in this room had an obligation as leaders in their community to project optimism despite the new turn of events. He was, however, losing his own grip on that rosy narrative. "With the recent spate of deaths, I don't know—it all seems so much more apocalyptic now. Like the story doesn't seem to have this relationship to effective treatment or a cure anymore. It now seems to have this relationship to death. It ends—it ends with everybody dying. *Will the last person alive in Chelsea please turn out the lights.*"

Gregg Bordowitz turned his video camera from face to face, freezing this moment in time. Cox was looking muscular and healthy in a sleeveless T-shirt. In fact, everyone in the room seemed robust, if understandably tired. The room was hot. Peter Staley removed his shirt.

Staley remained a lone defender of AZT. In low doses, it had kept him in good health for years in combination with ddI. But he was clear-eyed about the drug's long-term limitations.

"I felt forever now that I'm not going to outlive this epidemic. That I will—that I will die from this," he said. "The optimism that I'm feeling is that I'm gonna—I'm gonna have quite a few more years before that happens. . . . But I'm gonna die from this. This isn't going to be cured for years and years and years and years."

"Maybe that *is* our future, that we're gonna watch each other die," said Barr. Frustration drove his voice into a higher register. "That's not a new thought! We've been thinking that ever since we started the group. And that's going to be awful, if that's the case. It's already been awful, so there's not too much we can do about that." He inhaled deeply and leaned back on the sofa, thinking about this group of his friends, with whom he had argued, done battle, and posted bail. "I'm just—you know, I really honestly feel glad that I've got people to be with. Not many people have that," he said.

"It's better than having nobody to sit around watching you die," said Link.

Suddenly, Spencer Cox erupted in guttural laughter. "Does anyone ever look around and think to themselves, like: I'm twenty-five—or thirty or thirty-five—and I feel like an old widow sitting on Miami Beach!"

"That," Barr replied, "is because there's a sixty-five-year-old queen inside of you."

"I mean, really," Cox protested. "I'm in the gym the other night and Jim Baggett [another ACT UP activist] walks up to me and starts talking about how there's this memorial service, and there's this fight between two political factions over what to do with the body at the service. One group of people wants to decorate it in flowers and dance naked around it, and another group wants to carry it to downtown Manhattan. And I'm thinking, I'm twenty-five years old and this person is telling me that people are arguing over a corpse! Is this unnatural? Is this weird to anyone?"

"These political funerals," Link said, shaking his head. The artist David Wojnarowicz first proposed the idea that corpses should be carried in public protest to shock the public's conscience. Now they were almost commonplace. "I felt really ambivalent about them at first. But I'm having second thoughts. I'm not sure they're a bad thing."

David Barr had attended two political funerals, as had Harrington and Staley. Mark Fisher and Jon Greenberg both left instructions to parade their bodies through the streets of New York in anger. Comrades carried Greenberg from Reddens Funeral Home to Tomkins Square in the East Village for a respectful outdoor service, and hauled Fisher from his church funeral in Greenwich Village to Midtown, for a very political send-off in the rain outside George H. W. Bush's campaign headquarters.

"I think it's a powerful statement," he said.

"Dying is *not* a political act," Cox shouted. "It's something to be avoided at all costs!"

THE CLINTON YEARS were shaping up no more fortuitously than the dozen years before. We looked to Washington to change overnight, but it didn't. Clinton almost immediately retreated from his campaign commitment to integrate gays into the military, agreeing under sharply hostile resistance in Congress to sign off on "Don't Ask Don't Tell," which made it official U.S. policy that homosexuality was incompatible with military service. It took Clinton six months to tap an AIDS czar, settling on an unknown nurse and PhD student from Washington

State. Nothing like a Manhattan Project emerged. Meantime, the body count was unrelenting. The dancer Rudolf Nureyev died in January, the tennis star Arthur Ashe in February. There were obituaries for actors, musicians, ad execs, college administrators, and lawyers, including Richard Failla, named New York's first gay criminal court judge, and Rand Schrader, California's first gay municipal judge, at ages fifty-one and forty-eight respectively.

In June, ACT UP member Tim Bailey was dying. Bailey, who had been a top menswear designer until AIDS forced him into disability in his early thirties, was one of the movement's signal members, "as close to ACT UP royalty as anybody can get," as an article in the *Times* put it. In the hospital one night, he acknowledged his poor prognosis and asked Joy Episalla and Barbara Hughes, two of his closest friends in ACT UP, to carry his corpse to Washington and fling him over the White House gate.

The loss of so many friends had turned Episalla, a lesbian and an artist, into one of the group's most strident members. Hughes, in the same state, had no tolerance for anyone who could go about her ordinary life in the middle of such devastation, and while she worked as an executive chef most days, fighting the epidemic alongside her gay brothers was her primary commitment. Both women believed it was essential to put AIDS deaths on display.

They knew, though, that they couldn't comply with his request.

"We love you too much to treat your mortal remains that way," Episalla told him.

Bailey understood. "Alright," he said. "Do something formal and aesthetic in front of the White House. I won't be there anyway. It'll be for you."

Episalla agreed to develop a proposal for his approval. It was not long before Bailey sank into AIDS dementia, however. He sometimes thought his hospital room was a Parisian hotel suite or the backstage of a runway show, filled with lanky mannequins. Night after night, Episalla sat on his hospital bed, accompanying him on his dreamy pantomimed rounds, unsure how to proceed. Then one day his mind cleared miraculously, as if a sudden wind had chased off the storm. He opened his eyes and was fully lucid.

"I've been waiting for you," she said.

A smile pulled across his bony face. "Still here," Bailey said.

She didn't waste time. They talked about her plans and his, and the arrangements were sealed.

Bailey died at home two Mondays later. Episalla was lying next to him in bed and Ella Fitzgerald was on the stereo. By the time his doctor arrived to sign the death certificate, the apartment had filled with ACT UP friends, sipping martinis. A team from Reddens Funeral Home collected the body in due time, embalmed it, and laid it out in a simple pine box. His family said their goodbyes to him in a small service there.

Then on July 1, Episalla and Hughes backed a white panel van up to the funeral parlor and collected the casket. ACT UP members filled two charter buses and headed to Pennsylvania Avenue to eulogize Tim Bailey on the sidewalk in front of the White House. Bailey's executor, two of his brothers, and his employer, Patricia Field, were among them. Reddens agreed to receive the body again that afternoon.

But things went wrong from the start. The charter buses, accompanied by a coterie of reporters, arrived more than an hour ahead of the van. As they milled about the parking lot by the Capitol building, with their signs and bullhorns, they inadvertently attracted the attention of the local police. Dozens of officers, some in riot gear, materialized. By the time Hughes pulled into the parking lot under a light rain and Episalla stepped out of the van with an armload of white roses, the officers were twitching with uncertainty. When the Secret Service arrived, Episalla feared they were going to seize the body. She leaped to the driver's seat to fire up the engine, but an agent came through the passenger window and locked a bruising grip on her arm. The pain was so great she thought a bone had broken.

"Get your fucking hands off her," Hughes shouted from the back of the van, where she had been working to open the coffin in anticipation of a procession. But the officer prevailed, snatching the keys from Episalla's numb fingers.

"They're going to take him," Episalla shouted. "Save him!" She dove deep into the van to protect the casket.

Someone threw open the back door, exposing the body. Episalla grabbed the handle and tugged it closed.

"No, no, no," said a police officer, yanking the door back.

"This is not your property," she yelled.

"Easy. That's Tim," said Amy Bauer, one of the activists. "This is not a demonstration. This is a funeral procession. We are going to proceed with this coffin to the White House *as a funeral procession.*"

A detective attempted to mount the rear bumper, but was rebuffed by the crowd, which was worked up into a roiling explosion of anger. David Robinson, who in his trademark skirts and earrings was ACT

UP's lighthearted meeting facilitator, wore his street clothes as he stood squarely between the officers and the body. "Yeah, we have a dead body here," he seethed. "We have a corpse!" A lieutenant in a white shirt circled behind him and put him in a choke hold.

"Get your hands off of him," demanded Maxine Wolfe.

Robinson twisted free. His voice was shattered. "What the hell are you afraid of, that maybe ordinary citizens will see what our government is doing? Is that what you're afraid of, that maybe people are gonna see exactly what this government does?"

A canine unit arrived, ratcheting the tension even higher. Everyone looked to Amy Bauer at moments of danger. A small, boxy woman with a quiet masculinity, Bauer was ACT UP's longest-serving marshal, helping to assure the safety of protesters. This was a skill she had picked up in the women's movement and later studied at the War Resisters League. It helped that she had an MIT degree in traffic management. Yet as was typical in ACT UP, few people knew her background. What they knew was her mien, which was fiercely pacifistic, cool-headed, and disciplined. She directed everyone to surround the van and sit down.

"No violence. No violence," she chanted, and everyone joined in. Then something caught her eye that burst her usual Zen-like state. At the periphery of the fracas, a plainclothes cop in a Hawaiian shirt was cracking a joke.

She rose up in his face. "You're gonna fucking laugh at a funeral? Would you expect me to laugh at the funeral of a fucking police officer?"

Keith Cylar, his hair pinched into dreadlocks, joined her. "We have done everything you wanted us to do and now you are stopping us. Hell no. Get out the goddamn way."

"Back off," the officer warned. "Back off!"

Episalla decided it was now or never for the funeral. In pearls and a black spaghetti-strap dress, clutching the roses to her chest, she rose out of the back door of the van and began to deliver her planned eulogy, spitting out the words defiantly. Bailey's friends slowly levitated the open coffin and moved it toward the open air. The police pushed back with all the strength they had, and in a scene lifted from *Day of the Locust* the prow of the coffin surged skyward. Deafening screams filled the air as the box lurched and careened far above a welter of upraised hands. Bailey's coffin banged violently against the van, then spiraled sideways, revealing his silent face to the crowd. Episalla covered her mouth with both hands as the box slowly righted itself and settled back into the hands of the pallbearers, who slid Bailey back inside the vehicle without further incident.

The funeral would not take place. Police ordered the activists to leave town with the remains of Tim Bailey, and, feeling defeated, they did just that. A police escort of squad cars and motorcycles followed the caravan as far as Baltimore, an hour's drive.

THE CARGO had barely been unloaded at Redden's Funeral Home when another ACT UP member expired, and another, opening a period of death like nothing that had come before. In cumulative national numbers, the escalating figures were hard to fathom: on a pace to hit 42,000 dead in 1993 alone, 50,000 the following year. A new feeling of despair fell on the ranks of the activists, stripped even of the anger that once drove them. A number of the people who helped stage Bailey's chaotic funeral never returned to activism. The tussle over his body in Washington was a grotesque memory they could never shake. Many of ACT UP's oldest members also fell away. Larry Kramer declared activism dead and gone, and was sure he would follow close behind. By some unexpected turn of luck, he reconciled with David Webster, the love of his life, about whom he had angrily written *Faggots*. They retreated to a modest home in the country, where Kramer hoped to finish a last writing project, time permitting.

Garance Franke-Ruta shared Kramer's crushing conclusion that the activists had been defeated. Looking back at her young life, she struggled with the realization that her exhaustive efforts had been so futile. She could find no meaning in the suffering she witnessed, no life lessons worth contemplating in "this mass-death experience." She was not yet ready to give up the fight, though, so she decided instead to invest even more by pursuing a medical degree, though she had barely attended high school. She applied to Harvard, which, not surprisingly, suggested she prove herself at a lesser institution. Hunter College enrolled her on the basis of her GED. This kept her in New York City until Harvard finally relented, inviting her to that bubble of privilege as a twenty-three-year-old transfer student. If she raced through pre-med coursework and residencies, she might be back in the trenches in six years, at which point the global death toll would likely surpass fifteen million.

The only glimmer of hope on the horizon was the new drug class called protease inhibitors, which Merck had stopped studying after the terrorism attack in Lockerbie killed their project leader. Many pharmaceutical companies were at work developing them now. Human trials were being conducted by Hoffmann–La Roche, Abbott, Searle, Agouron, Kyoto, and Upjohn. On their heels, a half-dozen more laboratories had put protease inhibitors into early animal studies or else were, like Merck, well into preliminary laboratory work on competing versions. A new armamentarium of drugs was careening toward the market.

Swiss drugmaker Hoffmann–LaRoche was in the lead. Their protease inhibitor, which they called saquinavir, appeared to have shown minor impact on HIV—96 percent of it passed out of the body in the urine. Nonetheless, they moved it to a Phase II trial designed in three arms. About a hundred patients were randomly assigned to take AZT plus saquinavir, while equal numbers were given either AZT and ddC or a three-drug combination of AZT, ddC, and saquinavir. As the winter progressed, the triple-combination treatment regimen seemed to confer modestly better effects. Dr. Fauci, though, was telling the activists that protease inhibitors were proving no more durable in the body than AZT.

4

The Old Days

With the help of Richard Dworkin and Patrick Kelly—and massive doses of Doxil—Michael Callen managed to lay down vocal tracks for fifty-two songs. His voice had never sounded better. He was profoundly grateful to his collaborators for getting him this far, whatever his residual jealousy, and put it in their hands to finish the instrumental recordings and sound mix. His disease had worsened dramatically in recent weeks. Now his orange skin was tender and peeling. The lesions on his right leg had grown so numerous that there was almost no patch of flesh that wasn't involved. The whole limb had swollen and hardened and throbbed with pain. He walked with a cane. Still, it seemed he would live long enough to see the album completed.

He felt strong enough to travel that August, making his way to Provincetown, where the Flirtations had a booking, for final goodbyes. He bumped into Richard Berkowitz there. They had barely been in touch over the years. Berkowitz's own health odyssey had been quite traumatic. Beating back his drug addiction had been the most challenging thing he'd ever done, and his health reflected it. Here were two weathered warriors in steep decline. Being reunited buoyed both their spirits.

Berkowitz wanted to talk about their early history of writing together, the fun and the frustrations.

"We were political neophytes!" Callen hooted. Hanging on his bony frame was a black T-shirt with the word "DIVA" across the chest. "Reagan had just been elected and there was an ascendancy of right-wing—"

"Fascism!"

"—and this was the worst possible time to have a sort of serious, down-and-dirty discussion of the Mineshaft and what it might portend health-wise! But when I look back, it's almost embarrassing how upset we allowed ourselves to get about a handful of negative responses published in [the *New York Native*], a newspaper read by a thousand people maybe!"

It amazed Berkowitz how instantly connected they were, as though no time at all had passed. He remembered the evening they met, at a meeting of the world's first AIDS support group, and how immediately they had bonded. He mourned for their powerful partnership, for the sense of purpose and intellectual synergy that led to the invention of safe sex. He had never been so inspired as when working with Callen, nor as confident in himself and what he had to offer. Nobody believed in him the way Michael Callen did.

Like in the old days, he placed a tape recorder between them as they spoke. He wanted to write about the first dozen years of the epidemic, their epidemic. He filled two tapes that hot afternoon and returned to his apartment in New York to compose a vast history of their accomplishments and failures, perhaps at book length. He was determined to make sure their histories would survive them.

A couple of weeks later, with a draft taking shape, he called Callen in California with a progress report. Callen was animated, having gotten a bit of good news from his doctor. This came as a welcome relief to Berkowitz, who had been wrestling with how to handle the proximity of death's door in his piece. "I gotta tell you," Berkowitz said, "for a while, you were telling me you were dying—I can't even say the D word—and I worried that it was out of my own selfishness that I couldn't acknowledge it. Then I figured I owed it to you to acknowledge it and wrote that you were dying in the intro. But now you got back a clean bill of health from the tests—"

"Just say, during the writing of this article, I was given a death sentence twice and the difference is that for the first time in my twelve-year career, I accepted that death sentence. I'll die when I die. There's nothing I can do to prepare for it, more than I already have."

Now Berkowitz wanted to be the inspiring one. "You just don't know!" he pointed out.

"Right," Callen said, reconsidering. He hated the D word too. "In fact," he added, "I would be more comfortable if you—"

"I'm taking it out."

"Just say, 'The rollercoaster ride of AIDS has been particularly bumpy lately.'" They both laughed at this.

"You've been breaking all the AIDS rules for twelve years, so why give in now to what is expected?"

Berkowitz could hear Callen snicker faintly on the other end of the line. They fell silent for a time.

"I really appreciate everything, I want you to know that," Berkowitz said, his voice breaking.

"I want you to feel supported," Callen said. "Each article is a jewel—that's how to approach it and that's how you will get a book published, a deal. They'll say, 'This person can really write.'"

MERCK EXECUTIVES in Rahway, New Jersey, had been extremely quiet about their work with protease inhibitors, even though their renewed efforts had produced a drug that caused great excitement in their ranks. Their protease inhibitor, using the brand name Crixivan, was a single molecule specifically sculpted to interfere with the slicing action of the protease enzyme—a microscopic wrench to throw in the gears of HIV replication. It was the most complex molecule Merck had ever synthesized, requiring fourteen painstaking steps.

It had gone from the test tube to human trials with unusual speed. In fact, though the company would never reveal as much, they managed to do this by bypassing the usual animal studies, something no modern-day scientist was supposed to do. In the rules of pharmaceutical chemistry, once an experimental therapy proved itself in a test tube, scientists then introduced it in two animals—typically a rodent and a primate—to test its toxicity to the liver and availability in the bloodstream, the ultimate battlefield against HIV. This preliminary step could consume six months or a year. Only then would the drug go into human trials.

In this instance, the Merck scientists were convinced they had a game changer. In test tubes they saw Crixivan literally stop viral replication cold. Even without clinical data, Joel Huff, Merck's chief chemist, was so sure about Crixivan that he called Paul Reider, his colleague in charge of pharmaceutical production, urging him to prepare for full-scale commercial manufacturing. Reider was stunned.

"With no animal data, how do you know this one's good?" he asked.

After a period of evasiveness, Huff made an admission. "There was a 'big chimp' experiment."

Reider understood immediately what this meant: one of Merck's scientists—a "big chimp"—had taken the pill himself or herself. What went on behind Merck's closed doors would remain a secret. The results were good, that was the important thing. The "chimp" showed no toxic aftereffect, and large quantities of Crixivan made it from the stomach into the bloodstream. "It is very orally bioavailable," Huff reported.

That was enough for Reider. He cranked up the plant on the Rahway campus and in June had enough of the drug to enroll healthy, HIV-negative patients in a twelve-day Phase I safety study and another group of HIV patients in a proof-of-concept trial to look for signs of clinical improvements, also twelve days long.

The results of both studies were encouraging. This was the first really promising development in the company's long search for an anti-AIDS pill.

It was time for Dr. Emini to inform the community. In September, Merck invited Bill Bahlman, David Gold, and the other community advisory board members to Rahway to share their excitement. According to the scientists, all the patients experienced a strong antiviral effect. Using a new technique, they were able to prove this by counting the viral particles in the patients' blood. The question, they explained, was whether Crixivan's powers would wear off over time, like AZT's. To find this out, they were planning another trial, comparing Crixivan head to head with AZT, the disappointing benchmark. They hoped the activists would help speed enrollment by spreading the news through the AIDS community.

As energized as he was by the advances, Bahlman couldn't volunteer his own body for this study. He had recently taken part in a trial combining two nucleoside analogues—ddI and a new one called d4T—which left him with lasting and painful neuropathy, so he was now in another study examining a new therapy for nerve pain. But he agreed to help with recruiting, and the first Phase I Crixivan trial was up and running very quickly.

Within the first week, the very high expectations among researchers were exceeded. Using a brand new tool capable of counting the actual number of virus particles, they watched blood counts dipping so low in patient after patient that the new technology wasn't able to give accurate readings. This phenomenon had never been seen before with any drug.

The laboratory tests during the second week brought bad news: the virus rapidly mutated to evade the protease inhibitors. Viral loads shot back up to the millions per milliliter of blood. The promising drug was useless after no more than fourteen days. Emini shared the disappointing development at the next meeting of the community advisory board. Bahlman took it in stride. He had heard similar reports from activists working with Abbott and throughout the ACTG, where competing protease inhibitors were yielding disappointment after disappointment.

But there was an important anomaly, the Merck team added. A single patient in the study had sustained viral suppression past week two. In fact, Patient 142, as he (or she) was known, continued the successful run month after month. Rumors of this miracle patient's existence tore through the Merck campus, and even reached the company's offices in Europe and South America.

Emini didn't know what to make of this single patient's good fortune. Some at Merck were speculating that Crixivan may have cured Patient 142, but Emini was careful in the way he described the anomaly's significance. As he put it later, "That told us that it was possible. If it could happen in one, then by definition, it can happen in everyone. You just need to figure out how to do it." From then on, figuring out how to do it was the hectic work of Emini's team. As inspiration, someone had special mouse pads made up with a graph of Patient 142's viral load results. Results of the patient's monthly tests were delivered directly to Edward M. Scolnick, the Merck scientist overseeing all drug research. Patient 142 became the epidemic's holy grail.

CALLEN'S HEALTH began a rapid decline. His stomach ached, his intestines were a mess, and his weight fell precipitously. Severe anemia had him back in the hospital. Richard Dworkin redoubled his efforts to finish Callen's *Legacy* album, sensing that time was closing in. With Dworkin locked away in the studio, Patrick Kelly kept Callen company through the long hospital afternoons.

Callen experienced encroaching death in surprising ways. When his massively swollen leg throbbed, which it did almost without stop, he was fascinated to sense the entire length of his circulatory system sending rhythms from his heart to his feet. It felt almost *sensual,* he said. When he bit into a fresh tomato, the stimulation of his taste buds was so tactile it produced tears of pure joy. "It sounds so clichéd," he told a friend, "so trite, but my brain just repeats like a mantra: Life is good. Life is good."

After a few days, Dworkin and Kelly returned to New York to complete work on the album. They were not there long when Kelly was himself sent to the AIDS ward, with no precise diagnosis. His hospital stay stretched on without benefit. By early December, his breathing failed and he was intubated. Kelly's family rushed to his side. Callen wanted to come too, but he was wheelchair bound now and doctors were debating amputating his hardened leg. Amid his own cycle of discharges and readmittances, he sent his best wishes. On December 10, Dworkin and Kelly's parents, in keeping with his instructions, made the decision to pull the plug. Bereft, Dworkin sent Kelly to Redden's Funeral Home in the Village, stood at his graveside in Oregon, then caught a plane back to Los Angeles to be with Callen.

On Christmas Day, Dworkin arranged a small bedside party, which pleased Callen and brought to mind one of his last interviews, with the documentary crew that had followed him to Ohio. "I realize some people could look at my life and say, 'Oh, it was so sad. He died of AIDS and isn't that tragic.' But what I want to come through is that even after all the pain and all the torture, and even having AIDS, I can honestly say that being gay is the greatest gift I was ever given. I wouldn't change it for the world."

When his good friends had spoken their farewells that afternoon, Callen signed his last will and testament and then turned up the dial on his morphine drip, sliding into a deep and lasting sleep.

He died on a blindingly bright California afternoon, on December 27, 1993, just seventeen days after Patrick Kelly.

AFTER A YEAR of disappointments, the Clinton administration produced its first positive initiative in the epidemic. Washington released the first federal funding for safe sex education, finally producing a public health campaign that promoted condoms to prevent infections, abandoning the cryptic messages of past governmental anti-AIDS campaigns. Unveiled on television and radio in January 1994, the new spots featured celebrities, animated cartoon condoms, and young couples all speaking very specifically about HIV prevention. This represented a major sea change. But every one of the young couples was heterosexual. Even GMHC seemed bent on addressing the straight community in 1994, tempted by the administration's money. Officials placed posters in the city's subways and buses showing young straight couples as they kissed and handed one another foil-wrapped condoms. The sudden concern for heterosexuals seemed to some like the barricades were being moved further back. With no imminent news on the treatment horizon, attention had turned to the least likely to be infected, where success could be fairly guaranteed.

In the snowy stretch of mid-February came a stunning breakthrough in prevention research. Results were in for the study that had cleaved ACT UP in two, the one focused on blocking maternal transmission of the virus. Five hundred infected women were put on either AZT or placebo well along in their pregnancies. After giving birth, the infant received AZT syrup for eighteen weeks. The findings were incontrovertible. There were three times as many transmissions on placebo. In this setting, AZT was a true magic bullet—its transitory effect lasted long enough to block infections, in doses low enough to avoid harming child or mother. This finding promised to reduce the estimated two thousand new mother-to-child infections that took place in America every year, and would have an even more profound impact in developing countries, where perhaps a million children were born annually with HIV.

Mark Harrington couldn't appreciate the good news; on February 9, after a marathon vigil that lasted months, he watched Jay Funk, his former lover, succumb to the indignities of AIDS. Without a moment of self-pity, Funk had survived almost four years with just twenty-four CD4 cells. Then KS moved virulently into his lungs, and there was nothing that could be done. Harrington checked on him through the night and in the morning found him staring at the ceiling with a look of awe fixed on his lifeless face. It was the first time Harrington missed the old ACT UP. The group still functioned in dozens of chapters around North America and Europe, but because the local chapter had imploded he could not take his grief to the floor and speak Jay Funk's name there. Jay Funk had meant everything to Harrington, another gentle, beautiful, ravaged bolt of energy and life.

Harrington regressed for a few weeks, spending some time with family in San Francisco, then a week alone in Paris, writing his memories of Funk. Peter Staley tugged him back gently. He invited the HIVIPs to the British Virgin Islands, where his father kept a large sailboat. Staley and Harrington, Derek Link, Gregg Bordowitz, David Barr, and Spencer Cox swam hard in the choppy waters and put Joni Mitchell on the stereo as they prepared their evening meals in intensive harmony. A violent storm knocked the boat around through a long night, instilling a kind of animal fear, but they pulled through it and felt more bonded to one another, and to life, than ever.

Ten days later they were back to work. Harrington traveled frequently to Bethesda to monitor the Office of AIDS Research reorganization, once meeting with Fauci and Hill at another tense dinner. Gregg Gonsalves joined him on the TAG payroll, focusing on basic science policy, soon followed by Spencer Cox, who added responsibility for TAG's antiviral committee to his role in communications. Staley, still receiving a small annual severance package, continued on as the group's day-to-day director on a voluntary basis. In April, new health secretary Donna Shalala appointed him to the National Task Force on AIDS Drug Development, a kind of coordinating body to synch up the work of the FDA, NIH, and CDC.

There, all eyes were on protease inhibitors, but at a meeting in Hilton Head, South Carolina, everyone agreed that the protease inhibitors were as likely to trigger resistance as the older drugs after as little as tweve weeks. Harrington was disappointed, but not surprised. Much work remained to stabilize the research effort, and with Jay Funk in mind he would return to the battlefield and do what he could.

LARRY KRAMER spilled the dreaded capsules into his hand, the white ones with the blue bands and the prancing unicorns. He carried them to the guest bathroom, which flooded with the intense sunlight that bathed Malibu's white beaches. He was back in Barbra Streisand's world. She sent for Kramer, who soon resumed a routine of marathon sessions to help turn his stage play into a movie. He was no stranger to the medium, having written many scripts, one of which earned him an Oscar nomination (an adaptation of D. H. Lawrence's *Women in Love*) and another which earned him a handsome payday but much ridicule (*Lost Horizon*, the Liv Ullman musical, a dreadful flop).

Streisand had very specific ideas, many of which had no bearing on the actual history and struck Kramer as preposterous. Sharp in her focus was the wheelchair-bound physician, whom she intended to portray. In her view, the part needed to be bigger, more varied, more multidimensional. Did the doctor have a home life? Was she romantically involved? Kramer pushed back, typically choleric. Streisand was just as strong-willed.

In the middle of this struggle, Kramer was interrupted by an emergency telephone call from his New York gastroenterologist, Dr. Donald Kotler. Recent tests showed that Kramer's HIV infection had turned more virulent. His CD4s had fallen steeply. This was no surprise to Kramer. His belly ached and his gums bled constantly.

"You must start AZT as quickly as possible," Kotler told him. "Start at six hundred milligrams." So there Kramer was, in Streisand's guest bathroom, administering a first dose, hoping it bought him enough time to win over the diva to his vision. Dr. Jeffrey Greene, Kramer's infectious disease doctor, had also advocated for AZT, suggesting a somewhat lower dose, 500 milligrams. Kramer, always the contrarian, settled on 400.

Fortunately, the dose was tolerable and effective. His gums stopped bleeding and his intestines balanced out. And soon, his CD4 count lifted—not quite back to normal, but well above the level where he might have to worry about opportunistic infections. But he was not naïve. He knew AZT's impact was time limited.

HAVING FINALLY HELPED usher in the mandated reform measures at the Office of AIDS Research, Harrington and Gonsalves turned away from basic research—now safely in the hands of OAR director Dr. William Paul—and back to the drugs pipeline. Gonsalves was now a full member of the FDA's advisory board, charged with recommending whether new treatments should win approval. It's the kind of power AIDS treatment activists had sought from the onset. In May, the first new compound in years came before the panel.

Called d4T, the drug was another reverse transcriptase inhibitor, like AZT, ddI, and ddC. The Bristol-Myers Squibb Company had tested it thoroughly—more than ten thousand patients had been on d4T for eighteen months so far, with half assigned to 80 milligrams daily and the rest to half as much. There were serious side effect issues at either dose, including more severe neuropathy than had been seen in any previous antiretroviral. Still, the company called an early hearing at the FDA, requesting permission in May 1994 to halt the study and rush the drug to market. The company argued that compassion dictated a yes vote, a position that resonated with almost every activist across the country and most members of the FDA advisory board—except Gonsalves. He fiercely argued against approval, worried about repeating the mistakes made with AZT. And then he voted no, shocking other activists and stunning the drug company.

The application sailed through regardless, but the acrimony surrounding Gonsalves's vote only gained momentum and served to redraw the lines dividing the embattled AIDS movement—no longer West Coast versus East Coast, it was now everybody against TAG, condemned for abandoning the drugs-into-bodies philosophy at the core of AIDS activism. Marty Delaney at Project Inform drafted a statement protesting TAG's vote, signed by the movement's most influential leaders. "The community needs to say that we still believe in the accelerated approval process," the consensus statement declared.

Later that month, the Swiss company Hoffmann–La Roche requested early approval for its protease inhibitor, saquinavir, the first one to reach the regulators. The pharmaceutical company had completed a brief and difficult-to-interpret study comparing saquinavir in double and triple combinations. It appeared to fare marginally better than ddC in its weak ability to produce increases in CD4s and decreases in HIV levels. Most of it got chewed up in the liver—only 4 percent reached the bloodstream.

As TAG saw it, this was an especially fraught juncture. Saquinavir, as the first protease inhibitor to reach the FDA, had the potential to dominate the research agenda as AZT had, and slow down the development of other useful drugs. If the FDA acted out of the same misguided sense of compassion that had allowed AZT to flood the market, TAG protested, this could create a nightmare scenario, with tens of thousands of patients clamoring for saquinavir before its long-term effect was known. A large and lengthy trial was needed before approval. The TAG activists fanned out around the country in order to defend their position, which was, as Peter Staley wrote in an article for *POZ*, a new magazine for people living with AIDS, that the main goal of activists should be longevity, not "drugs into bodies." "If you accept the premise that our goal with antiretroviral research is to prolong life for as many people as possible, then our desire for early access to a promising treatment must be balanced with a desire for reliable information on the treatment's ability to prolong life," he wrote.

In June 1994, TAG alerted the FDA commissioner that the group would strenuously oppose saquinavir's application. The activists wanted the new drug to be put into an enormous trial involving eighteen thousand patients, far larger than anything in the history of AIDS. This was not an arbitrary number. For some time, TAG's members had been studying the research practices of various medical disciplines. Pharmacologists in cardiac research had long used a tool known as "large simple trials," which produced statistically reliable answers in a very short time. No one had ever tried such an approach in antiviral research. But Spencer Cox had drafted a protocol design showing how the trial could work. TAG forwarded Cox's proposal to FDA commissioner Kessler, imploring him to impose it on Roche and, in any case, to turn the company back until it had more impressive data. Early approval, they wrote, "would penalize people with AIDS/HIV by setting an inappropriately low standard" for protease inhibitors, they wrote. "We urge you not to invite Hoffman-LaRoche to apply for Accelerated Approval of Saquinavir until we can complete further discussion between FDA, its Advisory Committee, the company, and people with AIDS/HIV."

A few AIDS organizations cosigned TAG's letter. But Roche knew it did not represent the sentiments of the community. The company copied and faxed the letter to AIDS groups across the country. Project Inform and the national network of buyers clubs were outraged. So were ACT UP chapters by the dozens. "There's a space in my medicine cabinet I thought would be filled by a protease inhibitor by November," lamented Jeff Getty of ACT UP Golden Gate. In New York, Bill Bahlman and his colleagues working inside Merck were similarly incensed. "This is something we fought hard and long for," Bahlman said at a convulsive ACT UP meeting. "We've been arrested to get accelerated approval through—many of us in this room were arrested to get that.

We stormed the FDA! And we'll storm them again if they decide to accept these proposals." The fifty most powerful AIDS groups in the country signed a statement against TAG.

Harrington dismissed their concerns as "antiquated activist dogma." Most important, TAG had the FDA's ear. The saquinavir application for early approval was rejected handily. The company returned to the lab and doubled the size of its Phase II efficacy trial, from 1,500 to 3,000—not the large simple trial TAG advocated, but a significant improvement.

In the meantime, TAG produced a monograph, "Problems with Protease Inhibitor Development Plans," analyzing all the new protease inhibitors in the pipeline. It laid out the rationale for mandating a substantial increase in trial size. "Some individuals within the community of which I am a part, in their desperation, seem willing to forego any standards whatsoever, just for the opportunity of putting a new pill into their mouths," David Barr wrote in the introduction. "I, for one, am not willing to accept a standard of care based on desperation. I still want to know if the pill works. Not just for myself, but because there are tens of millions of people who will be faced with making those difficult treatment decisions long after I am gone."

THREE OF THE MOST vocal members of Merck's group of community advisers—Bill Bahlman, Marty Delaney, and Tom Blount, who joined from Atlanta—were obsessed not with large simple trials and eighteen thousand patients but with just one: Patient 142. A year after beginning on Crixivan, Patient 142 remained at undetectable viral levels, the only person in the world being treated for HIV in such a dramatic way. Hoping to learn 142's secrets, the company obtained permission to break the study code to find out who the patient was—a young man from San Francisco, it turned out. A Merck executive who reached him by phone found the patient to be smart, engaged, and, perhaps significantly, a stickler for taking his doses at precise intervals. When he first joined the study he was in quite good health, though his viral load was very significant, with substantial CD4s. And he had never taken any previous medicine for his HIV infection.

In the following weeks, the company began enrolling patients in a small study, attempting to replicate its success with Patient 142. Among the activist advisers, Tom Blount was the most enthusiastic about the research. He had quit his job as an architect and founded the Atlanta buyers club to acquire every experimental compound he could locate in his effort to save the man he loved, Jim Straley, who was quite sick. None of the country's buyers clubs had greater inventory, but nothing made a difference for Straley. Blount, born into a prominent and wealthy Republican family—his father had been Nixon's postmaster general—saw Crixivan as their last hope.

The study criteria were strict. Merck was looking for patients a lot like Patient 142: healthy upon admission, with high CD4s and a heavy burden of viral activity. Straley might have met those criteria, but not the final requirement, that the test subject be treatment naïve. Straley had tried nearly every available drug, experimental or not. He was rejected in June 1994. Blount ran an appeal all the way up to the principal investigator at the Birmingham, Alabama, enrollment site, an infectious disease specialist named Michael Saag, pleading for an exception to the rules, or at the very least access to the drugs on the parallel track. It didn't work. "I can't believe that Jim's life has such little value to everyone but me," Blount wrote in a bitter fax to Saag. "[T]he decision to not allow at least some compassionate use is completely immoral."

When the trial began that September at a handful of hospitals around the country, Blount tried a different tack. He flew from one participating hospital to another, hunting down the patients who had been accepted, and begging them for a few of their large, unmarked white capsules. Everyone donated some, such was the camaraderie in the plague's trenches. In total, he had amassed perhaps a month's supply. If he repeated his tour he might be able to double his cache, but he knew he was unlikely to contribute meaningfully to his lover's health as a beggar.

So he took a handful of the capsules to a shady outfit in Brooklyn that specialized in bootlegging prescription medication as unlicensed generics. Tom Blount was going rogue. He liquidated various portfolios and sold one of his homes, plowing $300,000 into his campaign to illegally replicate one of the most complex pharmaceutical compounds ever invented. He was prepared to do whatever it took.

WHEN THE PRELIMINARY results for Crixivan were in that winter, Emilio Emini convened the community advisory board, bringing the dozen or so activists to the company's modest conference room in Rahway. About fifteen company officials joined them. Emini spoke cautiously. There was no exact repeat of Patient 142, but the results were still impressive. For a small subset of fifty patients in the study, his team initiated combination therapy, adding in one of the nucleoside analogues like AZT or ddI.

Both approaches led to excellent results, at least for the short duration of the test. But the two-drug combination was better in every measure, especially in patients who hadn't taken one or the other of the drugs as monotherapy in the past. It was just as Mark Harrington had speculated years earlier: HIV mutated less when two different drug types were combined. Emini couldn't be sure resistance wouldn't eventually develop to cause the drug combinations to lose effectiveness. But the snapshot today was better than anything they had seen before.

Bahlman felt a chill of raw excitement. The other activists present felt similarly. This was the juncture that Jules Levin, a member from Brooklyn, had only dreamed of. A straight man with the disease, he hadn't been in the ACT UP trenches so he hadn't ridden the unhappy roller coaster of dashed hopes. This news looked like a gift from the heavens. His first thought was urgency. "We need a parallel track program right away," he said.

"We can stop the dying!" agreed Bahlman. "You have to implement those procedures as quickly as possible. And get the drug approved as quickly as possible. It's a humanitarian necessity."

Emini shook his head. The small study wasn't enough; the company needed to conduct a very large Phase II trial in order to know how well Crixivan performed. With a late-fall start date in mind, they gave sixty-seven medical centers in the U.S., Canada, Australia, and seven European countries approval to begin enrolling patients. But the drug was fiendishly difficult to make. It would be another year before Merck could produce enough, and then a year for the trial to reveal its secrets. If the results were good, then Merck would have to build a new plant to produce Crixivan in commercial quantities.

Emini didn't reveal that there was already a secret race to get the plant built. Joseph Vacca, a senior chemist, personally pressed the company's new chief executive, Ray Gilmartin, to check on Patient 142 himself. The experience moved him to give preliminary construction approval, a move the board of directors would be right to question. The plant would have a technically difficult task. Crixivan's complex production required fourteen painstaking steps, considerably more than any other drug. It took four months for Skip Volante, the unflappable head of process chemistry, and his team to manufacture enough for fifty patients. Hoping to cut production time, they devised a process for making the molecule in three prefabricated segments, then "snapping them together," like Lego pieces, but it was still painfully slow. Each patient in the Phase II study would need about one kilogram of Crixivan a year—fifty to one hundred times the dose of a typical drug.

To make that much, the company was running the Rahway plant at full capacity.

Emini told the CAB members it would be years before Crixivan could be released on a parallel track.

"It's my job to advocate for the PWA community," Bahlman said after a long silence. "We need this drug. How can I know that what you're telling me is true?"

Tom Blount was not so polite. "You're lying," he told the Merck officers.

Paul Reider, the company's VP, had listened to the pleadings silently. "Tom, you don't believe us? Why don't you come in and look. As long as you sign a secrecy agreement, we'll show you everything." No one could recall a time when a drugmaker had opened its doors to scrutiny from its customers. "Bring an expert with you," Reider insisted. "And if you can help us do it any better, let us know."

That afternoon, Blount was on the telephone with his Brooklyn contact asking him to recommend an expert. He knew just the man, an industry consultant in process chemistry based in London named Trevor Laird. Blount sent Laird an airline ticket.

NINETEEN NINETY-FIVE was the fourteenth year after the first cases of "gay cancer." It would be a year of partial vindication for Joe Sonnabend and his multifactorial theory of the plague. Granted, his early suspicions that cytomegalovirus caused the syndrome proved wrong, but he had always said that to save lives, researchers needed to look for multiple causes of the disease, not just a single virus. Researchers now recognized, as Sonnabend had surmised, that the skin cancer that claimed Michael Callen, Bob Rafsky, and so many others was not brought on by HIV—but like other opportunistic infections, took advantage of ravaged immune systems. It would take many years to identify the virus that caused Kaposi's sarcoma, a member of the herpes family transmitted through sex, and to determine that KS was not a cancer at all, but an opportunistic neoplasm—something for which an antiviral drug, not chemotherapy, might be needed.

But what by now was clear was that the KS caseload, first epitomized by the glamorous flight attendant from Quebec, was in fact a separate and parallel epidemic, one that began to recede soon after its mysterious arrival. In 1982, nearly half of all gay men diagnosed with AIDS were diagnosed with KS. Two years later, just 20 percent of newly diagnosed AIDS patients also had KS. Now, though the incidence of

HIV infection continued to rise, KS was rarely diagnosed in new AIDS patients. If Kaposi's sarcoma had been addressed separately instead of being lumped into HIV's arsenal, some deaths might have been prevented.

Sonnabend remained morose. There was still no remedy to offer KS patients, and now it was claiming its newest victim, Richard Berkowitz. After Michael Callen's death, Berkowitz plunged into a deep depression, the worst of his life. He published a heartbreaking eulogy in the gay papers for his old friend, cementing Callen's place in the pantheon of AIDS heroes. "[T]he father (he preferred 'Queen Mother') of the People with AIDS self-empowerment movement lives on in a million different ways," he wrote. "Every time gay men have sex safely, Michael Callen . . . is there. Every time a Person with AIDS takes prophylaxis medication to prevent PCP pneumonia . . . the speeches, the congressional testimony, the TV appearances, the protests, and the writing live on. And every time someone says 'Person with AIDS,' instead of 'AIDS victim,' Michael Callen's legacy of hope and grit continues."

Berkowitz could muster neither hope nor grit. Before winter was out he had tumbled back into crack cocaine, hammering his CD4s into the death zone. His first KS lesion appeared on the side of his nose that winter. He saw his friends and family stealing glances at it. It stared back at him every morning from the bathroom mirror, putting him face-to-face with his own mortality.

Then one morning Berkowitz had an epiphany and decided to honor Callen by entering rehab. After a year he was truly sober, the first time in memory.

His health never rebounded. There was a new KS lesion every two weeks. Then came the awful molluscum contagiosum, a rash of oozing bumps on his chest. His CD4 count fell, lower than anybody's he had ever known.

"I'm going down fast," he told Sonnabend. "I have only had safe sex from the time the booklet came out. For twelve years! I wasn't just teaching it, I was practicing it. I did a lot of work. I did my best to protect my health—the best I could. It wasn't enough. *I'm down to five CD4s!*"

Sonnabend was losing his oldest living patient. He thought he might never recover after Callen's death; the telephone call that would bring him to Berkowitz's bed one last time terrified him. He drew the usual blood samples. "Stop single-mindedly obsessing on the CD4 number," he said, reaching for something positive sounding to say. "There's also the CD8 numbers and yours are high." They both knew it wasn't enough.

TOM BLOUNT'S efforts to clone Crixivan progressed at an excruciating pace. The Brooklyn compounder, an orthodox Jew, lost some time around the Jewish high holy days. But he was able to break apart the three prefabricated segments of the molecule. One of them, the simplest, had already relinquished its secrets; he was halfway toward decoding the second. His methods were nefarious. He and his colleagues would dispatch agents around the country anytime a Merck scientist gave a technical presentation, scribbling notes and asking sharply detailed questions. They had been nearly discovered at Harvard recently. Dr. Reider was there to discuss the molecular properties of the HIV protease when a scruffy man in a trench coat caught his eye. The man slid into a front-row seat, "a place where nobody in their right mind sits," Reider said later, as the seating convention at Harvard was sacrosanct. No one but Nobelists and full professors took the front row. But this guy hunkered down there conspicuously, hunching over his notebook. Following his talk, Reider wanted to ask the intruder who he was, but he vanished without a clue.

Blount, meanwhile, was monitoring the official Merck trial through his sources at the various testing sites. By January, patients in Birmingham and Philadelphia fared so well on the Phase II trials that officials were hurrying to enter Phase III and quietly gave all final approvals to build large-scale production facilities. It looked as if Crixivan would be available by the end of the year. But this would be of no use to Jim Straley, who was now so weak he barely left bed. Blount pressed his man in Brooklyn to perform miracles. In a phone call in January, he reported that his team of chemists was getting close, but they still lacked key information. He wanted to talk about the upcoming meeting at Merck where the outside expert would evaluate the company's plant capacity.

"You have to take another person with you," said the bootlegger, in a thick Brooklyn accent.

This didn't seem possible. Merck had asked the activists to sign a nondisclosure agreement before returning to the facility. He worried about discovery.

"I don't know if we can," Blount said. He offered to get the information himself, but his compounder believed the task was too technical.

"Listen, there are some specific questions I have to ask in a specific way," he said. "I need to [send a specialist], and he's going to be wearing a wire," the drug cloner said.

To which Blount replied, "Oh."

When the day came, January 11, it was clear that Jim Straley could no longer wait for Crixivan. Blount went to the refrigerator to retrieve the thirty-day supply he had begged and borrowed. He had to help lift Straley's head onto a pillow so he could swallow his first capsule, not worrying for the moment what they would do when the supply was exhausted.

Blount tucked Straley back in bed and raced to the airport for a 6:50 flight. Jules Levin, his fellow CAB member, met his plane in Newark and drove him to the Merck plant, thirty minutes away. Along the way, Blount took Levin into his confidence for the first time. He confessed to his secret bootlegging work and revealed that a person with a wire would be joining them. Levin was furious at first, but he knew there was no stopping Blount. He agreed to stay silent.

"And I thought you were this simple architect from down south," he said finally.

Blount's spy met them at Merck's parking lot, dressed like an eager graduate student; the three were allowed inside without questions. Trevor Laird, the London expert Blount had hired to advise the activists, joined them in Merck's boardroom. John Doorley, Merck's head of its public relations team, opened the meeting with a few words meant to lower expectations about the tour and about the drug itself. Until that moment, Blount hadn't realized how raw his emotions were. He exploded, slamming a fist on the boardroom table. "You are so full of bullshit," he screamed. "I know what happened in Birmingham. I know what happened in Philadelphia." He glowered at the entire Merck team. "Not only do I know this is it. I know that *you* know this is it."

Nervously, Merck's Skip Volante, a short man with a stutter, talked fast and openly about the company's limits. Work was set to begin in March to retrofit two Merck plants in Elkton, Virginia, and in Flint River, Georgia, even without FDA approval. None of the company's other facilities were capable of producing Crixivan. The pilot plant in Rahway was operating at full capacity to meet the needs of the ongoing trials.

Volante explained each stage of the manufacturing process, and demonstrated how the prefabrication had saved time. It remained an onerous process, he said; it took 77 pounds of thirty raw materials to produce just 2.2 pounds of the drug, enough to supply one patient for a year. The company had to find a way to cut the time and increase yield dramatically.

Trevor Laird saw that one of the fourteen steps, coming toward the end of the syndication chain, was creating a bottleneck. This was not news to Merck. "We had been working on that step for four months, trying to improve the yield and the productivity of that step," Volante explained.

Laird was satisfied that Merck was doing all it could.

This upset Blount. He was near tears when he turned to Paul Reider. "Currently, how much can you make for an expanded-access program?"

"Tom, we're doing more than is possible already," Reider said. The pilot plant was running hard, from 8 a.m. to 4 p.m. every day. "If we did any more we'd jeopardize the whole program. Think about the risk. If we go back to the small equipment and run double shifts, that's nothing. That's like four hundred kilos."

Blount did a quick calculation. "Four hundred kilos is enough for four hundred people," he said bitterly. Tears filled his eyes as he turned to leave, stunned that Merck wouldn't automatically run the plant in multiple shifts. At the door he spun to fire a finger at the executives from Merck. "Four hundred people? That's like a fully loaded 747. You have the ability to save it and you're not doing it!" He was crying violently. "Every one of them is a human being," he said, then slammed the door behind him.

The room fell silent. Nobody said it, but it was impossible not to think of the 747 that had fallen from the sky over Lockerbie all those years ago, taking the life of Irving Sigel, their former team leader, and the man who first hypothesized the power of protease inhibitors. Emilio Emini would later say that this was the first time he clearly saw the end users for his products as individuals rather than market segments.

The next morning, Paul Reider called Blount.

"We'll do it," he said. "We'll get your four hundred kilos."

OVER THE NEXT few weeks, Tom Blount witnessed a miracle in Atlanta. His lover's turnaround was breathtaking, "like watering a wilted plant." Now he had to find pills to replenish his supply. At the pilot plant in New Jersey, frantic efforts were under way to add the necessary shifts for a parallel track distribution. Some four hundred employees were assigned to the task, a risky undertaking that had already cost Merck over a billion dollars. Skip Volante tried again to streamline the bottle-necked manufacturing process. It took another chemist, a young PhD whose mother ran a Greek diner in Queens, New York, to break the bottleneck. He did this by adding a dash of baking soda at a key point, changing the pH and doubling the output. ("Every cook knows you add baking soda," his proud mother boasted.) Meeting again with Levin and Blount a few weeks later at a hotel near Newark Airport, Merck's people committed to supplying enough Crixivan for 1,100 people in just a few weeks.

How to select the recipients became an immediate problem. Thousands and thousands of people were literally on the brink of death. Levin suggested a national lottery. The proposal revolted Bill Bahlman. He thought it was inhumane to make people with AIDS scramble for lifesaving pills as if they were candies spilled from a piñata. But as nobody had a better alternative, he accepted it with a proviso: that there would be no back-channel access for the rich or the connected. If Magic Johnson wanted Crixivan, he would have to go through the same lottery. The same for Jim Straley, whose secret stash was now gone.

"I could never ask you for a supply just for him," Blount told Reider.

"That's good," Reider replied, relieved.

At Merck's request, Bahlman and Levin agreed to set up the lottery mechanism and monitor it closely. Two million copies of a simple black-and-white brochure went out trying to identify patients with extremely low CD4s, under fifty. An 800 number was set up for people seeking registration forms, which needed to be signed by a doctor. In just six weeks doctors submitted the names of twelve thousand critically ill patients for inclusion in the lottery.

To avoid any appearance of favoritism, an outside company was retained to manage the selection process. Each patient was assigned an identifying number, and those numbers were sent to the Boston office of Ernst and Young, the same firm that counts secret ballots for the Oscars. A computer program was used to randomly select the lucky patients. Selections would be announced by summer.

While awaiting word if Jim Straley would make the cut, Blount was on the telephone almost daily with his contractor in Brooklyn. Using a clumsy but working formula, he had produced a small number of samples. Just then the underground team hit a wall. Manufacturing more compound required an ingredient that was sold by a single manufacturer, Nippon Soda in Japan, and Merck had cleaned them out.

By coincidence, Paul Reider was scheduled to give another technical briefing late in February at Emory College in Atlanta. The lab in Brooklyn was sending a secret representative. Blount decided to go along as well—and beg for the hoarded ingredient.

Inside the meeting, Reider was again shaken by a feeling of being followed. A technician in the audience pestered him with questions and then vanished before Reider could inquire about his interests in Crixivan. "That was eerie," he complained to Blount later that evening, over dinner at a Japanese restaurant in Atlanta. He was beginning to suspect corporate espionage. "The only way to ask those questions is if he actually had run the chemistry in his own hands."

Blount, who had had a little too much to drink, took another sip and turned to face Reider. He knew he would have to come clean sooner or later. Now he had no choice.

"Paul," he said. "Every now and then life brings you to a watershed. You come to the point where you realize it's all or nothing. Sometimes it's in a form where I'm in right now, where I have to trust you with something you can kill me with."

Reider smiled warmly. Over the previous year or more he had developed great affection for Blount and the other activists. "You can trust me, Tom," he said.

"Paul, it's me."

Reider caught his breath.

"It's me, Paul. I'm knocking off the drug."

A broad smile came across Reider's face. "I can't believe it," he said.

"Now there are two things I need from you. I need this element you've locked up at Nippon Soda. And I need you to test what we've made because I don't want to [have] a bad drug out there. That's my nightmare."

Reider shook his head in disbelief and begrudging admiration. "Send it to me," he said.

"You won't try to stop us?"

Reider waved away Blount's concerns. "It's unlikely you'll get the mix," he said. "It's more important you don't hurt anybody."

And in a day or two, the Brooklyn compounder called Blount with news. "I don't know what happened, but we have access to all this element now." With the chemical in hand, they quickly finished the assembly, breaking Crixivan's secret code.

"Good," Blount said. "Now I need you to send some of our compound anonymously for Paul Reider to test."

In a few weeks, Reider gave his opinion. "It's good," he said.

By this time, though, Blount was beginning to see the impossibility of his undertaking. Making Crixivan was one thing; making it in large enough batches even for one patient to maintain his dosage over time, relying on the erratic appearance of various ingredients, seemed like folly. He kept his doubts to himself, anxious to maintain pressure on Merck.

"I'm going to call it Stralevir," he said, an homage to Jim Straley.

"How much do you plan on making?" Reider asked.

"I figure about 30,000 the first year," he said. "My estimated cost is around $2,000 per person." Reider did the math: Blount's knockoff Crixivan could take away $60 million a year from Merck's bottom line. Reider couldn't let that happen—which was just the reaction Blount hoped for.

MICHAEL SEGGEV, Merck's junior community affairs specialist, was focused on enrolling the lottery winners as rapidly as possible. He received an onslaught of letters, many from mothers or lovers, which changed his plans. They began, "I am so grateful for what your company is doing. But sadly, he has passed away. I know that he would want someone else to get his medicine, so can you please pick the next person on the list?" Seggev was impatient. "Hurry up," he urged the fulfillment company. "Get the next person on the list. I mean, we have the drug—we'd better use it."

By summer, the 1,100 recipients had been chosen. Among them was a CAB member, Linda Grinberg, who had thirty CD4 cells left and was months past the date her doctors had predicted her demise. Too weak to travel, she had missed most of the board meetings in the past year. The drugs hit her like something from science fiction. Her immune cells shot up with Crixivan and her viral load plummeted. She felt marvelous for the first time in years. She discovered an inner peace that made her the envy of her friends. She even started dating again, in her forties, cautiously. Crixivan had brought Grinberg back to life.

When the letter for Jim Straley came, on August 18, Blount was relieved he had made the cut. But it was too late. Jim Straley died two days later, too far gone for the miracle pills. His relationship with Blount had lasted eighteen years, thirty days, and twelve hours. Blount was bereft. "I wanted twenty years," Blount said some time later. "I would have been satisfied with twenty."

EARLY IN JANUARY 1996, Spencer Cox packed his bags to attend the annual Conference for Retroviruses and Opportunistic Infections in Washington, D.C. He circled only two sessions on the schedule, where Abbott and Merck would separately report results. The buzz on the street was positive—Merck had dribbled out early findings suggesting that Crixivan seemed to chase HIV out of people's bodies. Cox was taking the gossip and rumors with ample skepticism.

Mark Harrington was even more doubtful. At a conference in the fall, an advance team for Abbott had promised great protease inhibitor data, but the data they presented instead struck Harrington as being irresponsible and unsubstantiated. The TAG team was hardened to the hype about protease inhibitors. Over their continued objections, saquinavir, the protease drug from Roche, had been cleared for release, the first one to appear at pharmacies. It had almost no impact on the epidemic. Its therapeutic benefits were modest at best, lasting only about sixteen weeks before resistance developed. Yet fifteen thousand patients were already taking the drug. Whether they might be resistant to better protease inhibitors was anyone's guess. Disgusted, Harrington stayed home in January.

Cox's trip to Washington was more arduous than usual, thanks to the fiercest nor'easter in a century. Two feet of snow fell in D.C., followed by a rapid rise in temperatures that caused massive flooding. Cox arrived late for the first of the scheduled talks. The room was surprisingly full. A phalanx of photographers stood in front of the podium. When the first slide appeared on the enormous screen behind the speaker, a gasp rose in the room. Crixivan, taken with two other drugs in combination, the slide indicated, had a lasting impact. The subsample of patients was small, just twenty-two in total. But over 90 percent of them had viral loads under detectable levels for two full years—the first long-term proof that scientists had outwitted HIV's mutation defenses long term.

One of these patients was Richard Berkowitz. Two weeks after taking his first dose, his CD4s started to rise. In four weeks, the rash of molluscum contagiosum vanished. At the end of eight weeks, his KS lesions melted away, even the one on his nose, forced into retreat by a rebounding immune system. The drug combination snatched him out of the coffin.

"These pills have to work on cytomegalovirus," he insisted to Dr. Sonnabend, still attached to the old theory.

Sonnabend shook his head. The evidence was irrefutable. "The molecule is designed to do only one thing," he said. "It knocks out HIV."

When Merck's presentation was complete the room erupted in applause and people raced to the rostrum. Cox, a stickler for "clinical end points," was not one of the celebrants. It didn't matter what the drug did in your bloodstream if people continued to die prematurely; that was the battle to be won. He was probably unduly pessimistic because of his own health, which had been in steady decline. Drug toxicity had recently led to emergency surgery. Then his doctor had started him on a series of anabolic steroid shots that left him exhausted. His patience, like his CD4 count, was in retreat. At a recent dinner party, where someone casually talked about "living with AIDS," he exploded, "I'm not *living* with AIDS! I'm *dying* of AIDS."

He attended Abbott's protease inhibitor presentation with the same negative attitude. A researcher was discussing results of Abbott's large trial, which had adapted Cox's trial design suggestions; it involved a placebo arm as well, which was also part of Cox's proposal. Cox's model showed that a very large study, enrolling very sick people, could produce reliable lifesaving information about the power of the therapy in a very short period of time. (The Abbott trial lasted just seven months.) He knew this would be controversial.

The results made Cox catch his breath. All the patients started with fewer than fifty CD4 cells per cubic milliliter of blood, and were allowed to stay on any drug their doctors thought necessary. Half were then assigned Abbott's protease inhibitor, called Norvir, plus AZT and ddI. The three-drug combination wasn't as powerful as Crixivan at pushing down viral load, but there was a stark survival benefit, as a gigantic grid shown on a slide made plain: the drugs were responsible for a 50 percent reduction in deaths during the time of the study. If Crixivan proved that it was possible to suppress the HIV virus for long periods of time, Norvir showed a correlation between suppression and longevity.

Tears filled Spencer Cox's eyes. "We did it," he whispered to the person sitting beside him. "We did it. We're going to live."

THAT AFTERNOON, I was at work when the receptionist sent a telephone call to my desk. I recognized the serious Brooklyn accent as Jules Levin's. "David, have you heard about the presentation here in Washington?"

I hadn't. "What's up?"

"I'm pulling together a community meeting to talk about it. Saturday morning, at NYU."

Two days later, after a heavy overnight snowfall, I set out for the NYU Medical Center on foot, as the trains and buses were not running. Levin had invited the virology chiefs from the three pharmaceutical giants involved in protease inhibitors research to speak directly to the infected community. Few people were out in the weather, but as I got closer to the lecture hall, on First Avenue and Thirty-second Street, I could tell it was going to be a massive event. More than 1,500 people pushed through the tall glass doors at the hospital, almost all of them gay men, cadavers with thin, straw-like hair folded and bent by their woolen caps.

This was far more than could be admitted. In a few weeks, Levin would stage a similar public meeting in Los Angeles, on the Paramount lot, with a large screen in an overflow tent to accommodate the crowds. But in New York, nearly half the people in the line—which choked the large foyer and popped out the door and down the block—would be turned away. When the last person was cleared to take a seat, many who remained in line pressed their ears against the heavy conference doors or waited in the lobby for news to dribble out.

I had a seat near the back. One by one, dusty-haired pharmaceutical executives presented findings from their newest studies, referenced in tall graphs projected on the screen behind them. Many of the words and phrases were brand new to most of the community members in the audience: "effective concentrations" and "viral loads" dropping in multiplication units they called "logs." We sat motionless in the hushed hall, unable for the most part to comprehend what we were being told.

Sensing our disorientation, one of the scientists interrupted his presentation abruptly. "Maybe you are not understanding what I am saying," he said, switching to plain English. "This is the biggest news ever in this epidemic. This stuff is actually clearing virus out of people's bodies. People are getting better! We don't know for sure yet, but we think these drugs—this whole class of drugs—might allow people to live a normal life."

I felt as though a hand had tightened around my throat. I had trouble breathing.

"This is what we've been working for all these years," he continued. "They're not a cure. We don't know what they are, in effect. But this is the first major piece of good news we have had in all these years. They're calling it the Lazarus effect. People who were in hospitals on their last breath are getting up and going back to work. We've never seen anything like it."

After years of "qualified optimism" and marginal advances that never dulled the blade of death, a decade and a half of scientists managing expectations, it was hard to retire skepticism and believe what he was saying. Yet here was a scientist grabbing us by the shirt collar, shaking us from our stupor. It had been many years since I had cried—maybe I hadn't shed a tear since Doug's memorial service—but now tears rolled down my cheeks. When I caught my breath again, it came in sobs. Was it over? Was the long nightmare passed? When the room emptied out, I found myself standing in the sun-creased lobby watching the men in the audience exchanging hugs and tears. I noticed how incongruously young everybody looked in the snow-whitened light. Most were, like me, not yet middle aged. I was thirty-five years old. I'd lived my entire adult life in the eye of unrelenting death. We all had. The feeling of relief overwhelmed me.

A man I did not know put his hand on my cheek, startling me. He turned my face toward his. He was perhaps in his mid-twenties, blue-eyed and radiant. He didn't speak. With a thumb, he wiped my cheeks, then kissed me on the lips, the kiss that Pericles gave Aspasia to awaken the Golden Age. It was not over. It would never be over. But it was over.

For Dear Life

Very quickly over the subsequent months, the number of commercially available protease inhibitors reached three, giving patients multiple options, depending on their resistance profiles. For many people it all came too late, and they became the last casualties of the last red-hot days of the plague. The total dead in our city was 100,000, almost one-third the national total. But for the rest, the physical impact of the drug combinations was joyous to observe. My friend Joe Westmoreland had been ready "to enter the past tense" when the medicine arrived. He swallowed the pills almost out of politeness. Within weeks, the KS lesions on his feet, which had been so bad they burst open, had closed and faded. A tenacious bout of CMV pneumonia slowly improved, and the retinitis, for which he took twice-daily infusions, resolved—in time, he was able to have the Hickman catheter removed from his chest. Similar miracles were taking place on AIDS wards across the Western world. In St. Vincent's, the plague's original epicenter, a remarkable proportion of patients lying on the AIDS ward rose unexpectedly and went home. In the first months of the new drug era, the census there dropped by 24 percent.

By the end of the first full year of the treatment era, no traces of the virus could be found in Staley, Harrington, Barr, or Cox. Their CD4 counts returned to near normal, proving what had only been hypothesized before: it is possible to regenerate a person's immune system. In the future, another medical breakthrough might eradicate HIV entirely and end the epidemic, but there was no denying that the plague was done. Within two years, the lasting power of these drugs was undeniable. The hospitals emptied and the AIDS ward signs were taken down. The epidemic that had wiped out a generation of gay men and then torn huge holes through African American and Latino families in most major American cities, the plague that burned through Europe, sub-Saharan Africa, Asia, and the Pacific, claiming millions and millions of lives worldwide, had been all but vanquished.

The Bay Area Reporter in San Francisco marked the occasion with the boldest screaming headline since the mass deaths started: "NO OBITS," it said.

The swing from before to after was even more profound in the developing world, especially in Africa. Thanks to a new generation of activists, the global price of AIDS drugs for a day's treatment has dropped to below a dollar, making it available (with humanitarian aid) to the most remote villages of the world. By 2011, 6 million people were taking the drugs ACT UP and TAG helped get released; by late 2016, more than 17 million. What the human community—with collaborators inside and outside of the pharmaceutical industry—have been able to accomplish is extraordinary.

But there was never a celebration, no parade in the streets. As 1996 receded into the past, the media went silent again, as did many of the survivors, who found themselves staggering into an unfamiliar land, exhausted, disoriented, and lost. An incomprehensible thing happens to the human mind when it is folded in fear and death for so long. It causes mysterious wounds and spurs unexplainable behaviors.

This describes no one more than Derek Link, who was still just twenty-seven when the plague years closed. It was thought that he was the sickest member of the HIVIP support group—he had testified as an AIDS patient under oath before Congress and issued a famous dictum to fellow activists, "HIV Negatives Get Out of Our Way"— but in fact he had never been infected at all. David Barr, the support group founder, pieced together the deception through inconsistencies in his stories, the vagueness about his doctor visits, his secrecy about lab results. I was incredulous when confronted with these facts. Some prominent survivors of the Holocaust have been revealed as liars, and it was so common for healthy people to claim illness, whether for sympathy or some other advantage, that the phenomenon had a name: "fictitious disorder" or, more familiarly, Munchausen syndrome. Derek Link was different. For almost a decade I watched him partake in some of the most instrumental skirmishes that revolutionized science and medicine. I watched his work save lives. He could have accomplished as much as an openly HIV-negative man; Jim Eigo and Martin Delaney were examples of that.

What drove him, I guessed, was a peculiar kind of thrill-seeking behavior. There was no more immediate battle in this epic war than the one to survive. For young men it was an almost romantic race against time. I can imagine, but not fully understand, a compulsion to feel those stakes very personally. The early 1990s produced very rare but disturbing stories of people who acquired their infections intentionally—"bug chasers," they were called. Some explained that the anxiety of becoming infected was far more difficult to bear than the diagnosis itself; others desired the community's support and collective love once they had been stricken. "Membership has its privileges," as Stephen Gendin, a leading HIV-positive activist, once put it.

"With the movement to try and de-stigmatize having HIV, the person with AIDS became a heroic figure in a community of people who were to some extent really lacking in models for heroic figures," said Garance Franke-Ruta. "And I think Derek probably just wanted that kind of community support and adulation."

Link offered another explanation to me, many years later. He said that what motivated him, as best as he could understand it himself, was self-preservation. By telling people he was infected he marked himself as untouchable, which kept him safe.

"I was scared all the time," he said tearfully. "That was my motivation."

"Everybody described your AIDS work as being heroic," I offered.

He threw his hands in the air. "I'm a forty-two-year-old gay man who survived the AIDS epidemic in New York City, you know. Am I a hero? Am I just lucky? Am I an asshole?"

After Derek Link's deceptions were uncovered, he never saw his closest friends again. "It was unforgivable," Staley said. Barr called it "a total betrayal of trust." Unconnected from his past, Link was adrift. He left New York City and made his career as a mapmaker, focused on the nation's decayed electrical grids. He was alone, crying often and convulsively, grieving for the friendships he squandered as much as the ones he lost to disease. The AIDS battle had been the most important part of his life, the place he was most authentically himself—but not himself at all.

THE OTHER NARRATIVES in the Protease Era were considerably less revelatory, but similarly disorienting. Joseph Sonnabend retired from medicine at seventy-two and relocated to London in 2005 to escape the horrid memories that haunted him in New York City. "Nearly everyone I knew and cared about is dead," he said. "They died right there in that battlefield, in those apartments—the streets of the Village and Chelsea reek of it." Richard Berkowitz, once healthy again, published a memoir and was the subject of a documentary on safe sex, but struggled financially, as did Bill Bahlman, who subsisted on disability insurance payments, volunteering a few hours a week on a cable news show covering gay issues. Chuck Ortleb, who had taken the *Native* into battle and then turned it against phantoms, left the public stage altogether.

Gregg Gonsalves and David Barr turned their attention to Africa, helping to mentor the drugs access movement there. Gregg Bordowitz, who recorded so much of the history on videotape, moved into academia. He taught filmmaking and new media, wrote and directed an opera on the work of Michel Foucault, and released numerous books. And Garance Franke-Ruta, after completing her pre-med studies, went on to a high-profile career in journalism instead.

Peter Staley lost a power struggle with Mark Harrington for control of the Treatment Action Group. While Harrington remained at TAG, and went on to win a MacArthur "genius" award for his work, Staley fell unexpectedly into the thrall of methamphetamine. He turned to the drug after his fortieth birthday, at a time when he felt most alienated from the community of activists that had nourished him. Meth seemed to restore him to a world of carefree sexual encounters, he thought. He disappeared for long stretches during a two-year addiction. A huge number of gay men went in the same direction. Drug addiction became a secondary epidemic, an aftershock in the community of HIV-positive survivors. Through multiple trips to rehab, Staley managed to return to sobriety. In 2004 he launched a campaign to fight methamphetamine addiction in New York's gay community, and for a time resumed his life as an activist. Thereafter, he receded as surely as the others, dispirited, retiring to his home in rural Pennsylvania and making his money in day-trades.

These were the heavy burdens of survival. Spencer Cox was the first of the activists to recognize the darkness that followed the plague. Immediately following the good news in 1996, he thought he'd return to college but never managed to find the funds to get his degree. Instead, he launched an initiative to address the epidemic of depression and drug addiction. He called it the Medius Institute for Gay Men's Health. It failed after a few years. That's when Cox turned to meth himself. He always denied being addicted, which was beside the point; meth fed his depression and undermined his reason.

When he died, because he had stopped taking the pills that were keeping him alive, the pills that had been the single-minded focus of his entire adulthood, there was much debate whether this could be classified as a suicide. What was clear was that living had proved more than he could handle. As was said about the great Holocaust writer Primo Levi after he plunged to his death, Spencer Cox had never left the camps.

Maybe none of us did.

Acknowledgments

Above anyone, I owe gratitude to Jonathan Segal, my editor at Alfred A. Knopf, for lifting me through the work of this book. He patiently waited many years as I struggled through a first draft, then peeled it and pampered it into a cogent whole. I have been fortunate to be his student, his project, and his friend. I am blessed to be published by a house headed by Sonny Mehta, whose faith in this book never wavered. Thanks to the entire Knopf team: Paul Bogaards, Nicholas Latimer, Kathy Zuckerman, Stephanie Kloss, Jess Purcell, Kevin Bourke, Amy Stackhouse, and Julia Ringo.

My work here, as throughout my body of AIDS writing, is driven by a profound and humble admiration for the men and women whose stories animate the present volume, and especially for those who did not live to see their contributions come to force, who never learned what a brilliant difference their efforts had made nor imagined what place history would accord them. I am in their debt in so many ways.

When assignments were handed out at the dawn of the plague, I raised my arm to enlist as a journalist, though I had neither experience nor innate ability—nothing, that is, but a hunger for answers. Sue Hyde, Cindy Patton, and the other collective members at Boston's legendary *Gay Community News* gave me my first assignments and bent my work into publishable news briefs, while Ellen Davidson and Jonathan Bennett at *The Guardian*, the radical newsweekly, schooled me in the politics of disease. But it was from Joe Nicholson at the *New York Post* that I learned how to wield journalism as an offensive weapon, and from Patrick Merla, the intrepid editor of the *New York Native* and a leading force in gay letters, that I learned how to think, to inform, and to agitate all in the same sentence. His ministrations, often delivered at piercing volume, still echo in my head decades after leaving his employ. Thanks to him, I had the opportunity to work with some of the singular reporters confronting the plague, especially Larry Kramer and Randy Shilts who both patiently mentored me in my early years.

Over the years, editors at numerous other publications have allowed my AIDS work to continue, including *The Village Voice*, the *East Village Eye*, *Grand Rapids Magazine*, *The New York Observer*, *New York Newsday*, *Lear's*, *Good Housekeeping*, *Mirabella*, *Glamour*, *Elle*, *New York*, *Details*, *Vanity Fair*, *The New Yorker*, and *GQ*. I owe special thanks to Linda Villarosa for giving me access to the science pages of *The New York Times* and to Mark Whitaker at *Newsweek*, who took a risk on a reporter of nontraditional lineage, letting me join my voice to the nation's chaotic dialogue.

This book is a work of research and reporting, aided only infrequently by my own memory. All errors and omissions are my own, of course. For research assistance and counsel, I owe a mountain of debt to Ron Goldberg. His meticulousness as a guardian of AIDS history is unmatched. I could not have completed this book without his tight focus, his generosity, and his friendship. Thanks also to Arielle de Saint Phalle, Hadass Silver, Reggie Ugwu, Jason Alarcon, Angela Flignor, Sam Tankard, Sam Donnenberg, Tara González, Oona Wallace, Nadine Levine, Cate Battey, Ali Kemal Güven, Jason Schwartz, Clare McKeown, Alex Wallace, Gastòn Yvorra, Clelia Simpson, and the other interns and assistants who lent their time and talents as researchers and transcribers. The blogger and ACT UP veteran Michael Petrelis was especially resourceful.

For opening up personal and family archives, thanks to Ferris Fain, Patrick Haggerty, Linda Godby, Garance Franke-Ruta, Richard Berkowitz, Richard Dworkin, Joseph Sonnabend, Bill Bahlman, Sara Rafsky, Ron Goldberg, Karen Hughes, Simon Watney, Iris Long, and Eleanor Burkett, who cleared her entire basement full of material into my car one sweltering afternoon. Of special historical significance is the vast personal archive of Mark Harrington. He organized much of the record of AIDS activism into scores of cartons, cramming them with original documents, drafts, audiotapes, and transcripts. Without his keen archivist inclination, the story of AIDS treatment activism could not be richly told. For the access he granted, including to his yet-unpublished memoir, which deserves a wide readership, I am in his lasting debt.

For guiding me through archives and collections: Polina E. Ilieva and Margaret Hughes of Archives and Special Collections at UCSF; Moira Fitzgerald from Yale's Beinecke Rare Book & Manuscript Library; Brandy Svendson with AIDS Vancouver; the official volunteer AmFAR archivist Harley Hackett; Rich Wandel, the founder and guiding star of the the Lesbian, Gay, Bisexual & Transgender Community Center National History Archive in New York; everybody at the ONE Archives at USC Libraries; Heather Smedberg at University of California, San Diego's Jonas Salk Papers; the rotating staff at the New York Public Library; the estimable Brent Phillips at the Fales Library and Special Collections, part of New York University; Tim Wilson of the Special Collections Center of the San Francisco Public Library; Dr. Ronald Bayer, co-creator of the Doctors and AIDS oral history archive housed at Columbia University; Brenda Marston, curator of Cornell University's Human Sexuality Collection; and Jim Hubbard, who is the original curator of the AIDS Activist Videotape Collection at New York Public Library and co-director (with Sarah Schulman) of the ACT UP Oral History Project at Harvard University Library—as well as a cherished friend, and my roommate through many of the years chronicled here. Additional, anonymous assistance was provided by the online archives at the University of Michigan, hosting the Jon Cohen AIDS Research Collection; La Guardia Community College's La Guardia and Wagner digital archives, keeper of the Edward I. Koch Collection; the Ronald Reagan Presidential Library and Museum; and the crack research assistants on the other end of the "ask a librarian" button at NYU's Bobst Library online portal. Also at NYU, deep gratitude to Perry Halkitis and his team at the Center for Health, Identity, Behavior, and Prevention Studies—Paris Mourgues and Staci Barton—for appointing me as a vising scholar there and aiding my research.

An immense trove of video footage helped remind me of these years, and provided remarkably visceral documentary evidence. Thanks to the videographers Tony Arena, Bill Bahlman, Gregg Bordowitz, David Buckingham, Jean Carlomusto, Vincent Gagliostro, Carl M. George, Catherine Gund, Robert Hilferty, Spencer Halperin, Jim Hubbard, Shraga Lev, Tim McCarthy, Mimi Plevin-Foust, John Schabel, Ellen Spiro, James Wentzy, Phil Zwickler, the members of two video collectives (DIVA TV and Testing the Limits), and many others.

I was lucky to count on the following for reading some or all of early drafts: Gail Griffin, Rolf Sjogren, Richard Dworkin, Jim Hubbard, Peter Staley, Scott McGehee, David Siegel, Ian Horst, Mark Blane, and thanks especially to Susan Thames and Barry Yeoman. Fond appreciation to my agents, Todd Shuster and Brian Lipson; to the writer Suki Kim, who encouraged me to move this history from my heart to the page, and to the late producer David Kennedy, who read and commented on every draft and whose untimely death has left a painful absence. My mother, who had always been the reader for whom I write, departed just as I began work on this volume. I was relieved to discover that her influence on me and my work lives on.

And finally to my family and friends who jogged my memories and excused my many absences through the pains of authorship. I'm lucky especially to count Doug Gould's siblings as my own: Jackie, Craig, and Jim, together with their spouses and children, have been a powerful presence in my life. Joy Tomchin, my filmmaking partner, deserves special praise. Her friendship, support, wisdom, and love sheltered me for the years of this book's gestation, and continue to sustain me every day. I am extremely lucky to have her in my life. But my deepest thanks go to Jonathan Starch, to whom I dedicate this book. His love, constancy, and friendship mean the world to me. It is for him, I know now, that I was spared.

Abbreviations Used in Notes

SOURCES (ARCHIVES, ORGANIZATIONS, ETC.)

AUOHP	ACT UP Oral History Project
BBA	Bill Bahlman Personal Archive
BBP	Bill Bahlman Papers, LGBT Community Center National History Archive
GF-RA	Garance Franke-Ruta Personal Archives
GMHCA	Gay Men's Health Crisis Archive, New York Public Library
JEA	Jim Eigo Personal Archive
JSNYP	Joseph Sonnabend Papers, New York Public Library
JSPG	Joseph Sonnabend Papers, LGBT Community Center National History Archive
LKA	Larry Kramer Archives, Yale University
MCA	Michael Callen Papers, LGBT Community Center National History Archive
MCUA	Michael Callen Unpublished Anthology
MHA	Mark Harrington Personal Archive
MHU	Mark Harrington Untitled Manuscript
PAOH	Physicians and Aids Oral History Project, Columbia University
PSA	Peter Staley Personal Archive
RBA	Richard Berkowitz Personal Archive
RDA	Richard Dworkin Personal Archive
RJGA	Ron Goldberg Personal Archive
TTLN	Testing the Limits Records, New York Public Library

PUBLICATIONS

JAMA	*Journal of the American Medical Association*
LAT	*Los Angeles Times*
MMWR	*Morbidity and Mortality Weekly Report*
NEJM	*New England Journal of Medicine*
NYN	*New York Native*
NYT	*New York Times*
PI	*Philadelphia Inquirer*
PI Perspective	*Philadelphia Inquirer Perspective*
SFC	*San Francisco Chronicle*

VV	*Village Voice*
WP	*Washington Post*
WSJ	*Wall Street Journal*

PEOPLE

AF	Anthony Fauci
AF-K	Alvin Friedman-Kien
BB	Bill Bahlman
BC	Bobbi Campbell
BR	Bob Rafsky
BS	Barbara Starrett
DB	David Barr
DW	Daniel William
EIK	Edward I. Koch
GF-R	Garance Franke-Ruta
HH	Harley Hackett
JC	James Curran
JE	Jim Eigo
JS	Joseph Sonnabend
LK	Larry Kramer
LM	Lawrence Mass
MC	Michael Callen
MH	Mark Harrington
MK	Mathilde Krim
PS	Peter Staley
RB	Richard Berkowitz
RD	Richard Dworkin
RG	Robert Gallo
RM	Rodger McFarlane

Notes

PROLOGUE: THE MEMORIAL SERVICE

3 Most had been: Intvs. Jim Hubbard, various.

5 By the following: Bruce Weber, "Spencer Cox, AIDS Activist, Dies at 44," *NYT,* December 12, 2012.

5 At the time of: "UNAIDS 2013 Global Fact Sheet," Joint United Nations Programme on HIV/AIDS (UNAIDS), 2013; see also C. McEvedy, "The Bubonic Plague," *Scientific American* 258, no. 2 (1988): 118–23.

5 In the United States: "HIV in the United States: At a Glance," Centers for Disease Control and Prevention, September 29, 2015.

5 In the early years: Judy L. Thomas, "Catholic Priests Are Dying of AIDS, Often in Silence," *Kansas City Star,* January 21, 2000.

5 The year Cox died: "HIV in the United States: At a Glance."

6 Cox had begun: In Gallup polls from March 14–18, 1987, and July 1–7, 1988, 55 percent and 57 percent, respectively, felt that homosexual relations "should not be legal."

6 "When we realized": Intv. David Barr, September 10, 2010.

7 "So for us": Primo Levi, *The Reawakening* (New York, NY: Simon & Schuster, 1995), 16.

8 When grieving friends: Intv. PS, March 17, 2009.

8 The camp sensibility: Nicholas Cox, email to author, March 21, 2014.

8 When Larry Kramer: Intv. LK, April 26, 2013; and intv. Chip Duckett, March 27, 2013.

8 "Love was always love": Gabriel García Márquez, *Love in the Time of Cholera* (New York, NY: Alfred A. Knopf, 1988), 345.

8 "If there was ever": Videotape of Spencer Cox memorial, retrieved from vimeo.com, transcript by author.

9 Minutes later came: Intvs. PS, October 14, 2009, and August 5, 2010.

9 He placed the pages: Videotape of Spencer Cox memorial.

PART I: WHEN IT RAINS, IT POURS

1. INDEPENDENCE DAY

13 "new City of Friends": Walt Whitman, "I Dream'd in a Dream," *Leaves of Grass* (Philadelphia: Rees Welsh & Co., 1882).

13   "Rare Cancer Seen": Lawrence K. Altman, "Rare Cancer Seen in 41 Homosexuals," *NYT,* July 3, 1981.

14   On the day: David Rothenberg, "Homophobia at the NYT," *NYN,* June 1–14, 1981; and Edward Hudson, "Rest Room Shut to Foreclose Use by Homosexuals," *NYT,* August 1, 1980.

15   A few months later: Leonard Budner, "Former Transit Officer Held as Slayer of Two in Village," *NYT,* November 21, 1980; and David Rothenberg, "Homophobia at the *NYT,*" *NYN,* June 1–14, 1981.

16   Moving through: See Edmund Bergler, *The Basic Neurosis, Oral Regression and Psychic Masochism* (New York, NY: Grune & Stratton, 1949); Charles W. Socarides, *Homosexuality: Psychoanalytic Therapy* (Lanham, MA: Jason Aronson, Inc., 1989); and *Diagnostic and Statistical Manual of Mental Disorders,* 2nd ed. (Arlington: American Psychiatric Association, 1968).

16   "With broadened parental": Introduction by Stanley F. Yolles in Peter Wyden, *Growing Up Straight: What Every Thoughtful Parent Should Know About Homosexuality* (New York, NY: Stein and Day, 1968), 8.

16   Inside a cramped: Intvs. JS, various.

16   Previously, Kaposi's sarcoma: "Follow-Up on Kaposi's Sarcoma and Pneumocystis Pneumonia," *MMWR* 30, no. 33 (August 28, 1981): 409–10.

17   "To me, this is": Intv. JS, July 28, 2009.

17   He had studied: Ibid.; and JS curriculum vitae, JSNYP.

17   His specialty was: Intv. JS, July 28, 2009; JS speech upon receiving amfAR's Award of Courage (2000), retrieved from amfAR.org.

17   He settled on Greenwich: Intv. JS, July 28, 2009.

18   He also developed: Intv. JS, July 9, 2013.

18   Then, in 1979: Intv. JS, July 28, 2009; Joseph Sonnabend, "AIDS Perspective," retrieved from aidsperspective.net; and JS curriculum vitae.

18   "unacknowledged minority": Donald Webster Cory, *The Homosexual in America* (New York, NY: Paperback Library, 1963), 17.

19   He soon had a: Intv. HH, March 16, 2014.

19   Unusual cases of protozoan: Matt Clark and Mariana Gosnell, "Diseases That Plague Gays," *Newsweek,* December 21, 1981.

19   There appeared to be: W. Lawrence Drew et al., "Prevalence of Cytomegalovirus Infection in Homosexual Men," *Journal of Infectious Diseases* 143, no. 2 (Febuary 1981): 189.

19   Sonnabend diagnosed: Intvs. JS, various.

20   Suspecting there might: Alvin Friedman-Kien, "The Reminiscences of Alvin Friedman-Kien, M.D.," *PAOH,* March 24, 1995.

20   Conant was unaware: Intv. AF-K, July 25, 2013.

20   He would start: Intv. HH, March 16, 2014.

20   He told Altman: Intv. JS, July 28, 2009; however, there is some dispute in memory between Sonnabend and Friedman-Kien about when it went out and to whom. AF-K says he had already sent numerous letters to physicians, in intvs. AF-K, July 25, 2013, and September 5, 2013; no copies of any letter could be located by author.

20   What did surprise him: A. Friedman-Kien et al., "Kaposi's Sarcoma and

Pneumocystis Pneumonia Among Homosexual Men—New York City and California," *MMWR* 30 (1981): 305–08; and intv. JS, July 28, 2009.

20 Had Friedman-Kien delayed: Friedman-Kien denies that he delayed, arguing that he had personally informed numerous doctors by this time; interview with F-K.

21 The gay bookstore: Andriote, *Victory Deferred.*

21 "a total invasion": Alex Witchel, "At Home With: Larry Kramer; When a Roaring Lion Learns to Purr," *NYT,* January 12, 1995.

22 He felt the burn: "Interview Larry Kramer," *Frontline,* January 22, 2005, retrieved from pbs.org.

22 There in Friedman-Kien's: Unsigned, "Donald J. Krintzman," *NYT,* November 12, 1981.

22 "Yes," Krintzman offered: LK, *Reports,* 12.

22 "We're only seeing the tip": "Interview Larry Kramer."

22 "We're applying to the NIH": Intv. AF-K, July 25, 2013.

22 But his mother: LK, intv. by Sarah Schulman, November 15, 2013, AUOHP.

23 "In the past": LK, *Reports,* 9.

23 About eighty people: Ibid., 39 and 13.

23 Friedman-Kien addressed: "Follow-Up on Kaposi's Sarcoma and Pneumocystis Pneumonia," 409–10; Walter T. Hughes, MD, "*Pneumocystis Carinii* Pneumonitis," *NEJM* 317, no. 16 (October 15, 1987): 1021; and Walter T. Hughes, "Successful Chemoprophylaxis for *Pneumocystis Carinii* Pneumonitis," *NEJM* 297 (December 22, 1977): 1381–83.

23 A treating doctor: Intv. Howard Grossman (date unknown).

23 "We think there might": Elizabeth Landau, "HIV in the '80s: 'People Didn't Want to Kiss You on the Cheek,'" retrieved from cnn.com, May 25, 2011.

23 "It was pandemonium": Intv. AF-K, July 25, 2013.

23 "Everybody looked": Landau, "HIV in the '80s."

23 Still, $6,635 was: "The History of the Gay Men's Health Crisis, Inc.," GMHC Circus Program, April 30, 1983, RJGA.

24 "Now, with Kaposi's": Over the next several weeks: LK, *Reports,* 16.

24 "Why is Bob Chesley": Ibid., 21.

2. EARLY THINKING

25 Through the week: LM, "KS: Latest Developments," *NYN,* August 24–September 6, 1981.

25 "The idea . . . is bizarre": Hilda Reiger, "The Riddle of Kaposi's Sarcoma," *Emergency Medicine* 13 (November 15, 1981): 155–56.

26 According to the CDC: "Follow-Up on Kaposi's Sarcoma and Pneumocystis Pneumonia," *MMWR* 30, no. 33 (August 28, 1981).

26 Leaving work late: Intv. JS, July 28, 2009.

26 There was one thing: See, e.g., Drew et al., "Prevalence of Cytomegalovirus Infection in Homosexual Men," *Journal of Infectious Diseases* 143, no. 2 (February 1981).

26   But there was an undeniable: Ibid.

27   For his tours: Intv. JS, July 28, 2009.

27   Military medical officers: Alan Brandt, *No Magic Bullet* (New York, NY: Oxford University Press: 1987), 112–13.

27   The evidence for its efficacy: "Penicillin for Prophylaxis," *NEJM*, November 25, 1948, 841–42; and Nicholas J. Fiumara et al., "Venereal Diseases Today," *NEJM*, April 23, 1959, 863–68.

27   The one time he forgot: Intv. JS, July 28, 2009.

27   hoping a relaxing: Ibid.

28   Next up was Michael: Ibid.

28   Adding to this overall: RB, *Stayin' Alive*, 113; and Will Grega, "Michael Callen Up Close," *Will Grega's Gay Music Guide* (New York, NY: Pop Front Press, 1994), 14–19.

28   What he loved even: RB, *Stayin' Alive*, 113.

28   As a child in Johannesburg: JS email to author, April 10, 2014.

29   It would be nearly: "Immigration," *Canadian Lesbian & Gay Archives*, retrieved from clga.ca.

29   "The rectum": Barry Adkins, "Look at AIDS in Totality: A Conversation with Joseph Sonnabend," *NYN*, October 7–13, 1985.

29   In a few short years: MC, *Surviving AIDS*, 40.

29   Sonnabend "moaned": RB audiotape transcript, "Callen in P-town—August 7, 1993," MCA.

29   "Move," he answered: MC audiotape, "75T—Michael Moves to NY and Gets Sick," MCA, transcript by author.

30   The results came back: Ibid.

30   That afternoon he called: Ibid.

30   Recovering from her: MC, *Surviving AIDS*, 75.

30   Of the men: Larry Mass, "Do Poppers Cause Cancer?," *NYN*, December 21, 1981–January 3, 1982.

30   Though she didn't know: BS, "The Reminiscences of Barbara Starrett, M.D.," *PAOH* (1999): 20.

31   In the brief obit: Unsigned, "Donald J. Krintzman," *NYT*, November 12, 1981.

31   Krintzman was Kramer's: LK, *Reports*, 11.

31   So had his *Native* article: LK, "A Personal Appeal from Larry Kramer," *NYN*, August 24–September 6, 1981.

31   "Two new cases of KS": LK, "A Letter from Larry Kramer," *NYN*, December 21, 1981–January 3, 1982.

31   The occasion was: Correspondence, Nathan Fain to LK, May 27, 1983, Randy Shilts Papers, San Francisco History Center of the San Francisco Public Library.

31   He had joined: LK, "A Letter from Larry Kramer."

32   Then Rapoport mused: "The History of the Gay Men's Health Crisis, Inc.," GMHC Circus Program, April 30, 1983, RJGA.

32   As Fain looked: Correspondence, Nathan Fain to LK, May 27, 1983.

32   A long East Coast: Michael Goodwin, "City's Water Shortage No Longer Emergency," *NYT*, January 19, 1982.

32   When the immensely: Larry Bush, "Heading Off the Gay Conspiracy," *NYN*, March 29–April 4, 1982.

33   Allen Ginsberg lived: Gary Indiana, "One Brief, Scuzzy Moment," *New York*, December 6, 2004.

34   As a congressman: See Alan H. Levy, *The Political Life of Bella Abzug, 1976–1998: Political Passions, Women's Rights, and Congressional Battles* (New York, NY: Lexington Books, 2013).

34   "I respect people": Brandon Judell, "Koch on Homophobia: It's a Matter of Conscience," *NYN*, May 16–31, 1981.

34   The NYPD refused: Brett Averill, "The Hot Spots," *NYN*, July 5–18, 1982; and sidebar, "The 15 Worst Danger Zones," *NYN*, July 5–18, 1982.

35   This was a lesson: Lawrence K. Altman, "In Philadelphia 30 Years Ago, an Eruption of Illness and Fear," *NYT*, August 1, 2006.

35   The death toll: According to "A Timeline of HIV/AIDS" on aids.gov, by the end of 1981 there were a total of 270 cases of severe immune deficiency among gay men reported and 121 deaths. The death total from the 1976 outbreak of Legionnaire's disease in Philadelphia was 34.

35   The agency's apathetic: Undated study of media coverage for an article by RM, LKA.

36   "We shouldn't jump": Intv. HH, March 16, 2014.

36   In a letter to a fellow: Letter from JS to Alexandra Levine, Professor of Hematology and Oncology at University of Southern California Medical Center, February 14, 1983, JSPNYP.

36   When he tested this: Intv. JS, July 9, 2013; and J. M. Richards et al., "Rectal Insemination Modified Immune Responses in Rabbits," *Science* 27 (April 1984): 390–92.

37   "I agree with capital": "Coalition in San Francisco to Fight Homosexuality," *NYT*, February 11, 1981.

37   "It could be the bugs": Matt Clark and Marina Gosnell, "Diseases That Plague Gays," *Newsweek*, December 21, 1981.

37   Others blamed amyl nitrite: LM, "Do Poppers Cause Cancer?"

37   Sonnabend kept all: JS, email to author, July 13, 2013.

37   "People who are promiscuous": LM, "Do Poppers Cause Cancer?"

38   "The term 'promiscuous'": JS, "Promiscuity Is Bad for Your Health," *NYN*, September 13–26, 1982.

38   He had been in and out: Intv. JC, September 23, 2013.

38   More than two hundred: BS, "The Reminiscences of Barbara Starrett, M.D.," 33–37.

38   Also attending was the new: Bruce Weber, "David J. Sencer Dies at 86, Led Disease-Control Agency," *NYT*, May 3, 2011; and BS, email to author, September 10, 2014.

38   When it was his time: Intv. JC, September 23, 2013; intv. BS, September 10, 2010.

39   "If this is a sexually": Intv. BS, September 10, 2010.

39   "It isn't going away": Shilts, *And the Band Played On*, 134.

39   "You're showing great": Intv. JC, September 23, 2013.

39   "Epidemics come": DW, "The Reminiscences of Daniel C. William, M.D., February 22–23, 1996, *PAOH* (1999).

39   Almost immediately after: Intv. JC, September 23, 2013.

39   Though both volunteered: DW, "The Reminiscences of Daniel C. William, M.D," 144–45; quotes from 66.

40   There was a curious: Intv. AF-K, July 25, 2013; and Shilts, *And the Band Played On,* 37–38.

40   "Gaëtan Dugas": Intv. AF-K, September 5, 2013.

40   He called the airline's: Ibid.

40   The two NYU Medical: Bruce Lambert, "Linda Laubenstein, 45, Physician and Leader in Detection of AIDS," *NYT,* August 17, 1992.

40   In Europe: Statistics from "History of HIV and AIDS Overview," retrieved from avert.org.

40   Using the tools: Intv. AF-K, July 25, 2013.

41   When she first employed: L. J. Laubenstein et al., "Treatment of Epidemic Kaposi's Sarcoma with Etoposide or a Combination of Doxorubicin, Bleomycin, and Vinblastine," *Journal of Clinical Oncology* 2 (October 1984): 1115–20.

41   "But Linda": Bayer and Oppenheimer, *AIDS Doctors,* 121.

41   The authorities at: JS, email to author, November 23, 2015.

41   But many of the city's: Intv. Howard Grossman, undated.

41   Nationwide, there were: Stats in *NYT* from May 1982.

41   Years later, once: G. J. van Griensven et al., "Epidemiology of Human Immunodeficiency Virus Type 1 Infection Among Homosexual Men Participating in Hepatitis B Vaccine Trials in Amsterdam, New York City, and San Francisco, 1978–1990," *American Journal of Epidemiology* 137, no. 8 (April 15, 1993): 909–15.

42   In Sonnabend's boutique: Intv. HH, March 16, 2014.

42   "You know, Mathilde": Intv. MK, March 25, 2011; and JS, email to author, July 17, 2013.

42   Born in Italy: MK biographical details from Ruth Schwartz Cowan, "Mathilde Krim," *Jewish Women: A Comprehensive Historical Encyclopedia* (Jewish Women's Archive, 2009); Deidre Carmody, "Painful Political Lesson for AIDS Crusader," *NYT,* January 30, 1990;

42   The Krims had played: Guest list gathered from online photos from John F. Kennedy Presidential Library and Museum, jfklibrary.org.

42   As she was setting: Intv. JS, July 9, 2013.

42   "And they're all young": Intv. MK, March 25, 2011.

43   Without a moment's: JS, email to author, July 17, 2013.

43   "It's rare": Intv. MK, March 25, 2011.

3 . COMPROMISED

44   Since getting the: MC audiotape, "75T—Michael Moves to NY and Gets Sick," MCA, transcript by author.

44   As the weather warmed: MC, "AIDS as an Identity," Part II, *Newsline,* undated (probably August/September 1986), transcript of a conversa-

tion between early PWA activists MC, RB, Bob Cecchi, and Bill Burke, May 20, 1986, RDA.

44 "if you didn't want to": MC, *Surviving AIDS,* 76.

44 "I'm a gay man": Ibid., 77.

44 "Once a whore": RB audiotape, "Conversation /Reminiscing—Callen March 11, 1993," transcribed by RB, MCA.

44 One humid June day: MC, *Surviving AIDS,* 1–2, including following story and quotes.

45 "Here's the number": MC, "AIDS as an Identity," Part I, *Newsline,* June/ July 1986.

45 In poetry and lyrics: MC, "Dredging the Hudson: On Being Gay, Promiscuity, Monogamous and MORE," unpublished, MCA.

45 "I only counted anal": RB audiotape transcript, "Callen and Berkowitz— The Interview," MCA.

45 Nonetheless, his statement cast him: MC, "Remarks of Michael Callen— American Public Health Association Annual Meeting—Las Vegas, Nevada 1986," MCA.

45 Richard Dworkin visited: MC Blue Cross/Blue Shield claim, June 19, 1982, MCA.

45 In a few months: RD email to author, June 16, 2014.

45 After his strength returned: MC, "I Know Malone Died at Sea," MCUA.

46 Afterward, he made: Entire account from JS office, with quotes, as recalled by MC in RB audiotape transcript, "SONY—60," MCA.

47 One early afternoon: MC datebook, RBA.

47 After formalities: Phone conversation between RB and MC from MC audiotape "100T—Save 95-232," transcribed by author, MCA.

47 An hour later: Entire account of support group meeting from RB, *Stayin' Alive,* 103–07.

48 "Every time he spoke": Intv. RB, September 4, 2013.

48 Following the meeting: RB, *Stayin' Alive,* 110–11.

48 "I have trouble": RB audiotape transcript, recalling the coffee with MC and his response, "Sony—60."

48 He had earned a: RB audiotape, "90T—From the First Week of February 1983 Telephone Conversations," transcript by author, MCA.

49 For his promotional: RB, *Stayin' Alive,* 59–60; with reference to food-stocking job at Krauszer's Food Store at 39.

49 "That's a swollen gland": Ibid., 75.

49 They didn't hurt: Ibid., 78.

49 He took to wearing: Ibid., 83.

49 On his way out: MC, "AIDS as an Identity."

49 When he made it back: RB, *Stayin' Alive,* 79–83.

49 "Previously found": Ibid., 115.

50 This was thanks: Correspondence between LK and his brother, and between his brother and his bank, LKA.

50 It was a time: LK, *Reports,* 23.

50 Committees were set up: "GMHC Board of Directors Minutes, April 12, 1982," GMHCA.

50   Rodger McFarlane: RM, Gay Men's Health Crisis Oral History, videotape, undated, GMHCA.

50   On the first day: Ibid.

50   They were "uniformly": Ibid.

50   McFarlane was twenty-seven: Ibid.

51   Instead they recognized: "GMHC Board of Directors Minutes, April 12, 1982."

51   Thanks to his steady charisma: Intv. LM, September 24, 2013.

51   Popham, who by day: Andrew Rosenthal, "Paul Popham, 45, Founder of AIDS Organization, Dies," *NYT*, May 8, 1987.

51   In fact, for the first: "GMHC Board of Directors Minutes, April 12, 1982"; and "GMHC Board of Directors Minutes, April 26, 1982," GMHCA.

51   In a goodwill gesture: "GMHC Board of Directors Minutes, April 12, 1982."

51   In the fall: Chambre, *Fighting for Our Lives*, 19.

51   When two more rooms: "The History of the Gay Men's Health Crisis, Inc.," GMHC Circus Program, April 30, 1983, RJGA.

51   He had in mind: Ibid.

51   Both McFarlane and Rosen: Chambre, *Fighting for Our Lives*, 17.

51   The board enthusiastically: "GMHC Board of Directors Minutes, August 31, 1982," GMHCA.

52   For their first major: "The History of the Gay Men's Health Crisis, Inc."

52   Rosen put them to work: *Lesbian and Gay Pride Guide*, New York, 1983.

52   "They come in the door": Jane Howard, "The Warrior," *Esquire* (December 1984).

52   He treated Rosen terribly: See LK, *Reports*.

52   Kramer's confessed inability: Intv. LM, September 24, 2013.

52   Still, much of Kramer's ire: Correspondence, Nathan Fain to LK, May 27, 1983.

52   "a top notch social": Mel Rosen, GMHC Oral History, videotape, November 1989, GMHCA.

52   Another board member: "GMHC Board of Directors Meeting Minutes, January 22, 1983," GMHCA.

53   "Every contact with": Bob Cecchi, GMHC Oral History, videotape, no date, GMHCA.

53   "As the number of cases": Robert Cecchi, "When the System Fails," *American Journal of Nursing* (January 1986).

53   "I should have shot": Michael Shnayerson, "Kramer vs. Kramer," *Vanity Fair*, September 30, 1992.

53   "the father of us all": Correspondence, LK to EIK, undated (presumably 1983), LKA.

53   "The rest of us thought": RM, GMHC Oral History, GMHCA.

54   to "have fewer partners": LM, "AIDS and What to Do About It," *GMHC Newsletter* (July 1982), GMHCA.

54   "the Elizabeth Taylor": DW, "Reminiscences of Daniel C. William," PAOH, 43.

54   But even the smallest: Correspondence, Nathan Fain to LK, May 27,

1983, including claims that LK considered himself to be the "mother" of GMHC; LK's belief that GMHC volunteers and clients were his "children" can be found in LK, *Reports,* 383.

54 The tensions were especially: Intv. LM, September 24, 2013.

54 One evening he admitted: Intv. Arnie Kantrowitz, September 25, 2013.

54 Mass wouldn't return: Intv. LM, September 24, 2013.

54 While working in London: Bayer and Oppenheimer, *AIDS Doctors,* 122.

55 As early as the mid-1970s: W. T. Hughes et al., "Successful Chemoprophylaxis for *Pneumocystis Carinii* Pneumonitis," *NEJM* 297 (1977): 1419–26.

55 Statistically, those: Michael N. Dohn and Peter T. Frame, "Clinical Manifestation in Adults," *Pneumocystis, Pneumonia,* 2nd ed. (CRC Press), 343–44. Before the wide use of PCP prophylaxis, over 60 percent of patients would have a recurrence of PCP within eighteen months. The one-year survival rate after a first bout of PCP was only 33 percent in 1981.

55 To be safe: Joseph A. Sonnabend, "Pneumocystis Pneumonia Can be Prevented: Why Did It Take So Long for Well Known Preventative Measures to Be Introduced in AIDS?," 2006, retrieved from aidsperspective.net.

56 In a succession of meals: Intv. MK, March 25, 2011.

56 She called a number: Ibid.

56 "It was not to be": Ibid.

56 When Friedman-Kien presented: Intv. AF-K, July 25, 2013.

56 "This," Friedman-Kien said: Ibid.

57 Through trial-and-error: Intv. Craig Metroka, September 5, 2013.

57 Krim had a tremendous: Intv. MK, March 25, 2011.

57 Before Israeli statehood: David B. Green, "This Day in Jewish History a Future AIDS Warrior Enters the World," *Haaretz,* July 9, 2013.

57 "A pretty girl on a bicycle": Intv. James Crowley, March 25, 2011.

57 In later years: Jane Perlez, "A Peek at Arthur Krim, Adviser to Presidents," *NYT,* April 14, 1986.

58 "come to my office after six": Intv. MK, March 25, 2011; and intv. Craig Metroka, September 5, 2013.

58 Thereafter, she convened: Intv. MK, March 25, 2011.

58 Among the 452 cases: *MMWR,* July 8, 1982.

58 The obvious explanation: Lawrence K. Altman, "Five States Report Disorders in Haitians' Immune Systems," *NYT,* July 9, 1982.

58 By mid-1982: "Opportunistic Infections and Kaposi's Sarcoma Among Haitians in the United States," *MMWR* 31, no. 26 (July 9, 1982): 353–54, 360–61.

58 The CDC hadn't: Intv. JC, March 22, 2014.

58 "Is this the same thing": Altman, "Five States Report Disorders in Haitians' Immune Systems."

59 Just before the CDC: All three cases were reported by the CDC in "Epidemiologic Notes and Reports *Pneumocystis Carinii* Pneumonia Among Persons with Hemophilia A," *MMWR* 31, no. 27 (July 16, 1982): 365–67.

60 Circulation soared to: Robin Pogrebin, "Controversial Gay Magazine Shuts Down," *NYT,* January 9, 1997.

60   The son of a meat: Alisa Solomon, "The Demise of the 'Native,'" *VV,* August 22, 1989. James Kinsella calls him "a pork-salesman's son" and reports of his pursuit of "the gay literati" in James Kinsella, *Covering the Plague: AIDS and the American Media* (New Brunswick: Rutgers University Press, 1989), 26.

60   While he was able: Intv. Michael Denneny, January 22, 2014.

60   Ortleb launched the *Native*: Ibid.

60   Once, during a: Katie Leishman, "The Outsider," *Rolling Stone,* March 23, 1989.

60   "It has now been a year": Charles L. Ortleb, "Editorial," *NYN,* August 16, 1982.

61   The disease agency had: LK, "Where Are We Now?," *GMHC Newsletter* (January 1983).

61   And the NIH: Figures from LK, *Reports,* 25.

61   So it was infuriating: There is some uncertainty about this fact. LK reports the tragedy and the foreign aid in the *GMHC Newsletter,* in various published articles, and in *Reports.* But while newspapers report deadly floods in Guatemala and El Salvador in September and October, the money apportioned by Washington was far below $25 million.

61   Though twice two: Statistics per James D'Eramo, "The Basics of AIDS—Understanding the Epidemic," *NYN,* October 25–November 7, 1982.

61   "The American people": LK, "Where Are We Now?"

61   Like Reagan: D'Eramo, "The Basics of AIDS."

61   The scabrous publisher: *SCREW,* December 5, 1983, as cited in Adam Nagourney and Dudley Clendinen, *Out for Good: The Struggle to Build a Gay Rights Movement in America* (New York, NY: Touchstone, 1999), 485.

61   With their doctors': MC and RB, "We Know Who We Are," *NYN,* November 8–21, 1982.

61   "This isn't a game": Ibid.

62   He and Berkowitz: MC, unpublished fourteen-page chapter-and-verse response to articles, letters to the editor, and other attacks in *NYN,* February 28, 1983, MCA.

62   "Confusing? Contradictory?": Untitled editorial, *NYN,* November 8–21, 1982.

63   All three knew: RB audiotape recalling pre-publication trip to the Mineshaft, RB audiotape, "Conversation/Reminiscing—Callen March 11, 1993," transcribed by RB, MCA.

63   "Call me naïve": RD, email to author, August 25, 2015.

63   "sex-negative" hysterics: MC and RB, unpublished letter, "Response to Attacks on We Know Who We Are," 1983.

63   The Toronto-based: Bill Lewis, "The Real Gay Epidemic: Panic and Paranoia," *Body Politic* (November 1982).

63   Being so brutally: "Callen and Berkowitz—The Interview."

63   They spent hours: Multiple MC and RB audiotapes, transcription by author.

64   "we could use the word *promiscuous*": "90T—From the First Week of February 1983 Telephone Conversations."

64   "We saw the light": "Conversation/Reminiscing."

64   On a crisp, fall-like: RB audiotape transcript, "13X Panasonic Side One at 50% . . . (M90)," dated "prob Aug/Sept 82," MCA; and additional quotes in RB audiotape transcript, "5X . . . Oct 82," MCA.

65   Such was the communication: Intvs with both men.

65   His experiments had shown: "100T—Save 95-232"; JS, email to author, March 22, 2014; and JS, "HIV Disease and Alpha Interferon," *AIDS Perspective*, March 21, 2009, retrieved from aidsperspective.net.

66   He had sent Callen: JS, email to author, March 22, 2014; and MC in MC audiotape "44—Mike and Richie Chat About Survival," November 2, 1987, MCA, transcribed by author.

66   Since his trauma-provoking: "44—Mike and Richie Chat About Survival"; and RB, email to author, February 8, 2016.

66   Consequently, he was: RB, email to author, September 11, 2013.

67   Nor did he have: RB had already begun work on his second article, RB, "Joseph Sonnabend," *Christopher Street* (December 1982).

67   That fall, Callen spent: Receipt from J&R Music World, MCA.

67   "I've got it on tape": "100T—Save 95-232."

67   "Let them say what": Intv. RB, September 4, 2013.

67   "I was never ashamed": Ibid.

67   "Gay men are dying": Ibid.

67   Berkowitz and Callen: MC and RB, "A Warning to Gay Men with AIDS," *NYN*, November 22–December 5, 1982.

68   After deliberating for a few days: Intv. RB, September 4, 2013.

68   Though timidly, the dominant: All by Lawrence K. Altman, "New Homosexual Disorder Worries Health Officials," *NYT*, May 11, 1982; "Clue Found on Homosexuals' Precancer Syndrome," *NYT*, June 18, 1982; and "Five States Report Disorders in Haitians' Immune Sytems." See also David W. Dunlap, "Having Claimed 558 Lives, AIDS Finally Made It to the Front Page," *NYT*, October 30, 2014.

69   My friend Andy Mosso: Andy Mosso, email to author, January 4, 2016.

69   Ermanno Stingo: See Ermanno J. Stingo Papers, ONE National Gay & Lesbian Archives, University of Southern California Libraries.

69   A courtly figure: Bruce Kogan, email to author, May 13, 2013.

69   If I needed proof: Andy Humm, "Midtown Cops Go Berserk in Gay Bar," *NYN*, October 11–24, 1982.

70   It took place on: James E. D'Eramo, "A Night at the AIDS Forum," *NYN*, December 20–January 2, 1983.

71   In San Francisco: David Perlman, "Mystery of S. F. Baby with 'Gay' Disease," *SFC*, December 10, 1982; and Arthur Ammann, email to author, March 26, 2014.

71   He suffered an enlarged: Intv. Arthur Ammann, September 18, 2013.

71   Recently there had been a number: See *MMWR*, December 17, 1982.

71   "heterosexual non-Haitians": A. Ammann et al., "Epidemiologic Notes and Reports Possible Transfusion-Associated Acquired Immune Deficiency Syndrome (AIDS)—California," *MMWR*, December 10, 1982.

72   Dr. Selma Dritz, the specialist in charge: "Editorial Note," *MMWR*, December 10, 1982.

72   Jaffe was the CDC's: JC curriculum vitae, archived at the Centre for AIDS Interdisciplinary Research at Oxford, retrieved from cairo.ox.ac.uk.

72   "We should report this": Intv. Arthur Ammann, September 18, 2013.

73   His *MMWR* letter: Ammann et al., "Epidemiologic Notes and Reports Possible Transfusion-Associated Acquired Immune Deficiency Syndrome (AIDS)—California."

4. DOUBT ALL THINGS

74   In a gesture of pity: Intvs. JS, various; and for apartment descriptions, MC and RB audiotapes, various.

74   "Joe, you're a doctor": RB audiotape, "Conversation/Reminiscing—Callen March 11, 1993," transcribed by RB, MCA.

74   After one visit: Intv. HH, September 5, 2013.

74   By early 1983: RB audiotape transcript, "AC-1—Reg Cassette—Side A—1982," MCA.

74   The IRS was preparing: Intv. HH, September 5, 2013.

74   On his own initiative: MC audiotape, "91B: Telephone Conversation Between Michael and Richard (B.)," no date (probably December 1982), MCA, transcribed by author; and confirmed by intv. HH, September 5, 2013.

74   Hackett had worked: Intv. HH, September 5, 2013.

74   Now he had come: Ibid.

74   He poured half of it: HH, email to author, March 25, 2014.

74   One low afternoon: "91B: Telephone Conversation Between Michael and Richard (B.)."

74   Hackett's stoicism finally: Intv. HH, September 5, 2013.

75   Nearly nine hundred: LK, "Where Are We Now?," *GMHC Newsletter* (January 1983).

75   "You're losing faith": "91B: Telephone Conversation Between Michael and Richard (B.)."

75   A little while later: Anecdote from RB audiotape transcript, "9X . . . Side A TDK MICRO . . . Page 1 (Jan 83???)," MCA.

76   In fact, Berkowitz: Intv. RB, September 4, 2013.

76   He had admitted: RB audiotape, "90T—From the First Week of February 1983 Telephone Conversations," transcript by author, MCA.

77   We can "come up": RB audiotape transcript, "6X . . . Micro . . . (11/82?)," MCA.

77   "The advice has to be": RB audiotape transcript, "14X . . . Side B . . . Page 1," February 1983, MCA.

77   "They're predisposed": Ibid.

77   Even in bed: MC audiotape, "102T—Callen 12-13," undated, transcribed by author.

77   He often claimed: Intvs. RD, various.

77   "*You* gave me this": MC audiotape, "75T—Michael Moves to NY and Gets Sick," undated, transcript by author, MCA.

78   "Michael, this is part": Intv. RB, September 4, 2013.

78   "Take him a copy": Ibid.

78   And the next day: George de Stefano, email to author, September 24, 2015.

78   "I'm like: I'm going": Intv. RB, September 4, 2013.

78   "Callen/Berkowitz/Sonnabend": See MC and RB, unpublished letter, "Response to Attacks on We Know Who We Are," 1983.

78   "It's not just an article": Intv. RB, September 4, 2013.

78   Callen, fresh from: MC datebooks for February 4–13, 1983, RDA.

78   "We're the Trotskys": "90T—From the First Week of February 1983 Telephone Conversations."

79   The winter weather: Robert D. McFadden, "20-Inch Snowfall Paralyzes Much of Mid-Atlantic Area," *NYT,* February 13, 1983.

80   Larry Kramer jumped: GMHC Board Minutes from April 12, 1982, and May 10, 1982.

81   The newsletter came: See "The History of the Gay Men's Health Crisis, Inc.," GMHC Circus Program, April 30, 1983, RJGA.

81   They held a tense: Correspondence, Ferris Fain to LM, December 19, 1982, GMHCA.

81   Some fifty thousand copies: There were two printings of 25,000 each, per "The History of the Gay Men's Health Crisis, Inc."

82   "If this article doesn't": LK, "1,112 and Counting," *NYN,* March 14–27, 1983.

83   For months they had been seeking: See "The History of the Gay Men's Health Crisis, Inc."

83   He quit in a tantrum: GMHC Board of Directors Minutes, April 18, 1983: "LK was not present having tendered his resignation from the board of GMHC inc verbally to the president on April 14, 1983," GMHCA.

83   When that failed: Shilts, *And the Band Played On,* 309–10.

83   "We need fighters": LK, *Reports,* 65.

84   "You use the tactics": Correspondence, Nathan Fain to LK, May 27, 1983, Randy Shilts Collection, San Francisco Public Library.

84   Gaëtan Dugas felt: Intvs. AF-K, July 25, 2013, and September 5, 2013.

84   After rejecting: Shilts, *And the Band Played On,* 147, revealed the CDC's belief he had infected forty people in ten cities.

84   He made friends: Intv. Brandy Svendson, date unknown; and Guy Babineau, "Gaëtan Dugas and the 'AIDS Mary' myth," *Daily Xtra,* November 8, 2007.

84   His T-cell count: AF-K, email to author, March 25, 2014.

84   In his calculus: Shilts, *And the Band Played On,* 247.

84   The frigid evening: Videotape, transcript by author, in AIDS Vancouver archive.

85   He turned the microphone: Andrew Rosenthal, "Paul Popham, 45, a Founder of AIDS Organization, Dies," *NYT,* May 8, 1987.

86   Confounding matters further: Anthony S. Fauci, "The Acquired Immune Deficiency Syndrome: The Ever-Broadening Clinical Spectrum," *JAMA* 249, no. 17 (1983): 2375–76.

86   "Please, if you don't get": Intv. Brian Willoughby, date unknown.

87   "With Gaëtan you get": Harry Reasoner, "Patient Zero," *60 Minutes,* November 15, 1987, transcript by author.

87   He called Dugas: Shilts, *And The Band Played On,* 439.

87   "Randy didn't want to": Intv. Michael Denneny, January 22, 2014.

88   After more than: "The History of the Gay Men's Health Crisis, Inc."

88   Curran, his hands tied: Intv. JC, September 23, 2013.

88   Mel Rosen, the executive: Correspondence, RD to Mel Rosen, January 31, 1983, MCA.

88   Including back taxes: MC audiotape, "113 T—Callen B1 + B2," transcript by author, MCA; and confirmed by Hackett, email to author, March 25, 2014.

88   She, as chairwoman: Nussbaum, *Good Intentions,* 89–92.

89   Through the family: JS, email to author, July 17, 2013.

89   She proposed a salary: HH, email to author, March 25, 2014.

89   Within a few weeks: JS, email to author, March 25, 2014.

89   Upon his return: JS, email to author, July 16, 2013.

89   "Too embarrassing": Intv. JS, July 28, 2009.

89   "When I am asked": Intv. MK, March 25, 2011.

90   "the kingdom of the sick": Sontag, *Illness as Metaphor,* 3.

90   It took two years: David W. Dunlap, "Having Claimed 558 Lives, AIDS Finally Made It to the Front Page," *NYT,* October 30, 2014.

90   The progressive *Village Voice:* Stephen Harvey, "Defenseless: Learning to Live with AIDS," *VV,* December 21, 1982; and James Kinsella, *Covering the Plague: AIDS and the American Media* (New Brunswick: Rutgers University Press, 1989), 29.

90   I know he saw the first: NBC News did the first report, a brief piece on June 17, 1982, featuring BC images; CBS News followed with another brief BC report, on December 26, 1982. Geraldo Rivera's feature-length segment on ABC's *20/20* aired May 19, 1983.

91   The plaza was crowded: Lindsey Gruson, "1,500 Attend Central Park Memorial Service for AIDS Victim," *NYT,* June 14, 1983.

91   In New York, there were: Ronald Sullivan, "Cases of AIDS in City Increase at Slower Rate Than Was Predicted," *NYT,* June 28, 1983; and Guillén and Perrow, *The AIDS Disaster,* 29. Of 1,450 cases nationwide, 43 percent were in New York City.

91   In May, the paper: Ronald Sullivan, "Prison's Food Shunned After AIDS Victim's Death," *NYT,* May 13, 1983, and "Sanitation Man from the Bronx Contracts AIDS," *NYT,* May 19, 1983.

92   Dr. Robert Gallo: Intv. RG, January 13, 2011.

92   In this environment: Bayer and Oppenheimer, *AIDS Doctors,* 4.

92   In *The Betrothed:* Alessandro Manzoni, *The Betrothed* (London: Ward, Lock, and Co., 1889), 400.

92   In New York at: Jane Gross, "Funerals for AIDS Victims: Searching for Sensitivity," *NYT,* February 13, 1987.

92   Peter Staley got: Intv. PS, March 17, 2009.

94   "I don't know": Ibid.

94   "It's plain weird": Intv. Tracey Tannenbaum, date unknown.

5. A MAN REAPS WHAT HE SOWS

95   "superior tone": Charles Jurrist, letter to editor, *NYN*, December 6–19, 1982. Quoted in MC and RB, unpublished letter, "Response to Attacks on We Know Who We Are," 1983.

95   For lessons in influencing: Intv. RB, September 4, 2013.

95   "Stand up and take": RB audiotape, "90T—From the First Week of February 1983 Telephone Conversations," transcript by author, MCA.

95   "Safe sex requires": MC and RB, *How to Have Sex in an Epidemic: One Approach* (New York, NY: News from the Front Publications, 1983), 16.

96   "How do I know that?": "90T—From the First Week of February 1983 Telephone Conversations."

96   "I think most gay men": Intv. JS, July 28, 2009.

96   In 1981, even despite: John Martin et al., "The Impact of AIDS on a Gay Community: Changes in Sexual Behavior, Substance Abuse, and Mental Health," *American Journal of Community Psychology* 17 (1989): 269–93.

96   There was universal: N. Himes, *Medical History of Contraception* (New York, NY: Gamut Press Inc, 1963), 186–206.

97   "I tried the experiment": Lesley Smith, "The History of Contraception," in *Contraception: A Casebook from Menarche to Menopause*, ed. Paula Briggs and Gabor Kovacs (Cambridge: Cambridge University Press, 2013).

97   "If we prevent": Intv. JS, July 28, 2009.

97   "I have become": *Sexual Medicine Today* (September 1982), MCA.

97   "You've written how": There is a dispute of memories over the speaker of this line. The conversation is not captured on audiotape. It is often attributed to JS, who recalls saying it, but I have privileged RD's claim to authorship here.

97   "If people approach": RB audiotape transcript, "4x—(NOV?) 1982 . . . TDK Micro . . . ," MCA.

97   "Temperamentally, we must": Intv. JS, July 28, 2009.

98   Berkowitz called: "90T—From the First Week of February 1983 Telephone Conversations."

98   They managed to pull: MC 1982 tax returns, in MCA.

98   Just before Memorial Day: Canceled check, May 20, 1983, MCA.

98   "the gay historical tradition": MC and RB, unpublished letter, "Response to Attacks on We Know Who We Are," 1983.

98   A second printing: Various receipts in MCA.

98   And then, to their great: Jonathan Lieberson, "Anatomy of an Epidemic," *New York Review of Books*, August 18, 1983, 17–22.

99   A television news: Correspondence, Gero von Boehm letter to MC, October 18, 1983, MCA.

99   "It was a lucky": RB audiotape transcript, "Callen in P-town—August 7, 1993," MCA.

99   Unbeknownst to Callen: Rebecca Reinhardt, Facebook message to author, March 5, 2014.

99   "promulgate universal joy": Unsigned, "Who Are the Sisters?," retrieved from thesisters.org.

99   He was also a registered: Randy Alfred, radio broadcast, *The Gay Life*, January 10, 1982, transcript by author, the Gay, Lesbian, Bisexual, Transgender Historical Society.

99   "Wrap it up": Unsigned, "Play Fair!," date unknown, retrieved from www .thesisters.org.

100   Gonorrhea diagnoses: Institute of Medicine, National Academy of Sciences, *Mobilizing Against AIDS: The Unfinished Story of a Virus* (Cambridge, MA: Harvard University Press, 1986), 24; and LM, "Some Good News: VD Rates are Down," *NYN*, April 11–24, 1983.

100   By then, more than half: Ann Giudici Fettner, "The All American Disease," *NYN*, October 22–November 4, 1984, quotes JC saying that 60 to 90 percent of gay men were exposed; "Antibodies to a Retrovirus Etiologically Associated with Acquired Immunodeficiency Syndrome (AIDS) in Populations with Increased Incidence of the Syndrome," *MMWR*, July 13, 1984, 377–79, says that 65 percent of the patients at one SF STD clinic were gay men; an article in *Epidemiology*, November 1, 1985, puts the figure at 67 percent. See also Harold W. Jaffe, MD, et al., "The Acquired Immunodeficiency Syndrome in Gay Men," *Annals of Internal Medicine* 103, no. 5 (1985): 662–64.

100   "Hopelessness kills": MC, *Surviving*, 10.

100   The study of viruses: See Dorothy Crawford, *The Invisible Enemy: A Natural History of Viruses* (Oxford: Oxford University Press, 2003).

100   "places where vegetable": Marlin Gardner and Benjamin H. Aylworth, *The Domestic Physician and Family Assistant* (Bedford, MA: Applewood Books, 1936), 79–80.

100   In 1683, using a microscope: J. R. Porter, "Antony van Leeuwenhoek: Tercentenary of His Discovery of Bacteria," *Bacteriological Reviews* 40, no. 20 (1976): 260–69.

100   Then, in 1876: Crawford, *The Invisible Enemy*; and Michael Worobey et al., "Point, Counterpoint: The Evolution of Pathogenic Viruses and Their Human Hosts," *Annual Review of Ecology, Evolution, and Systematics* 38 (2007): 515–40.

101   "organisms at the edge of life": Edward Rybicki, "The Classification of Organisms at the Edge of Life *or* Problems with Virus Systematics," *South African Journal of Science* 86 (April 1990).

101   It wasn't until 1935: R. Hausmann, *To Grasp the Essence of Life: A History of Molecular Biology* (Dordrecht, Netherlands: Kluwer Academic Publishers, 2003), 58; and W. Stanley, "Isolation of a Crystalline Protein Possessing the Properties of Tobacco-Mosaic Virus," *Science* 81 (1935): 644–45.

101   The second half of: Erling Norrby, "Nobel Prizes and the Emerging Virus Concept," *Archives of Virology* 153, no. 6 (2008): 1109–23.

101   In the 1960s, retroviruses: RG, *Virus Hunting*, 60–61.

101   That changed in December: Ibid., 132.

101   The disease was extremely rare: Nichols, *Mobilizing*, 65.

101   Instead, he stayed busy: A. Araujo and W. W. Hall, "Human T-lymphotropic Virus Type II and Neurological Disease," *Annals of Neurology* 56, no. 1 (July 2004): 10–19.

102   There could be many: RG, *Virus Hunting,* 135.

102   Gallo left the meeting: Ibid., 137; and Victoria A. Harden, Dennis Rodrigues, and Robert Gallo, MD, "In Their Own Words, NIH Researchers Recall the Early Years of AIDS," August 25, 1994, November 4, 1994, and June 8, 1995, retrieved from history.nih.gov.

102   There were just 59: As of June 30, 1983, per P. Ebbesen, "AIDS in Europe," *British Medical Journal* 287 (November 5, 1983): 1324–26.

102   His work began: Arno, *Against the Odds,* 12.

102   Brugière, a gay man: Crewdson, *Science Fictions,* 44–47; and Luc Montagnier, "A History of HIV Discovery," *Science* 298, no. 5599 (November 29, 2002): 1727–28.

102   In early February: Crewdson, *Science Fictions,* 48; and Grmek, *History of AIDS,* 64–65.

103   They appeared to be: Montagnier, *Virus,* 51–52.

103   It seemed that LAV: Montagnier, "A History of HIV Discovery."

103   He invited Montagnier: This is Montagnier's version of this history, in Montagnier, *Virus,* 23–55. See also RG, *Virus Hunting;* and Nikolas Kontaratos, *Dissecting a Discovery* (self-published, 2006). Both RG and Kontaratos, a retired police officer he worked closely with investigating this history, allege that Montagnier's submission had already been rejected by *Nature* and by *Science,* and that RG was offering to help him publish after repeat rejection. *Dissecting* shows RG memos to *Science* promoting the piece, but they make no mention of a previous submission.

103   In his haste: Both men agree that the article arrived without a summary, but RG says he read the abstract over the telephone to Montagnier, admitting his command of English may have caused a misunderstanding. Intv. RG, July 5, 2016; and Steve Connor, "AIDS: Science Stands on Trial," *New Scientist,* February 12, 1987.

104   "Indeed, we were": Montagnier, *Virus,* 56.

104   Jim Monroe, a public: New York City Department of Health AIDS Surveillance, "The AIDS Epidemic in New York City, 1981–1984," *American Journal of Epidemiology* 123, no. 6 (1986): 1013–25.

104   "If AIDS was something": MC, "AIDS as an Identity."

104   "a threat as horrible": John Rechy, "An Exchange on AIDS," letter to the editor, *New York Review of Books,* October 13, 1983. He continued, "The danger of AIDS cannot, must not be minimized. Our entire lives are being judged and condemned by heterosexuals, by doctors who know absolutely nothing about us. Sexual acts are being condemned as producing AIDS— acts which have occurred since before the time of Christ. We are under assault because AIDS just happened to strike us first."

105   Thanks to his newfound prominence: MC, "Remarks of Michael Callen to the New York Congressional Delegation," May 10, 1983, RDA.

105   He sat at his IBM: Karlyn Bowman et al., "Polls on Attitudes on Homosexuality & Gay Marriage," American Enterprise Institute for Public Policy Research, March 2013, 82.

105   "This is way too": Intv. RD, September 27, 2013.

105   He smoothed a stack: MC was the second PWA to offer congressional

testimony, following BC on April 13, 1982, retrieved from waxman.house
.gov/sites/waxman.house.gov/files/Gay_Cancer_Focus_of_Hearing.pdf.

105   "On the whole": *Congressional Record,* no. 69, May 19, 1983; and MC,
"The Trauma of Living with AIDS," May 10, 1983, MCA.

107   Though GMHC declined: MC and Dan Turner, "A History of the People
With AIDS Self-Empowerment Movement," *Body Positive* (December
1997). Originally published in 1988 in the *Lesbian and Gay Health Education Foundation Program Booklet.*

107   Those attending: Arthur Felson and Michael Shernoff, "AIDS Groups
Find Solidarity in Denver," *NYN,* July 4–17, 1983.

107   Among them was Dan: Burt A. Folkart, "Dan Turner; Offered Hope to
Those with AIDS," *LAT,* June 6, 1990.

107   With him was Bobby: Bettinita Harris, "An AIDS Victim Faces His
Future," *St. Petersburg Independent,* June 27, 1983.

107   Campbell posted Polaroids: Intv. Cleve Jones, January 22, 2014.

108   "How California": MC, *Surviving AIDS,* 177.

108   "like the dancing": MC, "AIDS as an Identity."

109   When they typed: Karla Jay, *Tales of the Lavender Menace: A Memoir of
Liberation* (New York, NY: Basic Books, 200), 137.

110   For many of the assembled: Felson and Shernoff, "Aids Groups Find Solidarity in Denver."

110   Early one morning: Unknown TV news report, captured on MC audiotape, "102T—Callen 12-83," transcript by author, MCA.

110   The firm had learned: Michael Daly, "AIDS Anxiety," *New York,* June 20,
1983.

111   By mid-August: Associated Press, "Heat Eases in Northeast; Storms Bat-
ter Gulf Coast," *NYT,* August 10, 1983.

111   Peter Staley, who: Intvs. PS, various.

112   "The discussion now": Recalled by author.

112   It made the cover: "Gay American: Sex, Politics, and the Impact of AIDS,"
Newsweek, August 8, 1983.

112   This was just: Randy Shilts, *Conduct Unbecoming: Gays & Lesbians in the
U.S. Military* (New York, NY: Ballantine Books, 1994), 227.

112   The magazine included: Tome Morganthau et al., "Gay America in Transition," *Newsweek,* August 8, 1983.

113   He was now caring: "News Summary: Saturday, October 1, 1983," *NYT,*
October 1, 1983.

113   Somehow he had: JS sworn affidavit, MCA.

113   He didn't have: Robert Abrams, Attorney General, "Complaint," September 30, 1983, MCA; and "People of the State of New York v. 49 West 12
Tenants Corporation," September 28, 1983, MCA.

113   "Please be advised": Correspondence, 49 West 12 Tenants Corporation to
JS, August 18, 2013, MCA.

113   When Sonnabend bumped: JS, "Affidavit," MCA.

113   He was busy: "News Briefs," *NYN,* January 2–15, 1984.

113   Those patients, according: "Stipulation of FACTS, People of the State of
New York, Joseph Sonnabend, et al V 49 WEST 12 TENANTS CORPO-
RATION," October 4, 1983, MCA.

114   He even got the GMHC: GMHC board meeting minutes, September 28, 1983, GMHCA; and RM in GMHC Oral History Interview, undated, GMHCA.

114   "irrational prejudice": Philip Shenon, "A Move to Evict AIDS Physician Fought by State," *NYT*, October 1, 1983.

114   "I'm just—it's": MC audiotape, "100T—Save 95-232," transcript by author, MCA.

114   Bobbi Campbell spent: Intv. Patrick Haggerty, February 11, 2014.

114   He managed this: BC personal diary, "July 28, 1983—Volunteer Park Tower," UCSF.

114   On August 17: BC personal diary, "August 17, '83—Board Rm NYC Dept of Health," UCSF.

115   WE DID IT!: BC personal diaries, ibid. and "Wed Aug 17, 1983—Mike & Sal's," UCSF.

115   He had just: BC personal diary, "July 28, 1983—Volunteer Park Tower."

115   In early October: BC personal diary, "Sunday Oct 9, 83, SFO Onboard PSA," UCSF.

115   On October 7: Color snapshot of BC, October 7, 1983, UCSF.

116   "maximum awareness": "Sunday Oct 9, 83—SFO Onboard PSA."

117   Callen's temperature rose: MC audiotape, "102T Callen 12-83," transcript by author, MCA.

117   In their first months: Intvs. RD, various.

117   "Now," he said: "102T Callen 12-83."

PART 2: INCURABLE ROMANTICS

1. LIFE, APPARENTLY

122   In the thirty months: Shilts, *And the Band Played On*, 380. This was disputed by the EIK aid Herb Rickman, who, in a letter to editor, *NYN*, April 11–24, 1983, argued that the administration had assigned a full-time staff of physicians and medical paraprofessionals to search out new AIDS cases; trained ninety infection control practitioners and nurses to help recognize and treat AIDS cases; and helped the municipal hospitals train all its directors of ambulatory and clinical services to recognize and treat AIDS cases, all at a cost of about $500,000. In a published reply, LK pointed out that the AIDS spending represented "existing funds being shifted around." A review of the Koch Papers at La Guardia reveals only surveillance studies.

122   In the same time frame: Shilts, *And the Band Played On*, 400.

122   That gap was even more: Ibid.

122   But even this contract: Carol Raphael, letter to the editor, "NYC AIDS Update," *VV*, July 17, 1984.

122   Nobody there had bothered: Shilts, *And the Band Played On*, 380.

122   "scientists of New York City": Herb Rickman, letter to the editor, *NYN*, April 11–24, 1983.

122   He made an unannounced: EIK, letter to the editor, "Off-the-Cuff Coverage," *NYN*, May 23–June 5, 1983.

122   He wrote a letter: EIK, letter to the editor, *NYN*, July 4–17, 1983.

122   "How much more manly": LK, letter to editor, "Larry Kramer Responds," *NYN*, April 11–24, 1983.

123   In a first: LM, "City Opens Gay Health Office," *NYN*, March 28–April 10, 1983.

123   "unsympathetic to the": Larry Bush, "The Politics of '84—The Year Ahead Will Test Gay Clout and Community," *NYN*, February 13–26, 1984.

123   Every year since 1971: David France, "Memories of Underdevelopment: A Brief History of the Gay Rights Bill," *VV*, March 25, 1986.

123   That was in the summer: Maurice Carroll, "Council Defeats Homosexual Bill by 22-to-19 Vote," *NYT*, May 24, 1974.

123   They did this with: France, "Memories of Underdevelopment."

123   "affectional preference": Joyce Purnick, "Court Overrules Order by Koch on Sexual Bias," *NYT*, June 29, 1985.

124   "insane": Maurice Carroll, "Bias by City Against Homosexuals Is Banned by Koch," *NYT*, January 24, 1978.

124   Anita Bryant's anti-gay: Dudley Clendinen and Adam Nagourney, *Out for Good: The Struggle to Build a Gay Rights Movement in America* (New York, NY: Simon and Schuster, 1999), 292.

124   "Someone once said": Cynthia Crosson, letter to the editor, "Homosexuality on Campus," *NYT*, April 16, 1978.

124   Besides the AIDS: Edward A. Gargan, "Rights Issue Perils City–Salvation Army Pact," *NYT*, December 22, 1983.

124   affecting about 1,100: Michael Goodwin, "Salvation Army Losing City Pacts for Stand on Hiring Homosexuals," *NYT*, March 3, 1984.

124   Their contracts totaled: Ari L. Goldman, "Archdiocese Clarifies Story on O'Conner and Pope," *NYT*, July 11, 1984.

124   "It would be totally": Goodwin, "Salvation Army Losing City Pacts for Stand on Hiring Homosexuals."

125   Derek Peterson, one-third: Intv. Ray Nocera, May 22, 2014.

125   A freelance writer named: Intv. Tom Steele and intv. Patrick Merla, confirmed by Merla in email; RG confirmed his clips.

125   Canteloupe made it: Obituary, *NYN*, March 26–April 8, 1984; obituary, *NYN*, April 9–22, 1984.

125   Wednesday he was: Intv. Tom Steele, November 5, 2013.

125   He spent more time: Katie Leishman, "The Outsider," *Rolling Stone*, March 23, 1989.

126   He solicited an article: Richard B. Pearce, "Parasites and AIDS," *NYN*, August 29–September 11, 1983.

126   He ran news: James E. D'Eramo, "New Strategies on AIDS: A Workshop at NIH," *NYN*, September 26–October 9, 1983; James E. D'Eramo, "Notables Come Out for AIDS Symposium," *NYN*, April 25–May 8, 1983; and James E. D'Eramo, "Looking for the Breakthroughs: The Academy of Sciences Conference," *NYN*, December 5–18, 1983.

126   He jokingly referred: Chuck Ortleb, editorial, "An Open Letter to: Dr. James O. Mason, Director of the Centers for Disease Control, et al.," *NYN*, January 16–29, 1984.

126   Jane Teas, a young: James E. D'Eramo, "Is African Swine Fever Virus the Cause?," *NYN*, May 23–June 5, 1983.

126   She had no personal: Ibid.

126   But she found the casual: Jane Teas, "Could AIDS Agent Be a New Variant of African Swine Fever Virus?," *Lancet* 321, no. 8330 (April 23, 1983): 923; also D'Eramo, "Is African Swine Fever Virus the Cause?"

127   Among the "Marielitos": Ethan Bronner, "Camp Personnel Deny Report of 20,000 Gay Refugees," *Miami Herald*, July 8, 1980; and "Cuba 1988," Voice of America–Radio Marti Program, Office of Research and Policy, United States Information Agency, 312.

127   "aliens afflicted with": The Immigration Act of 1917 excluded individuals from entering the United States who were found "mentally defective" or who had a "constitutional psychopathic inferiority," language that was used by the Public Health Service to denote gay people. The language changed in the 1952 Immigration and Nationality Act to include "aliens afflicted with a psychopathic personality, epilepsy, or a mental defect," but to clear up any potential confusion about where homosexuals stood, in 1965 Congress added "sexual deviation" as a cause for exclusion. See Margot Canaday, *The Straight State: Sexuality and Citizenship in Twentieth-Century America* (Princeton, NJ: Princeton University Press, 2009).

127   "an unequivocable": See Susana Peña, "'Obvious Gays' and the State Gaze: Cuban Gay Visibility and U.S. Immigration Policy During the 1980 Mariel Boatlift," *Journal of the History of Sexuality* 16, no. 3 (July 2007): 507, 510, and 512. According to "Cuban Refugees' Status Clarified by Immigration Service," a 1985 press release from the National Gay Task Force, the policy mutated in 1980 to state that only individuals making two affirmative declarations would be excluded; a 1985 clarification stated, "No alien will be considered ineligible for adjustment of status on the basis of sexual preference unless he/she makes or has made for the record an unequivocable [sic], unambiguous declaration that he/she is a homosexual."

127   "connect dots very easily": Leishman, "The Outsider."

127   James D'Eramo, who: James D'Eramo, email to author, October 18, 2013.

127   "a most uncommon": D'Eramo, "Is African Swine Fever Virus the Cause?"

127   They invited Teas: Intv. Tom Steele, November 5, 2013.

128   Not everybody was so: Jane Teas, "An AIDS Odyssey," *NYN*, December 17–30, 1984.

128   "It was like being": Ibid.

128   Three weeks after: J. Colaert et al., "African Swine Fever Virus Antibody Not Found in AIDS Patients," *Lancet* 321, no. 8333 (May 14, 1983): 1098.

128   "managed to set up": Teas, "An AIDS Odyssey."

128   "As a veterinarian said": Ibid.

128   Though they had only: BC journal, "1835, Saturday December 31, '83—Our House."; and BC journal, "0915, Wednesday, December 14, 1983—Our House."

128   It was the first: BC journal, "1030, Friday Dec 2, 1983—Our House."

128   They were complementary: BC journal, "1444, Tuesday Aug 30, '83—My Room" and "9099, Thursday Dec 22, 1983—Our House."

128   "You or a close friend": Archived in Box 1, Folder 2, MMS 96-33, Campbell Collection, UCSF Library & Center for Knowledge Management Archives & Special Collections Department; and BC journal, "1050, Wednesday Nov. 16, '83—Our House," "Two year anniversary of chemo! And I feel sickly."

128   They spent New Year's: BC journal, "0800, Tuesday Jan 3, 1984—Our House."

129   The chemo sapped: BC journal, "1000, Thursday Jan 19, 1983—Our House."

129   He spent his days: BC journal, "1300, Thursday January 26, '84—Our House" and "1015, Wednesday Dec 21, 1983—Our House."

129   But before the deviled: BC journal, "2315, Sunday January 29, 84—Our House."

129   Congress was hardly better: Intv. Tim Westmoreland, April 29, 2014.

129   On a dark Friday: MC audiotape "#109T," MCA, transcript by author.

129   His latest CD4: Ibid.

130   But a few months: James E. D'Eramo, "Informational Lightning Rod: The Office of Gay and Lesbian Health Concerns," *NYN*, November 21–December 4, 1983.

130   And it was true: Ibid. Enlow reveals that his budget is $120,000, and he mostly gives testimony.

130   He was given: D'Eramo, "Informational Lightning Rod."

130   "I'd like to see": Peg Byron and Steven C. Arvanette, "New York Shocked by Proposed S.F. Bath Ban," *NYN*, April 9–22, 1984.

131   show of unity: Ibid.

131   Enlow's coalition had: Draft text approved by GMHC, "11 Risk Reduction Guidelines for Healthier Sex."

131   He reached Enlow: "#109T."

132   In the end: Ibid.

132   On February 27: Robert Moroney, "State Grants $600,000 for AIDS Services," *NYN*, March 26–April 8, 1984.

133   Just the previous Sunday: The *60 Minutes* segment, called "Helen," first broadcast in February 1984, revealed that a three-year-old child born with AIDS had been held in quarantine since birth.

133   Lawmakers in Connecticut: George DeStefano, "Connecticut Assembly to Consider Quarantine Law," *NYN*, April 9–22, 1984.

133   "An Act Concerning": MC audiotape, "Panasonic," transcript by author, MCA.

134   it was a daily struggle: RB audiotape transcript, "Panasonic Microcassette—Side 1," MCA.

134   On another day: RB audiotape transcript, "SONY—60 Microcassette," MCA.

134   "Keep working out": "Panasonic Microcassette—Side 1."

134   But Berkowitz ditched: RB, emails to author, December 21, 2013, and January 18, 2014.

134   Despondent, Callen: Michael Paule, "GMHC, SIECUS Confer on Health," *NYN*, May 7–20, 1984.

134   "How fittingly ironic": MC correspondence ("personal & confidential") to "David," August 8, 1984, MCA.

134   Despite his efforts: Intvs. JS, 2008–2015, various.

2 . PARANOID FANTASIES

135   Chuck Ortleb came: James D'Eramo, email to author, October 18, 2013.

135   I was editing: Peg Byron and Steven C. Arvanette, "New York Shocked by Proposed S.F. Bath Ban," *NYN*, April 9–22, 1984.

135   Dr. James Mason: James D'Eramo, email to author, October 18, 2013.

136   Mason, a bishop: "Elder James O. Mason," official biography on the Church of Jesus Christ of Latter-Day Saints, retrieved from ldschurch-news.com; and James Mason, "Attitudes of the Church of Jesus Christ of Latter-Day Saints Toward Certain Medical Problems," in *Health and Medicine Among the Latter-Day Saints: Science, Sense, and Scripture*, ed. Lester E. Bush (New York, NY: Crossroad, 1993).

136   The church's anti-homosexual: Bush, ed., *Health and Medicine Among the Latter-Day Saints*, 173–74.

136   In fact, it was: Shilts, *And the Band Played On*, 399.

136   To his credit: *NYN*, January 2–15, 1984.

136   But any diplomatic: Shilts, *And the Band Played On*, 399.

136   He compounded: *NYN*, January 2–15, 1984.

136   As obstacles go: Letter from EIK to David Sencer, December 10, 1984, scolding him for ignoring queries from Councilman Joe Lisa.

136   In defending this: Lawrence K. Altman, "Fewer AIDS Cases Filed at End of 83," *NYT*, January 6, 1984.

136   AIDS, he decreed: Shilts, *And the Band Played On*, 310.

136   Mason and Sencer: Thomas Steele, "CDC Director Says Announcement of AIDS Case Is Forthcoming," *NYN*, April 8–22, 1984.

136   His voice was gentle: Ibid.

137   Mason said the Institut: Crewdson, *Science Fictions*, 98.

137   They had done so: Ibid., 91.

137   At the completion: Intv. JC, September 23, 2013.

137   They found LAV: Crewdson, *Science Fictions*, 106.

137   "This lead is": James E. D'Eramo, "Federal Health Officials Announce Cause of AIDS," *NYN*, May 7–20, 1984.

138   Given the stakes: For these statistics, see Shilts, *And the Band Played On*, 445.

138   "He was trying": James Kinsella, *Covering the Plague: AIDS and the American Media* (New Brunswick, NJ: Rutgers University Press, 1989), 42.

138   Lawrence Altman: Intv. Lawrence Altman, July 9, 2016.

138   He was impervious: Intvs. AF-K, July 25, 2013, and September 5, 2013.

138   "You haven't responded": Ibid.

138   "Federal Official Says": Lawrence K. Altman, "Federal Official Says He Believes Cause of AIDS Has Been Found," *NYT*, April 22, 1984.

139   But Gallo explained: Ibid.

139   None of this: Intv. JC, September 23, 2013; Montagnier, *Virus*, 68; and Crewdson, *Science Fictions*, 117–18.

139   He gave few: Montagnier, *Virus*, 68.

139   but bluntly declared: See ibid., 68, and RG, *Virus Hunting*, 189.

139   What's more, Gallo: Per RG, *Virus Hunting*, 190: The Pasteur team had developed a test, but they had trouble studying it because they had not been able to grow HIV in a cell line.

139   Gallo called his findings: Ibid., 188–90.

140   The French team: Montagnier, *Virus*, 68.

140   Gallo left the meeting: RG, *Virus Hunter*, 191.

140   "Today we add": Transcribed in "The following is the text of the statement made by Secretary of Health and Human Services Margaret Heckler, at a press conference concerning the cause of AIDS, held in Washington, D.C. on Monday, April 23, 1983," *NYN*, May 7–20, 1984.

141   In doing so: Crewdson, *Science Fictions*, 134.

141   "We are pleased": D'Eramo, "Federal Health Officials Announce Cause of AIDS," spelling corrected.

141   Gallo applied for: Patent Application Number PCT/US1985/000762, databased by Google, priority date April 23, 1984.

141   One, Cambridge Bioscience: Charles L. Ortleb, "Who Owns HTLV-3?," *NYN*, May 7–20, 1984.

141   And while he: J. A. Sonnabend and S. Saadoun, "HTLV-III and AIDS: What Does a Positive Test Mean?," *NYN*, September 24–October 7, 1984.

142   In a few weeks: Ann Giudici Fettner, "The Gazelle Paradigm," *NYN*, November 5–18, 1984.

142   "It takes much more": Email from JS, January 17, 2014.

142   "I watch all these things": Intv. JS, November 15, 2013.

142   "It's a huge stretch": From memory of author.

142   "You have to read this": Ibid.

143   The book, *Bad Blood*: James H. Jones, *Bad Blood: The Tuskegee Syphilis Experiment* (New York, NY: Free Press, 1981).

143   "Some of the same people": From memory of author.

143   When the study: Jones, *Bad Blood*, 193–98.

143   "They did it to": From memory of author.

143   "We're getting all": Intv. Ray Nocera, February 8, 2014.

143   "They *did* this to us": From memory of author.

143   He gave up eating: Intv. Tom Steele, November 5, 2013.

144   "Last night after Francis": From memory of author.

144   Shortly after sunrise: Email from PS, January 22, 2014.

145   This morning, as every: Intv. Lou Olivieri, January 13, 2014.

145   Acoustically, the trading: Intvs. PS, various.

146   Staley sat on: Ibid.

146   Even his older brother: Intv. PS, January 26, 2011.

147   Their desks were patched: Intv. Lou Olivieri, January 13, 2014.

148   In time, he wasn't: Donal Henahan, "Opera: Leontyne Price's Final Stage Performance," *NYT*, January 4, 1985.

148   This morning was like: August 16 or August 17, 1984, based on performance schedule for Huey Lewis.

148   "Huey Lewis": Intvs. PS, various.

150   "They have no idea": From memory of author.

150   I learned that he slid: Intv. Frances Chapman, February 16, 2014.

150   and it took him: There was no obituary, but he published a letter to the editor, *NYN*, December 1986.

152   Bobbi Campbell and: Randy Alfred, reports on Gay Life Radio, September 16 and 23, 1984.

152   On a gusty afternoon: David Lamble, "The National March: Chipping Away at Invisibility," *San Francisco Sentinel*, July 20, 1984.

152   "I have a message": "BC Speech (1984)," videotape archives of the GLBT Historical Society in San Francisco, retrieved from youtube.com, transcript by author.

153   A few days later: Intv. Cleve Jones, January 22, 2014.

153   "How many of this": Original in Michael Callen Papers, dated August 13, 1984; returned to sender, envelope stamped "NO LONGER HERE."

153   But Campbell never: Robert Campbell Sr. eulogy of BC, August 17, 1984, in "Bobbi Campbell Speech (1984)"; and intv. Robert Campbell Sr., February 14, 2014.

153   At precisely noon: Obituary, "Bobbi Campbell," *Gay Community News*, September 8, 1984.

153   Soon a sea of grief: Ibid.

154   "I have a message": Randy Alfred, reports on Gay Life Radio, September 16 and 23, 1984.

154   "It's important for us": Ibid.

154   Using conservative estimates: Estimating that 5 percent of the 1984 population total of 230 million were gay men.

154   I carefully smoothed: BC, untitled letter to the editor, *NYN*, September 10–23, 1984.

155   Nationally, the community's: Michael Callen, "Mike Goes to the Baths," unpublished and undated 1984 manuscript.

155   Management at St. Mark's: Jane Gross, "Bathhouses Reflect AIDS Concerns," *NYT*, October 14, 1985.

155   In the months since: Email from Richard Berkowitz, February 22, 2014.

155   "I won't dignify": Callen, "Mike Goes to the Baths."

155   When pressed, GMHC: Unsigned, "GMHC Update," *NYN*, June 18–July 1, 1984.

155   In fact, GMHC held: Per advertisement in *NYN*, June 18–July 1, 1984.

156   "I know it's not good": Transcript titled "Gallo Interview," from Ann Giudicci Fettner Papers, no date.

158   Late one night: MC audiotape, "Tape 116, Telephone Conversation Between Michael & Larry About Baths," MCA, transcript by author.

158   By July, three: Glenn Collins, "Impact of AIDS: Patterns of Homosexual Life Changing," *NYT*, July 22, 1985.

158   By October, Callen: MC, "Remarks of Michael Callen to the Annual Meeting of the American Public Health Association," Las Vegas, Nevada, 1986, MCUA.

159   Until recently: Thomas J. Jueck, "The Search for Herpes Drugs," *NYT,* May 26, 1983.

160   "There in the largest": MC, "Remarks of Michael Callen to the Annual Meeting of the American Public Health Association," Las Vegas, Nevada, 1986, MCUA.

160   The acyclovir did: MC datebook, RDA.

160   though not well enough: Ibid.

160   Regrettably, he canceled: Ibid.

160   Public Health Director: Matthew Crews, "S.F. Bathhouses Defy Closure Order: Health Dept. Expected to Seek Court Injunction, *NYN,* October 22–November 4, 1984.

160   Dr. Paul Cameron: "National News," *NYN,* November 5–18, 1984: "Fed Up Sex Expert Charges . . . Gays Are Worse Than Murderers," *Weekly World News* (October 1984).

160   In fact, in twenty-three states: Kevin Sack, "Georgia's High Court Voids Sodomy Law," *NYT,* November 24, 1998.

160   Even Mayor Ed Koch: David France, "Mayor Opposes Bathhouse Closure, Supports Gay Rights," *NYN,* June 17–30, 1985.

161   "Bathhouses don't cause": Editorial, "I Left My Towel in San Francisco," *NYN,* April 23–May 6, 1984.

161   Under his liberal: Honor Moore, "The Bishop's Daughter," *New Yorker,* March 3, 2008.

161   In response to: James E. D'Eramo, "Is African Kaposi's Sarcoma the Same as AIDS?," *NYN,* April 9–22, 1984.

161   But on the train ride: MC audiotape, "#111, Conv. About Politics, Rothenberg, Race, About Native," MCA, transcript by author.

161   This was all Callen: Ibid.

162   "Peter, I really": Ibid.

162   Though he now: Ibid.

162   After a year: Patrick Merla, "A Normal Heart: The Larry Kramer Story," in Mass, ed., *We Must Love One Another,* 42–44.

162   "I'd had two": Merla, "A Normal Heart," 44.

162   Callen found Kramer's: MC audiotape, "Tape 116, Telephone Conv. Between Michael + Larry About Baths."

3 . TESTING LIMITS

165   On a muggy August: David France, "Court Battle Begins on EO 50," *NYN,* August 27–September 9, 1984.

165   As the parties spilled: Ibid.

166   In late September: David France, "Court Declares Executive Order Banning Anti-Gay Discrimination Illegal," *NYN,* September 24, 1984.

167   Koch slumped imperiously: Ibid.

167   "What is outrageous": EIK, letter to the editor, *NYN,* January 28–February 10, 1985.

168   That December: Originally quoted in Jon Cohen, *Shots in the Dark: The Wayward Search for an AIDS Vaccine* (New York, NY: W. W. Norton and Company, 2001), 2–3, 15.

168   "What does the president": All quotes from Chip Brown, "Lester Kinsolving: Raising Cain in the Press Corps," *WP,* November 17, 1981.

168   That last part was: See Kathleen Kinsolving, *Gadfly: The Life and Times of Les Kinsolving—White House Watchdog* (New York, NY: WND Books, 2010).

169   With 7,699 reported: "Acquired Immunodeficiency Syndrome (AIDS) Weekly Surveillance Report—United States AIDS Activity," Center for Infectious Diseases, Centers for Disease Control, December 31, 1984.

169   As promised, Gallo: RG, *Virus Hunting,* 209; Shilts, *And the Band Played On,* 497; and Omar Sattaur, "How Gallo Got Credit for AIDS Discovery," *New Scientist,* February 7, 1985.

169   The French lab: Steve Connor, "AIDS: Science Stands on Trial," *New Scientist,* February 12, 1987.

169   "AIDS-associated": Shilts, *And the Band Played On,* 452.

169   The genomes: Crewdson, correcting Shilts, in *Science Fictions,* 588.

170   This was wholly: Montagnier, *Virus,* 77.

170   Still, such a coincidence: John Crewdson, "The Great AIDS Quest," *Chicago Tribune,* November 19, 1989.

170   As a result, their: RG, *Virus Hunting,* 177–79.

170   Nearly two years: Videotape of seminar for media hosted by the AIDS Medical Foundation, February 8, 1985, Randy Shilts Papers, James C. Hormel Gay and Lesbian Center, San Francisco Public Library, transcript by author.

170   To help clear: John C. Beldekas, "Face to Face: The Media and AIDS," *NYN,* February 25–March 10, 1985.

171   "I am therefore": Videotape of seminar for media hosted by the AIDS Medical Foundation, February 8, 1985.

171   Callen was equally: Intv. HH, February 12, 2014.

171   "He has something": Both quotes from RB audiotape transcript, "Callen in P-town—August 7, 1993," MCA.

171   "What has been": Ibid.

171   The hints were just: Ibid. RC amplifies his role, inaudible on the videotape.

172   "It was like dominoes": Ibid.

172   In a move that: Crewdson, *Science Fictions,* 18.

172   Somehow he managed: RG, *Virus Hunting,* 209.

173   "This rivalry stands": Videotape of seminar for media hosted by the AIDS Medical Foundation.

173   The whole matter: W. Rozenbaum, "Antimoniotungstate (HPA23) Treatment of Three Patients with AIDS and One Prodrome," *Lancet* 323, no. 8426 (February 23, 1985): 450–51.

173   Sonnabend personally: Email from Sonnabend, January 24, 2014.

173   The epidemic found: Brian Vastag, "Samuel Broder, MD, Reflects on the 30th Anniversary of the National Cancer Act," *JAMA,* December 19, 2001.

174   In his years of: Intv. Sam Broder, August 15, 2010.

174   The fact that the patient: Ibid.

174   But Broder's tiny: Victoria A. Harden, *AIDS at 30: A History* (Washington, DC: Potomac Books, 2012), 130; and "In Their Own Words: NIH

Researchers Recall the Early Years of AIDS," oral history interview of Sam Broder, conducted by Victoria Harden and Caroline Hannaway, February 2, 1997.

174   But late in the summer: "In Their Own Words: NIH Researchers Recall the Early Years of AIDS," oral history interview of Robert Yarchoan, conducted by Victoria Harden and Caroline Hannaway, April 3, 1998.

174   Excited by the results: Ibid.

175   Twelve patients: A. M. Levine et al., "Suramin Antiviral Therapy in the Acquired Immunodeficiency Syndrome," *Annals of Internal Medicine* 105, no. 1 (1986): 32–37.

175   When the study: All details in "In Their Own Words," April 3, 1998.

175   The only firm willing: "In Their Own Words," February 2, 1997.

175   Citing fear of contagion: Intv. Sam Broder, August 15, 2010.

175   His colleagues were: "In Their Own Words," February 2, 1997.

175   He had cultivated: Philip J. Hilts, "Experimental Drug AZT Was Designed for Tumors; Skill, Luck Led to Promising Tests on AIDS," *WP*, September 19, 1986.

176   For the next several: All details in "In Their Own Words," April 3, 1998.

176   "Everybody and their brother": Intv. Sam Broder, August 15, 2010.

176   The widespread use: George W. Rutherford et al., "The Epidemiology of AIDS-Related Kaposi's Sarcoma in San Francisco," *Journal of Infectious Diseases* 159, no. 3 (March 1989): 569–72.

176   Coming in third: B. S. Peters et al., "Changing Disease Patterns in Patients with AIDS in a Referral Centre in the United Kingdom: The Changing Face of AIDS," *British Medical Journal* 302, no. 6770 (January 26, 1991): 203–07; and Stephen D. Nightingale et al., "Incidence of *Mycobacterium Avium-Intracellulare* Complex Bacteremia in Human Immunodeficiency Virus-Positive Patients," *Journal of Infectious Diseases* 165, no. 6 (June 1992): 1082–85.

177   The story went: MC audiotape, "100T—Save 95-232," MCA, transcript by author.

177   "I'm their enemy": Ibid.

177   Finally, lawyers for: From the AG's formal complaint, MCA.

177   Conceding that their: Peter Frieberg, "N.Y. Doctor Granted New Lease in AIDS Eviction Case," *Advocate*, November 27, 1984.

177   Sonnabend was naturally: RB audiotape, "Tape 125," MCA, transcript by author.

177   "I haven't been": Ibid.

178   "What's going on": Ibid.

178   Through the winter: Intv. Sam Broder, August 15, 2010.

178   One morning in mid-February: *Burroughs Wellcome Co., Plaintiff-Appellee, v. Barr Laboratories, Inc., Defendant-Appellant, and Novopharm, Inc. and Novopharm, Ltd., Defendants-Appellants,* U.S. Court of Appeals, Federal Circuit, November 22, 1994; and "In Their Own Words," April 3, 1998.

178   It was as if: Philip J. Hilts, "Experimental Drug AZT Was Designed for Tumors; Skill, Luck Led to Promising Tests on AIDS," *WP*, September 19, 1986.

179   Unfortunately, it worked: Ibid.

179   Failure in the drug: Intv. Sam Broder, August 15, 2010.

179   Broder called Burroughs: *Burroughs Wellcome v. Barr Laboratories.*

179   At that time: Untitled chart, *NYN*, March 11–24, 1985.

179   The pharmaceutical giant: *Burroughs Wellcome v. Barr Laboratories.*

179   After Broder's call: Ibid.

180   In the summer of 1985: "In Their Own Words," April 3, 1998.

180   Yarchoan enrolled nineteen: Ibid.

180   The first patient: Ibid.

180   He was a furniture: per Mark Yarchoan, "The Story of AZT: Partnership and Conflict," thesis published on the website for Office of Medical and Scientific Justice, ca 2010.and ibid.

180   Yarchoan and Broder: "In Their Own Words," April 3, 1998.

180   He did not: Ibid.

180   Neither doctor could: Ibid.

180   At the end: Ibid.

180   But this turnaround: Ibid.

180   Over that time: Ibid.

180   "Not only were": Ibid.

180   "This is something": Ibid.

180   He began the study: Ibid.

181   A third patient: Ibid.

181   To Yarchoan: Ibid.

181   But he was excited: Ibid.

181   Broder called Burroughs: *Burroughs Wellcome v. Barr Laboratories.*

181   Many were gay: LM, email to author, March 8, 2014.

182   "Who are you?": LK, *Normal Heart,* 22.

182   Ned Weeks denounced: Ibid., 55.

182   "an awful sissy,": Ibid., 84.

182   The GMHC: Ibid., 78.

183   Audience members who: In Intv. LK, February 7, 2017, argues that Felix Turner is based on a real person who died in 1982, who has never been named because of "promises I made to him and legal problems created by his wife."

183   "Please learn": Ibid., 116.

183   "Don't lose that": Ibid., 117.

183   As a piece of art: See, for example, David Schechter, "'Hannah Senesh': Compelling Play About a Heroic Young Woman," *Christian Science Monitor,* April 29, 1985.

184   "My sexuality is": David France, "Koch Attends Gay Synagogue Benefit," *NYN,* June 17, 1985.

184   "It seems to me": Ibid.

184   By summer: Ronald Sullivan, "Approval of Blood Donor Test for AIDS Antibody is Expected," *NYT,* March 2, 1985; and David France, "Federal Gov't Allots $12 Million for Alternate HTLV-III Sites," *NYN,* March 25–April 7, 1985.

184   Handbills were passed: Sullivan, "Approval of Blood Donor Test for AIDS Antibody Is Expected."

184   as demonstrated in: Ann Giudici Fettner, "Blood Test 'Unacceptably' Inaccurate," *NYN*, July 1–14, 1985.

184   Their blood could: Ibid.

185   Equally troubling: Robert Pear, "AIDS Blood Test to Be Available in 2 to 6 Weeks," *NYT*, March 3, 1985; Sullivan, "Approval of Blood Donor Test for AIDS Antibody Is Expected."

185   Based on this percentage: David France, "HTLV-III Test Licensing Postponed: Controversy Over Effects of Test Reaches New Heights," *NYN*, February 25–March 10, 1985.

185   Considering that to date: Pear, "AIDS Blood Test to Be Available in 2 to 6 Weeks."

185   "Statistically," according: Matt Clark, "AIDS: The Blood-Bank Scare," *Newsweek*, January 28, 1985.

185   The New York State: Chuck Ortleb, "Politics of AIDS," *NYN*, February 25–March 10, 1985.

185   "To put it simply": Stephen S. Caiazza, "Why You Should Not Be Tested for HTLV-III," *NYN*, October 8–21, 1984.

185   Eighty percent of gay: L. McKusick, "AIDS and Sexual Behavior Reported by Gay Men in San Francisco," *American Journal of Public Health* 75, no. 5 (May 1985): 493–96.

185   They cut the average: Matthew Stadler, ed., "Study Finds Gay Men Have Decreased Sexual Activity," *NYN*, June 3–16, 1985; and ibid.

186   For this reason: Caiazza, "Why You Should Not Be Tested for HTLV-III."

186   Police officers in: Unsigned, "News Briefs," *NYN*, January 28–February 10, 1985.

186   Proposals for detention: Stuart Taylor Jr., "Supreme Court Hears Case on Homosexual Rights," *NYT*, April 1, 1986.

186   Atlanta's Metropolitan Vice Squad: Alexander Wallace, "Two Atlanta Bathhouses Closed by Vice Squad: Gay Groups Protest, but Most Gays Apathetic," *NYN*, February 25–March 10, 1985.

186   In Gainesville, Florida: David France, "Dumped AIDS Patient Dies in San Francisco," *Gay Community News*, November 5, 1983.

186   State health officials: Editorial, "Get Ready Folks. Especially in California," *NYN*, January 28–February 10, 1985.

186   This surprising news: Brian Jones, "Feds Quarantine Foreign Gays from Pacific Seaboard States," *NYN*, February 11–24, 1985.

186   "such extreme measures": David Talbot and Larry Bush, "At Risk," *Mother Jones* (April 1985).

187   The National Gay Task Force: Unsigned, "NGTF, AIDS Service Organizations Say Don't Take HTLV-III Test," *NYN*, January 28–February 10, 1985.

187   We were incensed: David France, "Federal Gov't Allots $12 Million for Alternate HTLV-III Sites," *NYN*, March 25–April 7, 1985; $60 million for blood bank: Sullivan, "Approval of Blood Donor Test for AIDS Antibody Is Expected."

187   which FDA commissioner: Pear, "AIDS Blood Test to Be Available in 2 to 6 Weeks."

187   For the eight million: Matthew Stadler, ed., "Reagan 1986 Budget Cuts AIDS Funding by $10 Million," *NYN*, February 25–March 10, 1985.

187   "This is a pernicious": Caiazza, "Why You Should Not be Tested for HTLV-III."

188   He did little to: Marianne Goldstein, "Stunned Friends Pray for Screen Idol," *NYP*, July 24, 1985.

189   "Just what *is*": Sue Simmons, "News 4 New York," WNBC, July 25, 1985.

189   He had raced: Ibid.

189   while there he took: Ibid.

189   We had also wished: Larry Bush, "First Blood: A Modest Proposal," *NYN*, July 1, 1985.

189   We prayed for: Unsigned, "DOCTORS: ROCK HAS AIDS," *NYP*, July 25, 1985.

189   The crush of reporters: Rock Hudson and Sara Davidson, *Rock Hudson: His Story* (New York, NY: William Morrow & Co, 1986), 30–31.

189   After a pause: Ibid.

189   His team produced: Ibid.

189   "Mr. Rock Hudson": Unsigned, "DOCTORS: ROCK HAS AIDS."

190   Reporters flew to Paris: Joe Nicholson, "New AIDS Rx May be Here Soon," *NYP*, July 26, 1985.

190   In the limelight: Ibid.

190   Without breaking his: Ransdell Pierson, "Federal Funding on AIDS Zooms," *NYP*, October 3, 1985.

190   "Associating his name": David France, "Rock Hudson: The Human Face of AIDS," *NYN*, August 12-25, 1985.

190   "Three of my close": Aljean Harmetz, "Hollywood Turns Out for AIDS Benefit," *NYT*, September 20, 1985.

191   "I felt it was": Ibid.

191   On September 17: Unsigned, "More H'wood Stars Dying of AIDS—Doc," *NYP*, August 2, 1985.

191   after the disease: Pat Wiles, "AIDS Now a Top Killer in NYC Men," *NYP*, August 18, 1985.

191   It came during: Count by author.

191   "I have been": Unsigned, "President's News Conference on Foreign and Domestic Issues," *NYT*, September 18, 1985.

192   next twenty-six days: Joy Cook, "Extra: Rock Hudson Dies," *NYP*, October 2, 1985.

192   Thereafter, he retired: Hudson and Davidson, *Rock Hudson*, 11.

192   "I am not happy": Stan W. Metzler, "AIDS-sufferer Rock Hudson, in a Message to Fellow Actors . . . ," UPI, September 20, 1985.

192   Only a few weeks: Jack Shermerhorn and Amy Pagnozzi, "Champagne and Caviar for His Friends at Funeral," *NYP*, October 3, 1985.

192   On a humid summer: AF, email to author, June 6, 2014; "In Their Own Words: NIH Researchers Recall the Early Years of AIDS," oral history interview of James C. Hill, conducted by Victoria Harden, October 4, 1988.

192   Wearing his trademark: "In Their Own Words: NIH Researchers Recall the Early Years of AIDS," oral history interview of AF, conducted by Vic-

toria Harden, DeWitt Stetten Jr., and Dennis Rodrigues, June 29, 1993. Context confirmed: AF, email to author, May 27, 2014.

192   Mike Goldrich was: AF, email to to author, May 27, 2014.

192   Sitting beside him: Ibid.

192   Fauci and his wife: Ibid.

192   When Fauci was: Ibid.

193   "You need to": Ibid.

193   "Jim, I knew": Ibid.

193   Reagan and Congress: Ransdell Pierson, "Federal Funding on AIDS Zooms," *NYP*, October 3, 1985.

193   More than $130 million: "In Their Own Words: NIH Researchers Recall the Early Years of AIDS," oral history interview of James C. Hill, conducted by Victoria Harden, October 4, 1988; AF, email with author, May 27, 2014.

193   Lowering his brow: AF, email with author, May 27, 2014.

193   "What could happen": "In Their Own Words: NIH Researchers Recall the Early Years of AIDS," oral history interview of James C. Hill, conducted by Victoria Harden, October 4, 1988; AF, email with author, May 27, 2014.

193   If they did: Ibid.

193   Fauci had considered: AF, email with author, May 27, 2014.

193   "I do not think": "In Their Own Words: NIH Researchers Recall the Early Years of AIDS," oral history interview of AF, conducted by Victoria Harden, DeWitt Stetten Jr., and Dennis Rodrigues, June 29, 1993. Context confirmed: AF, email to author, May 27, 2014.

194   Some of the younger: AF, email with author, May 27, 2014.

194   "Do you think": "In Their Own Words: NIH Researchers Recall the Early Years of AIDS," oral history interview of AF, conducted by Victoria Harden, DeWitt Stetten Jr., and Dennis Rodrigues, June 29, 1993.

194   He admitted he: Ibid.

194   "Brandt was very": Ibid.

194   In the coming days: AF, email with author, May 27, 2014.

194   The National Cancer: Ibid.

195   "It's much more": Intv. PS, February 4, 2014.

195   she often spent: Ibid.

195   They were "sisters.": Intv. Tracey Tanenbaum, undated.

196   "I'm like a nun": Ibid.

196   Homosexuality had: See, for instance: A. X. van Naerssen, ed., *Interdisciplinary Research on Homosexuality in the Netherlands* (New York, NY: Haworth Press, 1987).

196   the oldest gay bar: Intv. Peter Launy, March 13, 2012.

196   They were inseparable: Intv. Peter Launy, March 13, 2012.

196   His flight took Launy: Peter Launy, email to author, January 18, 2014.

197   He finally answered: Joe Nicholson, "Confessions of a Closeted Newspaperman," *NYN*, December 29–January 8, 1981.

197   Once he left the closet: Intv. Joe Nicholson, undated.

198   He once joined: Doug Ireland, "Rendezvous in the Ramble," *New York*, July 24, 1978.

198   "Tell me, Father": Intv. Joe Nicholson, undated.

198   Shilts, Zonana, and: Sam Howe Verhovek, "Responding to Gay Concerns, 10 on Council Abstain on Vote," *NYT*, September 11, 1987.

198   Papers across the: Dudley Clendinen and Adam Nagourney, *Out for Good* (New York, NY: Touchstone, 1999), 484.

198   In 1985, twenty states: Abigail Trafford and Gordon Witkin, "The Politics of AIDS: A Tale of Two States," *U.S. News & World Report*, November 18, 1985.

198   San Antonio's health: Ibid.

198   The mayoral race: Ibid.

199   By fall, the first: *Congressional Record*, 131 Cong Rec H 7984, House, October 1, 1985.

199   It had become perfectly: Clendinen and Nagourney, *Out for Good*, 521.

199   Terror-stricken students: Dirk Johnson, "Ryan White Dies of AIDS at 18," *NYT*, April 9, 1990.

199   Vandals broke: Jack Friedman and Bill Shaw, "Amazing Grace," *People*, May 30, 1988.

199   To Ray Kerrison: Ray Kerrison, "Finding an AIDS Scapegoat's Unfair," *NYP*, Sept 16, 1985.

200   He buckled on a towel: Richard Esposito, "The Case for Closing Bathhouses: Night Visit by *Post* Reporter Reveals Shocking Evidence," *NYP*, October 31, 1985.

200   When the weather cooled: Jack Peritz, "Rebel School Board Bigs Blast Move to Enroll AIDS Kids," September 5, 1985.

200   Next the paper: Joyce Purnick, "Koch Won't Put AIDS Patients in Queens Site," *NYT*, September 4, 1985.

201   "There is only": Unsigned editorial, "AIDS Kids Don't Belong in School," *NYP*, September 3, 1985.

201   The *Los Angeles Times*: Carol McGraw, "AIDS Epidemic; Trauma in the Gay Community," *LAT*, November 13, 1985.

201   "The silence only": Unsigned, "Gay Anti-Defamation League Formed," *NYN*, November 11–17, 1985.

201   They threatened legal: John A. Fall, "Gay and Lesbian Anti-Defamation League Changes Name," *NYN*, January 26–February 6, 1986.

201   More than seven hundred: John A. Fall, "The New Stonewall?," *NYN*, November 25, 1985.

201   It was the most: Ibid.

202   "Many of us had": Darrell Yates Rist, "No More Lies!," *NYN*, December 16, 1985.

205   She kept a great: John A. Fall, "Anti-Defamation League Zaps *New York Post*," *NYN*, December 16, 1985; and Barry Adkins, "Gays at the Post," *NYN*, January 20–26, 1986.

205   Richard Berkowitz returned: RB, email to author, January 18, 2014.

205   He thought of himself: Will Grega, *Will Grega's Gay Music Guide* (New York, NY: Pop Front Press, 1994), retrieved from michaelcallen.com.

205   who returned to: MC datebook, RDA.

206   "Maybe the men": Samir Hachem, "Rock 'n' Roll Lowlife with a Gay Conscience," *Advocate*, October 30, 1984.

206   The group was a marvel: MC datebook, RDA.

206   followed by a stretch: Ibid.

206   Finally taking his: Hachem, "Rock 'n' Roll Lowlife with a Gay Conscience."

206   He interspersed: RD, emails to author, various.

206   Their reputation spread: MC, "Mike Goes to the Baths: Notes for a Piece Never Written," undated, retrieved from michaelcallen.com.

206   He bowed to peer: MC datebook, RDA.

206   National Gay Task Force: Ibid.

206   and the Bathhouse: MC, "Mike Goes to the Baths."

207   His somewhat unexpected: From RB ad in *The Advocate*, undated, RBA.

207   Some 34 million: David Zurawik, "HBO's 'Normal Heart' is an extraordinary TV movie," *Baltimore Sun*, May 23, 2014; and Rodney Buxton, "An Early Frost," retrieved from museum.tv, the Museum of Broadcast Communications, no date.

207   The network lost: Edward Wyatt, "A Show That Trumpeted History but Led to Confusion," *NYT*, September 18, 2006.

208   It had become: Intv. Peter Launy, March 13, 2012.

208   A week-long vacation: Ibid.

208   Staley had not been: Intvs. PS, various.

208   And the end: Ibid.

208   Coincidentally, among: Ibid.

208   "AIDS: The Latest": John Langone, "AIDS: Special Report," *Discover*, December 1985.

208   "AIDS is incurable": Ibid., 31.

209   Sitting on the king-sized bed: Intv. PS, July 19, 2011.

209   The following Tuesday: Ibid.

209   Dr. William explained: PS spreadsheet showing his CD4 count on November 15, 1985.

209   well below a normal: Intv. PS, July 19, 2011.

209   It would be weeks: Ibid.

209   There now were: Untitled chart, *NYN*, December 9–15, 1985.

209   The virus Gallo: RG, *Virus Hunting*, 210.

210   Within the year: Crewdson, *Science Fictions*, 255.

210   Government policy: Ronald Reagan, "Executive Order 12591—Facilitating Access to Science and Technology," April 10, 1987, online by Gerhard Peters and John T. Woolley, the American Presidency Project, retrieved from presidency.ucsb.edu.

210   The second of these: RG, *Virus Hunting*, 209–10.

210   "The dinner was light": All above, ibid., 209.

210   Jacob, speaking: Per Crewdson, *Science Fictions*, 198.

210   If the matter landed: RG, *Virus Hunting*, 209–10.

210   He felt that: Ibid., 209.

210   Of little consequence: Crewdson, *Science Fictions*, 220.

210   Gallo returned home: RG, *Virus Hunting*, 211.

211   "I must impress": John Crewdson, "The Great AIDS Quest," *Chicago Tribune*, November 19, 1989.

211   In December, legal papers: RG, *Virus Hunting*, 211.

4 . WARFARE

212   One patient: "In Their Own Words: NIH Researchers Recall the Early Years of AIDS," oral history interview of Robert Yarchoan, conducted by Victoria Harden and Caroline Hannaway, April 3, 1998.

212   By January 1986: Ibid.

212   It meant that neither: Erik Eckholm, "Should the Rules Be Bent in an Epidemic?," *NYT,* July 13, 1986.

213   Two hundred and fifty: Ibid.

213   would be recruited: "In Their Own Words: NIH Researchers Recall the Early Years of AIDS," oral history interview of Robert Yarchoan, conducted by Victoria Harden and Caroline Hannaway, April 3, 1998.

213   in San Deigo: M. A. Fischl et al., "The Efficacy of Azidothymidine (AZT) in the Treatment of Patients with AIDS and AIDS-Related Complex," *NEJM* 317, no. 4 (July 1987): 185–91.

213   The point person: Elinor Burkett, "The Queen of AZT," *Miami Herald,* September, 23, 1990.

213   with a fierce intelligence: Ibid.

213   She had authored: M. A. Fischl et al., "Tuberculous Brain Abscess and Toxoplasma Encephalitis in a Patient with the Acquired Immunodeficiency Syndrome," *JAMA* 253, no. 23 (1985): 3428–30.

213   Her training was: Margaret A. Fischl "Biographical Sketch," submitted with research application, undated.

213   "God have mercy": Intv. Samuel Broder, August 15, 2010.

213   His arguments were: Bruce Nussbaum, *Good Intentions,* 137.

213   "Do we have the right": Eckholm, "Should the Rules Be Bent in an Epidemic?"

214   The Burroughs Wellcome: "In Their Own Words: NIH Researchers Recall the Early Years of AIDS," oral history interview of Robert Yarchoan, conducted by Victoria Harden and Caroline Hannaway, April 3, 1998.

214   The FDA agreed: Fischl et al., "The Efficacy of Azidothymidine," 185–91.

214   This was the high: Nussbaum, *Good Intentions,* 151.

214   It had many fans: Anne-Christine d'Adesky, "AIDS Treatment: A Guide to Antivirals and Immune Boosters," *NYN,* January 6–12, 1986.

214   The belated U.S. trials: Ibid.

214   Early studies were: Ibid.

214   It was AZT: Ann Guidici Fettner, "The Promise of Compound S," *NYN,* April 14, 1986.

214   Five years into: Montagnier, *Virus,* 81.

214   of eminent scientists: Ibid.

214   It was an American: Ibid.

214   or HIV, and: Steven Epstein, *Impure Science: AIDS, Activism, and the Politics of Knowledge* (Berkeley: University of California Press, 1996), 77.

214   Montagnier and the: Montagnier, *Virus,* 81.

215   Though he had no vote: Ibid.; and Crewdson, *Science Fictions,* 236.

215   As the body count: 15,948 at the end of 1985, per CDC surveillance web page.

215   In his own defense: Intv. RG, July 5, 2016

215   Finally, in February: Crewdson, *Science Fictions*, 226–28.

215   But the distributors: Ibid.

215   The CDC would soon: In mid-June 1986.

215   one confirmed case: Crewdson, *Science Fictions*, 252–53.

215   For their part: Intv. RG, July 5, 2016

215   Kids were removed: Alex Michelini and Mike Santangelo, "Fate of AIDS Pupils Weighed," (New York) *Daily News*, August 28, 1985.

216   Its peculiar physical: Mirko D. Grmek, *History of AIDS: Emergence and Origin of a Modern Pandemic* (Princeton: Princeton University Press, 1990), 77.

216   Nothing like this: Ibid., 77.

216   "the arguments stale": RG, *Virus Hunting*, 213.

216   After all that: Crewdson, *Science Fictions*, 382.

216   "Around here we say": Ibid., 329.

216   Dr. Broder: John Crewdson, "Even Outside of Science, Robert Gallo Is a Celebrity," *Chicago Tribune*, November 19, 1989.

216   Whether this was: Crewdson, *Science Fictions*, 382.

216   They identified a second: See Lawrence K. Altman, "Third AIDS Virus Found in Sweden," *NYT*, November 20, 1986.

216   where HIV-2: Erik Eckholm, "Heterosexuals and AIDS: The Concern Is Growing," *NYT*, October 28, 1986; and Thomas C. Quinn, Jonathan M. Mann, James W. Curran, and Peter Piot, "AIDS in Africa: An Epidemiologic Paradigm," *Science*, November 21, 1986, 955.

217   In the fifth year: John Fall, "Reagan Slashes AIDS Funding," *NYN*, March 3, 1986.

217   "offensive . . . to a majority": Robert D. McFadden, "Judge Overturns U.S. Rule Blocking 'Offensive' Educational Material on AIDS," *NYT*, May 12, 1992.

218   When William F. Buckley: Joseph Sobran, "The Politics of AIDS," *The National Review*, May 23, 1986.

218   and demanding that its: Intv. BB, March 26, 2011.

218   "It becomes a little": Ibid.

218   Though admitting that: Barry Adkins, "Battle for 'Gay Rights Bill' Begins in City" and "City Desk," *NYN*, January 27–February 1, 1986.

218   Jewish: Editorial, "Homosexuals' Rights Need Protection," *NYT*, January 24, 1986.

218   and Protestant leaders: Editorial, "The Christian Disease Center (CDC)," *NYN*, May 19, 1986.

218   Thereafter, the *Native*: Ibid.

219   The first fifty people: Guy Trebay, "Voice Vote: The Gay Rights Bill Takes the Floor," *VV*, April 1, 1986.

219   "I am opposed": Ibid.

219   "Nothing makes me": Ibid.

219   The longest-debated: David France, "Memories of Underdevelopment: A Brief History of the Gay Rights Bill," *VV*, March 25, 1986.

219   Victory, limned with: Rolf Sjogren, email to author, December 4, 2015.

219   "Soon after the gay": Ray Kerrison, "Closet? Heck, They're All over the House!," *NYP*, March 22, 1986.

223   Vacations in Tahiti: Intv. Peter Launy, March 13, 2012.

223   The best Japanese: Ibid.

223   The fact was: Ibid.

224   Learning he was: Ibid.

224   He withdrew physically: Ibid.

224   Staley thought they: Ibid.

224   Back at J. P. Morgan: Intv. PS, March 3, 2009.

224   He could see it: Intv. Peter Launy, March 13, 2012.

224   Finally, in late April: PS credit card statement, April 1986, PS emails to author, various.

224   Staley packed up: Intv. PS, March 3, 2009.

224   Then an unpredictable: Ibid.

224   Staley was given: Intv. Peter Launy, March 13, 2012.

224   He loved the UK: Ibid.

224   Germany and France: Ibid.

224   Flummoxed and increasingly: Intv. PS, March 3, 2009.

224   They certainly could not: Intv. Peter Launy, March 13, 2012.

224   "I'm going to": Ibid.; and intv. PS, March 3, 2009.

225   "But, Peter, what": Intv. Peter Launy, March 13, 2012.

225   For only the second: Intv. PS, March 3, 2009.

225   When he got: Intv. Peter Launy, March 13, 2012.

225   a few weeks later: PS credit card statement, in PS emails to author; and intv. Peter Launy, March 13, 2012.

225   Gallo arrived late: Crewdson, *Science Fictions*, 248–49.

225   So was Lowell Harmison: Ibid.

226   There at the table: Ibid., 249. Montagnier said the source of the money was "not really said in proper words."

226   It was now: Ibid., 44; and Arno, *Against the Odds*, 12.

226   In the early 1950s: See Debbie Bookchin and Jim Schumacher, *The Virus and the Vaccine* (New York, NY: Macmillan, 2004); and David M. Oshinsky, *Polio: An American Story* (Oxford: Oxford University Press, 2005).

226   These were grave: Correspondence, Jonas Salk to President Ronald Reagan, November 6, 1986.

226   He invited: Crewdson, *Science Fictions*, 288–89.

226   Numerous Nobel Prize: Jonas Salk, correspondence to President Ronald Reagan, November 6, 1986, included letters forwarded from David Baltimore, Paul Berg, Renato Dulbecco, Robert Holley, Salvador Luria, Daniel Nathans, Howard Termin, Lewis Thomas, and Rosalyn Yallow.

226   It did little good: Jonas Salk, correspondence to James Watson, February 19, 1987.

226   Montagnier and Gallo: Robert C. Gallo et al., "First Isolation of HTLV-III," *Nature* 321, no. 6066 (May 1986): 119–20. RG claims to have isolated the AIDS virus in December 1982, three months before Pasteur isolated LAV from BRU.

227   Privately, Salk called: Crewdson, *Science Fictions*, 295.

227 In the following year: Michael Specter, "U.S., France Settle AIDS-Study Feud; Credit for Virus' Discovery to Be Shared by Two Labs," *WP*, April 1, 1987.

227 Like weary parents: Marlene Cimons and James Gerstenzang, "U.S., France to End Legal Dispute, Share in Patent Rights for AIDS Test," *LAT*, April 1, 1987.

227 Their unseemly squabble: Andy Coghlan, "Was Robert Gallo Robbed of the Nobel Prize?," *New Scientist*, December 16, 2008.

227 Koch signed it: Heritage of Pride Records, LGBT Community Center National History Archive, retrieved from gaycenter.org/community/archive/collection/086.

227 Up in front: RD, email to author, February 6, 2016.

227 He now knew: RD, emails to author, various.

228 Dworkin and Callen: MC, quoted in "Lowlife, 'Where the Boys Are,' at an Outdoor Concert During NYC Gay Pride 1986," a videotape by Nelson Sullivan, retrieved from 5ninthavenueproject's YouTube channel.

228 They called this: Intv. BB, March 26, 2011.

228 In one memorable: Unsigned, "The Advocate and the Academy," AIDS Clinical Trials Group Network, undated, retrieved from actgnetwork.org.

229 Included were the: Per phone call with Bahlman, they were: David Axelrad, William F. Buckley, Paul Cameron, Noach Dear, Jerry Falwell, Adolph Hitler, Lyndon LaRouche, Yehuda Levin, Rupert Murdoch, Eddie Murphy, Cardinal O'Connor, Pat Robertson, and Donna Summer.

229 "It doesn't matter": Unsigned, "The Advocate and the Academy."

229 "We are on": BB, email to author, May 24, 2014.

229 The march barely: Larry Rohter, "Marchers Laud City's New Law Prohibiting Bias," *NYT*, June 30, 1986.

229 Some thirty thousand: Robert D. McFadden, "Nation Rekindles Statue of Liberty as Beacon of Hope," *NYT*, July 4, 1986.

229 Police officers in: Martin Garbus, *Courting Disaster: The Supreme Court and the Unmaking of American Law* (New York, NY: Times Books, Henry Holt and Company, 2002), 111.

229 named Michael Hardwick: Unsigned, "Arrest in Man's Home Began Test of Georgia Law," *UPI*, July 1, 1986.

229 Police took both: From *Bowers v. Hardwick*, June 30, 1986; Justice White opinion retrieved from law.cornell.edu.

229 As the case: Unsigned, "Arrest in Man's Home Began Test of Georgia Law."

230 "a heinous act": From *Bowers v. Hardwick*, June 30, 1986; Justice White opinion retrieved from law.cornell.edu.

230 A friend with: BB intv. by Sarah Schulman, AUOHP, March 10, 2010.

230 "Sheridan Square": Ibid.

230 Well over a thousand: Ibid.

230 including Michael Callen: Intv. RD, various.

230 The police, perhaps: BB intv. by Sarah Schulman, AUOHP, March 10, 2010.

230 The sit-in lasted: Ibid.

230   Bahlman felt a: Ibid.

231   "That's appalling": Intv. RD, May 29, 2013.

231   "Did you hear": John H. Bunzel, "Hope's Joke," letter to the editor, *LAT,* July 30, 1986.

231   There was a scattering: Ibid.

231   After the first: John Rhodes, "A Miracle of Miracles," (New York) *Daily News*, March 29, 1987.

231   "What We All Want": Anonymous, "Publisher," *NYN,* December 29, 1986.

232   During June: Originally T4, but changed here and throughout this letter for consistency.

233   Those who could: JS, "Data Sheet for Persons Interested in AL 721," JSNYP.

233   The *Native*'s anonymous: JS, email to author, April 14, 2014.

233   a chorus and orchestra: Rhodes, "A Miracle of Miracles."

233   The compound was: Bruce Nussbaum, *Good Intentions*, 49.

233   under the guidance: M. Lyte and M. Shinitzky, "A Special Lipid Mixture for Membrane Fluidization," *Biochimica et Biophysica Acta—Biomembranes* 812, no. 1 (1985): 133–38, retrieved from sciencedirect.com.

233   His interest was in: Ibid.; Unsigned, "AL 721: Experimental AIDS Treatment," *Documentation of AIDS Issues and Research Foundation* (April 1986), retrieved from AIDS.org.

234   But in vitro: Lyte and Shinitzky, "A Special Lipid Mixture for Membrane Fluidization."

234   This led one: Nussbaum, *Good Intentions*, 51.

234   Their idea was: Ibid., 54.

234   He noted positive: See P. S. Sarin et al., "Effects of a Novel Compound (al 721) on HTLV-III Infectivity in Vitro," *NEJM*, November 14, 1985.

234   but was unable: Nussbaum, *Good Intentions*, 62.

234   His story was: John James, "AL721—Experimental AIDS Treatment," *AIDS Treatment News*, April 11, 1986.

234   Callen found a: Intv. JS, July 28, 2009.

234   Sonnabend and Callen: Intv. JS, July 28, 2009; and David Meiren and Gregg Bordowitz, directors, *PWAHG: AL 721,* perf. by Michael Callen and Thomas Hannan, PWAHG, 1987. DVD.

235   But she reluctantly: Intv. Tracey Tanenbaum, undated.

235   After work one: Per PS datebook, PSA.

235   "I'm not ashamed": PS emails to author, various.

235   "If folks freak out": Ibid.

235   Staley was mesmerized: Ibid.

235   In Gold, he saw: Intv. PS, March 3, 2009.

235   "Everybody in the room": Intv. PS, March 3, 2009.

235   Gold crinkled his: Photos in Michael Lesser personal archives.

236   "I've got money": Intv. PS, March 3, 2009.

236   Within a week: PS emails to author, various.

236   One day in November: BB, Marty Robinson, and Henry Yaeger, "Conversation," December 13 (probably 1987), transcript in BBA, 3.

236   None of the panelists: Editorial, "Don't Panic, Yet, Over AIDS," *NYT*, November 7, 1986.

236   "Well over fifteen": Unsigned, "The Lavender Hill News," *Newsletter of the Lavender Hill Mob* (January 1987).

237   Gold, who knew: Intv. PS, March 3, 2009.

237   "Think of me as": Ibid.

237   The AZT Phase II: Fischl et al., "The Efficacy of Azidothymidine."

237   Most were turned: D. Richman et al., "The Toxicity of Azidothymidine (AZT) in the Treatment of Patients with AIDS and AIDS-Related Complex," *NEJM* 317 (July 1987): 192–97.

237   Others were excluded: Medical Officer Review of NDA 19-655; Date Submitted: Dec 2, 1986; Date Rec'd: Dec 3, 1986; MOR Completed: March 9, 1987.

237   Slightly more than: Fischl et al., "The Efficacy of Azidothymidine"; and JS, "Review of AZT Multicenter Trial Data," self-published, October 1987, retrieved from AIDSPerspective.net. The number of patients taking AZT was 144, with 137 on placebo.

237   One of the first: Cohn's participation in the study is author's conclusion based on analysis of multiple sources, but unconfirmed by any of his doctors. See, e.g., Nicholas von Hoffman, "The Snarling Death of Roy M. Cohn," *Life* (March 1988).

237   "There's nothing more": Author has surmised that the patient Broder discussed, in Intv. Samuel Broder, August 15, 2010, was Cohn; Broder declined to reveal the identity of this (or any) patient, describing him only as "famous."

238   "faster and better": Medical Officer Review of NDA 19-655.

238   Even when five: "In Their Own Words: NIH Researchers Recall the Early Years of AIDS," oral history interview of Samuel Broder, conducted by Victoria Harden and Caroline Hannaway, February 2, 1997.

238   Nearly half the people: Richman et al., "The Toxicity of Azidothymidine."

238   Fischl's view: Burkett, "The Queen of AZT."

238   Patients on AZT: Richman et al., "The Toxicity of Azidothymidine."

238   A handful withdrew: Fischl et al., "The Efficacy of Azidothymidine."

238   When they checked: Medical Officer Review of NDA 19-655.

238   Two more died: Ibid.

238   Their proposal presented: Ibid.

239   "We must stop: "In Their Own Words: NIH Researchers Recall the Early Years of AIDS," oral history interview of Samuel Broder, conducted by Victoria Harden and Caroline Hannaway, February 2, 1997.

239   The death toll: Nussbaum, *Good Intentions*, 158–59.

239   The drug was no: Fischl et al., "The Efficacy of Azidothymidine."

239   "There really is": Barry Adkins, "AZT Available to 6500 AIDS Sufferers," *NYN*, October 13, 1986.

239   She took the restraints: James H. Kim and Anthony R. Scialli, "Thalidomide: The Tragedy of Birth Defects and the Effective Treatment of Disease," *Journal of Toxocological Sciences* 122, no. 1 (2011): 1–6.

239   Cooper's predecessor: Ibid.

239   But on December: Medical Officer Review of NDA 19-655.

240   By its own estimate: Erik Eckholm, "Test Group for AIDS Drug Is Broadened to Include 7,000," *NYT*, October 1, 1986.

240   Concerned that lives: Intv. Ellen Cooper, October 1, 2010; and see Mark Carl Rom, "Gays and AIDS: Democratizing Disease," in *The Politics of Gay Rights*, ed. Craig A. Rimmerman, Kenneth D. Wald, and Clyde Wilcox (Chicago: University of Chicago Press, 2000).

240   The news touched off: Nussbaum, *Good Intentions*, 156.

240   On the first weekend: AP, "Thousands Ask About AZT Treatment," *Boston Globe,* September 23, 1986; and see Eve Nichols, *Expanding Access to Investigational Therapies for HIV Infection and AIDS* (Washington, D.C.: National Academy Press, 1991).

240   Cooper still had: Intv. Ellen Cooper, October 1, 2010.

241   "The main thing": Leo Tolstoy, *Sevastopol Sketches,* trans. David McDuff (London: Penguin Classics, 1986) (originally published as *Sevastopol in December* [1855], *Sevastopol in May* [1855], and *Sevastopol in August* [1856]), 45-46.

242   Officially, the National: *Report on Carcinogens,* 13th ed. (Research Triangle Park, NC: U.S. Department of Health and Human Services, Public Health Service, 2014).

244   Three thousand of these: Avram Finkelstein intv. by Sarah Schulman, AUOHP, January 23, 2010.

244   For a full month: Ibid.

PART 3 : AN OUNCE OF PREVENTION

1. THE BARRICADES, 1987

247   On those afternoons: Michael Shnayerson, "Kramer vs. Kramer," *Vanity Fair* (October 1992).

247   His stage play: Don Shewey, "Theatre; AIDS on Stage: Comfort, Sorrow, Anger," *NYT,* June 21, 1987.

248   The organization's budget: Krishna Stone, email to author, September 2, 2014.

248   The volunteer army: Ibid.

248   "separate and individual": LK, *Reports,* 135.

248   "the great unwashed radicals": Ned Weeks in LK, *The Normal Heart,* 25.

248   "I think it must": LK, *Reports,* 103.

248   "Get off your fucking": Ibid., 102.

248   Her hilarious novel: Mervyn Rothstein, "Hollywood and Literature: An Uneasy Romance," *NYT,* July 13, 1986.

249   "an adamant and abrasive": Darrell Yates Rist, "Antibody-Testing Wars," *NYN,* March 16, 1987.

249   "Auschwitz on the Hudson": Intv. Michael Petrelis, April 22, 2014.

249   Kramer came to: Ibid.

249   "Bring people": Ibid.

249   Sawyer had recently: Intv. Eric Sawyer, March 19, 2012.

249   "I'm going to try": Ibid.

250   Someone placed a: Bradley Ball, "It Started with Nora Ephron," unpublished manuscript about the origins of ACT UP, Bradley Ball Papers, New York Public Library.

250   I later learned: Charlotte Kidd, "Forum for Aids Center Has a Sheen," *PI*, September 28, 1988.

250   "If my speech tonight": LK, *Reports*, 127–36.

251   The current executive: Bradley Ball, intv. by Ron Goldberg, June 19, 1994, RJGA.

251   Earlier in the month: Ibid.

251   Dressed as Nazi: Michael Petrelis, email to author, May 1, 2014; and untitled and unsigned history of ACT UP, distributed at ACT UP meetings, RJGA.

251   As conservative as: Bradley Ball, intv. by Ron Goldberg, June 19, 1994, RJGA.

251   Next, the film historian: Ibid.

251   The author of: Ibid.

252   Consensus formed around: ACT UP Meeting Minutes, March 12, 1987, Bradley Ball Papers, New York Public Library.

252   Almost 350 people: Mike Salinas, "Kramer, Mob, Others Call for Traffic Blockade," *NYN*, March 30, 1987; Ball, "It Started with Nora Ephron."

252   Chuck Ortleb was there: Untitled and unsigned history of ACT UP, distributed at ACT UP meetings, RJGA.

252   So were Andy Humm: Avram Finkelstein, intv. by Sarah Schulman, AUOHP, January 23, 2010.

252   He revealed that he: Ibid.

252   In the interest: Untitled and unsigned history of ACT UP, distributed at ACT UP meetings, RJGA.

252   "It's not about": Bradley Ball, letter to Donald Luxton, April 3, 1987, Bradley Ball Papers, New York Public Library.

252   The first item: ACT UP Meeting Minutes, March 3, 1987, RJGA.

252   Specific actions were: Ibid.

253   conversation pivoted to: Intv. Vivian Shapiro, April 30, 2014.

253   But the group: ACT UP Meeting Minutes, March 3, 1987, RJGA.

254   "When abstraction sets": Albert Camus, *The Plague; The Fall; Exile and the Kingdom and Selected Essays* (New York, NY: Everyman's Library, distributed by Random House, 2004), 79.

254   Six hundred people: Untitled and unsigned history of ACT UP, distributed at ACT UP meetings, RJGA.

254   Larry Kramer arrived: Bradley Ball, intv. by Ron Goldberg, June 19, 1994, RJGA.

254   The posters were handsomely: Ibid.

254   "FDA, YOU SLAY ME": Videotape of Wall Street demonstration, March 24, 1987, filmmaker unknown, author's transcript.

254   He took one: Bradley Ball, intv. by Ron Goldberg, June 19, 1994, RJGA.

254   Banks of cameras: Untitled and unsigned history of ACT UP, collected at ACT UP meetings, RJGA.

254   It was a story: Ibid.

254   "Why is the FDA": "Why We Are Angry," flyer distributed at Wall Street demonstration, March 24, 1987, RJGA.

254   "There is no question": LK, "The FDA's Callous Response to AIDS," *NYT*, March 23, 1987.

255   It sparked an: PS email to author, May 6, 2014.

255   "Well, if you ask me": Intv. PS August 5, 2010.

255   He leaned deeply: Intv. PS, August 5, 2010.

255   Sonnabend studied the: JS, "Remembering The Original AZT Trial," *POZ*, January 29, 2011.

255   What Sonnabend wanted: Nussbaum, *Good Intentions*, 246.

255   Mathilde Krim put: MK, correspondence with AF, May 4, 1987.

256   "moral thing": Nussbaum, *Good Intentions*, 247.

256   Once he had full: Ibid., 248.

256   "If you don't": Ibid., 247.

256   Then one frigid: Ibid., 245.

256   They spoke to: Intv. Claire Klepner, October 8, 2015.

256   But it was even more: Nussbaum, *Good Intentions*, 249.

257   Besides struggling to: Ibid., 250.

257   Between his duties: MC datebook, 1987.

257   Callen was also: Intv. RD, April 18, 2014; Nussbaum, *Good Intentions*, 250; and MC datebook, January 8–12, 1987.

257   In between: For example, MC attended Michael Calvert's memorial, January 7, 1987, MC datebook; MC visited sick patients Wednesday, April 15, 1987, MC datebook; and RD, email to author, July 8, 2014.

257   And then there was: MC datebook, January–April, 1987.

257   "walker": John Tierny, "The Big City: The Sound of Non-Music," *NYT Magazine*, March 13, 1994.

257   Someone at the union: Intv. RD, April 18, 2014.

257   Another leadership role: Bruce Nussbaum, *Good Intentions*, 250.

257   But as a favor: MC, undated draft of a speech, MCA.

258   "Who could sue": Nussbaum, *Good Intentions*, 251.

258   Thereafter, they might: MC, undated draft of a speech, MCA.

258   Word spread quickly: Videotape of the People With AIDS Health Group press conference, May 4, 1987, TTLN, transcript by author; and "Remarks of Michael Callen, PWA Health Group, May 4, 1987," JSNYP.

258   People from Texas: MC, undated draft of a speech, MCA; and videotape of the People With AIDS Health Group press conference, May 4, 1987, TTLN, transcript by author.

258   More than five hundred: Nussbaum, *Good Intentions*, 251.

258   "Please do this": MC, undated draft of a speech, MCA.

258   As spring approached: MC datebook, April 13, 1987.

258   Still wary: MC, Undated draft of a speech, MCA.

258   Not only did: "Howard Moody Obituary: Howard R. Moody, Influential Minister-Activist, 91," retrieved from judson.org/howard-moody-obituary.

258   The substance arrived: Intv. RD, April 18, 2014.

259   Over strenuous objections: MC, undated draft of a speech, MCA; JS sent the original back to the company, JS, email to author, October 9, 2015.

259   Reporters shot looks: MC, undated draft of a speech, MCA.

259   The next morning: Ibid.

259   A friendly *New York Times*: Ibid.

259   It was two more: MC datebook, April 24, 1987, RDA; "Adam Laboratory Report, April 29, 1987," MCA; and ibid.

259   A distribution was: MC datebook, April 24, 1987; and MC, "Remarks of Michael Callen, PWA Health Group, May 4, 1987," JSNYP.

259   The line outside: MC, "Remarks of Michael Callen, PWA Health Group, May 4, 1987," JSNYP.

259   Peter Staley took: PS, correspondence with author, various.

260   It featured Michael Callen: Unlabeled videotape, RDA.

260   At 9 p.m.: MC datebook, April 24, 1987, MCA.

260   Several more times: MC, undated draft of a speech, MCA.

261   he ordered a: Donna Mildvan et al., "An Open-Label, Dose-Ranging Trial of AL721 in Patients with Persistent Generalized Lymphadenopathy and AIDS-Related Complex," *Journal of Acquired Immune Deficiency Syndromes* 4, no. 10 (October 1991): 945–51.

261   "no indication of": Ibid.

261   With that, Fauci: Nussbaum, *Good Intentions*, 260; and MC, undated draft of a speech, MCA.

261   Reluctantly, Fauci finally agreed: Intv. Tim Westmoreland, April 29, 2014.

261   Waxman, who represented: Ibid.

261   He called his first: Ibid.; Tim Westmoreland, "Henry Waxman, the Unsung Hero in the Fight Against AIDS," *Politico Magazine*, February 4, 2014, retrieved from politico.com.

261   "look for research": Ibid.

261   When the morning: Obituary, "Nathan Kolodner, 38, Ex-AIDS Group Head," *NYT*, August 30, 1989.

262   They crowded on one side: Nussbaum, *Good Intentions*, 119.

262   "It's useless": MC, undated draft of a speech, MCA.

262   Fauci smiled: Ibid.

262   "Look": Ibid.

262   Instead, with the road: Intv. Claire Klepner, October 8, 2015.

263   Callen's agenda: MC, *Surviving*, 31.

264   Since up to 75 percent: MC, "AIDS Research: Missed Opportunities and Misplaced Priorities," unpublished editorial, undated, MCUA.

264   "Look, Dr. Fauci:" Nussbaum, *Good Intentions*, 121.

264   "I am here": MC, *Surviving*, 31.

264   "There isn't a doctor": Kahn, *Winter War*, 60.

264   "I can't do that": Nussbaum, *Good Intentions*, 121; and AF, email to author, May 16, 2014.

264   "Why not?": Nussbaum, *Good Intentions*, 121.

264   Callen knew the data: MC, *Surviving*, 31.

264   If Bactrim were rolled: Intv. AF, September 27, 2010.

264   At the NIH: AF, email to author, May 16, 2014.

264   *Primum non nocere:* Ibid.

264   "Please, I *beg* you": Nussbaum, *Good Intentions*, 121; and MC, "AIDS Research."

265   "I can't do that": Nussbaum, *Good Intentions*, 121.

267   The committee: Michael Nesline, intv. by Sarah Schulman, AUOHP, March 24, 2003.

2. THINGS FALL APART

269   On June 5, 1987: *MacNeil/Lehrer NewsHour*, PBS, June 5, 1987.

269   Ultimately he resigned: Edward Barnes and Anne Hollister, "The New Victims: AIDS Is an Epidemic That May Change the Way America Lives," *Life* (July 1985); and HH, correspondence with author, March 25, 2015.

269   "posed . . . [a] threat": Barnes and Hollister, "The New Victims."

269   "The Washington meeting": Jim Lehrer, *MacNeil/Lehrer NewsHour*, PBS, June 5, 1987, corrected for sense in author's transcription.

269   Sonnabend stared: JS, emails to author, various.

270   One, a drug: Walter T. Hughes, "*Pneumocystis Carinii* Pneumonitis," *NEJM* 317, no. 16 (October 1987): 1021. Hughes's article cites Craig Metroka et al., "Successful Chemoprophlylaxis for *Pneumocystis Carinii* Pneumonia with Dapsone in Patients with AIDS and ARC," presented at the Third International Conference on AIDS, Washington, D.C., June 1–5, 1987.

270   "From a medical point": Jim Lehrer, *MacNeil/Lehrer NewsHour*, PBS, June 5, 1987.

270   "[T]he reality for many": JS, undated letter, JSPG.

270   In typical fashion: JS, email to author, March 13, 2015.

270   While traveling: Andrew Rosenthal, "Paul Popham, 45, a Founder of AIDS Organization, Dies," *NYT*, May 8, 1987.

270   In recent weeks: LK, *Reports*, 160; intv. Larry Mass, September 24, 2014.

271   "intimates other than": MC, "AIDS: The Linguistic Battlefield," in *The State of Language*, ed. Christopher Ricks and Leonard Michaels (Berkeley: University of California Press, 1990), 179.

271   "longtime companion": Rosenthal, "Paul Popham, 45, a Founder of AIDS Organization, Dies."

271   "keep fighting": LK, *Reports*, 161.

271   Kramer soon turned: Ibid., 176 and 162.

271   "I don't think you are": Ibid., 162–63.

272   Kramer charged $1,000: Ibid., 176.

272   "I would much rather": LK, memo, "To All the Members of ACT UP," June 8, 1987, RJGA.

272   Three weeks later: Michael Nesline, intv. by Sarah Schulman, AUOHP, March 24, 2003; Gerald M. Boyd, "Reagan Urges Abstinence for Young to Avoid AIDS," *NYT*, April 2, 1987; and Philip M. Boffey, "Reagan Urges Wide AIDS Testing but Does Not Call for Compulsion," *NYT*, June 1, 1987.

272   His few comments: Richard Pearce, PhD, "Co-Factors and AIDS," *NYN*, May 5–19, 1987.

272   "When it comes to": Boyd, "Reagan Urges Abstinence."

272   Now, under mounting: Philip M. Boffey, "Reagan Names 12 to Panel On AIDS," *NYT*, July 24, 1987.

272   He charged the commission: Ibid.

272   To chair the commission: Ibid.

273   To fill out the commission: Philip M. Boffey, "The AIDS Commission," *NYT*, September 9, 1987.

273   "blood terrorism": Ibid.

273   "recalcitrant carriers": Dirk Johnson, "Woodrow Augustus Myers Jr.; A Commissioner Who Knows Strife," *NYT*, January 20, 1990.

273   Theresa Crenshaw: Josh Getlin, "Protesters Say Reagan Commission Lacks Expertise," *LAT*, September 10, 1987; and Sandra G. Boodman, "Top Officers of AIDS Panel Step Down Over Infighting; Chairman Told Officials He Was Undermined," *WP*, October 8, 1987.

273   The nation's most: Sandra G. Boodman, "AIDS Commission's New Chairman Earns High Marks for Leadership," *WP*, April 17, 1988.

273   The ACLU prepared: Philip M. Boffey, "Washington Talk: The AIDS Commission; First Meeting Is Today, but Not the First Criticism," *NYT*, September 9, 1987.

273   Dr. Frank Lilly: David W. Dunlap, "Frank Lilly, a Geneticist, 65; Member of National AIDS Panel," *NYT*, October 16, 1995.

273   "As far as I know": Boffey, "Reagan Names 12 to Panel On AIDS."

274   "impressionable youth": Ibid.

274   He placed an ad: MC, "Not Everyone Dies of AIDS: Michael Callen's Story of Survival," *VV*, May 3, 1988, 34.

274   Dozens of people: Ibid.

275   "Now that published reports": Ibid.

3. TERMINAL VELOCITY

276   Brian Gougeon started: Susan Wild Bernard, correspondence with author, May 24–July 2, 2013, and May 2–5, 2014.

277   Norma Gougeon laid: Brian Gougeon's funeral service program, September 9, 1987.

277   She kept the cause: Susan Wild Bernard, correspondence with author, May 24–July 2, 2013, and May 2–May 5, 2014.

278   She had taken: Intv. Iris Long, July 29, 2010.

278   Her chosen specialty: Ibid.

278   Money was not: Ibid.

279   "They're very interesting": Intv. Michael Long, October 27, 2014.

279   "Shut up and listen!": Intv. JE, August 5, 2010.

279   "Nobody, if they succeeded": Ibid.

280   The role AIDS: Ibid.

280   A few months: Ibid.

280   When Marty Robinson: JE, email to author, May 16, 2014.

280   "Don't worry": Intv. JE, August 5, 2010.

280   "I'm starting a study group": Ibid.

280   "sustained protest": "Committee to Protest the AIDS Commission," leaf-
        let, August 17, 1987, RJGA.

281   She had a medical degree: Sandra G. Boodman, "Top Officers of AIDS
        Panel Step Down Over Infighting; Chairman Told Officials He Was
        Undermined," *WP*, October 8, 1987.

281   she traveled the country: Sandra G. Boodman, "Views of 4 US AIDS Pan-
        elists Hit," *WP*, August 26, 1987.

281   For the September: Bradley Ball, letter to *Washington Blade*, September
        21, 1987, RJGA; announcement, *NYN*, September 14, 1987; speech by
        Rebecca Cole, *NYN*, September 28, 1987, 16; Rebecca Cole, intv. by Sarah
        Schulman, AUOHP, June 30, 2008; videotape of testimony, retrieved from
        footage.net, transcript by author; and speech by Marty Robinson reprinted
        in *NYN*, September 28, 1987, 14–16.

281   Nearly one hundred: Bradley Ball, letter to *Washington Blade*, Septem-
        ber 21, 1987, RJGA.

281   The chairman: Sally Squires, "Setting the Course on AIDS; How an
        Admiral Turned Around the AIDS Commission," *WP*, June 7, 1988.

281   What happened over: Ibid.

281   A number of appointees: Philip M. Boffey, "Washington Talk: Presidential
        Commissions; Can the AIDS Panel Now 'Pull It Together'?," *NYT*, Octo-
        ber 16, 1987.

282   While it was true: Ibid.; and Sandra G. Boodman and Michael Specter,
        "Extent of AIDS Infection in U.S. Remains Uncertain," *WP*, December 3,
        1987.

282   By sorry comparison: Boffey, "Washington Talk: Presidential Commis-
        sions."

282   "We are really worried": Squires, "Setting the Course on AIDS."

282   Even on a starvation budget: Ibid.

282   Staggered, Mayberry: Sandra G. Boodman, "AIDS Panel Chairman to Be
        Replaced; White House Expected to Pick Retired Admiral Watkins as Suc-
        cessor," *WP*, October 7, 1987; and "Setting the Course on AIDS; How an
        Admiral Turned Around the AIDS Commission," *WP*, June 7, 1988.

282   "this administration's blatant": Flyer from ACT UP AIDS Commission
        demonstration outside National Press Building, Washington, D.C., Sep-
        tember 9, 1987, RJGA.

282   "But sometimes the challenge": Speech by LK, *NYN*, September 28,
        1987, 17.

283   Petrelis touched on: Michael Petrelis, "AIDS Commission Faces Criti-
        cism," September 9, 1987, Washington, D.C., videotape 327545, CONUS
        Archive, transcript by author.

283   "I can assure you": Ibid.

283   "To criticize this": Sandra G. Boodman, "First Meeting Puts AIDS Panel
        on Rocky Path," *WP*, September 10, 1987, A3.

283   "We believe we have": Ibid.

283   But what most: Bradley Ball, letter to *Washington Blade*, September 21,
        1987, RJGA.

283   "We need to deliver": Ibid.

284 "CONGREGATION: I am": Order of worship, Brian Gougeon's memorial service, September 19, 1987.

286 There now were: MH, *Testing the Limits*, "Tape 1828," TTLN, transcript by author.

286 It occupied a large: Derek Hodel, email to author, August 5, 2014.

286 A banged-up elevator: Garance Franke-Ruta, correspondence with author, December 18, 2014; and Derek Hodel, email to author, August 5, 2014.

287 "In the absence": Derek Hodel, "People With AIDS Health Group/ Coalition," videotape, Testing the Limits Records, New York Public Library.

287 "equal or better than": A. Bruce Montgomery et al., "Aerosolized Pentamidine as Sole Therapy for *Pneumocystis Carinii* Pneumonia in Patients with Acquired Immunodeficiency Syndrome," *Lancet* 2, no. 8557 (August 29, 1987): 480–83.

287 Some doctors built: Nussbaum, *Good Intentions*, 231; and R. A. Mciver et al., "An Effectiveness Community-Based Clinical Trial of Respirgard II and Fisoneb Nebulizers for *Pneumocystis Carinii* Prophylaxis with Aerosol Pentamidine in HIV-Infected Individuals," Toronto Aerosol Pentamidine Study Group, *Chest* 110, no. 1 (July 1996): 141–46.

287 The mist sat inside: T. Flannigan et al., "Prophylaxis Against *Pneumocystis Carinii* Pneumonia in Patients Receiving Azidothymidine," *NEJM* 317, no. 18 (1987): 1155; and Warren E. Leary, "F.D.A. Approves Drug That Fights Leading Killer of AIDS Patients," *NYT*, June 16, 1989.

288 NIAID never: Philip M. Boffey, "Official Blames Shortage of Staff for Delay in Testing AIDS Drugs," *NYT*, April 30, 1988.

288 he "just didn't": Arno and Feiden, *Against the Odds*, 95.

288 With the help: Sally Smith Hughes et al., *The AIDS Epidemic in San Francisco: The Response of Community Physicians, 1981–1984*, vol. II, San Francisco AIDS Oral History Series (Berkeley: University of California, Regional Oral History Office, 1996).

288 Rather than creating: MC, MK, Ron Najman, and JS, "Community Research Initiative (CRI): A Proposal for the Prevention of AIDS," November 12, 1986.

288 They called their: MC, essay, "Remarks of Michael Callen at PAAC Teleconference," New Orleans, May 17–18, 1989.

288 In little time: JS, "Origin and Need for CRI," sample letter for fundraising, circa April 1988, JSNYP.

289 News of these: Walter T. Hughes, "*Pneumocystis Carinii* Pneumonitis," *NEJM*, October 15, 1987.

289 But Fauci still refused: AF, email to author, May 16, 2014.

289 "I would go for": Boffey, "Official Blames Shortage of Staff for Delay in Testing AIDS Drugs."

290 "I like the guy": Sandra G. Boodman, "AIDS Panel Chairman to Be Replaced; White House Expected to Pick Retired Admiral Watkins as Successor," *WP*, October 7, 1987.

290 "competent": Boffey, "Washington Talk."

290   Public opinion was: Cartoon by Tom Darcy, *New York Newsday*, November 13, 1987.

290   On October 6: Sandra G. Boodman, "Top Officers of AIDS Panel Step Down Over Infighting; Chairman Told Officials He Was Undermined," *WP*, October 8, 1987.

291   Watkins, a staunch: Squires, "Setting the Course on AIDS."

291   "I'm a sailor": T. Rees Shapiro, "Admiral Led 1980s AIDS Commission," *WP*, July 28, 2010.

291   Watkins inherited an office: Boodman, "Top Officers of AIDS Panel Step Down."

291   Unopened mail was: Squires, "Setting the Course on AIDS."

291   In quick succession: "Public Hearing Schedule as of February 22, 1988," published by the Presidential Commission on the Human Immunodeficiency Virus Epidemic, RJGA.

292   Peter Staley had been: Intv. PS, January 6, 2014.

292   He helped organize: RG, "ACT UP: An Activist's Timeline (1987–1994)," RJGA.

292   He spent that night: PS, email to author, May 14, 2014.

292   He convinced local: ACT UP Coordinating Committee Meeting Minutes, October 18, 1987, RJGA.

292   But it was still: Ibid.

292   With Kramer on: PS, email to author, June 12, 2014.

293   Sean Strub, a co-owner: ACT UP Coordinating Committee Meeting Minutes, November 3, 1987, RJGA.

293   But before the night: Ibid.

293   "first-class accommodations": "Fundraising Letter," undated, ACT UP Meeting Notes March 31–June 22, 1987, RJGA.

293   After a weeks-long: Intv. PS, January 6, 2014.

293   His CD4 count: PS spreadsheet showing his CD4 count on September 22, 1987.

293   Tracey Tanenbaum: Tracey Tannenbaum, intv. PS and Tracey Tannenbaum, January 6, 2014.

294   There on a slight knoll: Anne-Christine d'Adesky, "Civil Disobedience and the Wedding," *NYN*, October 26, 1987.

294   "I'm going to ask you": Ibid.; and Andy Humm, videotape, "1987 Gay Rights March on Washington," *Gay USA*, October 11, 1987, retrieved from youtube.com, transcript by author.

295   Begun just months: Sandra G. Boodman, "Giant Quilt Names 1,920 AIDS Victims," *WP*, October 10, 1987.

296   Though the Parks Service: Lena Williams, "200,000 March in Capital to Seek Gay Rights and Money for AIDS," *NYT*, October 12, 1987; and Humm, "1987 Gay Rights March on Washington."

296   Groups of Broadway: Gloria Campisi, "Gays March in Washington," *Philadelphia Daily News*, October 12, 1987.

296   For a mile or so: Rober Getso, "ACT UP/ New York," videotape, June 23, 2008, retrieved from youtube.com.

296   "How many must die": Humm, "1987 Gay Rights March on Washington."

296   Almost four thousand: Lena Williams, "600 in Gay Demonstration Arrested at Supreme Court," *NYT*, October 14, 1987.

296   "Every day in our lives": Douglas Jehl, "600 Gay Rights Activists Arrested in Capital Protest," *LAT*, October 14, 1987.

296   By noon, 840 people: Police said 600. Ibid.

296   "Your gloves don't match": Williams, "600 in Gay Demonstration Arrested at Supreme Court."

297   He began: BB, correspondence with author, July 8, 2014.

297   Editorial writers quickly: Maggie Mahar, "Pitiless Scourge," *Barron's*, March 13, 1989.

297   Independent analysts put: Nussbaum, *Good Intentions*, 181.

297   Burroughs Wellcome's profit: William Alpert, "Good News/Bad News: Many Potential AIDS Drugs in View, but Much Testing Needed," *Barron's*, March 9, 1987.

297   On December 17, 1987: Intv. BB, various.

298   The commissioners liked: Ibid.

298   "They're not particularly": ACT UP Meeting Minutes, April 11, 1988, RJGA.

298   Fauci's national AIDS: BB, intv. by Sarah Schulman, March 10, 2010, AUOHP.

298   "I like your flyer": Intv. BB, various.

298   "No, it's 475": Ibid.

298   One of them was Hill: Ibid.

299   Fauci soon invited: AF, correspondence with author, June 6, 2014.

299   "Fauci: Space Isn't": AF, "Dinner with Anthony Fauci and James Hill," December 17, 1987, transcribed by BB, BBA.

299   Hoping to reset relations: Intv. PS, various.

299   "arbitrarily and capriciously": Marilyn Chase, "AIDS Patient Advocates, US Square Off for Hearing on Drug Development Suit," *WSJ*, December 11, 1987.

299   Bahlman did not: BB, correspondence with author, June 2, 2014.

299   "To be honest": AF, "Dinner with Anthony Fauci and James Hill."

300   "The fact is": Ibid.

300   "We want clinical": Ibid.

301   This kind of argument: Mark Schoofs, "The Placebo Question Is a Moot Point," *Windy City Times*, December 1, 1988.

301   "I don't complain": AF, "Dinner with Anthony Fauci and James Hill."

302   "We're talking over": Ibid.

302   "You got a little carried": Ibid.

303   They met weekly: Jonathan Ned Katz, "Herbert Spiers: November 8, 1945–March 2, 2011," undated, retrieved from outhistory.org.

303   David Z. Kirschenbaum: David Z. Kirschenbaum, intv. by Sarah Schulman, October 19, 2003, AUOHP; and Daniel Wolfe, intv. Sarah Schulman, February 27, 2010, AUOHP.

303   David Barr was: DB, intv. by Sarah Schulman, May 15, 2007, AUOHP.

303   Long answered question: Herb Spiers, intv. by Sarah Schulman, July 2, 2008, AUOHP.

303   He did the same: DB, intv. by Sarah Schulman, May 15, 2007, AUOHP.

304   Through this effort: JE, Gary Kleinman and Iris Long, letter to Dr. Fred
       T. Valentine, April 8, 1988.

304   But a strange: Ibid.

304   In the whole: Chart from December 21, 1987, *NYN*, January 4–10, 1988.

304   "an unrecognized scandal": JE, Gary Kleinman and Iris Long, letter to Dr.
       Fred T. Valentine, April 8, 1988.

304   Any NYU physician: Ibid.

304   This made little: Krishna Stone, email to author, September 2, 2014.

304   That, Valentine explained: JE, Gary Kleinman and Iris Long, letter to Dr.
       Fred T. Valentine, April 8, 1988.

305   In preparation: Intv. JE, August 5, 2010; and PS, "JE's Remarks for the
       Panel: AIDS Activism NOW, the LGBT Center, New York City, April 11,
       2012," April 18, 2010, retrieved from blogs.poz.com.

305   She put sixty: M. Fischl et al., "Safety and Efficacy of Sulfamethoxazole
       and Trimethoprim Chemoprophylaxis for *Pneumocystis carinii* Pneumonia
       in AIDS," *JAMA* 259, no. 8 (1988): 1185–89.

4. AGAINST NATURE

306   It seemed that his: Intv. PS, various.

306   Later in the month: PS spreadsheet showing his CD4 count on Febru-
       ary 23, 1988.

306   Six months to the day: "Agreement," March 10, 1989, PSA.

307   The struggle cost: PS spreadsheet showing his CD4 count on Septem-
       ber 27, 1988.

307   The best he could: "Agreement," March 10, 1989, PSA.

307   Staley fell in: Intv. PS, various.

308   "Welcome to ACT UP": MH, "Chapter 1," MHU.

308   "If there are any": "ACT UP Facilitator's Guide," prepared October 10,
       1990, RJGA.

308   Besides his work: ACT UP Meeting Agenda, April 5, 1988, RJGA.

308   These supplemented: Ibid.

308   "MEN USE CONDOMS": Alexandra Juhasz, intv. by Sarah Schulman,
       January 16, 2003, AUOHP.

309   "burn-out workshops": ACT UP Meeting Minutes, June 6, 1988, RJGA.

309   To deal with: ACT UP Meeting Minutes, May 30, 1988, RJGA.

309   The sole and towering: Ibid.

310   He had just: "An Open Letter to Dr. Anthony Fauci," *VV,* May 31, 1988,
       reprinted in LK, *Reports,* 193–99.

310   "ACT UP has to": ACT UP Meeting Minutes, May 30, 1988, RJGA.

310   Drugs, she argued: Ibid.

310   "Being out on the streets": Ibid.

310   As a member: Ibid.

310   Like Bahlman: Ibid.

310   Ortez Alderson: "Ortez Alderson: Inducted 1991 [Posthumous]," Chicago

Gay and Lesbian Hall of Fame, undated, retrieved from glhalloffame.org; and ibid.

311   But it was the newest: MC, "AIDS Research: Missed Opportunities, and Misplaced Priorities," unpublished editorial, undated, MCUA.

311   The Olympic diving champ: Sharon Robb, "Louganis Not About to Belly Flop," *Sun Sentinel*, August 16, 1987.

311   Elton John sent: Jack Friedman and Bill Shaw, "Amazing Grace," *People*, May 30, 1988.

311   "Despite all the attention": Ibid.

312   Callen couldn't believe: MC, correspondence to Ryan White, January 19, 1988, MCA.

312   Callen grabbed a phone: MC, "AIDS Research: Missed Opportunities, and Misplaced Priorities," unpublished editorial, undated, MCUA.

312   He asked if: Ibid.

312   "If world-famous Ryan": "Aids and Passive Genocide: 30,534 Unnecessary Deaths from PCP Due to Scandalous Failure to Prophylax: Testimony Given at FDA Hearing Concerning the Approval of Aerosol Pentamidine as Prophylaxis Against PCP," first published in *AIDS Forum* 2, no. 1 (1989).

312   "It is a national": MC, "AIDS Research: Missed Opportunities, and Misplaced Priorities."

313   Ronald Reagan was: Frank Newport et al., "Ronald Reagan from the People's Perspective: A Gallup Poll Review," Gallup, June 7, 2004.

313   he and Dworkin: Email from RD to author, June 16, 2014.

313   Sometimes it seemed: MC, "Gay Pride Rally Speech, June 29, 1991," MCUA.

313   On Saturday, June 25: Phil Zwickler, "Lesbian and Gay Pride 1988," *NYN*, July 11, 1988.

314   We live in wartime: MC, "Gay Pride Rally Speech, June 25, 1988," MCUA.

315   The physician tried: Untitled and unsigned eulogy for Griffin Gold, JSNYP.

315   "I have to ask": Ibid.

315   She thought he seemed: Ibid.

315   He was a thirty-two-year-old: Obituary, "Griffin Gold, AIDS Worker, 33," *NYT*, March 8, 1989.

315   "He won't make it": Intv. Michael Lesser, undated.

315   A massive regimen: Email from Michael Lesser to author, August 5, 2014.

315   A few days later: PS, email to author, November 8, 2015; Leland M. Roth, "Ernest Flagg: Beaux-Arts Architect and Urban Reformer," *Journal of the Society of Architectural Historians* 46, no. 4 (1987): 420–22.

315   "Why weren't you": Intv. PS, March 17, 2009.

316   In February: ACT UP Meeting Minutes, June 21, 1988, RJGA.

316   ACT UP sent an army: Sally Chew, "ACT UP Zaps AIDS Commission," *NYN*, February 29, 1988.

316   Sonnabend, Tom Hannan: "Hearings Agenda," February 18–20, 1988, RJGA.

316 "Lipid research": MC, "Testimony of Michael L. Callen," before the Presidential AIDS Commission on the Human Immunodeficiency Virus Epidemic, Research Findings, February 19, 1988, MC estate.

316 "pulled me into": Philip M. Boffey, "FDA Budget for AIDS Called Too Low," *NYT,* February 20, 1988.

316 "We are not ready": Sally Squires, "Setting the Course on AIDS; How an Admiral Turned Around the President's AIDS Commission," *WP,* June 7, 1988.

317 In the end: Sandra G. Boodman, "Commission's Chief Faults AIDS Response," *WP,* June 3, 1988.

317 "the key to the entire": Julie Johnson, "Reagan, Spurning Tougher Move, Orders Anti-Bias Rules on AIDS," *NYT,* August 3, 1988.

317 "I am very much": Boodman, "Commission's Chief Faults AIDS Response."

317 No reporters were: Julie Johnson, "Report by AIDS Panel Gets Muted Reaction by Reagan," *NYT,* June 27, 1988.

317 If Watkins felt: Intv. Monsignor Watkins, May 12, 2014.

318 More than six hundred: *Star-Ledger,* February 5, 1988.

318 "There are certain": Kenneth B. Noble, "Company Halting Health Plan on Some 'Life Style' Illnesses," *NYT,* August 6, 1988.

318 As the AIDS: Bruce Lambert, "US Confronting AIDS with Sense of Realism," *NYT,* February 17, 1988.

318 The Southern Baptists: Peter Steinfels, "Southern Baptists Condemn Homosexuality as 'Depraved,'" *NYT,* June 17, 1988.

318 Similarly inimical views: Ibid.

318 Given the increasing: Laurence Zuckerman, "Open Season on Gays: AIDS Sparks an Epidemic of Violence Against Homosexuals," *Time,* March 7, 1988.

318 Nationally, anti-gay: John T. McQuiston, "1,000 Protest Attacks Aimed at Homosexuals," *NYT,* August 31, 1988; and Constance L. Hays, "2 Men Beaten by 6 Youths Yelling 'Fags,'" *NYT,* August 24, 1988.

319 "When we": Handout, "The Lesbian and Gay Freedom Ride, Summer 1988," RJGA.

319 Convention organizers were not: Rex Wockner, "ACT UP Clashes with Atlanta Cops," *NYN,* August 1, 1988.

319 dressed in black boots: Barbara O'Dair, "Jesus Lived with His Mom," *VV,* undated.

320 ACT UP staged: Rex Wockner, "Riot Squad Turns Kiss-in into Bash-in in Atlanta," *Bay Area Reporter,* July 28, 1988.

320 The Gay and Lesbian: Rex Wockner, "Acting Up in Alabama," *NYN,* August 29, 1988.

320 Lloyd Bentsen became: John Ward, "Coming Out," *VV,* July 26, 1988.

320 The Riders needed: Wockner, "Acting Up in Alabama"; and Heidi Dorow, intv. by Sarah Schulman, April 17, 2007, AUOHP.

320 The Riders headed: Wockner, "Acting Up in Alabama."

320 "I have zero": Rhonda Pines, "Freedom Ride not Welcome, Says Folmar," *Montgomery Advertiser,* July 19, 1988.

320   Progressing through: Ron Goldberg, "Freedom Ride, 1988," RJGA; and Wockner, "Acting Up in Alabama."

320   By morning: ACT UP Meeting Minutes, August 1, 1988, RJGA.

321   Eleven people were: Ron Goldberg, email to author, July 24, 2014.

321   "No God-given right": Rex Wockner, "Outsiders in the Big Easy," *NYN*, September 5, 1988.

321   While in New Orleans: ACT UP Coordinating Committee Meeting Minutes, August 2, 1988; and Rich Magill, "Civil Disobedience and Arrest Expected in N.O.," *Big Easy Times*, August 12, 1999.

321   The last stop: Rick Buck, "Gay Rights Protesters Given Escort," *Tampa Tribune*, August 26, 1988.

321   About a hundred: Ibid.

321   In response to: Philip Boffey, "Unproven AIDS Drug to Be Given Wider Use," *NYT*, August 15, 1988.

322   "This opens": Ibid.

322   His ginger hair: MH, email to author, December 24, 2014.

322   His degree from Harvard: MH, intv. by Sarah Schulman, March 8, 2003, AUOHP.

322   He dabbled in: Peter Kurth, "Marked Man," *POZ* (Febuary 1998).

322   He was drafted: MH, MHU.

322   Afterward, Johnson spoke: Ibid.; and Kurth, "Marked Man."

322   He presented a: MH, JE, IL, and David Z. Kirschenbaum, *A Glossary of AIDS Drug Trials, Testing & Treatment Issues*, reference manual, undated.

322   "Taking control": MH, MHU.

322   The committee passed: Ibid.

322   The crushing heat: Jerry Cheslow, "Mosquito Infestation Expected in June," *NYT*, June 5, 1988; Walter Sullivan, "Experts Issue Warning About Dengue Fever," *NYT*, March 8, 1988.

323   David Barr and Mickey: Intv. Mickey Wheatley, July 22, 2014.

323   On a hot summer night: Ibid.

323   A twenty-three-year-old: Bordowitz, *The AIDS Crisis*, 87.

323   associate named Gregg: Gregg Bordowitz, intv. by Sarah Schulman, December 17, 2002, AUOHP; and Gregg Bordowitz curriculum vitae (2012), retrieved from greggbordowitz.com.

323   He conducted: ACT UP Coordinating Committee Meeting Notes, August 16, 1988, RJGA.

323   "just sort of by word": DB, intv. by Sarah Schulman, May 15, 2007, AUOHP.

323   "And it's global": Ibid.

323   Barr and Wheatley: ACT UP Meeting Minutes, May 23, 1988, RJGA.

324   The PWA Health Group: MC, videotape, "Testimony of Michael L. Callen, Before Presidential Commission on Human Immunodeficiency Virus Epidemic, in Extemporaneous Remarks Following His Prepared Statement," 1988, BBA.

324   Now lawyers for: Gina Kolata, "An Angry Response to Actions on AIDS Spurs F.D.A. Shift," *NYT*, June 26, 1988.

324   "They're not following": Intv. DB, September 10, 2010.

324   "Look": Gregg Bordowitz, intv. by Sarah Schulman, December 17, 2002, AUOHP.

324   This made perfect: Intv. DB, September 10, 2010.

324   "Gregg, you're becoming": Gregg Bordowitz, intv. by Sarah Schulman, AUOHP, December 17, 2002.

324   When the din: Intv. DB, September 10, 2010.

324   "a major action": ACT UP Meeting Minutes, June 13, 1988, RJGA.

324   "We need to seize": ACT UP Meeting Minutes, June 13, 1988, RJGA.

325   Members subsequently: ACT UP Meeting Minutes, June 21, 1988, RJGA; Robert Garcia Papers, 1988–1993, Cornell University Library; and Karen Ramspacher, intv. Sarah Schulman, July 2, 2008, AUOHP.

325   Because the first: Sean Strub, email to author, July 22, 2014.

325   Benefit soirees were: ACT UP Meeting Minutes, August 22, 1988, RJGA.

325   Staley plunged: ACT UP Coordinating Committee Meeting Minutes, July 12 and September 20, 1988, RJGA.

325   Sonnabend's study: JS, "Egg Yolk Lipids: Monitoring Five Patients Receiving Egg Yolk Lipids," JSNYP; and Kahn, *AIDS: The Winter War*, 96.

325   At a second meeting: ACT UP Coordinating Committee Meeting Minutes, August 30, 1988, RJGA.

326   He was methodical: ACT UP Coordinating Committee Meeting Minutes, September 6, 1988, RJGA.

326   Taking charge: Intv. Michelangelo Signorile, April 2011.

326   The issues of women: "Ortez Alderson: Inducted 1991 [Posthumous]," Chicago Gay and Lesbian Hall of Fame, undated, retrieved from glhalloffame.org.

326   Staley and Bordowitz: MH, MHU.

326   When the six: Ibid. Same source for all below.

327   "You're totally beautiful": Michael Musto, *La Dolce Musto* (New York, NY: Carroll & Graf, 2007), 239.

327   "Seize control!": Kiki Mason, "FDA: The Demo of the Year," *NYN*, October 24, 1988.

328   Maxine Wolfe, Maria: The Costas, letter to the Mulberry Group, March 2, 1991, including a history of the Costas entitled "A Costa Her/History."

328   Proving that ACT UP: Musto, *La Dolce Musto*, 239.

328   The FDA Building: Dan Bellm, "Storming the FDA: A Power-and-Passion Play," *VV*, October 25, 1989.

328   The activists streamed: Mason, "FDA: The Demo of the Year."

328   "Anybody with AIDS": Beatriz da Costa and Kavita Philip, eds., *Tactical Biopolitics: Art, Activism, and Technoscience* (Cambridge, MA: MIT Press, 2008), 336.

328   "AZT is not enough": Documentary, *How to Survive a Plague*, transcript by author.

328   "I Got the Placebo": Da Costa and Philip, eds., *Tactical Biopolitics*, 336.

328   The Delta Queens: Ibid.; and Bellm, "Storming the FDA."

328   The Forget-Me-Nots: Chris Bull, "Seizing Control of the FDA," *Gay Community News*, October 16–22, 1988.

329   "FDA—Fucking Disaster": Mason, "FDA: The Demo of the Year."

329   And then from below: Intv. Michelangelo Signorile, April 2011.

330   "Excuse me": Intv. PS, August 5, 2010.

330   By 4 p.m.: Mason, "FDA: The Demo of the Year."

330   The protest and mass: Bordowitz, *The AIDS Crisis,* 238; "FDA Action Media Report," ACT UP Media Committee, RJGA.

331   "The poor homosexuals": Patrick Buchanan, "Is Catholicism Now 'Unacceptable'?," *NYP,* May 24, 1983.

332   "In the long war": Mason, "FDA: The Demo of the Year."

332   ACT UP followed: Warren Leary and David Binder, "Washington Talk: Briefing; Making Amends," *NYT,* November 3, 1988; and "Why I Demonstrated at the FDA," emphasis in original, RJGA.

333   It opened at: "WPA Theatre," list of productions, Lortel Archives, retrieved from lortel.org; and Patrick Merla, "A Normal Heart: The Larry Kramer Story," in Mass, ed., *We Must Love One Another,* 56.

333   "Imagine the worst": Mel Gussow, "Skewers for the Political in Kramer's 'Just Say No,'" *NYT,* October 21, 1988.

333   "an exercise in churlishness": John Beaufort, "New Comedy by Gurney Ranks as His Most Entertaining Play," *Christian Science Monitor,* November 2, 1988.

333   The anxiety triggered: Nussbaum, *Good Intentions,* 329.

333   A chronic active: David France, "The Angry Prophet Is Dying," *Newsweek,* June 11, 2011.

333   Kramer was also: Ibid.

333   Certain minor health: Karen Heller, "It's Decision Time for an AIDS Activist Playwright: Larry Kramer Knows He Doesn't Have That Much Time Left. Should He Write or Fight?," *PI,* May 1, 1991.

333   He immediately started: LK, "Checking In: My Chart," *POZ* (August/September 1994).

333   His gums bled: Ibid.

333   His infectious disease: Ibid.

333   As an atheist: Andrew Sullivan, "LK, with Sugar on Top," *POZ,* May 12, 1995.

333   "Always wear something": France, "The Angry Prophet Is Dying."

334   Although they had: LK, "Checking In."

334   one of the coldest: Intv. PS, March 17, 2009; obituary, "Griffin Gold, AIDS Worker, 33," *NYT,* March 8, 1989.

335   That same week: Handwritten phone call memos for MC, March 18, 1989, MCA.

335   he was memorialized: Michael Lesser, email to author, April 15, 2014.

335   "Celebration of Life": Program for "Celebration of Life, March 13, 1989," Judson Memorial Church.

335   He chose a heartbreaking: PS, email to Ron Goldberg, August 12, 2014.

335   The first scientific: Intv. PS, October 14, 2009.

336   Cox came out: Intv. Spencer Cox, September 10, 2010.

337   Iris Long had: Iris Long, "AZT Windfall; Profits on PWAs' Bodies Report Provided at ACT UP Meeting," September 14, 1988, RJGA.

337 "obscene": Ibid.

337 Weiss determined that: Ted Weiss, from Weiss press release.

337 "The American people": Ibid.

338 "the party of homosexuals": AP, "Hatch Says Democrats 'Party of Homo-sexuals,'" *NYT,* September 2, 1988.

338 "anyone whose life style": Julie Johnson, "Washington Talk: Lobbies; Homosexual Groups and the Politics of AIDS," *NYT,* October 6, 1988.

338 Two of them filled: MC, "Living with AIDS," speech made in late 1988 at a forum organized by Alvin Friedman-Kien, MCUA.

338 "The saddest thing": Ibid.

338 In his spare time: MC, "How to Run a Successful PWA Singles' Tea," in *Surviving,* 169–73.

338 Six and a half years: MC, "Living with AIDS."

338 "Never": Intv. Richard Dworkin, December 30, 2014.

338 There on the back: MC, "Living with AIDS."

339 He let his finger: Intv. Richard Dworkin, June 2014.

5. DENIAL

340 Peter Staley and Mark: Intv. PS, August 5, 2010.

340 Lisa Behrens: MH audiotape transcript, "Peter & Mark Talk About Drugs and Money at Burroughs-Wellcome," January 23, 1989, MHA.

340 Behrens, a short: MH, email to author, June 2, 2014; Lisa Behrens, "Lisa Behrens LinkedIn," retrieved from linkedin.com; and MH, "Peter & Mark Talk About Drugs and Money at Burroughs-Wellcome."

340 After a time: MH, MHU.

341 "punk formalwear": Ibid.

341 "Our goal": MH, "Peter & Mark Talk About Drugs and Money at Burroughs-Wellcome."

341 Matching his provocation: MH, MHU.

341 Harrington rattled off: For this figure, see "The Toll: Bad News for Women and I.V. Users," *Newsweek,* November 2, 1987.

341 "You have a fig leaf": MH, "Peter & Mark Talk About Drugs and Money at Burroughs-Wellcome."

341 "If you can give": Ibid.

342 He snubbed out: MH, MHU.

342 "I think it's really": MH, "Peter & Mark Talk About Drugs and Money at Burroughs-Wellcome."

343 Tom Kennedy: Tom Kennedy audiotape transcript, "Tom Kennedy, VP Production Engineering," April 19, 2001, Wellcome Library Archives and Manuscripts, retrieved from archives.wellcomelibrary.org.

343 "That's right": MH, "Peter & Mark Talk about Drugs and Money at Burroughs-Wellcome."

344 The FDA still: Frank Young, correspondence with MH, March 2, 1989, MHA.

344 The numbers of patients: Gina Kolata, "In AIDS, Virus Forces Choice Between Longer Life or Eyesight," *NYT,* December 8, 1987, and "Despite

Promise in AIDS Cases, Drug Faces Testing Hurdle," *NYT,* December 13, 1988.

344   Syntex Corporation: JE, BB videotape of the DHPG demonstration, "Tape 20002," BBA.

344   When the details: "Tape 20002."

344   The study required: JE, "T+D Update, Delivered to the Meeting," May 8, 1989, JEA.

344   Treatment + Data sent: Ibid.

344   Unwilling to consider: Frank Young, correspondence with MH, March 2, 1989, MHA.

345   He was now: BB, email to author, June 16, 2014.

346   This was not: BB, "Tape 1b," January 12, 2011.

346   "Obviously, they think": "Tape 20002."

347   "Ellen Cooper has ice": "The Treatment and Data Digest," no. 77, January 12, 1991, RJGA.

347   The following Monday: Gina Kolata, "FDA Said to Be Re-evaluating Order for More Studies on an AIDS Drug," *NYT,* February 6, 1989.

348   He even invited: Frank Young, correspondence with MH, March 2, 1989, MHA.

348   Suramin, a fifty-year-old: Richard Goldstein and Robert Massa, "Compound Q: Hope and Hype," *VV,* May 30, 1989.

348   He was at work: LK, *Reports,* 225.

348   For many months: Ibid., 277–78.

348   Recently he had made: Ibid., 227.

349   Democracy, Kramer: Ibid., 304.

349   He demanded to know: Ibid., 277–78.

349   Thereafter he clipped: Ibid., 220.

350   Nobody from T+D: MH, MHU.

350   Accounts in the community: Goldstein and Massa, "Compound Q."

350   "It's possible": Ibid.

350   In addition, she had: BS, "The Reminiscences of Barbara Starrett, M.D.," *PAOH,* 1999.

350   Even if the power: Ibid.

351   But his newfound: Peter B. Flint, "Barry Gingell, 34, Medical Expert on Treating AIDS Patients, Dies," *NYT,* May 30, 1989.

351   "Dr. Barry was": Intv. PS, August 5, 2010.

351   She also said: Ibid.

351   "I think that's": Ibid.

351   At sunrise: PS, Burroughs-Wellcome action report to ACT UP, undated, RJGA.

351   To them it seemed: ibid.

351   They rose with: Ibid.

352   Lee Arsenault, a forty-one-year-old: Gregory Childress, "4 Activists Storm Burroughs Wellcome in Protest over Cost of AIDS Drug," *Durham Morning Herald,* April 26, 1989.

352   Staley opened: PS, "After Three Weeks of Planning."

352   "They sent us back": Intv. PS, August 5, 2010.

353   A guard shouted: PS, "After Three Weeks of Planning."

353   The doors closed: Intv. PS, August 5, 2010.

353   It was small: PS, "After Three Weeks of Planning."

353   "Ma'am," said Lee: Videotape of Hal Bramson, "Hal Bramson Interview (Part 2 of 4)," retrieved from youtube.com.

353   "There's a situation": Intv. PS, August 5, 2010; and PS, "After Three Weeks of Planning," Burroughs Wellcome action report to ACT UP, undated.

353   The other men: PS, "After Three Weeks of Planning." Same source for all below.

354   "Burroughs Wellcome is": Transcript of WRDC Raleigh news report in documentary, *How to Survive a Plague*.

355   Dr. Frank Young: Unsigned, AP, "FDA Acts on AIDS Drugs," *New York Newsday*, June 27, 1989; and JE, "A Turning Point for AIDS Treatments/Victories for AIDS Activism," memorandum, May 8, 1989, JEA.

355   "the entire map of AIDS": MH, *Testing the Limits*, "Tape 1828," TTLN, transcript by author.

356   A group of five: Ibid.

356   A physician in Europe: Terence Monmaney, "Preying on AIDS Patients," *Newsweek*, June 1, 1987; Janny Scott and Lynn Simross, "AIDS: A Search for Options—Underground Cures," *LAT*, August 16, 1987.

356   Across San Francisco: Jim Beal press statement, "Compound Q," June 10, 1991, GF-RA.

356   There was no strong: Joseph Palca, "Trials and Tribulations of AIDS Drug Testing," *Science* 247 (March 1990): 1406.

357   Many people reported: Jim Beal press statement, "Compound Q."

357   But the consortium leadership: Palca, "Trials and Tribulations of AIDS Drug Testing."

357   They were the perfect pair: Intv. Vera Beyers and Alan Levin, May 27, 2010.

357   A script was readied: Intv. Curtis Ponzi, May 27, 2010.

357   Delaney then turned: Project Inform, "Compound Q—The Real Story," *PI Perspective* 7 (November 1989), retrieved from projectinform.org.

357   At a fractious board: Stephan Pardi, "Death, Hypocrisy, and Imbroglio in New York," *San Francisco Sentinel*, October 12, 1989.

357   "I have AIDS": Gina Kolata, "AIDS Drug Tested by Group Critical of F.D.A.," *NYT*, June 28, 1989.

358   Once a month: Intv. Risa Denenberg, undated.

358   To run the New York: Intv. Barbara Starrett, September 10, 2010.

358   Starrett assembled: Ibid.

358   Nothing was known: Intv. Barbara Starrett, September 10, 2010; and MH, MHU.

358   "We're not talking": Laurie Garrett, "FDA Probes AIDS Research: Unsanctioned Drug Experiment Seen as a Challenge to Agency," *New York Newsday*, July 3, 1989.

359   "You're just like Ellen": MH, MHU.

359   Alarmed when: Robert Steinbrook and Victor Zonana, "FDA Asks AIDS Group to Halt Test of Chinese Drug," *LAT*, August 9, 1989.

359   Sixty-six patients: Gina Kolata, "Critics Fault Secret Effort to Test AIDS Drug," *NYT*, September 19, 1989; and Project Inform, "Compound Q—The Real Story."

359   The doctors invited: Intv. Vera Beyers and Alan Levin, May 27, 2010.

359   "Hi Jim": BS videotape recording, transcript by BS.

360   Some patients had: Intv. Barbara Starrett, September 10, 2010.

6. MADNESS

364   Bachardy, whose life partner: Don Bachardy, correspondence with author, May 21, 2006.

364   Barbier mounted a one-man: Mark Gevessier, "Local Heroes," *7 Days*, June 22, 1988.

364   Sonnabend submitted: MC, "Remarks of Michael Callen, a Gay Man with AIDS and President of the Board of Directors of Community Research Initiative (New York) at FDA Hearings, Rockville, Maryland, May 1, 1989," HSA.

364   Cooper was still: Laurie Garrett, "AIDS Drug Gets FDA Approval," *New York Newsday*, February 7, 1989.

364   "AIDS and Passive Genocide": MC, "AIDS and Passive Genocide: Unnecessary Deaths from PCP to a Scandalous Failure to Prophylax, Testimony Given at a FDA Hearing Concerning the Approval of Aerosol Pentamidine as Prophylaxis Against PCP," May 1, 1989, MCUA.

365   In May 1989: Arno and Feiden, *Against the Odds*, 118.

365   Finally, there was an approved: Robin Eisner, "Doctors' Group Lobbies for Insurance Coverage of Cheaper and Better AIDS Treatment," *New York Doctor*, October 3, 1988.

365   In a case of inexcusable: JS, "Pneumocystis Pneumonia Can be Prevented. Why Did It Take so Long for Well Known Preventative Measures to Be Introduced in AIDS?," September 2006, retrieved from aidsperspective .net.

365   It took another forty-five: Warren E. Leary, "FDA Approves Drug That Fights Leading Killer of AIDS Patients," *NYT*, June 16, 1989.

365   Soon, a quarter of a million: Laurie Garrett, "Parasite Kills AIDS Patient Despite Use of Special Drug," *New York Newsday*, October 17, 1989.

365   "The AIDS community": MC, "Remarks of Michael Callen."

365   "Everybody is out to make": Phil Zwickler, "C-FAR Occupies FDA Regional Office," *NYN*, July 4, 1988.

365   "deplorable": Editorial, "The Storming of St. Pat's," *NYT*, December 12, 1989.

366   "virus-like": S-C. Lo et al., "A Novel Virus-Like Infectious Agent in Patients with AIDS," *American Journal of Tropical Medicine and Hygiene* 40, no. 2 (February 1989): 213–28; and transcript in "The VV Interview with the Publisher of the *Native*," *NYN*, July 10, 1989.

366   Those ads had helped: Transcript in "The VV Interview with the Publisher of the *Native*; and Alisa Solomon, "The Demise of the 'Native,'" *VV*, August 22, 1989.

366 But when Ortleb's piece: Katie Lieshman, "The Outsider," *Rolling Stone*, 1988.

367 "rhyme": Ibid.

367 "We have to say": Solomon, "The Demise of the 'Native.'"

367 "A boycott by gay people": Editor's note, letters section, *NYN*, June 5, 1989.

367 Dubbed *Le Manifeste de Montreal:* "History," AIDS Action NOW, retrieved from aidsactionnow.org.

367 When they reached: Randy Shilts, "The Era of Bad Feelings," *Mother Jones* 14, no. 9 (November 1989): 32.

368 "on behalf of people living": Tim McCaskell, "Taking Our Place," *CATIE* (summer 2011), retrieved from catie.ca.

368 The highlight came: MH, *Testing the Limits,* "Tape 1828," TTLN, transcript by author.

368 Speaking from a makeshift: "Video tape #1103b," BBA.

369 "The reasons I can't get": Ibid.

369 "No, no; they don't": Intv. Susan Ellenberg, October 27, 2010.

370 Hoping to reset: Transcript, "ACT UP Talks with Anthony Fauci, MD, Bethesda, MD, 6.20.89," RJGA.

370 He was convinced: AF, intv. Victoria Harden, March 7, 1989, "In Their Own Words: NIH Researchers Recall the Early Years of AIDS," Office of NIH History, transcript retrieved from history.nih.gov.

371 "The July ACTG meeting": BB, intv. Sarah Schulman, March 10, 2010, AUOHP. Quote attributed to Iris Long by author.

371 "If I close my eyes": Intv. AF, September 27, 2010.

372 "Nobody wants to be": Intv. Michael Long, October 27, 2014.

372 He was quoted: MH, correspondence with Mr. Thomas McAn, VP Corporate Communications, Bristol-Myers Company, June 26, 1989, RJGA.

372 "It makes sense": Marilyn Chase, "Scientist Promotes Two-Track System for Testing, Distributing AIDS Drugs," *WSJ*, June 26, 1989.

372 On July 7, 1989: MH, "ACT UP/NIAID/II," memorandum to ACT UP, July 7, 1989, RJGA.

372 "What we say here": Ibid.

373 In fact, they had: Ibid.; "Ellen Cooper—7.9.89," RJGA, and "Remarks on Parallel Track, Ellen Cooper, MD, Director, Division of Anti-viral Drug Products, FDA, to ACT UP, June 21, 1989," RJGA.

373 "It must be": MH, "ACT UP/NIAID/II."

373 He would appoint: Ibid.

373 "None of what we did": Intv. JE, August 5, 2010.

374 "make ddI available": MH, MHU.

374 "The summer of treatment": Ibid.

374 Barbara Starrett was settling: Ibid.

374 Sefakis, an ACT UP: MH, MHU.

374 recognized the psychosis: Intv. Barbara Starrett, September 10, 2010.

375 She reached Sheaffer's: Ibid.

375 "You're having a reaction": Ibid.

375 "He just needs support": Ibid.

375 After a rough night: MH, MHU.

375 By the following Tuesday: Intv. Barbara Starrett, September 10, 2010.

375 Starrett was ecstatic to see him: Ibid.

375 She made an announcement: Ibid.

375 For people with relatively: Unsigned, "Life-Stretching Drug," *Economist*, August 26, 1989.

375 This meant that: B. D. Colen, "AIDS: The Mounting Drug Bill," *New York Newsday*, August 29, 1989.

375 from the current 40,000: Editorial, "AZT's Inhuman Cost," *NYT*, August 28, 1989.

375 The company's profits: Marilyn Chase, "Burroughs Wellcome Reaps Profits, Outrage from Its AIDS Drug," *WSJ*, September 15, 1989.

376 triggering dozens of biting: Philip J. Hilts, "Wave of Protests Developing on Profits from AIDS Drug," *NYT*, September 16, 1989.

376 Three others from ACT UP: "Treatment and Data Committee Digest," September 11, 1989, RJGA.

376 who brought leaders: Unsigned, "Drug Maker Rejects Pleas," *NYT*, September 6, 1989.

376 He scolded ACT UP: "The Treatment and Data Digest," September 11, 1989, RJGA.

376 Lisa Behrens: MH audiotape transcript, "Peter & Mark Talk About Drugs and Money at Burroughs-Wellcome," January 23, 1989, MHA.

376 On a night early: MH, MHU.

376 After eighteen months: MH, intv. Sarah Schulman, March 8, 2003, AUOHP.

376 It was John Sefakis: MH, letter to *NYT*, undated, GF-RA.

376 Sheaffer had died: Gina Kolata, "Critics Fault Secret Effort to Test AIDS Drug," *NYT*, September 19, 1989.

376 The death came forty days: MH, untitled, ACT UP and the birth of AIDS treatment activism, MHU.

377 Over the next month: PS, email to author, November 12, 2015.

377 "If we are going to support": MH, untitled, ACT UP and the birth of AIDS treatment activism.

377 "People always die": Correspondence with LK, various.

377 He knew Scott: MC, "A Farewell to Smarm," undelivered speech, 1990.

377 had joined the trial: "T+D Update 10-02-89," RJGA.

377 The bottom line: MC, "A Farewell to Smarm."

377 After the meeting: MH, untitled, ACT UP and the birth of AIDS treatment activism.

378 "His decline was so": Kolata, "Critics Fault Secret Effort to Test AIDS Drug."

378 she barely managed: Intvs. Howard Grossman, various.

378 The group's coordinating: ACT UP Coordinating Committee Meeting Minutes, September 19, 1989, RJGA.

378 "The difference of how": Intv. Vera Beyers and Alan Levin, May 27, 2010.

378   Though CD4 cell counts: Vera S. Byers et al., "A Phase I/II Study of Trichosanthin Treatment of HIV disease," *AIDS* 4, no. 12 (1990): 1189–96.

378   "mixed but intriguing": Project Inform, "Compound Q—The Real Story," *PI Perspective* 7 (November 1989), retrieved from projectinform.org.

378   Marty Delaney called: Dennis Wyss, "The Underground Test of Compound Q," *Time*, October 9, 1989.

378   Some five hundred men: Ibid.

378   When Delaney was finished: Ibid.

378   And then a surprising: Jesse C. Dobson, "Compound Q Revisited, Again," February 14, 1991, GF-RA.

378   With the trial completed: Jim Corti, correspondence with GF-R, February 22, 1991, GF-RA.

378   Large groups formed: GF-R, handwritten undated notes, GF-RA.

378   as well as in Holland: Jim Beal, press statement, June 10, 1991, Folder "Q," GF-RA.

378   "from Maine to Baja": GF-R, handwritten undated notes, GF-RA.

378   An organization called: Celia Farber, "AIDS," *SPIN* (June 1989): 90.

379   Many of its HIV-positive: Intv. Eugene Fedorko, August 25, 2012.

379   Aloe vera juice: Bob Lederer, "AIDS," *SPIN* (June 1989): 91.

379   "If it's suboptimal": Intv. PS, August 5, 2010.

379   But his CD4s: PS spreadsheet showing his CD4 count on October 6, 1989.

380   "There," Staley said: Intv. PS, August 5, 2010.

381   When Staley saw: Michelangelo Signorile, "AIDS Activists Storm Stock Exchange, Halting Trading: High Price of Burroughs' AZT Under Fire," *OutWeek*, September 24, 1989.

382   The following Monday: Intv. PS, August 5, 2010; and Philip J. Hilts, "AIDS Drug's Maker Cuts Price by 20%," *NYT,* September 19, 1989.

382   "in the interests of justice": Unsigned, "People v. James McGrath, Scott Robbe, and Peter Staley, defendants," *New York Law Journal,* May 25, 1990.

382   The Provincetown affiliate: BB videotape, "TAPE 20194," undated, BBA, transcript by author.

382   Others had demanded: Ibid.; and correspondence with Derek Link.

383   Fauci accepted: BB videotape, "TAPE 20194."

383   Inside, the worn linoleum: Bill Snyder, "Anthony Fauci: Unfinished Business," *Lens* (April 2004).

383   About fifty activists: MH, correspondence with AF, November 3, 1989, MHA.

383   Richard Elovich: Richard Elovich, intv. Sarah Schulman, March 14, 2007, AUOHP.

383   "Bill! How you doin'?": BB videotape, "TAPE 20194." Same source for all below.

386   "We've exhausted our patience": MH, MHU.

386   "All they think is guys": AF, phone conversation with MH, November 2, 1989, MH notes, MHA.

386   "It is vital that": MH, letter to AF, November 3, 1989, MHA.

386   Their delegation would: Letter says Ken Wiley, but Fornataro used both names.

387   Some eight hundred: MH, "7th AIDS Clinical Trials Group Meeting," November 6–8, 1989, Bethesda, MD, MHA.

387   Dr. Hoth took the rostrum: Ibid.

387   "They will not be permitted": Ibid.

387   This included every: MH, correspondence with Dan Hoth, November 14, 1989, BBA.

387   Despite the sting: Correspondence, T+D memo to "AIDS Activist Groups," July 7, 1989, p. 2, describes meetings on June 24, 1989; and ibid.

388   "the iceberg effect": MH, untitled, ACT UP and the birth of AIDS treatment activism.

388   They heard interesting: "Cytomegalovirus Retinitis: New Approaches," Johns Hopkins AIDS Service, March 1996.

388   Dr. Larry Corey: MH, MHU.

388   This threatened to trigger: MH, correspondence with Dan Hoth, November 14, 1989, BBA.

388   Dr. Corey announced: MH, "Belly of the Beast," OutWeek, November 26, 1989.

388   "an apocalypse": Simon Watney, "Missionary Positions: AIDS, 'Africa,' and Race," Critical Quarterly 31, no. 3 (September 1989): 45–62.

389   Having survived that: MH, correspondence with author, June 13, 2014.

389   presumably associated: MH, email to author, June 13, 2014.

389   In PWAs: Phillip Zakowski et al., "Disseminated Mycobacterium Avium-Intracellulare Infection in Homosexual Men Dying of Acquired Immunodeficiency," JAMA 248, no. 22 (1982): 2980–82.

389   The condition was: Stephen D. Nightingale et al., "Incidence of Mycobacterium Avium-Intracellulare Complex Bacteremia in Human Immunodeficiency Virus–Positive Patients," Journal of Infectious Diseases 165, no. 6 (June 1992): 1082–85.

389   "It's too late for me": MH, MHU.

389   "We had some useful": Intv. MH, September 9, 2010.

389   The year drew to: ACT UP Coordinating Committee Meeting Minutes, September 19, 1989, RJGA.

390   The group's battlefronts: ACT UP Coordinating Committee Meeting Minutes, April 18 and June 19, 1989, RJGA; and Owen Fitzgerald, "No Gay Weddings, City Hall Rejects Proposal Made by 30," New York Daily News, June 24, 1989.

390   "Warning: This Tells Lies": ACT UP, "The Weekly Report," week of September 11, 1989, RJGA.

390   "This is true!": Michel Guibert-Lassallel, letter, 1989, RJGA.

391   "What we are entitled to": LK, Reports, 300.

391   "I'm concerned": ACT UP Coordinating Committee Meeting Minutes, November 28, 1989, RJGA.

391   "in a pluralistic society": Videotape of local news coverage in How to Survive a Plague, documentary, transcript by author.

391   He invented a scientific: Andrew Hacker, "The Priest, the Politician and the Party Line," NYT, March 26, 1989.

392 "This is Jesus Christ": Ray Navarro, videotape, private collection, in *How to Survive a Plague,* documentary, transcript by author.

393 Forty-three people were: Jason DeParle, "111 Held in St. Patrick's Protest," *NYT,* December 11, 1989.

393 "Somewhere in that Cathedral": JE, emails to author, various.

PART 4 :
REVOLT OF THE GUINEA PIGS

I. NEW BEGINNINGS

397 "It is too brutal": MC, "Yale Speech," undated, RDA.

397 He and Griffin Gold: MC audiotape, "Mike on Quitting PWAC," transcript by author, MCA.

397 "That's $2 million": Ibid.

397 It was true: He mentions "this particular financial crisis" in ibid.

398 He charged the medical: Unsigned, "CRI Review Committee, 9.25.90: Research Issues in Brief," MCA.

398 Soon, Larry Kramer piled: Correspondence, LK to Board of Directors, February 4, 1991, MCA.

398 "mad as the Ayatollah": Paul Taylor, "AIDS Guerrillas," *New York,* November 12, 1990.

398 The board ignored: Correspondence, Richard Mack Jr., PhD, and Gregg L. Broyles to LK, January 24, 1991, MCA.

399 "one more lowly": MC audiotape, "Mike on Quitting PWAC."

399 At the very least: Callen, *Surviving AIDS,* 237.

399 Until then, a new: MC audiotape, "Mike on Quitting PWAC."

399 He begged Dworkin: Intv. RD, December 30, 2014.

399 For more than two years: Ibid.

399 "If you had said": Robert Vasquez, intv. MC, "Sex1," undated, transcript by MC, RDA.

399 At Callen's urging: Intv. RD, December 30, 2014.

399 Throughout, Dworkin: Intv. RD, December 30, 2014.

399 "as a partner": Duberman, *Hold Tight Gently,* 247.

400 Mark Harrington bluntly: Correspondence, MH to Daniel Hoth, November 14, 1989, MHA.

400 "It is never": GF-R, "Criteria for the Development of a More Humane ACTG," memo for the Women's Action Committee, March 5, 1990.

400 "all the AIDS organizations": Correspondence, JE to AF & Daniel Hoth, December 31, 1989, MHA.

400 Its budget had: MH, MHU; and Kenneth H. Bacon, "National Institutes of Health Faces Host of Ills as Demand for Research Surges," *WSJ,* May 22, 1990.

400 By painful comparison: John Noble Wilford, "Space Shuttle Poised to Begin Mission to Retrieve a Satellite," *NYT,* January 7, 1990.

400 "With a past & present": Correspondence, JE to AF & Daniel Hoth, December 31, 1989, MHA.

400   Not even a flurry: Correspondence, various, GF-RA.

400   The rest of the OIs: MH, "VIII AIDS Clinical Trials Group Meeting," meeting notes, March 5–7, 1990, MHA.

401   "a genteel form": MH, "Eating Where They . . . ," *OutWeek*, February 18, 1990.

401   "[T]he privacy or other interests": MH, MHU.

401   In what they hailed: Jack Killen, "Note to the Record, Subject: Patient/ Advocate Participation in ACTG Meetings," January 31, 1990, GF-RA.

401   When invitations went: Ibid.

402   They dispatched Harrington: Intv. Brenda Lein, date unknown.

402   After returning to New York: MH, untitled, ACT UP and the birth of AIDS treatment activism," MHU.

402   But when they arrived: GF-R, "8th AIDS Clinical Trial Group Meeting: Data and Drama," March 5–7, 1990, GF-RA; and MH, "VIII AIDS Clinical Trials Group Meeting," meeting notes.

402   To respond to this affront: MH, "VIII AIDS Clinical Trials Group Meeting."

402   "Are you going": MH, "ACT UP and the Birth of AIDS Treatment Activism."

402   Garance Franke-Ruta: GF-R, "8th AIDS Clinical Trial Group Meeting: Data and Drama."

402   One T+D member: MH, "VIII AIDS Clinical Trials Group Meeting"; and William Snow, correspondence with author, February 4, 2015.

403   combination therapy: MH, "VIII AIDS Clinical Trials Group Meeting."

403   "That's not the point": Ibid.

404   She scurried off: GF-R, "8th AIDS Clinical Trial Group Meeting: Data and Drama."

404   The ACTG critique: Unsigned, *History of the Discovery and Development of Crixivan,* a publication of Merck & Co., 1996.

404   It called the ACTG's: MH, *A Critique of the ACTG,* May 1, 1990, 48, MHA

404   He offered a blueprint: Ibid., 39.

404   "And the theme": MH, telephone conversation with Jack Killen, March 13, 1990, transcript by MH, "Responses to *Critique,*" MHA.

404   "Anatomy of a Disaster": MH, "Anatomy of a Disaster: Why Is Federal AIDS Research at a Standstill?," *VV,* March 13, 1990.

404   Upon publication: MH, telephone conversation with Jack Killen, March 13, 1990.

404   One ACTG official: Gina Kolata, "Advocates' Tactics on AIDS Issues Provoking Warnings of a Backlash," *NYT,* March 11, 1990.

404   "They should be afraid": Ibid.

405   "I get nothing": MH, telephone conversation with anonymous, "Remarks of a Frustrated ACTG Researcher," March 22, 1990, transcript by MH; author confirmed with anonymous.

405   "Why not more": MH, "Anatomy of a Disaster."

405   Harrington had seen: MH, email to author, October 15, 2014.

406   Miles was a high-ranking: Steve Miles, emails with author, various.

406   Derek Link, who: See Dale Peck, *Visions & Revisions: Coming of Age in the Age of AIDS* (New York: Soho Press, 2015).

406   He had a CD4 count: Chapter 2 of MH, unpublished, MHA.

407   David Barr was just: David Barr, intv. by Sarah Schulman, May 15, 2007, AUOHP.

407   He had the telltale: Ibid.

407   "One must have": Spencer Cox, "Darling, He Said That You're Going to Die!," undated circular.

407   Already strapped: Nina Reyes, "Doing What GMHC Does," OutWeek, October 17, 1990.

407   There was now one: ACT UP press release, "Massive AIDS Demonstration to Descend on National Institutes of Health," April 16, 1990.

407   Burton, and the actor: Obituaries, various, NYT, January 6, 1, and 8, 1990, and February 17, 1990.

407   The tiny Bay Area: Online Searchable Obituary Database from Bay Area Reporter, Archive of the GLBT Historical Society, retrieved from obit .glbthistory.org.

407   A spokesman for AIDS: Seth Mydans, "Man with AIDS Is Shot to Death by Friend, Who Commits Suicide," NYT, January 4, 1990.

408   Inspired by something: MH, videotape, "1767: NIH MTG," DTV; and ACT UP press release, "Massive AIDS Demonstration to Descend on National Institutes of Health."

408   On March 17: PS datebook, PSA; and Charlie Franchino, intv. with Sarah Schulman, January 11, 2010, AUOH.

408   Hill agreed to set: Intv. Charlie Franchino, June 3, 2014.

408   Posing as tourists: Ibid.

408   They were surveying: MH, MHU.

408   This should not have: ACT UP Coordinating Committee Meeting Minutes, May 1, 1990, RJGA.

408   "See ya later": Intv. Charlie Franchino, June 3, 2014.

409   The evening began: MH, MHU.

409   Hill's dinner was: Charlie Franchino, intv. with Sarah Schulman, January 11, 2010, AUOHP.

409   Staley turned: Ibid.

409   "ACT UP is planning": MH, MHU.

409   He locked his fingers: Intv. Charlie Franchino, June 3, 2014; and intvs. PS, various.

409   "Don't you think there": Ibid.

409   "We've tried everything": MH, MHU.

409   "These are our demands": Charlie Franchino, intv. with Sarah Schulman, January 11, 2010, AUOHP.

410   "Medical apartheid": Unsigned, "ACT UP Demands for N.I.H. Action," OutWeek, May 30, 1990.

410   Fauci struggled to maintain: Charlie Franchino, intv. with Sarah Schulman, January 11, 2010, AUOHP; and MH, MHU.

410   "A lot of people": MH, MHU.

410   Harrington was savoring: MH, telephone conversation with Jack Killen, March 13, 1990, transcript by MH, MHA.

410   Every Wednesday: Charlie Franchino, email to author, October 2, 2014.

410   Most were white men: GF-R, email to author, August 14, 2015.

411   Just one member: Paul Schindler, "Keith Cylar, 45, AIDS Activist Co-founded Housing Works," *Villager*, March 14–20, 2004.

411   Two years earlier: Intv. Charles King, October 18, 2013.

411   Over six weeks: Dirk Johnson, "Ryan White Dies of AIDS at 18; His Struggle Helped Pierce Myths," *NYT*, April 9, 1990; ACT UP Coordinating Committee Meeting Minutes, May 1, 1990, RJGA.

411   They convinced the country's: Cliff O'Neill, "Demonstrators Rain Fire and Brimstone on NIH Headquarters," *OutWeek*, June 6, 1990.

411   Monday after Monday: *TITA*, February 5, 1990, RJGA.

411   A subcommittee was: ACT UP Coordinating Committee Meeting Minutes, January 30, 1990, RJGA.

411   Money was pouring: Statement of Income, ACT UP, January-February 1990, RJGA.

411   The assailant was: ACT UP Coordinating Committee Meeting Minutes, February 25, 1990, RJGA.

412   Shouting matches erupted: LK, "From Larry Kramer, 16 Apr 90," memorandum, RJGA.

412   Some messages were: *TITA*, September 17, 1990, RJGA.

412   "Who elected Peter Staley": *TITA*, March 12, 1990, RJGA.

412   "His eyes never met": Ibid.

412   "in ACT UP": David Robinson, "To the Membership of ACT UP, 4/9/90," memorandum, RJGA.

412   With the May 21: JE, "Open Letter to Fauci," May 28, 1990, JEA.

412   He authorized publication: "NIAID AIDS Agenda," May 1990, MHA; and "ACT UP Responds to NIAID's Allegations and Evasions," May 21, 1990, MHA.

412   "Federal officials": Jim Baggett, "An Open Letter to All N.I.H. Employees Concerning the May 21 AIDS Demonstration," May 1990, RJGA.

413   When they finally: Lou Chibbaro Jr., "1,000 Demonstrators Storm the NIH," *Washington Blade*, May 25, 1990.

413   Infection rates per capita: CDC chart reproduced in *Piss & Vinegar*, April 1990, BBP.

413   Some 1,200 activists: Mary O'Connor et al., "NIH Says AIDS Rally Did Not Affect Business," *Bethesda Gazette*, May 17, 1990.

413   "Ten Years": Cliff O'Neill, "Demonstrators Rain Fire and Brimstone on NIH Headquarters," *OutWeek*, June 6, 1990.

413   A group of twenty-one: Correspondence, Walter Armstrong et al. to "Mulberry Group," March 2, 1991, GF-RA.

414   "Just doing my job": Intv. PS, August 15, 2010.

414   "It was interesting theater": O'Neill, "Demonstrators Rain Fire and Brimstone."

414   "I think Fauci understands": Ibid.

414   "This is the Middle":Wachter, *The Fragile Coalition*, 75.

414   "a gangster group": Gina Kolata, "Advocates' Tactics on AIDS Issues Provoking Warnings of a Backlash," *NYT*, March 11, 1990.

414   Worldwide, 386,588: LK, "A 'Manhattan Project' for AIDS," *NYT*, July 16, 1990.

415   "Never again could": Intv. JE, August 5, 2010.

415   "the very *heart*": Unsigned, "An Open Letter to ACT UP from the Treatment + Data Committee," undated, MHA.

415   "remarkable mainly for": Wachter, *The Fragile Coalition*, 115.

415   Compounding matters: Tracy J. Davis, "Opening the Doors of Immigration: Sexual Orientation and Asylum in the United States," *Human Rights Brief,* American University, undated, retrieved from american.edu.

415   They were quickly: Wachter, *The Fragile Coalition*, 114.

416   Soon, more than eighty-five: Marilyn Chase, "Demonstrations and Boycott over Travel Curbs Threaten to Disrupt International AIDS Meeting," *WSJ,* May 8, 1990.

416   "More information about": Unsigned, "An Open Letter to ACT UP from the Treatment + Data Committee."

416   They asked ACT UP: Wachter, *The Fragile Coalition*, 69.

416   "Joining the Boycott": Unsigned, "An Open Letter to ACT UP from the Treatment + Data Committee."

416   By a show of hands: ACT UP New York press release, "New York's ACT UP to Attend San Francisco AIDS Conference," June 8, 1990; and unsigned, "Proposal for ACT UP/NY's Participation in Sixth International AIDS Conference in San Francisco & Related Events, June 17–24," by "Ad Hoc San Francisco Conference Planning Committee of ACT UP/NY," no date.

417   Staley returned: See unsigned, "Proposed Budget for San Francisco Week of Activities," presented to the May 7, 1990, ACT UP meeting.

417   The media operation: GF-R handwritten notes, GF-RA.

417   It would be a large: Unsigned, "Funding Proposals for ACT UP Participation in San Francisco AIDS Conference," undated, GF-RA.

417   This year's "Drugs": "AIDS Treatment Research Agenda," ACT UP Treatment & Data Committee, June 1990, 9.

417   Protease inhibitors: Ibid., 11.

417   "We have lost the war": Ibid., 1.

417   "a loose cannon": Wachter, *The Fragile Coalition*, 70.

418   "Everyone had hoped": Ibid., 72.

418   As consolation: "Interview with Larry Kramer," *Sentinel,* June 7, 1990.

418   "The same Doctor": LK, "A Call to Riot," *OutWeek,* March 14, 1990.

418   "By any means": Wachter, *The Fragile Coalition*, 200.

418   "We are up against a wall": *MacNeil/Lehrer NewsHour,* date unknown, transcript by author, retrieved from home recording, PSA.

419   Vito Russo had come: Rex Wockner, "AIDS Activists Seize Center State at World AIDS Conference," *OutWeek,* July 4, 1990.

419   "You need to tell them": Intv. PS, October 22, 2014.

420   Additionally, an anarchist: Wachter, *The Fragile Coalition*, 172.

420   The San Francisco Police: Ibid., 177.

420   Wild rumors wafted: Unsigned, "Security Discussion," internal ACT UP memorandum, GF-RA; and Wachter, *The Fragile Coalition*, 178.

420   Some five thousand: Wachter, *The Fragile Coalition*, 180.

420   Hulking bodyguards: Ibid., 193.

420   Dr. Fauci was talking: *Nightline,* date unknown, transcript by author, retrieved from home recording, PSA.

421   "Nobody but you can": Intv. PS, October 21, 2014.

421   When his eyes adjusted: PS emails, various.

421   *This is because:* Intv. PS, October 21, 2014.

421   "But first, I would": Rex Wockner, "ACT UP Dominates S.F. AIDS Conference, Science Shoved into Background," *Philadelphia Gay News,* June 29–July 5, 1990.

424   Tensions never went: Wachter, *The Fragile Coalition,* 173.

424   "For the 1990s": Laurie Garrett, "Discord Among the Researchers," *New York Newsday,* June 26, 1990.

424   In fact, the epidemic: Ibid.

424   Dr. Robert Yarchoan: Ibid.

424   A line of passing criticism: See *TITA,* July 9, 1990.

424   He wandered over: MH, "9th AIDS Clinical Trials Group (ACTG) Meeting, July 10–13, 1990," MHA.

425   "Science thrives on": MH, "Political Science: Let My People In," *Out-Week,* August 8, 1990.

425   "I've never come closer": MH, "9th AIDS Clinical Trials Group (ACTG) Meeting, July 10–13, 1990."

425   "None of this could": MH, "Political Science."

425   "*We* don't have access": See letters to the editor by Heidi Dorow and Linda Meredith, *OutWeek,* August 22, 1990.

425   "criminal negligence": Maxine Wolfe, "A Short Herstory of Women and AIDS Activism," *ACT UP Reports* (fall/winter 1990), RJGA.

426   He had since: S. E. Krown et al., "Kaposi's Sarcoma in the Acquired Immune Deficiency Syndrome: A Proposal for Uniform Evaluation, Response, and Staging Criteria," *Journal of Clinical Oncology,* September 1, 1989, 1201–07.

428   Only one hundred: Nina Reyes and Duncan Osborne, "Swamped by Surge in AIDS, GMHC Forced to Curtail Caseload," *OutWeek,* October 17, 1990.

428   At the end of: Ibid.

429   "It's not trying": Ibid.

429   Now there was: LK, "Kramer vs . . . ," *OutWeek,* June 20, 1990.

429   "If I had to describe": MC, "Not Everyone Dies of AIDS," *VV,* May 3, 1988.

429   New KS lesions: MC, *Surviving AIDS,* 242.

429   "soul-weary": Ibid.

429   Though Dworkin's affair: Intv. RD, December 30, 2014.

429   Right after Labor Day: Ibid.

429   That those men: Peter Applebome, "Helms Kindled Anger in Campaign, and May Have Set Tone for Others," *NYT,* November 8, 1990.

430   "If I am ever brave": Douglas Crimp, *Melancholia and Moralism: Essays on AIDS and Queer Politics,* (Cambridge: MIT Press, 2002), 171.

430   That December: GF-R, "Summary of Our Knowledge of L-697,639 & L-697,661 (through 3.1.91)," GF-RA.

430   Though infected: Intv. BB, October 30, 2014.

430   He wanted to learn: Ibid.

430   Under his guiding hand: Edwin Durgy, "Drug Kingpin," *Forbes*, May 4, 2013.

431   Emini far outscored: Intv. Emilio Emini, May 20, 2011.

431   One hundred experts: Correspondence, John Doorley to BB et al., March 22, 1991, BBP.

431   They quickly synthesized: Ibid.; and GF-R, "Summary of Our Knowledge."

431   None of the patients: Intv. BB, October 30, 2014.

432   "We want a seat": Intv. BB, March 26, 2011.

432   That study would: Correspondence, John Doorley to BB et al., March 22, 1991, in BBP.

433   When the meeting: Intv. BB, October 30, 2014.

433   "Our discussions": Correspondence, John Doorley to BB et al., March 22, 1991.

433   When he pointed out: BB et al., correspondence with Gordon Douglas, May 1, 1991, BBP; John Doorley, correspondence with BB et al., May 24, 1991, BBP.

434   "It's a common": JE, "Cambridge Speech 120190," December 1, 1990, JEA.

434   The drugs had: MH, "9th AIDS Clinical Trials Group (ACTG) Meeting, July 10–13, 1990."

434   He still had not: MH, untitled, ACT UP and the birth of AIDS treatment activism, MHU.

435   Calling themselves: All above from Paul Rykoff Coleman, "ATAC's Renegades," *OutWeek*, November 28, 1990.

435   Marty Delaney at Project: Correspondence, Martin Delaney to Ellen Cooper et al., August 16, 1990, MHA.

435   "My situation in": Marilyn Chase, "Cooper Resigns Post as Top Regulator for AIDS Drugs, Citing Stress, Fatigue," *WSJ*, December 26, 1990.

435   "She's been like": Gina Kolata, "Citing Stress, F.D.A Aide Wants Out," *NYT*, December 22, 1990.

436   In the major cities: "Treatment and Research Agenda for Women with HIV Infection," ACT UP, revised May 1991 edition.

436   Some 1,500 researchers: Ibid.

436   Tensions remained high: Maxine Wolfe, "Of Meetings and Moratoria: Reality vs. Rumor, an Open Letter to NY ACT UP," undated, RJGA.

436   In protest one morning: Ibid.

436   With his remaining: Correspondence, David Byar, "To the Members of ACT UP," undated, MHA.

436   From a nearby phone: Tracy Morgan, intv. by Sarah Schulman, October 12, 2012, AUOHP.

436   "Mrs. O'Leary's cud-chewing": Patrick Giles, letter to *TITA*, April 22, 1991.

437   In a rejoinder threaded: Tracy Morgan, annotated copy of David Byar, "To the Members of ACT UP," undated, RGA.

437   ACT UP was numbed: Mark Harrington, "Life Among the Ruins," *OutWeek*, October 3, 1990.

437   Half the Division: GF-R handwritten note, December 6, 1990, GF-RA.

437   Had they thought: GF-R, "Agenda for Meeting at NIAID," December 27, 1990, GF-RA.

438   Franke-Ruta had reports: No author, "British Drug Firm's Profit Gained 28% in Six Months," *WSJ*, May 4, 1990.

438   When the members: Intv. PS, August 5, 2010.

438   ACT UP gave them: Event invitation, dated November 7, 1990, RJGA.

438   The Countdown volunteers: *T&D Digest* 72, December 10, 1990.

438   Link and San Francisco's: Derek Link's handwritten notes, "Genentech Conference Call Jan 11 5pm," MHA.

438   "Committee after committee": C-SPAN videotape, retrieved from c-span.org, transcript by author.

438   Although punctuated by: "Countdown 18 Months," *T&D Digest* 71: November 26, 1990.

439   "Science isn't done": Derek Link, "Countdown 18 Months Meeting with Fauci," undated, MHA.

439   She brought Staley: "Ansamycin/Rifabutin," *T&D Digest* 71, November 26, 1990.

439   Luckily, rifabutin proved: Vassil St. Georgiev, *Infectious Diseases in Immunocompromised Hosts* (Washington, DC: CRC Press), 331.

439   In combination with: P. M. Sullam, "Rifabutin Therapy for Disseminated *Mycobacterium Avium* Complex Infection," *Clinical Infectious Diseases* (April 1996): supplement 1, S37–41.

2. DAYS OF DESPERATION

440   "The AIDS Crisis": *TITA*, October 22, 1990, RJGA.

440   Teams of three: Intvs. Ron Goldberg, various.

441   He had decided: MC, "Are You Now, or Have You Ever Been?," *PWA Newsline* (January 1989).

441   Late in March: Per Maxine Wolfe, "Of Meetings and Moritoria: Reality vs. Rumor, an Open Letter to NY ACT UP," undated, RGJA.

441   "concentration camp": William G. Niederland, "The Problem of the Survivor," *Journal of the Hillside Hospital* 10 (1961): 233.

441   High on the agenda: Maxine Wolfe, intv. by Jim Hubbard, February 19, 2004, AUOHP.

442   The proposal passed: Wolfe, "Of Meetings and Moritoria."

442   "It's not like it's": Derek Link, "HIV Negatives: Get Out of Our Way," undated, MHA.

442   Larry Kramer opened: Mass, ed., *We Must Love One Another*, 63.

442   Tracy Morgan changed: Nina Reyes, "ACT UP Lesbians Spooked by Threats and Harassing Calls," *OutWeek*, May 22, 1991.

442   Reports were made: Ibid.

442   This, of course: See "Report: General Meetings, Dec 17–Jan 7," *Newsletter*, January 14, 1991, RJGA.

442   The internecine battles: PS spreadsheet showing his CD4 count.

443   "A final real management": MH audiotape transcript, "Peter & Mark Talk

About Drugs and Money at Burroughs-Wellcome," January 23, 1989, MHA.

443   The next time: PS spreadsheet showing his CD4 count, March 6, 1991.

443   "As far as I'm": PS memo, "To ACT UP," undated, RJGA.

443   Franke-Ruta was: GF-R, emails to author, various.

444   Swelling of the brain: GF-R, "Coming of Age Amid Grief, Death and AIDS," in *The Vaccine Handbook: Global Perspectives,* ed. Patricia Kahn (New York, NY: AIDS Vaccine Advocacy Coalition, 2005), 282.

444   He asked Dr. Sonnabend: Intvs. JS, various.

445   "to spend one penny": C-SPAN, Senate Session, April 27, 1988, retrieved from c-span.org, transcript by author.

445   "We've got to call": EIK, "Senator Helms's Callousness Toward AIDS Victims," *NYT,* November 7, 1987.

445   To many of Helms's colleagues: No author, "Conservatives; Third Men," *Economist,* February 22, 1975.

445   They passed his: EIK, "Senator Helms's Callousness Toward AIDS Victims."

445   "the only weapon": Kevin J. Hayes, *The Road to Monticello: The Life and Mind of Thomas Jefferson* (New York, NY: Oxford University Press, 2008), 586.

446   "They don't like me": C-SPAN footage in *How to Survive a Plague,* documentary, transcript by author.

446   But within months: McFadden, "Judge Overturns U.S. Rule Blocking 'Offensive' Educational Material on AIDS."

447   Between the spats: MH, intv. by Sarah Schulman, March 8, 2003, AUOHP.

447   As he arrived at the: MH memo, "Strategy and Actions Meeting—Oct 22," RJGA.

447   "I don't want any": Simon Watney audiotape, undated, transcript by author.

449   He began to recede: JE, intv. by Sarah Schulman, March 5, 2004, AUOHP.

449   The unhappy task: Intv. Charlie Franchino, undated.

3 . LIFE

450   They didn't get: Merck draft statement for the Berlin conference.

450   Marty Delaney from Project: Intv. BB, March 26, 2011.

451   "It may sound strange": Intv. Emilio Emini, May 20, 2011.

451   "It's not good, Bill": Intv. BB, March 26, 2011.

452   His CD4 count: BB, emails to author, various.

452   "Look," Bahlman said: Intv. BB, October 30, 2014.

452   "the world's most famous": *Why Am I Gay?,* HBO, August 10, 1993, transcript by author.

452   It's not that they: Barry Callen, email to author, November 21, 2014.

452   Later, every Sunday: Ibid.

453   Growing up in the: MC audiotape, "#170 Dad 2/26/92," transcript by author, MCA.

453   Michael's skin was a deep: Barry Callen, email to author, November 21, 2014.

453   Michael made it known: Ibid.

455   He remembered: MC audiotape, "#169 Mom 2-25-92," transcript by author, MCA.

455   But nobody under: Barry Callen, email to author, November 21, 2014.

456   "We're *dying* in this state": BR, in *How to Survive a Plague,* documentary, transcript of local newscast by author.

457   "It looks like what": DIVA TV videotape, undated, transcribed by author, DTV.

457   One weekend: MH, "Larry Kramer's Nostalgia for the 1980s," unpublished article, MHA. LK doesn't recall this weekend, but doesn't deny MH descriptions.

457   "Spoiled children": Intv. LK, October 27, 2010.

457   When he first: Michael Shnayerson, "Kramer vs. Kramer," *Vanity Fair* (October 1992).

458   However, in deference: Mark Milano, "Conference Call," letter to the editor, *Advocate,* unknown date, RJGA.

458   Mark Milano, a film: Mark Milano, intv. with Sarah Schulman, May 26, 2007, AUOHP.

458   Harrington had studied: MH, MHU.

459   "foolish, grandiose, and absurd": Ibid.

459   Since early in the: Derek Link, Facebook messages to author, various.

460   Since his first blood: MH remarks to International AIDS Conference in Amsterdam, July 21, 1992, MHA.

460   "My tissue samples": MH, MHU.

461   The slides also: Intvs. MH, February 2015.

462   "I noticed that": TAG videotapes #10 and #11, transcript by author.

462   While in Amsterdam: In email November 11, 2014, Dworkin says Callen called him with the pulmonary KS diagnosis on May 23, 1992.

462   Back in California: MC, "In My Time of Dying," *QW,* August 30, 1992.

462   When an answering: RD, emails to author, various.

463   To Callen's surprise: Duberman, *Hold Tight Gently,* 259.

463   "Re-read your own": MC, "In My Time of Dying."

463   "It's begun to": MC, "Dinosaur's Diary," *QW,* August 30, 1992.

464   Thus began what: BR, "Diversionary Tactics," *QW,* August 2, 1992.

464   "To all within": Michael Kelly, "A Delicate Balance: Issues—AIDS; AIDS Speech Brings Hush to Crowd," *NYT,* August 20, 1992.

472   By then he had: Intv. Craig Metroka, September 5, 2013.

472   No concrete action: Correspondence, Jack Killen to MH and Gregg Gonsalves, July 28, 1992, MHA.

473   On the Senate side: Intv. Tim Westmoreland, April 29, 2014.

473   On January 8: MH chronology, "S. 1: Genesis of a Legislative Initiative," MHA.

473   Besides her obvious: MH, MHU.

473   Next, a group of TAG: Ibid.; and MH chronology, "S. 1: Genesis of a Legislative Initiative."

474   "I'm working on S.1": MH chronology, "S. 1: Genesis of a Legislative Initiative."

474   Clinton finally gave him: Natalie Angier, "Scientist Is Named to Head AIDS Research Office," *NYT*, February 17, 1994.

474   Leading his agenda: Andrew Pollack, "US Official to Shift Funds Toward Basic AIDS Research," *NYT*, August 10, 1994.

474   "I know you have": BR, "Confession to Sara," Sara Rafsky personal archive.

475   "[N]ow comes the reign": Ibid.

475   After a long weekend: MC, "To Do List, 3/25/93," MCA.

475   He was down to: Correspondence, MC to "Dear, DEAR friends," September 22, 1993, MCA.

475   Painful ulceration of: Fax, MC to Deborah Tannen, MCA.

475   Thrush had invaded: Correspondence, MC to "Flirts," June 23, 1993, MCA.

475   But he was being: Correspondence, MC to "Cris Williamson & Tret Fure," March 24, 1993, MCA.

475   "A miracle drug": Correspondence, MC to Anthony Roberts, February 16, 1993, MCA.

475   He had a car: Correspondence, MC to "Flirts," June 23, 1993; and correspondence, MC to Pacific Oaks Medical Group, attn. Karen Pike, March 1, 1993, MCA.

475   "It's gross": Correspondence, MC to "Cris Williamson & Tret Fure," March 24, 1993, MCA.

476   "Look," he said: Intv. RD, December 30, 2014.

476   On April 8: Correspondence, MC to David Corkery, April 8, 1993, MCA.

476   In Europe, a huge: Lawrence K. Altman, "New Study Questions Use of AZT in Early Treatment of AIDS Virus," *NYT*, April 2, 1993.

476   He drafted an article: MC, "The Emperor Has No Clothes," a typescript for an article, undated, MCA.

476   "Given that nine": MC, "DOXIL: A New Miracle Drug," a typescript for an article, undated, MCA.

476   In the end: Altman, "New Study Questions Use of AZT in Early Treatment of AIDS Virus."

477   "It's been a huge": PS, videotape of NBC News report, undated, in *How to Survive a Plague*, documentary, transcript by author.

477   Mark Harrington cast: MC, "The Crisis in Clinical AIDS Research," TAG, December 1, 1993.

477   "A couple of doctors": Gregg Bordowitz videotape, undated, in *How to Survive a Plague*, documentary, transcript by author.

477   In fact, two years: MH, memo to ACT UP, "14 February 1991, Day of Desperation (Results from VA298)," MHA.

477   That erased any: Gina Kolata, "Federal Study Questions Ability of AZT to Delay AIDS," *NYT*, February 15, 1991.

480   There were obituaries: Bruce Lambert, "R. C. Failla, Justice and Leader on Gay Rights Issues, Dies at 53," *NYT*, April 12, 1993; and "Rand Schrader, Judge and Gay Advocate, 48," *NYT*, June 15, 1993.

480   "as close to ACT UP": Jeffrey Schmalz, "Whatever Happened to AIDS?,"
       NYT, November 28, 1993.

480   "Alright," he said: Joy Episalla eulogy, retrieved from actupny.org.

480   He sometimes thought: Intv. Joy Episalla and Barbara Hughes, July 21,
       2011.

480   "I've been waiting": Ibid.

481   But things went: DIVA TV videotape, #1227A, transcript by author,
       DVT.

482   This was a skill: Amy Bauer, intv. by Sarah Schulman, March 7, 2004,
       AUOHP.

483   In cumulative national: CDC, "HIV/AIDS Surveillance Report, U.S.
       HIV and AIDS cases Reported Through December 1994," year-end edi-
       tion, vol. 6, no. 2, retrieved from cdc.gov; and "Update: Trends in AIDS
       Incidence, Deaths, and Prevalence—United States, 1996," *MMRW* 46,
       no. 8 (February 28, 1997): 165–73.

483   A number of the people: Intv. Joy Episalla and Barbara Hughes, July 21,
       2011; and Hughes, email to author, November 15, 2015.

483   By some unexpected: Mass, ed., *We Must Love One Another*, 68.

483   Hunter College enrolled her: GF-R, email to author, November 21, 2014.

483   Human trials were: D. Gold and R. Loftus, "Protease Inhibitors: Where
       Are They Now?," *GMHC Treatment Issues* 9, no. 1 (January 1995): 1–7.

484   About a hundred: MH, "Update & Commentary on Protease Inhibitor
       Development Plans," in D. Barr et al., "Problems with Protease Inhibitor
       Development Plans," TAG, February 23, 1995, MHA.

484   As the winter: Ibid.

4. THE OLD DAYS

485   He was profoundly: Intv. RD, December 30, 2014.

485   Now his orange skin: MC and RB, "The Last Word," *New York Press*,
       September 2, 1993.

485   The whole limb: RB, email to author, December 26, 2014.

485   They had barely: Ibid.

485   Beating back his drug: Intv. RB, January 8, 2015.

485   Berkowitz wanted: RB audiotape transcript, "Callen & Berkowitz—The
       Interview: Edited Version," in MCA.

487   Merck executives: David Gold, "Merck Protease Trial to Begin," *GMHC*
       Treatment Issues 7, no. 9 (October 1993).

487   It was the most complex: Merck & Co., "History and the Discovery and
       Development of Crixivan"; intv. Joe Vacca, May 20, 2011; and Collins and
       Vedantam, "8 Years and $700 Million Later."

487   This preliminary step: Intv. Paul Reider, undated.

487   "With no animal data": Ibid.

488   The results of both: Merck & Co., "History and the Discovery and
       Development of Crixivan," 1996, Jon Cohen AIDS Research Collection,
       retrieved from umdl.umich.edu; and ibid.

488   It was time for: Gold, "Merck Protease Trial to Begin."

488   He had recently: Intv. BB, October 30, 2014.

488   Viral loads shot: "Understand Your Test Results: Viral Load," retrieved from aids.gov.

488   In fact, Patient 142: Paul Reider, correspondence with author, November 17, 2014. Reider sent a slide with Patient 142's blood values.

489   Results of the patient's: Huntly Collins and Shankar Vedantam, "A New Drug in the Race with Death," *PI*, March 18, 1996.

489   "It sounds so clichéd": Celia Farber, "AIDS: Words from the Front," *SPIN* (April 1994).

489   They were not there: Intv. RD, December 30, 2014.

489   "I realize some": *Why Am I Gay?*, HBO, August 10, 1993, transcript by author.

490   There were three: Lawrence K. Altman, "In Major Finding, Drug Curbs H.I.V. Infection in Newborns," *NYT*, February 21, 1994.

491   Without a moment: MH, MHU.

491   Then KS moved: MH, intv. by Sarah Schulman, March 8, 2003, AUOHP.

491   He invited the HIVIPs: MH, MHU.

491   Ten days later: "TAG at Ten," MHA.

491   Gonsalves joined him: MH, MHU.

491   In April, new health: "TAG at Ten," MHA; and unsigned, "National AIDS Drug Development Task Force to Meet in Early 1994, HHS' Lee Cites Intercompany AIDS Collaboration as Spur to Formation of New Panel," *Pink Sheet*, December 6, 1993.

491   There, all eyes: "TAG at Ten."

492   "You must start": LK, "Checking In: My Chart," *POZ* (August/September 1994).

492   Fortunately, the dose: Ibid.

493   The Bristol-Myers Squibb: Unsigned, "F.D.A. Panel Recommends AIDS Drug Despite Incomplete Data," *NYT*, May 21, 1994.

493   The application sailed: "TAGline 1994: August 94," retrieved from treatmentactiongroup.org.

493   "The community needs": David Thomas, "TAG, ACT UP in Hot Fax War," *POZ*, October 1, 1994.

493   Most of it got chewed: "TAGline 1995: December 95," retrieved from treatmentactiongroup.org.

494   "If you accept the premise": PS, "Start Making Sense," *POZ*, August 1, 1995.

494   A few AIDS organizations: MH, MHU.

494   "There's a space": David Thomas, "TAG, ACT UP in Hot Fax War," *POZ*, October 1, 1994.

494   "We've been arrested": Video tape: JW0082_1actupTAGaccelerate, James Wentzy Archive.

495   The fifty most powerful: Tim Horn, "Protease Inhibited," *POZ*, April 1, 1996.

495   "antiquated activist": MH, MHU.

495   Hoping to learn: Intv. Paul Reider, undated.

495   Among the activist: Intv. Tom Blout, November 14, 2014.

495   He had quit his job: Ibid.

496   "I can't believe": Michael Saag, *Positive: One Doctor's Personal Encounter with Death, Life, and the US Healthcare System* (Austin, TX: Greenleaf Book Group Press, 2014).

496   There was no: Huntly Collins and Shankar Vedantam, "8 Years and $700 Million Later, How a Better Drug Was Found," *PI*, March 17, 1996.

497   Bahlman felt a chill: Intv. BB, various.

497   "We need a parallel": Intv. BB, October 30, 2014.

497   "We can stop the dying!": Intv. BB, March 26, 2011.

497   If the results were: Lawrence Altman, "A New AIDS Drug Yielding Optimism as Well as Caution," *NYT*, February 2, 1996.

497   Joseph Vacca, a senior: Michael Seggev, email to author, various.

497   The experience moved: Ibid.

497   Crixivan's complex production: Merck & Co., "History and the Discovery and Development of Crixivan"; intv. Joe Vacca, May 20, 2011; and Collins and Vedantam, "8 Years and $700 Million Later."

497   to manufacture enough: Intv. Skip Volante, May 20, 2011. Same source for below.

498   "It's my job to advocate": Intvs. BB, Various.

498   "You're lying": Intv. Paul Reider, undated.

498   "Tom, you don't believe": Intv. Paul Reider, undated.

498   "Bring an expert": Intv. Emilio Emini, May 20, 2011.

498   But what by now: J. G. Dore et al., "Declining Incidence and Later Occurrence of Kaposi's Sarcoma Among Persons with AIDS in Australia: The Australian AIDS Cohort," *AIDS* 10, no. 12 (October 1996): 1401–06.

498   Two years later: Valerie Beral et al.,"Kaposi's Sarcoma Among Persons with AIDS: A Sexually Transmitted Infection?," *Lancet*, January 20, 1990, 123–28.

499   "[T]he father": RB, "Truth Be Told," *Boston Phoenix*, January 7, 1994.

499   Berkowitz could muster: Intv. RB, January 8, 2015. Same source for all below.

500   "a place where nobody": Intv. Paul Reider, undated.

500   By January, patients: Merck & Co., "History and the Discovery and Development of Crixivan."

501   Blount tucked Straley: Tom Blount, email to author, December 27, 2014.

501   John Doorley, Merck's: Intv. Tom Blount, November 14, 2014.

501   Work was set: Merck & Co., "History and the Discovery and Development of Crixivan."

501   None of the company's: Collins and Vedantam, "8 Years and $700 Million Later."

501   It remained an onerous: Elyse Tanouye, "Medicine: Success of AIDS Drug Has Merck Fighting to Keep Up the Pace," *WSJ*, November 5, 1996.

502   Trevor Laird saw: Intv. Skip Volante, May 20, 2011.

502   This upset Blount: Intv. Paul Reider, undated.

502   "Every one of them": Intv. Tom Blount, November 14, 2014.

502   The next morning: Intv. Paul Reider, undated.

502   "like watering a wilted": Intv. Tom Blount, November 14, 2014.

502   Some four hundred: Tanouye, "Medicine."

503   He did this: Intv. Paul Reider, undated.

503   "Every cook knows": Ibid.

503   Meeting again: Number per Michael Seggev, email to author, November 3, 2014.

503   Levin suggested: Intv. Jules Levin, November 3, 2014.

503   He thought it was: Intv. BB, October 30, 2014.

503   "I could never ask": Intv. Paul Reider, undated.

503   Two million copies: Intv. Michael Seggev, May 20, 2011.

503   An 800 number: Huntly Collins and Shankar Vedantam, "A New Drug in the Race with Death," *PI*, March 18, 1996.

503   In six weeks: Intv. Michael Seggev, May 20, 2011; and Michael Seggev, email to author, November 3, 2014.

503   A computer program: Merck & Co., "History and the Discovery and Development of Crixivan."

504   "That was eerie": Intv. Tom Blount, November 14, 2014.

504   He was beginning: Intv. Paul Reider, undated.

504   "The only way to ask": Ibid.

504   "Now there are two": Intv. Tom Blount, November 14, 2014.

504   "You won't try": Intv. Paul Reider, undated.

504   "It's good": Ibid.

505   "How much do you": Ibid.

505   "I am so grateful": Intv. Michael Seggev, May 20, 2011.

505   By summer: Ibid.; and Angelo Ragaza, "Back to Life, Back to Reality: Linda Grinberg," *POZ*, April 1, 1999.

505   Too weak to travel: Intv. Michael Seggev, May 20, 2011.

505   Jim Straley died two days: Collins and Vedantam, "A New Drug in the Race with Death."

506   At a conference: MH and Michael Marco, with Spencer Cox and Tim Horn, "TAG Does ICAAC," 1995.

506   Its therapeutic benefits: Tim Horn, "Protease Inhibited," *POZ*, April 1, 1996.

506   Yet fifteen thousand: Ibid.

506   Two weeks after: Intv. RB, January 8, 2015. Same source for all below.

507   The three-drug combination: Lawrence Altman, "A New AIDS Drug Yielding Optimism as Well as Caution," *NYT*, February 2, 1996.

508   More than 1,500 people: Intv. Jules Levin, November 3, 2014.

EPILOGUE: FOR DEAR LIFE

511   The total dead: 319,849 total deaths, per amfAR: "Thirty Years of HIV/ AIDS: Snapshots of an Epidemic," retrieved from amfAR.org.

511   "to enter the past": Joe Westmoreland, "Near Dead Again," *POZ*, May 1, 2006.

511   A tenacious bout: Joe Westmoreland, correspondence with author, various.

511   In the first months: Ramón A. Torres and Michael Barr, "Impact of Combination Therapy for HIV Infection on Inpatient Census," *NEJM* 336 (May 1997): 1531–33.

511   The epidemic that had: "A Brief Timeline of AIDS," retrieved from factlv .org.

512   "NO OBITS": David Klingman, "For Once, No AIDS Obits in Gay Paper," AP, August 15, 1998.

512   David Barr, the support: Intv. David Barr, September 10, 2010.

513   "Membership has": Stephen Gendin, "Riding Bareback," *POZ*, June 1, 1997.

513   "And I think Derek": Interview with GF-R, September 28, 2010.

513   "I was scared": Intv. Derek Link, March 25, 2011.

513   "It was unforgivable": Intv. David Barr, September 10, 2010.

513   Joseph Sonnabend retired: JS, email to author, November 2, 2015.

Bibliography

Andriote, John-Manuel. *Victory Deferred: How AIDS Changed Gay Life in America*. Chicago: University of Chicago Press, 1999.

Arno, Peter S., and Karyn L. Feiden. *Against the Odds: The Story of AIDS Drug Development, Politics, and Profits*. New York, NY: HarperCollins, 1992.

Banzhaf, Marion, and ACT UP New York Women AIDS Book Group. *Women, AIDS, and Activism*. Boston: South End Press, 1990.

Bayer, Ronald, and Gerald M. Oppenheimer. *AIDS Doctors: Voices from the Epidemic, An Oral History*. New York, NY: Oxford University Press, 2000.

Berkowitz, Richard. *Stayin' Alive: The Invention of Safe Sex, A Personal History*. Boulder, CO: Westview, 2003.

Bordowitz, Gregg. *The AIDS Crisis Is Ridiculous and Other Writings: 1986–2003*. Cambridge, MA: MIT Press, 2004.

Brier, Jennifer. *Infectious Ideas: U.S. Political Responses to the AIDS Crisis*. Chapel Hill: University of North Carolina Press, 2009.

Burkett, Elinor. *The Gravest Show on Earth: America in the Age of AIDS*. Boston: Houghton Mifflin, 1995.

Callen, Michael. *Surviving AIDS*. New York, NY: HarperPerennial, [1990] 1991.

Chambre, Susan M. *Fighting for Our Lives: New York's AIDS Community and the Politics of Disease*. New Brunswick, NJ: Rutgers University Press, 2006.

Corless, Inge B., and Mary Pittman. *AIDS: Principles, Practices & Politics*. New York, NY: Hemisphere Publishing Corporation, 1988.

Crewdson, John. *Science Fictions: A Scientific Mystery, a Massive Cover-Up, and the Dark Legacy of Robert Gallo*. Boston, MA: Little, Brown and Company, 2002.

Duberman, Martin. *Hold Tight Gently: Michael Callen, Essex Hemphill, and the Battlefield of AIDS*. New York, NY: New Press, 2014.

Engel, Jonathan. *The Epidemic: A Global History of AIDS*. New York, NY: Smithsonian Books/Collins, 2006.

Epstein, Steven. *Impure Science: AIDS, Activism, and the Politics of Knowledge*. Medicine and Society. Berkeley, CA: University of California Press, 1996.

Fettner, Ann Giudici, and William A. Check. *The Truth About AIDS: Evolution of an Epidemic*. New York: Henry Holt and Company, [1984] 1986.

Gallo, Robert C. *Virus Hunting: AIDS, Cancer, and the Human Retrovirus: A Story of Scientific Discovery*. New York: BasicBooks, 1991.

Gould, Deborah B. *Moving Politics: Emotion and ACT UP's Fight Against AIDS*. Chicago: University of Chicago Press, 2009.

Grmek, Mirko D. *History of AIDS: Emergence and Origin of a Modern Pandemic*. Princeton, NJ: Princeton University Press, 1990.

Guillén, Mauro F., and Charles Perrow. *The AIDS Disaster: The Failure of Organizations in New York and the Nation.* New Haven, CT: Yale University Press, 1990.

Jonsen, Albert R., and Jeff Stryker. *The Social Impact of AIDS in the United States.* Washington, DC: National Academy Press, 1993.

Kahn, Arthur D. *AIDS: The Winter War—A Testing of America.* Lincoln, NE: IUniverse, Inc., [1993] 2005.

Kalichman, Seth, and Nicoli Nattrass. *Denying AIDS: Conspiracy Theories, Pseudoscience, and Human Tragedy.* New York, NY: Copernicus/Springer, 2009.

Kapstein, Ethan, and Joshua Busby. *AIDS Drugs for All: Social Movements and Market Transformations.* Cambridge, UK: Cambridge University Press, 2013.

Kwitny, Jonathan. *Acceptable Risks.* New York, NY: Poseidon Press, 1992.

Lauritsen, John. *The AIDS War: Propaganda, Profiteering, and Genocide from the Medical-Industrial Complex.* New York, NY: Asklepios, 1993.

Lewes, Kenneth. *The Psychoanalytic Theory of Male Homosexuality.* New York, NY: Simon and Schuster, 1988.

LK. *Reports from the Holocaust: The Making of an AIDS Activist.* New York: St. Martin's Press, 1989.

———. *The Normal Heart and the Destiny of Me.* New York: Grove Press Edition, 2000. (Original published 1985.)

Long, Thomas. *AIDS and American Apocalypticism: The Cultural Semiotics of an Epidemic.* SUNY Series in the Sociology of Culture. Albany, NY: State University of New York Press, 2005.

Lupton, Deborah. *Moral Threats and Dangerous Desires: AIDS in the News Media. Social Aspects of AIDS.* London, UK, and Bristol, PA: Taylor & Francis, 1994.

Ma, Pearl, and Donald Armstrong. *AIDS and Infections of Homosexual Men.* Stoneham, MA: Butterworths, 1989.

Mass, Lawrence D., ed. *We Must Love One Another or Die: The Life and Legacies of Larry Kramer.* New York: St. Martin's Press, 1997.

Mayer, Kenneth, and Hank Pizer. *The Emergence of AIDS: The Impact of Immunology, Microbiology, and Public Health.* Washington, DC: American Public Health Association, 2000.

Montagnier, Luc, and Stephen Sartarelli. *Virus: The Co-discoverer of HIV Tracks Its Rampage and Charts the Future.* New York, NY: W. W. Norton, 2000.

Nelkin, Dorothy, David Willis, and Scott Parris. *A Disease of Society: Cultural and Institutional Responses to AIDS.* Cambridge, UK, and New York, NY: Cambridge University Press, 1991.

Nichols, Eve K. *Mobilizing Against AIDS: The Unfinished Story of a Virus.* Cambridge, MA: Harvard University Press, 1986.

Nussbaum, Bruce. *Good Intentions: How Big Business and the Medical Establishment Are Corrupting the Fight Against AIDS.* New York, NY: Atlantic Monthly Press, 1990.

Price, Mark de Solla. *Living Positively in a World with HIV/AIDS.* New York: Avon Books, 1995.

Rueda, Enrique. *The Homosexual Network: Private Lives and Public Policy.* Old Greenwich, CT: Devin Adair, 1982.

Shilts, Randy. *And the Band Played On: Politics, People, and the AIDS Epidemic.* New York, NY: St. Martin's Press, 1987.

Sontag, Susan. *Illness as Metaphor and AIDS and Its Metaphors.* 2nd ed. New York, NY: Farrar, Straus and Giroux, 1988.

Teal, Donn. *The Gay Militants.* New York, NY: Stein and Day, 1971.

Triechler, Paula A. *How to Have Theory in an Epidemic: Cultural Chronicles of AIDS.* Durham: Duke University Press, 1999.

Wachter, Robert. *The Fragile Coalition: Scientists, Activists, and AIDS.* New York, NY: St. Martin's Press, 1991.

Index

Musto, Michael, 328
Mycobacterium avium-intracellulare
(MAI), 71, 176, 389, 400, 405, 417,
438, 439
Myers, Woodrow, 273
Myerson, Bess, 14

NAC, 350
naltrexone, 214
Nasrallah, Tom, 107
Nation, The, 398
National Academy of Sciences, 317
National AIDS Treatment Research
Epidemic, 368–9
National Association of People With
AIDS (NAPWA), 108, 110, 115,
116, 152, 312
National Cancer Institute, 17, 76, 141,
253
National Gay Rights Advocates, 299
National Gay Task Force, 83, 110, 132,
187, 206, 320
National Institute of Allergy and
Infectious Diseases (NIAID), 173,
181, 192, 193, 194, 287–8, 298, 302,
303, 365, 386, 423, 439, 461–2
National Institute on Drug Abuse, 194
National Institutes of Health (NIH), 22,
61, 65, 89, 115–16, 139, 173, 176–7,
181, 192, 194, 215, 237, 253, 261–2,
264, 273, 300–1, 303, 316, 370, 373,
401, 408, 409–10, 411, 425, 432,
437, 442, 450, 458, 459, 461–2, 473,
491
National Press Club, 280, 438–9
National Public Radio, 326
National Review, 218, 228
National Task Force on AIDS Drug
Development, 491
National Women and HIV Infection
Conference, 435–7
Nation of Islam, 382
Nature, 103, 172
Navarro, Ray, 429
NCI, 173–4, 178–9, 180, 213, 238, 405–6
Near, Holly, 153–4
Nesline, Michael, 267, 281, 292
New England Journal of Medicine, 289
new germ model, 36–7
New Jersey, 318
New Orleans, La., 321
New Scientist, 211

Newsweek, 112, 153, 154, 185
New York, N.Y., 6, 33, 42, 58, 122, 213,
220, 287
number of AIDS cases in, 91, 142
New York, 110, 398
New York AIDS Network, 107
New York Civil Liberties Union, 131
New York Daily News, 123, 197, 204,
229–30, 234
New Yorker, 60
New York Gay Men's Chorus, 33, 228
New York Native, 23, 24, 31, 34, 35, 37,
44, 46–7, 50, 53, 60, 63, 65, 67–8,
70, 90, 99, 111, 117, 121–2, 124,
125, 126, 137, 138, 142, 150, 154,
156, 160–1, 166, 182, 184, 186–7,
190, 197, 201, 202, 205, 252, 332,
366, 485
AZT trials in, 214
Berkowitz's ads in, 207
bizarre headlines of, 265, 268
CDC mocked by, 218
food supplement study in, 231–3
Petrelis criticized in, 249
New York Newsday, 290, 355, 424
New York Observer, 290
New York People with AIDS
(PWA-NY), 130, 132, 133, 134
New York Physicians for Human Rights,
38–9, 83
New York Police Department (NYPD),
34, 69–70
New York Post, 188, 189–90, 197, 198,
199, 200–1, 204, 219–20, 223
New York Review of Books, 98–9
New York State, 132
money for AIDS in, 161
New York State AIDS Advisory Council,
206, 257
New York Stock Exchange, 380
New York Times, 13–15, 20–1, 22, 31,
34, 53, 68–70, 90, 91–2, 125, 138–9,
180, 181, 182, 198, 204, 229, 236,
249, 253, 254, 259, 270–1, 276, 324,
338, 341–2, 345, 359, 365–6, 377–8,
382, 390, 404, 456, 480
Nicaragua, 223, 240–2
Nicholson, Joe, 197–8, 199–200
Nichols, Stuart, 45
Nightline, 152
Nixon, Richard, 173, 191
Nocera, Ray, 126

Photographic Credits